Early Detection and Rehabilitation Technologies for Dementia:

Neuroscience and Biomedical Applications

Jinglong Wu
Okayama University, Japan

Medical Information Science Reference

Senior Editorial Director: Kristin Klinger
Director of Book Publications: Julia Mosemann
Editorial Director: Lindsay Johnston
Acquisitions Editor: Erika Carter
Development Editor: Myla Harty
Production Coordinator: Jamie Snavely
Typesetters: Mike Brehm, Jennifer Romanchak and Deanna Jo Zombro
Cover Design: Nick Newcomer

Published in the United States of America by
Medical Information Science Reference (an imprint of IGI Global)
701 E. Chocolate Avenue
Hershey PA 17033
Tel: 717-533-8845
Fax: 717-533-8661
E-mail: cust@igi-global.com
Web site: http://www.igi-global.com/reference

Library of Congress Cataloging-in-Publication Data

Early detection and rehabilitation technologies for dementia: neuroscience and biomedical applications / Jinglong Wu, editor.
p. ; cm.
Includes bibliographical references and index.
Summary: "This book provides a comprehensive collection for experts in the Neuroscience and Biomedical technology fields, outlining various concepts from cognitive neuroscience and dementia to neural technology and rehabilitation"--Provided by publisher.
ISBN 978-1-60960-559-9 (hardcover) -- ISBN 978-1-60960-560-5 (ebook) 1. Dementia--Diagnosis. 2. Neurologic examination. I. Wu, Jinglong, 1958-
[DNLM: 1. Dementia. 2. Brain--physiopathology. 3. Diagnostic Techniques, Neurological. 4. Early Diagnosis. WM 220]
RC521.E27 2011
616.8'3--dc22
2010054442

British Cataloguing in Publication Data
A Cataloguing in Publication record for this book is available from the British Library.

Table of Contents

Section 2

Detailed Table of Contents

We examined the relationship between leukoaraiosis (LA) and visual interpolation ability (VIA) in healthy subjects using a novel method that involves the quantitative measurement of VIA. In the chapter, the bilateral extent of LA was significantly associated with a decline in VIA. This result demonstrates the clinical importance of mild LA in addition to moderate and severe LA. It also indicates a useful possible application of our method for the early detection of cognitive impairment.

We introduce a newly developed integrative fMRI-MEG method combined with a spatial filtering (beamforming) technique as a non-invasive neuroimaging method to reveal dynamic processes in the brain. One difficulty encountered when integrating fMRI-MEG analyses is mismatches between the activated regions detected by fMRI and MEG. To overcome this difficulty, we devised a spatial filter based on a generalized least squares (GLS) estimation method. The filter can achieve accurate reconstruction of MEG source activity even when a priori information obtained by fMRI is insufficient. In addition, we describe the feasibility of a newly developed optically pumped atomic magnetometer as a magnetic sensor to simultaneously measure MEG and MR signals.

In humans, functional imaging studies have found a homolog of the macaque motion complex, MT+, that is suggested to contain both the middle temporal (MT) and medial superior temporal (MST) areas in the ascending limb of the inferior temporal sulcus. In the macaque, the motion-sensitive MT and MST areas are adjacent in the superior temporal sulcus. In this chapter, we tentatively identify these subregions as the human homologs of the macaque MT and MST areas, respectively. Putative human MT and MST areas were typically located on the posterior/ventral and anterior/dorsal banks of a dorsal/posterior limb of the inferior temporal sulcus. These locations are similar to their relative positions in the macaque superior temporal sulcus.

Visual orienting attention is best studied using visual cues. Spatial and temporal attention has been compared using brain-imaging data. We developed a visual orienting attention tool to compare auditory when a visual target was presented. We also designed a control task in which subjects had to click on the response key consistent with a simultaneous spatial task. The reaction time for spatial location attention was faster than that without an auditory stimulus. Brain-imaging data showed that the inferior parietal lobe (IPL) and anterior cingulated cortex (ACC) were activated in the visual-spatial attention task and that the activation was enhanced during the task with the auditory stimulus.

Recent event-related fMRI studies suggest that a left-lateralized network exists for reading Chinese words (to contrast two-character Chinese words and figures). In this chapter, we used a 3T fMRI to investigate brain activation when processing characters and figures in a visual discrimination task. The results showed that discrimination of Chinese characters is performed by a bilateral network that processes orthographic, phonological, and semantic features. Significant activation patterns were observed in the occipital region (BA17, 18, 19, and 37), temporal region (BA22 and 38), parietal region (BA7, 39, and 40), and frontal region (BA4, 6, 10, and 46) of the brain and in the cerebellum. We conclude that a constellation of neural substrates provides a bilateral network that processes Chinese subjects.

We studied behavioral performance and brain activities associated with word priming using a Japanese Word Stem Completion (WSC) task. As seen in the fMRI results, the bilateral middle and inferior frontal gyrus were active with a right hemispheric prevalence. In addition, the superior and inferior parietal gyrus and the supplementary motor area were activated. The prefrontal-parietal network observed in our study is consistent with the areas that were activated during an English word stem task. These results suggest that the facilitatory effects observed in the WSC test were successful for implicit memory retrieval.

We examined the neural mechanisms of face perception using event-related potentials (ERPs). Face stimuli of different spatial frequencies were used to investigate how low-spatial-frequency (LSF) and high-spatial-frequency (HSF) components of the face contribute to the identification and recognition of the face and facial expressions. The results suggested that LSF is important for global processing of facial expressions, whereas HSF handles featural processing. There were significant amplitude differences between positive and negative LSF facial expressions in the early time windows of 270-310 ms. Subsequently, the amplitudes among negative HSF facial expressions differed significantly in the later time windows of 330–390 ms. Discrimination between positive and negative facial expressions precedes discrimination among different negative expressions in a sequential manner based on parallel visual channels.

Previous studies about localization ability in the vertical plane have reported contradictory results. One is that the sound source from an upper direction is perceptually superior for a subject, and the other is that a lower direction is superior. The purpose of this study is to clarify sound localization ability in the vertical plane and to detect dementia in the early stage using the aging tendency of aural characteristics.

Hidenori Hiraki, Graduate School of Natural Science and Technology, Okayama University, Japan
Satoshi Takahashi, Graduate School of Natural Science and Technology, Okayama University, Japan
Jing long Wu, Graduate School of Natural Science and Technology, Okayama University, Japan

In a previous study involving a normal person, the area of the kinetic visual field was shown to become smaller with increased target brightness and advancing age. However, the exact relationship between this contrast and their visual fields is unknown. In this chapter, we estimated quantitatively on normal people as a fundamental study of the early detection of dementia in patients. These results were reported using an improved Goldmann perimeter, which has an electric slider to operate targets at constant speeds.

Qi Li, Graduate School of Natural Science and Technology, Okayama University, Japan & School of Computer Science and Technology, Changchun University of Science and Technology, China
Naoya Nakamura, Graduate School of Natural Science and Technology, Okayama University, Japan
Jinglong Wu, Graduate School of Natural Science and Technology, Okayama University, Japan
Yasuyuki Ohta, Graduate School of Medicine, Dentistry, and Pharmacological Sciences, Okayama University, Japan
Koji Abe, Graduate School of Medicine, Dentistry, and Pharmacological Sciences, Okayama University, Japan

In this chapter, we investigated the effects of modality-specific selective attention on audiovisual integration using simple visual and auditory stimuli in healthy human subjects. Our results showed that significant bimodal enhancement was present only in the divided attention condition, which is similar to the results of a previous study using complex semantic stimuli. Therefore, we conclude that stimulus complexity does not influence the modality-specific selective attention effects of audiovisual integration.

Previous studies have demonstrated that the cognitive deficits of AD can be detected during a pre-clinical period with neuropsychological tests. In the present chapter, we introduce the development of two tactile pattern delivery devices. The first delivery device is MRI-compatible and can serve to investigate the underlying neural mechanisms of active and passive tactile pattern discrimination. The second delivery device is designed to investigate the characteristics of passive shape discrimination for psychological experiments. These devices may contribute to the early detection of AD with neuropsychological approaches.

We studied the prospective memory (PM) performance of 20 older people using the message task in delayed recall from the Rivermead Behavioral Memory Test (RBMT) Nine of the subjects had mild cognitive impairment (MCI), while the remaining 11 were healthy subjects (HS). The retrievals in PM were divided into two components: remembering to remember and remembering the content. We administered neuropsychological tests corresponding to each of these stages to investigate the impairment process. Ten subjects showed impairment in remembering to remember and had low performance in encoding, recognition and retrieval in both the auditory verbal memory test and the fluency test, which requires divergent thinking and semantic memory. The other ten subjects were unimpaired, but they

Alzheimer's disease (AD) is a constantly progressive and highly complex neurodegenerative disease, and there are many ways to molecularly characterize the various stages. Homologous to BACE1, BACE2 was a recent discovery, and together these two enzymes make up a new family of transmembrane aspartic proteases. The key enzyme, BACE1, initiates the formation of Aβ, represents a candidate biomarker, as well as a drug target for AD, exhibit all the functional properties of β–secretase. We will review the biology of BACE1 and focus attention to BACE1 as a candidate biomarker for the early detection, prediction, and biological activity in AD.

We identified a novel APP mutation (E693delta; referred to as the Osaka mutation) in a pedigree with probable Alzheimer's disease (AD), resulting in a variant Aβ lacking glutamate at position 22. Based on theoretical predictions and in vitro studies on synthetic mutant Aβ peptides, the mutated Aβ peptide showed a unique and enhanced oligomerization activity without fibrillization. This was further confirmed by PiB-PET analysis on the proband patient. Collectively, we concluded that the Osaka mutation is the first human evidence for the hypothesis that oligomeric Aβ is involved in AD.

This study aimed to evaluate the usefulness of a statistical assessment of cortical activity using electroencephalograms (EEGs) with normative data and the ability of such an assessment to contribute to the diagnosis of Alzheimer's disease (AD). We studied 15 patients with AD and 8 patients with mild cognitive impairment (MCI). The selected EEGs from each subject were analyzed by standardized Low Resolution Electromagnetic Tomography (sLORETA) and statistically compared with the age-matched normal data sets at all frequencies. These results were in agreement with evidence from statistical neuroimaging using MRI/SPECT. Submission of normal EEG data sets to sLORETA might be useful for the detection of diagnostic and predictive markers of AD and MCI in individual patients.

Apraxia is the inability to perform skilled and/or learned movements, not explainable on the basis of more elemental abnormalities. There are several types of apraxia of which the most commonly recognized are (1) limb kinetic apraxia, the loss of hand and finger dexterity; (2) ideomotor apraxia, deficits in pantomiming tool use and gestures with temporal and spatial errors, but with knowledge of the tasks still present; (3) ideational apraxia, the failure to carry out a series of tasks using multiple objects for an intended purpose; and (4) conceptual apraxia, loss of tool knowledge, when tools and objects are used inappropriately. Apraxia can be a feature of both frontotemporal dementia and Alzheimer disease, and even a rare presenting manifestation of both. How sensitive apraxia measures would be in early detection is not well known.

Neuronal transcytosis was observed at the stage when no neurotransmitter was released after the injection of wheat germ agglutinin-conjugated horseradish peroxidase (WGA-HRP; WGA = 22 kDa, HRP = 40 kDa) into the vagus nerve. The co-injection of Rab3A-siRNA with WGA-HRP into the vagus nerve was performed to further examine this phenomenon. This co-injection resulted in the transcytosis of WGA-HRP, both of the passing type, by which it crossed the synapses, and of the secretion type followed by endocytosis of postsynaptic membranes. These findings raised the possibility in vivo that WGA plays an important role in the transcytosis of protein. Therefore, WGA may be a valuable tool for therapeutic drug targeting via transcytosis. These studies suggested that WGA-Aβ could be localized to solitary neurons via transcytosis.

Olfactory dysfunction is a frequent non-motor symptom in Parkinson's disease (PD). This symptom is considered to be an early manifestation of the disease. The aim of this study was to establish the cortical basis of olfactory function in patients with PD. This study was conducted on ten healthy, normosmic subjects and seven patients with PD (one with subjective olfactory dysfunction and nine without subjective olfactory dysfunction). The result indicates that subjective symptoms are different from objective test results in patients with PD. These activated areas may be related to the orbitofrontal cortex corresponding to the olfactory cortices. This study suggests that normosmic subjects with PD already have damage to their olfactory function.

The current knowledge base on circulating serum and plasma risk factors of the cognitive decline of degenerative Alzheimer's Disease is linked to cholesterol homeostasis and lipoprotein disturbances and apolipoprotein E. Lipoprotein lipase (LPL). We have generated an LPL-deficient mouse model that was rescued from neonatal lethality by somatic gene transfer. The levels of the presynaptic marker synaptophysin were reduced in the hippocampus while the levels of the post-synaptic marker PSD-95 remained unchanged in the LPL-deficient mice. The decreased frequency of mEPSC in LPL-deficient neurons indicated that the number of presynaptic vesicles was decreased, which was consistent with the decreases observed in the numbers of total vesicles and docking vesicles. These findings indicate that LPL plays an important role in learning and memory function, possibly by influencing presynaptic function.

Alzheimer's disease (AD) and many other neurodegenerative disorders belong to the family of protein misfolding diseases. To evaluate PET amyloid-imaging tracer [11C]BF-227 as an agent for in vivo detection of various kinds of misfolded protein, a [11C]BF-227 PET study was performed in patients with various protein misfolding diseases, including AD, frontotemporal dementia (FTD), dementia with Lewy bodies (DLB), sporadic Creutzfeldt-Jakob disease (sCJD) and Gerstmann-Sträussler-Scheinker disease (GSS). We confirmed that BF-227 can selectively bind to α-synuclein and prion protein deposits using postmortem brain samples. Based on these findings, [11C]BF-227 is not necessarily specific for β-amyloid in AD patients. However, this tracer could be used to detect various types of protein aggregates in the brain.Noninvasive Detection of Misfolded Proteins in the Brain using Amyloid PET Probe [11C]BF-227.

Positron emission tomography (PET) is a sensitive technique for functional and molecular imaging. In vivo detection of amyloid beta (Aβ) deposits could be useful for early diagnosis of Alzheimer's disease (AD). In this chapter, a novel imaging probe, 2-[2-(2-dimethylaminothiazol-5-yl)-ethenyl]-6-[2-(fluoro)ethoxy]benzoxazole ([11C]BF-227), is reported. A significantly higher distribution volume ratio (DVR) value was observed in AD patients in cortical regions, e.g., the cingulate, frontal, temporal, parietal and occipital regions, than in control subjects. Satisfactory correlation of these values to the semiquantitative standardized uptake values (SUV) was obtained. These findings suggest that [11C] BF-227 is a promising PET probe for clinical evaluation of early Aβ deposition in AD patients.

Positron emission tomography (PET) using the tracer 18F-FDG revealed findings specific to Alzheimer's disease (AD)—mainly the posterior part of the brain and the association cortices of the parietal and occipital lobes were affected by a reduction in glucose metabolism. Recent clinical interests on dementia have focused on the early detection of AD and variation of Parkinson's disease, namely de-

In this chapter, we investigate the effects of Japanese music on the alleviation of dementia symptoms in Japanese patients as compared to the effects of classical music. We collected 87 volunteers including 79 dementia patients, 2 people under 65 years of age, 10 early-stage senior (65-74), and 66 late-stage seniors (>75). We observed their responses in two ways: the physiological response as determined by Near-Infrared Spectroscopy (NIRS), which measures changes in blood flow, and the subjective response as determined by questionnaires. Our results show that dementia patients tend to judge Japanese music as being played in a major key, while healthy subjects judged these songs as being in a minor key. Our results reveal characteristic responses of dementia patients to the Japanese music and provide evidence for the improvement of using music therapy for dementia patients by accounting for their Japanese culture.

To elucidate the mechanism of transcranial magnetic stimulation (TMS) with maximum voluntary muscle contraction (MVC) (used to facilitate motor neuron function), the effects of magnetic stimulation at the foramen magnum level with MVC were tested by recording motor evoked potentials (MEPs) and the maximum muscle force. Three MEPs in the first dorsal interosseus (FDI) muscle elicited by TMS to the motor cortex or foramen magnum stimulation were recorded before and then at 15 minutes intervals for 1 hour after 4 MVCs (while subjects maximally pinched a strain-gauge transducer for 2 seconds). Foramen magnum stimulation with MVC significantly decreased MEP amplitudes after TMS with MVC for 1 hour. Oxy-Hb concentration of the left M1, subtracting the right M1, tended to increase after TMS with MVC. The present results suggest that TMS during MVC induces increased cortical motor neuron excitability.

In this chapter, we report the development of novel tactile display devices. These devices can be used to stimulate the skin of the subject's hand to produces both pressure and movement stimulation. The

We developed a novel portable device, consisting of two grips, that allows the patient to perform exercises at home. While a patient grasps both grips with one hand, the driving grip reciprocates at several speed adjustments. The relative distance between the movable and fixed grip enables the hand to open. In addition, a master-slave system that measures the surface EMG on the healthy arm is proposed for self-controlled rehabilitation therapy. This portable device is not complex and can be used without assistance.

The purpose of this study was to develop a finger display device that has a four-degree-of-freedom (4DOF) length. This device was designed for rehabilitation and cognitive experimentation. The device can change the finger span between the thumb and four fingers, and the distance between digits is controlled by four motors. Each finger is controlled independently, and rehabilitation is performed on each individual finger. The device can be used for not only rehabilitation but also basic tactile studies.

This chapter proposes a new nonlinear model, called a log-linearized viscoelastic model, to estimate the dynamic characteristics of human arterial walls. The validity of the proposed method is determined by demonstrating how arterial wall impedance properties change during arm position testing in the vertical direction. The results indicated that stiffness and viscosity decrease when the arm is raised and increase when it is lowered, in the same pattern as mean blood pressure. This result suggests that our proposed nonlinear arterial viscoelastic model is less affected by changes in mean intravascular pressure during arm position changes.

The purpose of this study is to develop a simple system to recognize the movement of a patient's hand using measurements of EMG signals from only the most characteristic points on the forearm to replace similar, but more complex, research such as multi-channel measurement and wave analysis by FFT. We specified the optimum measuring points on the palm and back sides of the forearm for the recognition of hand motion by the experimental system. Our system successfully recognized hand motion through the analysis of the surface EMG signals measured from only two optimum points to allow arbitrary control of the rehabilitation device based on the recognition results.

In this chapter, a new method based on the "Person-Centered Care" concept is proposed for eliciting the support needs from, and determining their priorities for people with early-stage dementia who are eager to maintain their social living despite coping with various difficulties. First, all of the actual and potential tasks of social living in their daily life are determined. Support needs are then extracted systematically from those tasks by paying attention to what factors are bothering these people or are confusing to them rather than directly asking the individuals what type of support they want or need. Finally, the support needs are prioritized by taking the degree of the individuals' confusion and task frequency into consideration. Some interviews were conducted based on the proposed method to confirm that support needs can be determined systematically from people with early-stage dementia.

Preface

Dementia is a progressive neurodegenerative disease, of which Alzheimer's disease (AD) is the most frequent cause. AD is characterized by the progressive formation of insoluble amyloid plaques and vascular deposits of amyloid beta peptide in the brain. AD patients suffer from a loss of neurons and synapses in the cerebral cortex and certain sub-cortical regions. Numerous researchers in pathophysiology and molecular neurology have focused on the cause of AD in an effort to identify clinical markers, such as the beta-site amyloid precursor protein-cleaving enzyme 1, which can be used to diagnose AD. However, until recently, there were no medical tests capable of conclusively diagnosing AD pre-mortem. The mini-mental state examination (MMSE), a brief, 30-point questionnaire, as well as the clinical dementia rating (CDR), a five-point numeric scale, are the standard tests used to help the physician determine whether a person suffering from memory impairments has AD. Both of these tests include simple questions and problems in a number of areas, such as arithmetic, memory and orientation, used to quantify the severity of dementia symptoms. However, the sensitivity of the MMSE test is approximately 80%, and it has very limited use in screening for patients with mild cognitive impairment (MCI), a major risk factor for the development of AD.

The application of neuroimaging technology to the study of AD has been steadily increasing over the last two decades. To date, the majority of neuroimaging reports that have contributed to the understanding of the pathophysiology and clinical course of AD have utilized structural magnetic resonance imaging (MRI) and positron emission tomography (PET). In addition, functional MRI (fMRI) has been used as a research tool to study AD since 1999. The fMRI studies of AD have focused on two overlapping objectives: understanding the basic biological mechanisms and pathophysiology of AD and developing an effective diagnostic tool or clinical biomarker. The development of biomarkers via fMRI is anticipated to influence the clinical management of AD in three significant ways: differentiating healthy aging from AD, enhancing diagnostic specificity when evaluating a patient with dementia, and monitoring the biological progression of AD for the purposes of drug development and drug testing.

Recent fMRI studies have used spatial attention tasks to study the different neural substrates activated in adults with AD and in normal age-matched adults. These reports found that the most pronounced differences between the two groups were found in the superior parietal lobule (SPL), which was more highly activated in controls, and the frontal and occipitotemporal (OCT) areas, which showed greater activity in AD patients. Differentiating between default networks in AD and normal age-matched adults is another approach and typically uses independent component analysis. A third kind of study uses functional connectivity MRI and focuses on the identification of hubs within the human cerebral cortex, determining the stability of hubs across subject groups and task states and exploring whether the locations of hubs can be correlated with one component of AD pathology.

In the very early stages of AD, altered cognitive symptoms involve mild impairments in learning, memory, or planning. Several researchers use cognitive tasks, including memory tasks, visuospatial tasks, and language tasks, in order to identify differences in cognitive function between AD patients and normal controls. These studies have convincingly demonstrated that it is possible to use cognitive tasks to detect deficits in AD patients during a preclinical period spanning several years. For instance, some researchers have found high levels of pathological lesions in the primary visual areas and certain visual association areas within the occipito-parieto-temporal junction and posterior cingulate cortex in AD patients.

Language is succinctly defined as a "human system of communication that uses arbitrary signals, such as voice sounds, gestures, or written symbols". This system is used to encode and decode information. In the literature on dementia, the presence or absence of language deficits has come to occupy a pivotal position with respect to certain nosological and nosographical issues. Simply using the correct language engenders trust. This is especially true of the language we use when talking about medical issues-particularly AD. Media reports on AD contribute significantly to the public's awareness and knowledge of the condition. Increasing the general understanding of dementia makes seeking diagnosis or support easier for people with concerns about memory loss. The more that other people understand about their experience, the better the quality of life will be for people living with dementia. Language appears to be affected in the early stages of dementia, but the effect is often seen only in selected areas and with significant individual variability. It would appear that impairments in transcribing dictated information and in the pragmatic use of language can be detected early if sensitive tasks are employed. Performance transcribing dictations may indicate a partial lexical knowledge of written words, suggesting that some features of the words' specification in the brain's lexical stores are either absent or inaccessible as a result of brain degeneration.

New efforts have been made to find a preclinical marker for the early detection of AD using tactile discrimination procedures. In order to discriminate different objects by touch alone, humans need to store the spatial information from the first object in their working memory and then compare that spatial construction to the second object. This procedure activates a widely distributed cerebral network, which includes areas for the initial processing of skin indentations, the computation and elaborate reconstruction of shapes and the processing of tactile working memory. The abnormal processing of somatosensory information in AD patients is thought to contribute to a functional decline in tactile shape discrimination compared to normal controls.

Dyslexia is a learning disorder that manifests itself as a difficulty with reading, decoding, comprehension, and/or fluency. It is separate and distinct from reading difficulties resulting from other causes, such as non-neurological deficiencies in vision or hearing, or from poor or inadequate reading instruction. It is estimated that dyslexia affects between 5-17% of the U.S. population. Dyslexia is thought to be the result of a neurological defect/difference, and while it is not an intellectual disability, it is variously considered to be a learning disability, a language disability and a reading disability, among other categories. Persons with dyslexia may have an Intelligence Quotient (IQ) that ranges anywhere from 70 to well above average. Dyslexia is a condition that is neurological in origin and is thus not attributed to factors such as socio-economic background, a lack of motivation to learn, or IQ level. Research using brain-imaging techniques indicates that physiological differences in the brains of dyslexics underlie differences in cognitive functioning and development. At the cognitive level, these deficits may occur in visual processing, linguistic processes (such as phonological representation), and memory.

Another group of neurological deficits stem from motor neuron disease (MND). MNDs are a group of neurological disorders that selectively affect motor neurons, the cells that control voluntary muscle activity including speaking, walking, breathing, swallowing, and general movement of the body.

Rehabilitation robotics is a special branch of robotics that focuses on machines that can be used to help people recover from severe physical trauma. Rehabilitation robotics has only recently begun to make serious inroads in the world of physical therapy, but in many cases, the results are miraculous.

There is increasing interest in using robotic devices to provide rehabilitation therapy following neurological injuries, such as stroke and spinal cord injury. The general paradigm uses a robotic device to physically interact with the participant's limbs during movement training, although there are also paradigms in which the robot "coaches" the participant without making physical contact.

Biomechatronics is an applied interdisciplinary science that aims to integrate mechanical elements, electronics and parts of biological organisms. It also encompasses the fields of robotics and neuroscience. Three main areas are emphasized in current Biomechatronics research.

Following the original demonstration that electrical activity generated by ensembles of cortical neurons can be employed directly to control a robotic manipulator, research on brain-machine interfaces (BMIs) has experienced impressive growth. BMIs provide a digital channel between the brain and the physical world. Electrophysiological measurements of brain activity, such as electromyography (EMG), electroencephalograms (EEGs) and electrooculograms (EOGs) can provide a non-muscular channel through which external devices can be controlled. Previous research recently presented a survey on EEG based brain-machine interfaces (BMIs) and the feasibility of a brain interface to control wheel chairs.

Recent advances in the analysis of brain signals, training patients to control these signals, and improved computing capabilities have enabled people with severe motor disabilities to use their neural signals for both communication and control of objects in their environment, thereby bypassing their impaired neuromuscular system. Non-invasive, EEG-based brain-computer interface (BCI) technologies can be used to control a computer cursor or a limb orthosis, for word processing and accessing the Internet, as well as other functions, such as environmental control or entertainment. With the advent of non-invasive electrodes, EEG research has been directed towards the development of BMIs to replace damaged motor nerves.

Clearly, these developments hold promise for the restoration or replacement of limb mobility in paralyzed subjects. In the future, however, several hurdles will have to be passed. These include designing a fully implantable biocompatible recording device, further developing real-time computational algorithms, introducing a method for providing the brain with sensory feedback from the actuators, and designing and building artificial prostheses that can be controlled directly by brain-derived signals

Dementia is a serious loss of cognitive ability in a previously unimpaired person beyond what might be expected from normal aging. It may be static, as in the case of a unique global brain injury, or progressive, resulting in long-term decline due to damage or disease in the body. Although dementia is far more common in the geriatric population, it can occur in any stage of adulthood. Similar sets of symptoms due to organic brain syndromes or dysfunction are given different names when they occur before adulthood. Until the end of the nineteenth century, dementia was a much broader clinical concept.

The diseases that can cause dementia include Alzheimer's disease, vascular dementia, Lewy body dementia, fronto-temporal dementia, Huntington's disease, and Creutzfeldt-Jakob disease. Doctors have identified other conditions that can cause dementia or dementia-like symptoms, including reactions to medications, metabolic problems and endocrine abnormalities, nutritional deficiencies, infections, poisoning, brain tumors, anoxia or hypoxia, and heart and lung problems.

While there is no cure for dementia, advances have been made toward developing medications that can slow down the process. Cholinesterase inhibitors are often used early in the course of the disease. Cognitive and behavioral interventions may also be appropriate. Educating and providing emotional support to the caregiver are also important. There is some evidence that the regular, moderate consumption of alcohol and a Mediterranean diet may reduce the risk of developing dementia. In addition, a recent study has shown a link between high blood pressure and developing dementia. The study, published in the Lancet Neurology Journal in July 2008, found that medications that lower blood pressure reduced dementia by 13%.

Neurological rehabilitation is often used to reduce physical and cognitive impairments and related disabilities. It has also been shown to increase independence, so patients can participate in daily self-care and other activities to improve their health-related quality of life (QOL). Learning skills after a stroke, a traumatic brain or spinal cord injury or other diseases target the neural networks for movement, sensation, perception, memory, planning, motivation, reward, language, and other aspects of cognition that remain undamaged to compensate for those that were lost.

The rehabilitation of sensory and cognitive functions typically involves retraining neural pathways or training new neural pathways to regain or improve the neurocognitive functioning that has been diminished by disease or traumatic injury.

Speech therapy, occupational therapy and other methods that "exercise" specific brain functions are used. For example, eye-hand coordination exercises may rehabilitate certain motor deficits, while well-structured planning and organizing exercises might help rehabilitate certain frontal lobe "executive functions" following a traumatic blow to the head.

Jinglong Wu
Okayama University, Japan

Section 1

Chapter 1
The Relationship between Visual Interpolation Ability and Leukoaraiosis in Healthy Subjects

Kaechang Park
Brain Check-up Center, Kochi Kenshin Clinic, Japan

Yinlai Jiang
Department of Intelligent Mechanical Systems Engineering, Kochi University of Technology, Japan

Shuoyu Wang
Department of Intelligent Mechanical Systems Engineering, Kochi University of Technology, Japan

ABSTRACT

This chapter examines the relationship between leukoaraiosis (LA) and visual interpolation ability (VIA) in healthy subjects using a novel method that involves the quantitative measurement of VIA. LA has been found through neuroimaging studies and is caused by demyelinization and degenerative changes in arterioles that are related to atherosclerosis (Breteler et al., 1994). Moderate and severe LA have been regarded as surrogate markers for stroke and cognitive impairment. In the present study, the bilateral extent of LA was significantly associated with a decline in VIA. This result demonstrates the clinical importance of mild LA in addition to moderate and severe LA. It also indicates a useful possible application of this method for the early detection of cognitive impairment.

INTRODUCTION

In both natural and artificial environments, because of factors such as occlusion and darkness, it is impossible to visualize the complete details of objects. Thus, the recognition of an object from its separate visible fragments, defined as visual interpolation, is a fundamental ability of the visual system.

Psychological studies have divided visual interpolation into two types, according to their differences in phenomenology. These two types

DOI: 10.4018/978-1-60960-559-9.ch001

are modal interpolation and amodal interpolation (Michotte, Thines & Crabbe, 1964/1991). In modal interpolation, objects that are interpolated have a sensory presence in areas that lack local specification. Modal interpolation occurs when portions of an object are camouflaged by an underlying surface that happens to project the same luminance and color as a nearer object, as shown in Figure 1A. In amodal interpolation, one perceives or registers unspecified parts of objects even though the relationships among the parts are hidden. The most ordinary amodal interpolation occurs when portions of an object are occluded by another object (Figure 1B). No matter which type of interpolation occurs in the early processing of visual cognition, images are recognized in late visual processing based on scattered and incomplete information. For example, as shown in Figure 1C, a letter "A" that is partially erased can be perceived using the precondition that it is an alphabetical image. However, it is unclear whether modal or amodal interpolation occurs in this case.

We previously found that cortical activation in the frontal cortex and occipital cortex during incomplete-letter recognition was compared with complete-letter recognition using fNIRS (functional near-infrared spectroscopy). The findings demonstrated that the oxygenated hemoglobin concentration during the incomplete-letter recognition task was larger than the concentration during the complete-letter recognition task. Furthermore, significant differences in the oxygenated hemoglobin concentration were observed in the lateral prefrontal and occipital areas. These findings indicate that the lateral frontal cortex plays an important role in the recognition of incomplete objects.

We had previously used a quantitative method to measure visual interpolation ability (VIA) with partially erased letters (Jiang & Wang, 2007; 2008). This method may be used to evaluate the subtle decline in visual function of healthy subjects who show no cognitive impairment in conventional examinations. Leukoaraiosis (LA) has been found through neuroimaging and is caused by pathological changes such as demyelinization, gliosis, vessel lipohyalinosis, and disturbed blood-brain exchange (Breteler et al., 1994). Postmortem studies have indicated that LA is associated with degenerative changes in arterioles that are related to atherosclerosis (Hachinski, Potter & Merskey, 1987). This finding suggests that cerebral arteriosclerosis of the penetrating vessels is the main factor responsible for LA pathogenesis. However, a small extent of LA is frequently can be diagnosed in young people, although the pathogenic implications of these diagnoses remain unclear (Moody, Thore, Anstrom, Challa & Langefeld et al., 2004; Park, Yasuda, Toyonaga, Yamada & Nakabayashi et al., 2007). On the other hand, a large extent of LA diagnosed in elderly patients is well known to be caused by near infarcts that result in recurrent stroke and cognitive impairment, especially of the frontal lobe (Moody et al., 2004). In the present study, we used a novel VIA measurement

Figure 1. Illustrations of visual interpolation. (A) Modal interpolation (Kanizsa triangle). A white triangle is perceived even though it is not drawn. (B) Amodal interpolation. A triangle is perceived despite partial occlusion by a disk. (C) Common incomplete object. The letter A is perceived from its fragments despite partial erasure.

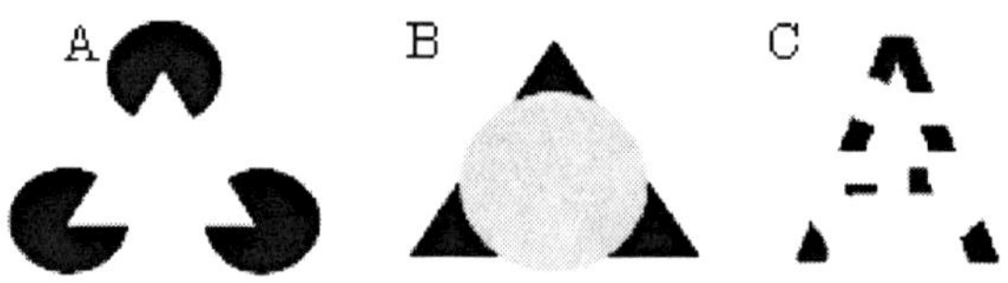

method to determine whether the small extent of LA diagnosed in healthy middle-aged individuals affects visual cognitive function.

EXPERIMENT

Subjects

A total of 296 subjects were involved in this study (118 men and 178 women; average age 52.0±7.7). Each subject underwent MRI as part of a health check-up study in the Brain Check-up Center of Kochi Kenshin Clinic, had normal visual acuity without glasses and had no medical history of neurological or psychiatric disorders.

Measurement of Visual Interpolation Ability

VIA was measured using a previously reported quantitative measurement procedure (Jiang et al., 2008). Letters were extracted from the Microsoft Paint program that was installed in a Windows 2000 environment. The font was MSP Gothic, and the font size was 72. The letter color was black, and the background color was white. Letters were presented in the center of bitmap images that were 128 x 128 pixels in size. A program developed in Microsoft Visual C++ was used to produce partially erased letters. According to the program, black pixels in an alphabetic letter image were erased with rectangles, simulating the procedure used to erase a letter by hand with an eraser. First, the position and gradient of each rectangle over the letter image were randomly determined. Then, the black letter pixels covered by the rectangles were erased until the ratio of the number of erased pixels to the number of black pixels in the original image reached a set value. Examples of partially erased letters are shown in Figure 2. There were five erasure ratios: 0.7, 0.8, 0.86, 0.9 and 0.92. Erasure was categorized into three groups, according to rectangle size. In the first group, the rectangle size was one pixel × one pixel. Thus, letters were erased one pixel at a time. In the second group, the rectangle length was 4-8 pixels, and its width was 2-4 pixels. In the third

Figure 2. Partially erased letter "R" (L and W denote the length and width of the rectangle)

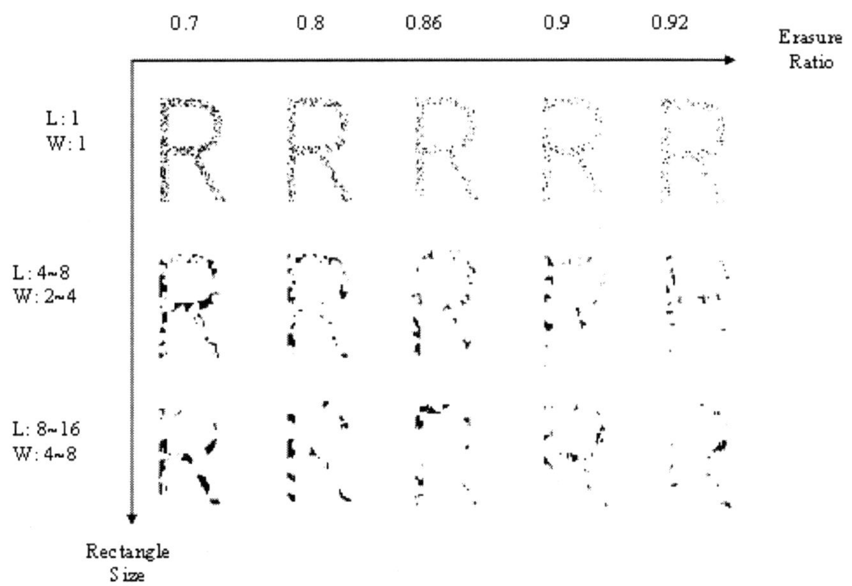

group, the rectangle length was 8-16 pixels, and the width was 4-8 pixels. As shown in Figure 2, the erased letters were more difficult to recognize at higher erased:black ratios, and the remaining parts of the letters became farther away from one another at larger rectangle sizes.

Humans recognize and remember objects according to their features (Bjork & Bjork, 1998). When a partially erased letter is recognized, the features of the image are sampled and compared with the memorized features, and a decision is made based on similarity (Pelli, Burns, Farell & Moore, 2006). Therefore, with increasing erasure ratios, fewer and fewer features are left, making the erased letter more difficult to recognize. The features of an object are generally correlated, and the correlation between features plays an important role in their recognition (Singer & Gray, 1995). In the present study, the larger we set the erased rectangle, the farther apart the remaining parts of the erased letter became (Figure 2), which reduced the correlations between the remaining features. Therefore, the erased letter became more difficult to recognize with an increase in rectangle size.

In a previous study, the results of an incomplete-letter recognition experiment showed that the rate of correct letter identification decreased as the erasure ratio and rectangle size increased. The features and correlations between those features played important roles in letter recognition, as shown Figure 2. Features that differentiate objects and the importance of these features varied for different objects. The fewer objects with which a feature is associated, the more important the feature becomes. Pixels are the elementary features used by computers to represent objects. Letters are composed of black pixels. Taking black pixels as the basic feature of a letter, an algorithm based on the idea of information entropy was proposed to calculate the amount of information associated with a single black pixel. Thus, based on this information, the VIA is quantitatively defined. The importance of the pixels was evaluated based on the associated information. This algorithm could evaluate the VIA more accurately than using the correct identification rate because the importance of the erased parts of a letter was taken into consideration in this algorithm (Jiang et al., 2008).

In the present study, each of 26 partially erased alphabets was presented at the erased ratios of 0.7, 0.86 and 0.9. The rectangle lengths and widths were also randomly chosen from 8 to 16 pixels and 4 to 8 pixels, respectively. The display duration for each incomplete letter was 200 ms. These parameters were determined according to our previous study results (Jiang et al., 2008).

LA Diagnosis and Grading

Magnetic resonance imaging (MRI) examinations were performed using a 0.4 T open MRI (APERTO, Hitachi Medical Corporation, Tokyo, Japan). The imaging protocol parameters consisted of T2-weighted images (repetition time/echo time [TR/TE] = 5800/105 ms), T1-weighted images (TR/TE = 350/13.6 ms), and fluid-attenuated inversion recovery (FLAIR; TR/TE = 9000/105 ms; inversion time = 2200 ms) images. Images were obtained as 27 transaxial slices per scan. The slice thickness was 5 mm with no interslice gaps. LA was defined as a focal lesion 3 mm in diameter with hyperintensity in T2-weighted and FLAIR images and without prominent hypointensity in TI-weighted images. LA grading was performed according to a modified method from the Atherosclerosis Risk in Communities (ARIC) Study. The gradation included the following: no white matter signal abnormalities (grade 0, none); minimal "dots" of subcortical white matter in the lateral cerebral hemisphere (grade 1, minimal); multiple dots of subcortical white matter hyperintensity (WMH) in the bilateral cerebral hemisphere (grade 2, mild); continuous periventricular rims with scattered patches of subcortical WMH in the bilateral cerebral hemisphere (grade 3, moderate); and thick, shaggy periventricular hyperintensity (PVH) with subcortical WMH, which may have confluent PVH in the bilateral cerebral hemisphere (grade 4, severe).

RESULTS

The number of subjects with each LA grade included 236 subjects with G0, 27 with G1, 28 with G2, 4 with G3 and 1 with G4; thus, the percentages of G0, G1, G2, G3, and G4 patients were 79.7%, 9.1%, 9.5%, 1.4% and 0.3%, respectively. The percentage of subjects with a lateral extension of LA was 88.9%, while the percentage with a bilateral extension was 11.1%. The distribution of VIA in the present study was Gaussian, with some differences in the distribution peaks between bilateral and lateral LA, as shown in Figure 4. A receiver operator characteristic (ROC) curve shows that the optimal cutoff value was 0.587 when the condition variable was bilateral LA (data not shown).

The VIA was divided by the cutoff value. Then, the VIA was considered high if it fell above the cutoff value and low if it fell below the cutoff value. We calculated the age-adjusted odds ratios using the G0 group as the reference group. Table 1 shows the significant association between VIA decline and bilateral lesions of LA. The adjusted odds ratio of this observation was 2.506 (95% CI, 1.127-5.574) (p-value < 0.024).

DISCUSSION

The term leukoaraiosis is derived from the Greek *leuko* (white) and *araiosis* (rarefaction) and refers to lesions of altered signal intensities on CT scans and MRIs in the periventricular and subcortical white matter of elderly people (Hachinski et al., 1987). Traditionally, LA findings have been thought to have no clinical significance because many individuals with LA are asymptomatic. However, there is accumulating evidence from population-based studies that LA is associated with an increased risk of stroke and recurrent stroke, depending on the severity of LA present (Inzitari,

Figure 3. Grading of leukoaraiosis

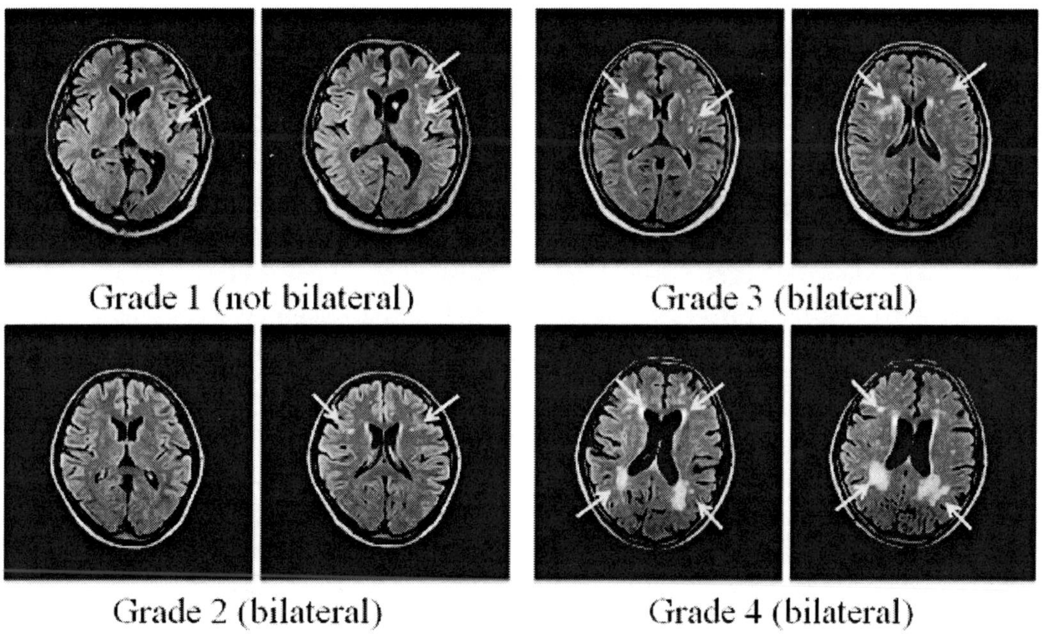

Figure 4. LA distribution. The X-axis corresponds to the VIA, and the Y-axis corresponds to the number of subjects. The upper and lower panels show the distribution curves of bilateral and lateral LA, respectively.

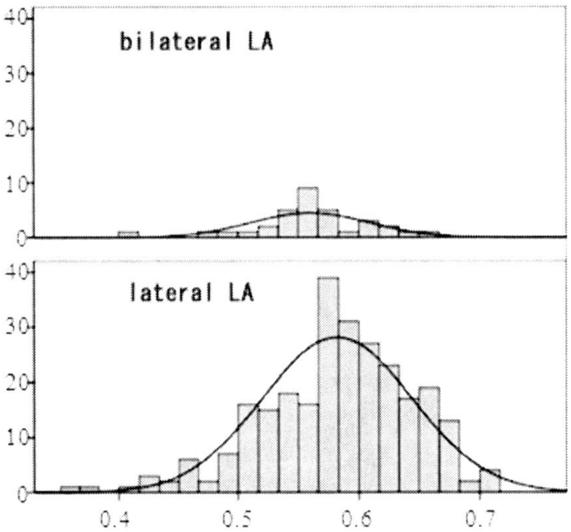

Giordano, Ancona, Pracucci & Mascalchi et al., 1990). Furthermore, cases of moderate and severe LA are also significantly associated with cognitive impairments and dementia of the Alzheimer type (Brun & Englund, 1986). The relationship between cognitive function and LA was examined in 1,077 elderly subjects who were randomly sampled from the general population and subjected to a Rotterdam scan study (de Grout et al., 2000). This study reported that patients with severe LA performed nearly one standard deviation below average on tasks involving psychomotor speed. Furthermore, it was found that LA progression in the elderly was more strongly associated with psychomotor speed than with memory performance and global cognitive function. Thus, LA could be considered as an intermediate surrogate of brain dysfunction, including cerebrovascular damage. The prevention of LA occurrence and progression may contribute to avoiding these serious diseases. On the other hand, the effects of minimal or mild LA, which occur often in middle-aged healthy individuals, have not been studied to determine if they decrease cognitive function. Our results show that the bilateral extent of LA significantly decreases VIA, even in minimal or mild cases. Minimal LA has been reported to be associated with metabolic syndrome and is a symptom of early-stage atherosclerotic organ damage (Park et al., 2007). When LA exists in the brain, however mild it may be, cerebral blood flow decreases in normal brain tissues surrounding the LA (Moody et al., 2004). An fNIRS study showed that cortical activation during visual interpolation was observed in both the occipital area of the primary visual field and the extensive frontal area, including

Table 1. Age-adjusted odds ratios between LA grading and visual interpolation ability

	adjusted OD	95% CI	p-value
G0	1.000	reference	(-)
G1	0.392	0.348-1.036	0.059
G2 + G3 + G4	2.506	1.127-5.574	0.024

the dorsolateral prefrontal cortex (DLPF), which plays a central role in visual working memory and decision making (data not shown). These fNIRS experimental results may explain the VIA decline that is associated with the bilateral extent of mild LA (grade 2). A small extent of LA should be an indicator that an individual could develop moderate or severe LA with cognitive impairment implications. Our method may be a useful tool for the early detection of mild cognitive impairment in healthy subjects.

ACKNOWLEDGMENT

This study was supported in part by a research grant (Research for Promoting Technology Seeds 2006) from the Japan Science and Technology Agency.

REFERENCES

Bjork, E. L., & Bjork, R. A. (1998). *Memory*. New York, NY: Academic Press.

Breteler, M. M. B., Van Swieten, J. C., Bots, M. L., Grobbee, D. E., Claus, J. J., & van den Hout, J. H. (1994). Cerebral white matter lesions, vascular risk factors, and cognitive function in a population-based study: The Rotterdam Study. *Neurology*, *44*, 1246–1252.

Brun, A., & Englund, E. (1986). *A white matter disorder in dementia of the Alzheimer type: A pathoanatomical study*. (pp. 253-262).

de Groot, J. C., de Leeuw, F. E., Oudkerk, M., van Gijn, J., Hofman, A., Jolles, J., & Breteler, M. M. (2000). Cerebral white matter lesions and cognitive function: The Rotterdam scan study. *Annals of Neurology*, *47*, 145–151. doi:10.1002/1531-8249(200002)47:2<145::AID-ANA3>3.0.CO;2-P

Hachinski, V. C., Potter, P., & Merskey, H. (1987). Leukoaraiosis. *Archives of Neurology*, *44*, 21–23.

Inzitari, D., Giordano, G. P., Ancona, A. L., Pracucci, G., Mascalchi, M., & Amaducci, L. (1990). Leukoaraiosis, intracerebral hemorrhage, and arterial hypertension. *Stroke*, *21*, 1419–1423.

Jiang, Y., & Wang, S. (2007). The human visual recognition ability for incomplete letters. *International Journal of Innovative Computing. Information and Control*, *3*, 1183–1192.

Jiang, Y., & Wang, S. (2008). Measurement and quantitative analysis of human visual interpolation ability for partially erased objects. *ICIC Express Letters*, *2*, 7–13.

Michotte, A., Thines, G., & Crabbe, G. (1964/1991). Amodal completion of perceptual structures. In Thines, G., Costall, A., & Butterworth, G. (Eds.), *Michotte's experimental phenomenology of perception*. Hillsdale, NJ: Lawrence Erlbaum Associates.

Moody, D. M., Thore, C. R., Anstrom, J. A., Challa, V. R., Langefeld, C. D., & Brown, W. R. (2004). Quantification of afferent vessels shows reduced brain vascular density in subjects with leukoaraiosis. *Radiology*, *233*, 883–890. doi:10.1148/radiol.2333020981

Park, K., Yasuda, N., Toyonaga, S., Yamada, S. M., Nakabayashi, H., & Nakasato, M. (2007). Significant association between leukoaraiosis and metabolic syndrome in healthy subjects. *Neurology*, *69*, 974–978. doi:10.1212/01.wnl.0000266562.54684.bf

Pelli, D. G., Burns, C. W., Farell, B., & Moore, D. C. (2006). Feature detection and letter identification. *Vision Research*, *46*, 4646–4674. doi:10.1016/j.visres.2006.04.023

Singer, H. W., & Gray, C. M. (1995). Visual feature integration and the temporal correlation hypothesis. *Annual Review of Neuroscience*, *18*, 555–586. doi:10.1146/annurev.ne.18.030195.003011

KEY TERMS AND DEFINITIONS

Cognitive function: An intellectual process by which one becomes aware of, perceives or comprehends ideas. It involves all aspects of perception, thinking, reasoning and remembering.

Cognitive Impairment: Unusually poor mental function that is associated with confusion, forgetfulness and difficulty concentrating.

Leukoaraiosis: The rarefaction of white matter that can be detected by CT and MRI in elderly individuals.

Magnetic Resonance Imaging (MRI): It is primarily a medical imaging technique that is most commonly used in radiology to visualize detailed internal structures.

Partially Erased Letters: Incomplete letters whose recognition information is partially erased.

Visual Interpolation: The human ability to recognize an object based on its parts.

White Matter: One of the two components of the central nervous system consisting largely of myelinated axons.

Chapter 2
Integrative fMRI–MEG Methods and Optically Pumped Atomic Magnetometers for Exploring Higher Brain Functions

Tetsuo Kobayashi
Department of Electrical Engineering, Graduate School of Engineering, Kyoto University, Japan

ABSTRACT

This chapter introduces a newly developed integrative fMRI-MEG method combined with a spatial filtering (beamforming) technique as a non-invasive neuroimaging method to reveal dynamic processes in the brain. One difficulty encountered when integrating fMRI-MEG analyses is mismatches between the activated regions detected by fMRI and MEG. These mismatches may decrease the estimation accuracy, especially when there are strong temporal correlations among activity in fMRI-invisible and -visible regions. To overcome this difficulty, a spatial filter was devised based on a generalized least squares (GLS) estimation method. The filter can achieve accurate reconstruction of MEG source activity even when a priori information obtained by fMRI is insufficient. In addition, this chapter describes the feasibility of a newly developed optically pumped atomic magnetometer as a magnetic sensor to simultaneously measure MEG and MR signals.

INTRODUCTION

What is the mind? What mechanisms in the brain are associated with visual awareness? An important step toward answering these questions is obtaining precise knowledge about the dynamic brain processes involved in these functions. Although recent neuroimaging techniques such as magnetoencephalography (MEG) (Hämäläinen,

DOI: 10.4018/978-1-61960-559-9.ch002

Hari, Ilmoniemi, Knuutila, & Lounasmaa, 1993), positron emission tomography (PET), near-infrared spectroscopy (NIRS), and functional magnetic resonance imaging (fMRI) (Frackwiak, Berkinblit, Fookson, & Poizner, 1998; Murata & Iwase, 2001; Augustyn, & Rosenbaum, 2005; Adam, Mol, Pratt, & Fischer, 2006; Kovacs, Buchanan, & Shea, 2008) have become powerful tools for exploring higher brain functions (Kobayashi, Ozaki, Nagata, 2009), each technique has limited spatial and/or temporal resolution that hamper our understanding of dynamic brain processes.

To overcome these limitations, neuroimaging methods that fuse multimodal techniques are being developed (Dale, Liu, Fischi, Buckner, Belliveau, Lewine, & Halgren, 2000; Schulz, Chau, Graham, McIntosh, Ross, Ishii, & Pantev, 2004; Okamoto, Dan, Shimizu, Takeo, Amita, Oda, Konishi, Sakamoto, Isobe, Suzuki, Kohyama, & Dan, 2004; Carrie, Reynolds, Goodyear, Ponton, Dort, & Eggermont, 2004). However, at present, there is no applicable technique that can provide sufficiently high spatial and/or temporal resolution. We have developed an integrative fMRI-MEG neuroimaging method to analyze the dynamic activation of multiple cortical areas (Innami, Kobayashi, Jung, Ohashi, Hamada, Nagamine, Fukuyama, Azuma, & Tsutsumi, 2004; Ohashi, Innami, Jung, Hamada, & Kobayashi, 2006; Okada, Ohashi, Jung, Hamada, & Kobayashi, 2007). Here, we introduce the latest version of the fMRI-MEG integrative neuroimaging method.

MEG (with superconducting quantum interference devices, SQUIDs) and high-field MRI (with superconducting magnets that require cryogenic cooling) are difficult to measure simultaneously. Optically pumped atomic magnetometers (OPAMs) are currently expected to overtake SQUIDs, and the possibilities for using OPAMs for biomagnetic field measurements and MRI have been demonstrated. We have developed a highly sensitive atomic magnetometer as a magnetic sensor to measure both MEG and MR signals. We describe the principles of the atomic magnetometer and the results of biomagnetic field measurements.

INTEGRATIVE fMRI-MEG NEUROIMGING

Methods

The procedure of integrating fMRI-MEG (Innami, et al., 2004; Ohashi, et al., 2006; Okada, et al., 2007) consisted of sequential steps. First, activated neocortical regions were determined by statistical analysis of the fMRI data, using statistical parametric mapping software (SPM). In the SPM, the imaging time series was realigned, spatially normalized to the stereoscopic space of the Montreal Neurological Institute (MNI) template, and smoothed with a Gaussian kernel with a 6 mm full width at half maximum (FWHM).

Second, the orientations of equivalent current dipoles (ECDs) placed at the center of gravity in individual activated voxels were estimated by a procedure that maximized the inner product of the lead field and the measurement field vectors. Third, the time courses of the regional dipole moments were obtained by projecting the spatial filter vector onto the measured neuromagnetic fields. The spatial filter vector was obtained based on a linearly constrained beamforming technique, in which the center of gravity of each fMRI activated cluster was treated as the location of the linear constraints.

One of the possible problems in fMRI-MEG integrative analysis is mismatches between the activated regions detected by fMRI and MEG. These mismatches cause serious degradation of the estimation accuracy, especially when fMRI-invisible activity has high temporal correlations to activity detected by fMRI. We developed a spatial filter that can achieve accurate reconstruction of MEG source activity even when a priori information from fMRI is insufficient (Okada, et al., 2007). The filter is based on the generalized least squares (GLS) estimation method. The GLS method requires the determination of the noise covariance matrices, and the filter utilizes the measured MEGs for this determination. Principal component analysis (PCA) is applied to the measured MEGs to determine the noise covariance matrices. Simulation results using conditions in which fMRI-invisible MEG sources are present demonstrated that the proposed filter could reconstruct MEG source activity more accurately than could methods based on either the ordinary least squares method or minimum variance beamforming. The validity of the proposed method was also discussed along with measured data from an experiment using an apparent motion visual stimulus. The results demonstrated that the proposed method could reconstruct reasonable time courses of activations.

Demonstration of the Method

To demonstrate the capability of the integrative fMRI-MEG method, it was applied to measured data obtained during two visual perception tasks. One was an apparent motion perception task, in which multiple cortical areas (not only the primary and secondary visual areas (V1/2), but also cortical areas related to processing visual motion, such as the fifth visual area (hMT+/V5) and the intraparietal sulcus (IPS)) are known to activate simultaneously (Okada, et al., 2007). We also applied the method to data obtained during a visually-guided saccade task and could successfully reconstruct reasonable time courses of dynamic neural activity in multiple visual areas (such as IPS, hMT+/V5, V1/V2).

An experimental paradigm in the fMRI measurement was designed to compare brain activity during apparent visual motion perception and control conditions, each block lasting 30 s. Data from blood oxygenation level dependent (BOLD) contrast under the two different conditions were compared. A pair of visual stimuli presented in the apparent visual motion perception experiment is shown in Figure 1. Under control conditions, a fixed point at the center of the screen was presented.

Seven healthy subjects (21-33 years old) with normal and corrected-to-normal visual acuity participated in the experiments. All subjects gave written informed consent after the purpose and procedure of the experiments were explained to them.

Upper-right and lower-right white circles in a pair of stimuli in Figure 1 were switched every 500 s in the apparent motion perception block. The diameter of the white circle was 1 degree and it was presented in the upper right visual field 1 degree away from the fixation point. One

Figure 1. A pair of visual stimuli used in the experiments

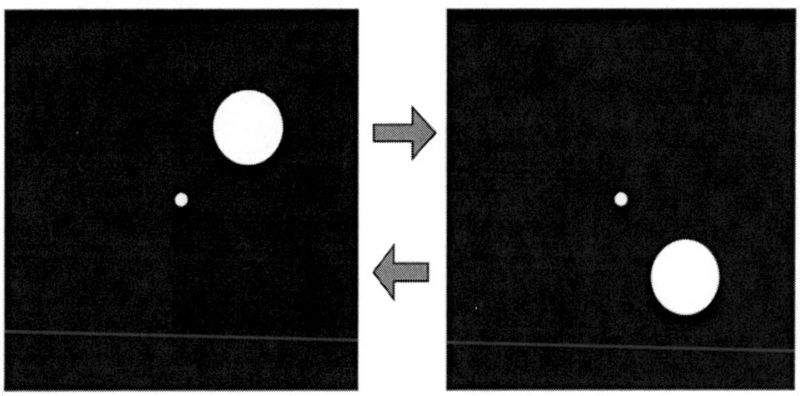

experiment consisted of 10 blocks. Stimuli were projected onto a screen using an LCD projector.

In the MEG measurements, the upper-right and lower-right white circles shown in Figure 1 were switched every 1.3 s. The switching time was treated as a trigger for averaging to obtain event-related responses.

Acquisitions of MRI and MEG Data

A Signa Horizon (GE) operated at 1.5 T was used with the standard fMRI procedure (gradient echo EPI; TR = 3 s, TE = 40 ms, FA = 90 degree, FOV = 22 cm, 25 5-mm-thick slices, spacing = 1 mm, image matrix = 64 x 64). We scanned 100 functional images for each slice. After the experiment, T1-weighted anatomical images (0.86 x 0.86 x 1.5 mm voxel size) were acquired for co-registration with the functional mean images.

In the MEG experiments, a 306-channel whole-cortex MEG system (VectorView, Neuromag), with 204 first-order planer gradiometers and 102 magnetometers, was used. The sampling frequency of the data acquisition was 500.8 Hz. In the present study, event-related neuromagnetic fields (ERFs) were measured for 300 trials. The ERFs with 204 gradiometers were used in the present integrative analysis.

Results and Disucssion

Figure 2 shows a representative result of fMRI-MEG integration analyses during apparent motion conditions in a representative subject. Significant differential activations (corrected, $p<0.001$) are overlaid onto three axial planes. In this subject, three clusters were activated: the ipsilateral V5, contralateral V5 and contralateral V1/V2 (as seen in the MRIs in Figure 2). The left graphs in Figure 2 represent time courses of reconstructed activations of all voxels in each cluster.

Since activations obtained during the pre-trigger time duration are considered to be noise, we calculated the standard deviation (SD) of the noise in each voxel using the pre-trigger data. Subsequently, activations stronger than 4 SD

Figure 2. The results of fMRI analyses in a representative subject (right). Significant differential activations (corrected, p<0.001) during apparent motion conditions are overlaid onto three axial planes. The time courses of reconstructed activations of all voxels in three clusters: the ipsilateral V5, conralateral V5 and contralateral V1/V2, are shown in the left.

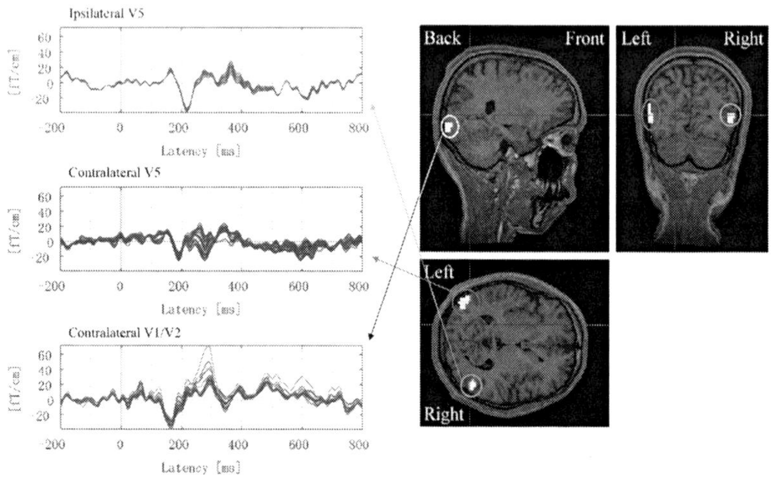

($p<0.0001$) were extracted to determine the significant activation latencies in each voxel. Finally, we visualized the dynamic activations in multiple clusters.

Although there were individual differences, the present fMRI-MEG integrative neuroimaging method successfully estimated dynamic cortical activity during apparent motion perception in all seven subjects. Repetitive and/or simultaneous activations in the same cortical areas (such as V5 and V1/2) were confirmed, providing evidence for the involvement of feedback mechanisms in apparent visual motion perception. These results demonstrate that the present method is promising for revealing the dynamics of multiple cortical activity changes associated with higher cognitive brain functions.

HIGH-SENSITIVITY ATOMIC MAGNETOMETERS

Principles

Optically pumped atomic magnetometers (OPAMs) using alkali metal vapors contained in glass cells are capable of measuring extremely small magnetic fields. OPAMs are based on the detection of Larmor spin precession in the alkali atoms contained in the glass cells. In recent years, OPAMs operating under spin-exchange relaxation-free (SERF) conditions have reached sensitivities comparable to and even surpassing those of SQUID-based magnetometers. The most sensitive atomic magnetometer has sensitivity in the subfemtotesla range (Kominis, Kornak, Allred, & Romalis, 2003). In addition, OPAMs have the intrinsic advantage of not requiring cryogenic cooling.

Methods

One of our experimental magnetometer setups is shown in Figure 3. The magnetometer's sensor head was a cubic Pyrex glass cell, 30 mm on each side. The cell contained potassium metal and He and N2 as buffer gases at a ratio of 10 to 1 for slowing the diffusion of potassium atoms to the cell walls and for quenching.

Potassium atoms were spin-polarized by a circularly polarized pump laser beam supplied by a laser diode with an external cavity (Tiger, Sacher Lasertechnik), tuned to the center of the pressure-broadened D1 line of potassium atoms (770.1 nm). A linearly polarized probe laser beam supplied by the other laser diode (Lion, Sacher Lasertechnik) was slightly blue-detuned from the D1 resonance (769.9 nm) and crossed the pump beam at a right angle in the cell. Both the pump and probe laser beams were 30 mm in diameter.

The polarization rotation of the probe beam was measured as a change in the intensity differences between the vertical and horizontal polarization components split by the polarized beam splitter. Changes in the intensity differences were detected by a balanced amplified detector. The cell was heated to approximately 450 K by hot flowing air in an oven to increase the atomic density and was placed at the center of three-layer-μmetal magnetic shields with a shielding factor of 104 at 30 Hz.

Weak external DC magnetic fields passing through the magnetic shields were canceled by three-axes Helmholtz coils set up around the cell. The sensitivity of the magnetometer was 10-100 fT/Hz1/2 at frequencies below several hundred Hz.

Measurements

We made a phantom that models the human head (taking into account the distributed electric currents) to evaluate the atomic magnetometer. The diameter of the phantom was 100 mm. The dipole electrode was 6 mm long and was positioned 5 mm from the bottom of the phantom.

Subsequently, we scanned the phantom on a plane and used the atomic magnetometer to measure the field distributions generated by the dipole electrode in the phantom. The phantom was

Figure 3. Schematic of the experimental setup: Atomic spins of K are polarized to y direction by a circularly polarized pump beam. The polarized spins evolving in a a-directed magnetic field rotate the polarization direction of the probe beam.

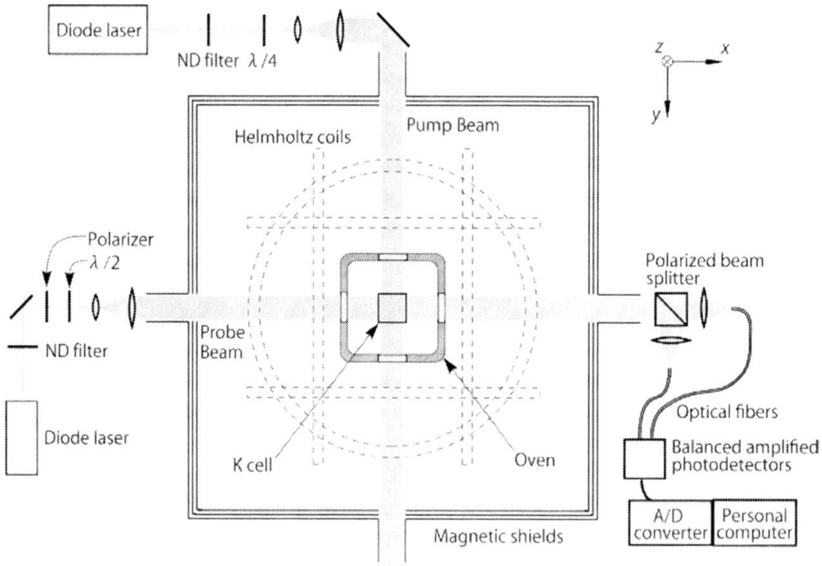

placed in a basket above the oven and scanned two-dimensionally on an x-y plane by a gearing mechanism composed of plastic components and operated by wires leading out from the shields. The distance from the center of the cell to the dipole electrode was about 60 mm.

To verify the accuracy of the measurements, the measured magnetic field distribution was compared with the theoretical distribution obtained by Sarvas's equation (Sarvas, 1987). Figure 4(a) and 4(b) are the measured and theoretical magnetic field distributions from the dipole electrode, respectively. The goodness of fit value for this localization was 97.9%.

Finally, measurements of magnetocardiographies (MCGs) in a small rat (female Wistar rat that was 4 weeks old and weighed 86 g) were performed (Taue, Ichihara, Sugihara, Ishikawa, Sugioka, Mizutani, Liu, Hirai, Tabata, & Kobayashi, 2008). The anesthetized rat was laid in

Figure 4. (a) Measured and (b) theoretical magnetic field distributions generated from the phantom

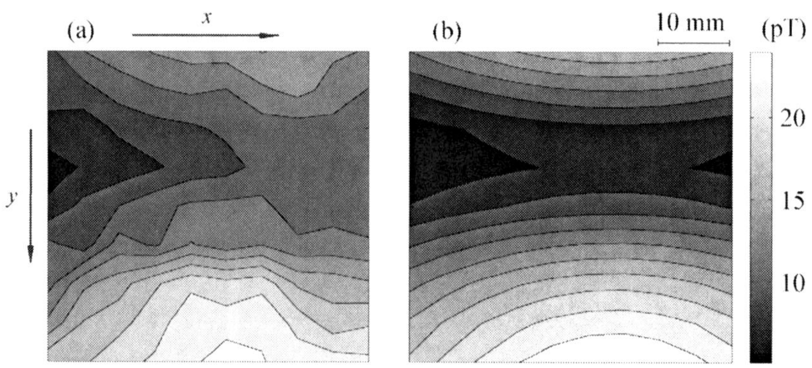

a container on the oven with its stomach down. Figure 5 shows a representative MCG waveform measured from the small rat. Figure 5 (b) is a MCG waveform averaged over 5 cardiac cycles triggered by each peak, indicated as arrows in Figure 5 (a).

CONCLUSION

We introduced a novel neuroimaging method by integrating fMRI and MEG to analyze spatial and temporal aspects of multiple cortical activities. In addition, we described the principles of the atomic magnetometer and the results of biomagnetic field measurements.

The applicability of new neuroimaging methods and sensors as described in the present paper might provide important advancements in cognitive brain research and improve the clinical diagnosis and management of neurological and psychiatric disorders.

ACKNOWLEDGMENT

The author thanks all of the members of his group in Kyoto University for their cooperation. The author also appreciates Dr. Ishikawa at the University of Hyogo and Mr. Ichihara at Canon, Inc. Some of the results introduced in this paper were obtained by the Innovative Techno-Hub

Figure 5. Measured MCG signals: (a) A representative measured MCG waveform. Peaks (arrows) of heartbeats are observed. (b) A waveform averaged over 5 heartbeats.

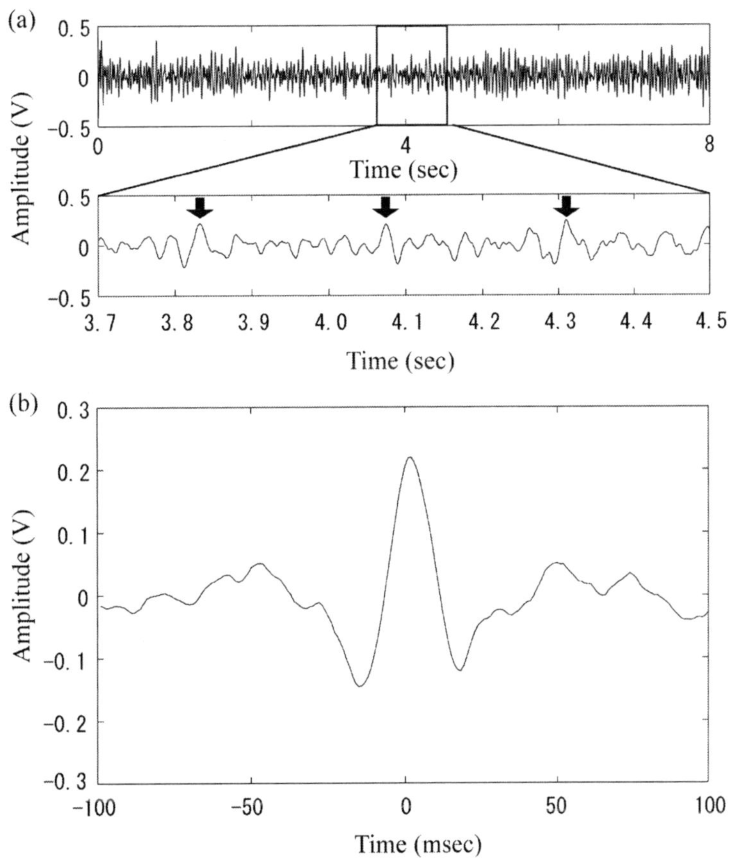

for Integrated Medical Bio-imaging Project of the Special Coordination Funds for Promoting Science and Technology, supported by the Ministry of Education, Culture, Sports, Science and Technology (MEXT), Japan.

REFERENCES

Carrie, J. S., Reynolds, A., Goodyear, B. G., Ponton, C. W., Dort, J. C., & Eggermont, J. J. (2004). Simultaneous 3-T fMRI and high-density recording of human auditory evoked potentials. *NeuroImage*, *23*, 1129–1142. doi:10.1016/j.neuroimage.2004.07.035

Dale, A. M., Liu, A. K., Fischi, B. R., Buckner, R. L., Belliveau, J. W., Lewine, J. D., & Halgren, E. (2000). Dynamic statistical parametric mapping: Combining fMRI and MEG for high-resolution imaging of cortical activity. *Neuron*, *26*, 55–67. doi:10.1016/S0896-6273(00)81138-1

Frackowiak, R. S. J., Friston, K. J., Frith, C. D., Dolan, R. J., Price, C. J., & Zeki, S. … Penny, W. (2003). *Human brain function*, 2nd ed. Amsterdam, The Netherlands: Elsevier Academic Press.

Hämäläinen, M., Hari, R., Ilmoniemi, R. J., Knuutila, J., & Lounasmaa, O. V. (1993). Magnetoencephalograph-theory, instrumentation, and applications to noninvasive studies of the working human brain. *Reviews of Modern Physics*, *65*, 413–497. doi:10.1103/RevModPhys.65.413

Innami, Y., Kobayashi, T., Jung, J., Ohashi, S., Hamada, S., & Nagamine, T. (2004). An fMRI-MEG integrative method for dynamic imaging of multiple cortical activities [in Japanese]. *Transactions of the Japanese Society For Medical Biological Engineering*, *44*, 777–784.

Kobayashi, T. (2009). Basics and applications of functional MRI [in Japanese]. *Human Interface*, *11*, 39–44.

Kobayashi, T., Ozaki, I., & Nagata, K. (Eds.). (2009). *Brain topography and multimodal imaging*. Kyoto, Japan: Kyoto University Press.

Kominis, I. K., Kornak, T. W., Allred, J. C., & Romalis, M. V. (2003). A subfemtotesla multichannel atomic magnetometer. *Nature*, *422*, 596–599. doi:10.1038/nature01484

Ohashi, Y., Innami, Y., Jung, J., Hamada, S., & Kobayashi, T. (2006). A study on the application of a linearly-constrained adaptive beamformer to fMRI-MEG integrative analysis [in Japanese]. *Transactions of the Japanese Society for Medical and Biological Engineering*, *44*, 722–727.

Okada, Y., Ohashi, S., Jung, J., Hamada, S., & Kobayashi, T. (2007). An fMRI-MEG integrative neuroimaging method: Improvements of its accuracy and robustness by suppression of fMRI-invisible coherent activities [in Japanese]. *Transactions of the Japanese Society for Medical and Biological Engineering*, *45*, 275–284.

Okamoto, M., Dan, H., Shimizu, K., Takeo, K., Amita, T., & Oda, I. (2004). Multimodal assessment of cortical activations during apple peeling by NIRS and fMRI0. *NeuroImage*, *21*, 1275–1288. doi:10.1016/j.neuroimage.2003.12.003

Sarvas, J. (1987). Basic mathematical and electromagnetic concepts of the biomagnetic inverse problem. *Physics in Medicine and Biology*, *32*(1), 11–22. doi:10.1088/0031-9155/32/1/004

Schulz, M., Chau, W., Graham, S. J., McIntosh, A. R., Ross, B., Ishii, R., & Pantev, C. (2004). An integrative MEG-fMRI study of the primary somatosensory cortex using cross-modal correspondence analysis. *NeuroImage*, *22*, 120–133. doi:10.1016/j.neuroimage.2003.10.049

Sekuler, R., & Blake, R. (2002). *Perception* (4th ed.). Boston, MA: McGraw-Hill Higher Education.

Taue, S., Ichihara, S., Sugihara, Y., Ishikawa, K., Sugioka, H., & Mizutani, N. … Kobayashi, T. (2008). Measurement of biomagnetic fields in small animals by use of an optical pumping atomic magnetometer. In R. Kakigi, et al (Eds.), *Biomagnetism*. (pp. 9-11). Hokkaido University Press.

KEY TERMS AND DEFINITIONS

Apparent Motion: The phenomenon in which the human visual system can be fooled into perceiving continuous motion by presenting a sequence of stationary images at the proper rate.

Beamforming: A signal processing technique used in sensor arrays for directional signal transmission or reception. This spatial selectivity is achieved by using adaptive or fixed receive/transmit beam patterns.

Functional Magnetic Resonance Imaging (fMRI): A type of specialized MRI scan. It measures the hemodynamic response (change in blood flow) related to neural activity in the brain or spinal cord of humans or other animals. It is one of the most recently developed forms of neuroimaging.

Magnetocardiography (MCG): A technique to measure the magnetic fields produced by electrical activity in the heart using extremely sensitive devices.

Magnetoencephalography (MEG): A non-invasive technique used to measure magnetic fields generated by small intracellular electrical currents in neurons of the brain. MEG provides direct information about the dynamics of evoked and spontaneous neural activity and the location of sources in the brain.

Optically Pumped Atomic Magnetometer (OPAM): Devices that measure magnetic fields by using lasers to detect the interaction between the magnetic field and alkali metal atoms in a vapor.

Principal Component Analysis (PCA): A mathematical procedure that transforms a number of possibly correlated variables into a smaller number of uncorrelated variables called principal components. The first principal component accounts for as much of the variability in the data as possible, and each succeeding component accounts for as much of the remaining variability as possible.

Superconducting Quantum Interference Devices (SQUIDs): Very sensitive magnetometers used to measure extremely weak magnetic fields, based on superconducting loops containing Josephson junctions.

Chapter 3
Location and Functional Definition of Human Visual Motion Organization using Functional Magnetic Resonance Imaging

Tianyi Yan
Graduate School of Natural Science and Technology, Okayama University, Japan

Jinglong Wu
Graduate School of Natural Science and Technology, Okayama University, Japan & International WIC Institute, Beijing University of Technology, China

ABSTRACT

In humans, functional imaging studies have found a homolog of the macaque motion complex, MT+, which is suggested to contain both the middle temporal (MT) and medial superior temporal (MST) areas in the ascending limb of the inferior temporal sulcus. In the macaque, the motion-sensitive MT and MST areas are adjacent in the superior temporal sulcus. Electrophysiology has identified several motion-selective regions in the superior temporal sulcus (STS) of the macaque. Two of the best-studied areas include the MT and MST areas. The MT area has strong projections to the adjacent MST area and is typically subdivided into the dorsal (MSTd) and lateral (MSTl) subregions. While MT encodes the basic elements of motion, MST has higher-order motion-processing abilities and has been implicated in the perception of both object motion and self motion. The macaque MST area has been shown to have considerably larger receptive fields than the MT area. The receptive fields of MT cells typically extend only a few degrees into the ipsilateral visual field, while MST neurons have receptive fields that extend well into the ipsilateral visual field.

DOI: 10.4018/978-1-60960-559-9.ch003

This study tentatively identifies these subregions as the human homologs of the macaque MT and MST areas, respectively (Fig. 1). Putative human MT and MST areas were typically located on the posterior/ventral and anterior/dorsal banks of a dorsal/posterior limb of the inferior temporal sulcus. These locations are similar to their relative positions in the macaque superior temporal sulcus.

INTRODUCTION

The human visual area V5, also known as the MT (middle temporal) visual area, is a region of the extrastriate visual cortex that is thought to play a major role in motion perception, the integration of local motion signals into global percepts and the guidance of some eye movements. MT is connected to a wide array of cortical and subcortical brain areas. Its inputs include the visual cortical areas V1, V2 and dorsal V3 (dorsomedial area), the koniocellular regions of the LGN and the inferior pulvinar. The pattern of projections to the MT area changes somewhat between the representations of the foveal and peripheral visual fields, with the latter receiving inputs from areas located in the midline cortex and retrosplenial region.

A standard view holds that V1 provides the "most important" input to the MT area. Nonetheless, several studies have demonstrated that neurons in the MT are capable of responding to visual information, often in a direction-selective manner, even after the V1 area has been destroyed or inactivated. Moreover, studies by Semir Zeki and collaborators have suggested that certain types of visual information may reach the MT area before they reach the V1 area. The MT area sends its major outputs to areas located in the cortex immediately surrounding it, including the FST, MST and V4t (the middle temporal crescent) areas. Other MT projections target the eye movement-related areas of the frontal and parietal lobes (frontal eye field and lateral intraparietal area).

In primates, a motion-sensitive area in the occipitotemporal visual cortex was identified both functionally and anatomically. It was named the V5 area or MT area, after its middle temporal location in the owl monkey (Duffy and Wurtz, 1991b). Recently, it has been renamed the MT+ area, indicating that it probably comprises functionally segregated subregions (Albright and Desimone, 1987; Ha¨ndel et al, 2007). In the macaque, it is now accepted that the preference of V5/MT+ for motion stimuli is rooted in the receptive field properties of retinal M ganglion cells, which project exclusively to neurons of the magnocellular subdivisions of the dorsal lateral geniculate nucleus (Huk et al, 2002). This magnocelluar pathway has been shown to project to V5/MT+ (Huk et al, 2002). With the advent of non-invasive brain imaging tools, such as positron emission tomography (PET) and functional magnetic resonance imaging (fMRI), human motion processing has been investigated more directly than was possible in the past (Tianyi et al, 2009).

Several neuroimaging studies have localized the human homolog of the monkey motion complex that is often referred to as MT+ and includes the middle temporal (MT) and other adjacent motion-sensitive areas, such as the medial superior temporal (MST). The monkey MST area has been shown to have considerably larger receptive fields than the MT area. The receptive fields of MT cells typically extend only a few degrees into the ipsilateral visual field, while MST neurons have receptive fields that extend well into the ipsilateral visual field (Tootell et al, 1995). Raiguel et al. (1997) recorded neurons in the MST whose receptive fields extended 30–40° into the ipsilateral field (Ha¨ndel et al, 2007), whereas MT receptive fields protruded only 10–15° into the ipsilateral field.

No study has been able to distinguish the MT area from the MST area in humans. Although previous experiments have assessed ipsilateral responses within human MT and thus offer some evidence for large receptive fields within a region of the MT area, our experiments are unique in that they provide conclusive evidence for a double-dissociation of the human MT and MST areas. A previous study of MT subdivisions defined a putative MT area as the region of MT that did not exhibit ipsilateral responses (Smith et al, 2006; Boussaoud et al, 1992). Our experiments use two complementary measurements, one measuring relatively large receptive fields and the other measuring relatively small receptive fields. In addition to providing positive evidence for the existence of human MT and MST areas, our measurements revealed a retinotopic organization in human MT that was similar to proposals that have been previously documented in macaque MT. This evidence further strengthens the case for homology between these cortical motion-processing structures in humans and macaques. Here, we show that, similar to the results found in monkeys, the two areas are adjacent and can be functionally separated in humans.

EXPERIMENT

Subjects and Stimuli

Nine healthy subjects with no previous neurological or psychiatric disorders (age range 19–31 years, mean age 25 years; five women, four men) participated in the study. The subjects had normal or corrected-to-normal vision and were all right-handed. We obtained written informed consent from all subjects before the start of the experiment. The study was approved by the Institutional Research Review Board of ShengJing Hospital, China. Visual stimuli were created on a display using a resolution of 800 × 600 pixels.

MT+ Localizer Stimulus

All subjects were experienced psychophysical observers, were practiced at maintaining fixation, and had participated previously in other functional magnetic resonance imaging (fMRI) studies. Consent was obtained, and all procedures were in compliance with safety procedures for magnetic resonance research. Each subject participated in two scanning sessions: one to obtain high-resolution anatomical brain images and one to measure the contralateral versus ipsilateral responses (one for each visual hemifield). In all sessions, subjects were instructed to watch the motions of dots while maintaining fixation on a 0.5°, full-contrast fixation point. Area MT+ localizer stimulus was functionally identified based on responses to stimuli that alternated in time between moving and stationary dot patterns (Figure 1A). These methods were also used in the study by Huk et al. (2002). Moving dots traveled toward and away from their fixed positions (8°/sec) within a 120° diameter circular aperture. They alternated direction once per second (white dots on a black background; dot diameter of 0.25°).

Ipsilateral Stimulus

Ipsilateral stimulation is a complementary test used to distinguish MST from MT. We tested for ipsilateral responses using stimuli restricted to the left or right hemifield. The stimuli alternated every 18 sec for 7 cycles between a field of moving dots and a similar field of static dots (Figure 1B). The dots were restricted to a peripheral circular aperture (120° diameter) with its closest edge located 15° from fixation. These peripheral moving stimuli were expected to evoke neuronal activity in the contralateral hemisphere in the macaque MT and MST areas, but they would be expected to evoke activity in the ipsilateral hemisphere only in the MST area, where the receptive fields are sufficiently large to extend into the ipsilateral hemifield. The ipsilateral scans were repeated 6–12 times in each hemifield for each subject.

Figure 1. Moving versus stationary (see stimuli parts), localizing MT. The MT area was identified based on responses to stimuli that alternated in time between moving (radially inward and outward from a fixation point, alternating direction every second for 18 sec) and stationary (18 sec) dot patterns. Subjects fixated on a small high-contrast square in the center of the dot field. B, Ipsilateral stimulation identifying MST. Responses to ipsilateral stimulation were assessed by presenting a peripheral dot patch in the left or right visual field. The 15° diameter field of dots alternated between moving (18 sec) and stationary (18 sec).

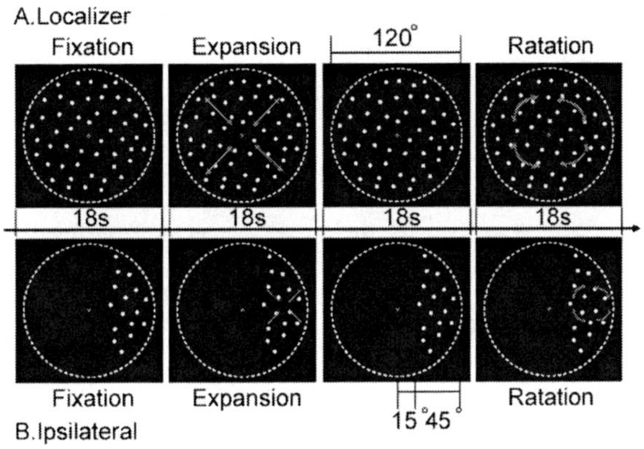

RESULTS

Identifying MT+

The MT area was identified separately for each subject, based on a combination of anatomical and functional criteria. Specifically, a contiguous region was marked by hand to include voxels on the lateral surface of the occipital lobe, where the fMRI time series correlated strongly with the moving/stationary stimulus alternations (r>4.00, chosen separately for each subject). The two subjects shown in Figure 2 further suggest that the ipsilateral response tended to mirror the anterior part of the MT+ area rather than the entire complex. Indeed, corroborating the results of Smith et al. (2006), the ipsilateral response was located slightly anterior to the contralateral response, i.e., the MT+ area (Table 1). The average locations of the activations of the putative human homolog of the MT+ area in left hemispheres were -45, -68 and 3 and in the right hemispheres were 45, -61 and 3.

First, this activity was often found in a different sulcus (or sulci), with MT clearly on the other side of an intervening gyrus. This fact was somewhat obscured on the flat-map representation but was more evident when the data were viewed in sagittal slices of the three-dimensional (3D) brain volume. Second, the application of a high correlation threshold (higher than that used in the figures) to the MT+ localizer responses revealed a clear distinction between MT+ and this posterior–ventral activity. In fact, the MT+ localizer stimulus elicited activity throughout much of the occipital lobe; the responses were simply stronger (withstanding a higher correlation threshold) in the MT+ area.

Position of MT+ Subregions

To better evaluate the relative positions of these areas in the 3D cortical volume, we transformed the regions corresponding to MT and MST from the flat map to the corresponding gray matter in the high-resolution anatomy images of each subject's brain. In all of the right hemispheres in which we were able to define MT and MST, we observed that MT fell primarily on the posterior

Figure 2. Activations observed by comparing right hemifield visual motion using a t-value threshold of four (P < 0.000099). Responses were superimposed on axial and sagittal anatomical slices of two exemplary participants (subjects BRB and WNN).

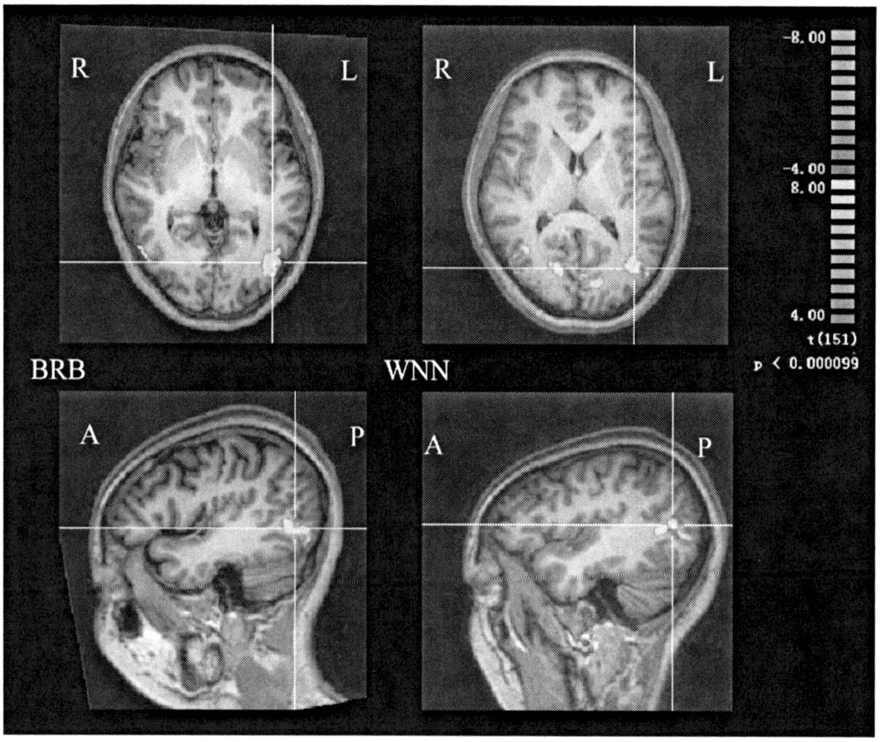

Table 1. V5/MT+ coordinates in this study compared to other studies. Data are given in coordinates (middle columns).

Years	Author		Talairach Coordinates					
			Left hemisphere			Right hemisphere		
1993	J. D. G. Watson	PET/ MRI	-44	-70	0	40	-68	0
1995	Roger B. H. TooTell	FMRI	-45	-76	3	45	-76	3
1997	Patrick Dupont	PET/ MRI	-40	-70	-4	40	-64	4
1997	Michael S. Beauchamp	FMRI	-42	-70	3	42	-70	3
1998	Andrew T. Smith	FMRI	-46	-70	4	46	-70	4
1999	Stefan Sunaert	FMRI	-42	-66	2	42	-62	6
2000	Serge O. Dumoulin	FMRI	-47	-76	2	44	-67	0
2001	Sean P. Dukelow	FMRI	-	-	-	44	-67	2
2005	Marcus Wilms	FMRI	-43	-67	8	49	-64	9
Mean location in present study			-45	-68	3	45	-61	3

(-ventral) bank of a sulcus, whereas MST fell on an anterior (-dorsal) bank. This sulcus could usually be identified as a dorsal/posterior limb of the inferior temporal sulcus (ITS). Although this dorsal/posterior continuation of the ITS was the clearest anatomical landmark, we also observed that MT+ sometimes continued posteriorly into the lateral occipital sulcus and/or onto the lateral occipital gyrus.

Identifying MST: Ipsilateral Stimulation

The MST area was defined separately for each subject to include a contiguous subregion of MT that was distinct from the retinotopically defined MT that responded strongly to peripheral ipsilateral stimulation. Figure 3B shows the ipsilateral responses in the right hemisphere of one subject. Although the ipsilateral responses were relatively weak compared to the contralateral responses, a subregion of ipsilateral activity was clearly identifiable, marked by the cyan curve drawn on the inflated map.

In defining MST, we note that our conservative criteria sometimes left some MT regions unclassified (neither MT nor MST). MST, in the right hemispheres in which it was identified, was always anterior and often dorsal to MT, although there was some degree of variability across subjects. In these eight hemispheres, MST typically abutted MT; when some degree of separation was apparent, the areas were still within 5 mm of one another along the gray-matter surface. However, in one subject, we did not observe a clear double dissociation between the two MT subregions.

Figure 3. A, activation observed by comparing wide-field optic flow minus stationary correlation (P < 0.05) in subject 5 on both the inflated brain and an axial slice. Activation is observed in the MT area in the ascending limb of the inferior temporal sulcus (ITS, outlined on the inflated brain with a dashed white line).

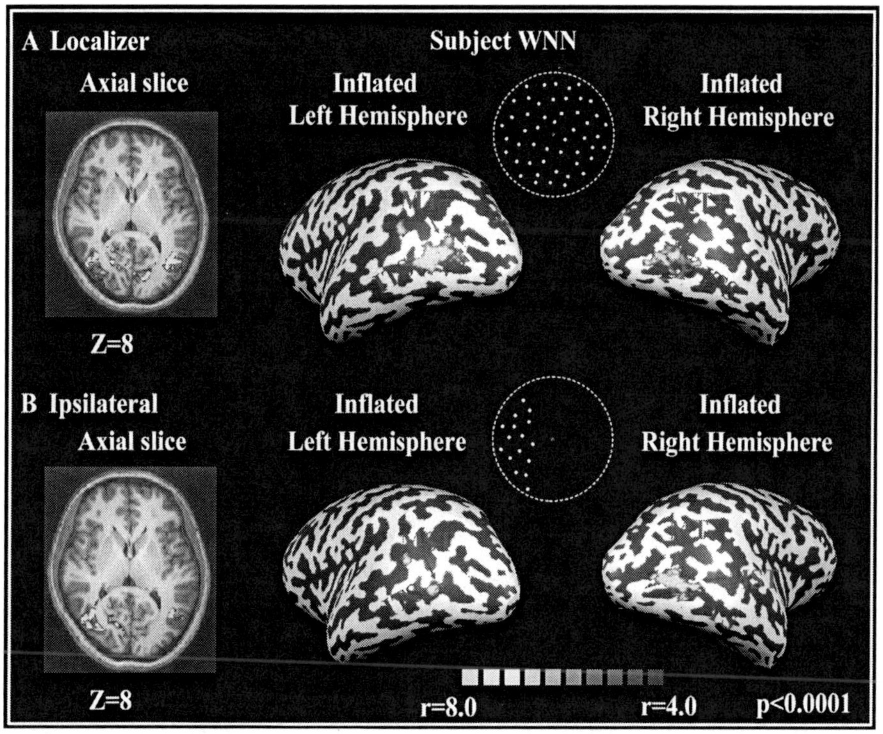

DISCUSSION

Several studies have shown that moving visual stimuli preferentially activate an area in the lateral occipito-temporal cortex in humans. This area has been named MT+ because it likely represents a complex of distinct areas that include the human homologs of the MT and MST areas found in monkeys. Our study shows that this assumption was correct. We demonstrated that MT, which typically lies in the ascending limb of the inferior temporal sulcus, is made up of two parts: MT and the more anterior but immediately adjacent MST. MST, in turn, can be separated into two adjacent parts, a posteromedial part that is activated by ipsilateral visual field and an anterolateral part that is activated in the peripheral visual area (Boussaoud et al, 1992).

One central goal of neuroscience is to describe the neuronal mechanisms underlying the transformation of sensory information, which is often unreliable, ambiguous or contaminated by disturbing signals. Some of the most intriguing insights have been gained from monkey studies aimed at addressing visual motion perception. To perform such studies, paradigms requiring the animal to extract a global motion signal embedded in noise have been used widely to acquire psychophysical measurements of visual motion processing (Sean et al, 2001). This approach, combined with single-cell recordings, has yielded intriguing insights into the mechanisms underlying global visual motion processing. Whereas studies of non-human primates have contributed substantially to our current knowledge of the neurophysiological responses underlying global motion perception, human studies measuring brain activity based on the responses of large neuronal populations are lacking. There are many reasons for this lack of information. First, a major difference between human and monkey studies are that it is only possible to adjust the stimuli to the preferences of the neuron under study in animals. Furthermore, non-invasive functional imaging of the human brain encompasses the responses of myriad neurons that potentially differ with respect to a number of important properties, including response fields (RF) size and preference for distinct motion directions and speeds (Dubowitz et al, 1998). A second major problem is that the spatial resolution of imaging techniques such as fMRI may not be sufficient to functionally separate cortical areas that lie in immediate proximity to each other.

These results also indicate that psychophysical comparisons of stimuli in the two visual fields must avoid the vertical meridian by significantly more than 15° (eccentricity angle) for maximum independence. Complete interhemispheric independence may be impossible to achieve throughout the visual cortex. The ipsilateral visual representation is thus a highly organized system, and it is topographically well integrated with other aspects of human visual cortical organization. The communication across the inter-hemispheric "seam" in higher visual areas is presumably related to the construction of a unitary visual percept, uniting the two hemifield maps that are present in lower-tier areas. Although in this study, we focus on this inter-hemispheric seam in the visual cortex, a similar approach using different stimuli should make it possible to map the interhemispheric seam in other cortical systems.

CONCLUSION

The results presented here contribute to observations that have established the notion of two distinct motion-sensitive areas in the MT+ area. As in the monkey brain, the human MST area has a greater specificity for global motion than does the MT area, and the latter responds equally well to wide field visual stimuli and random motions. However, given the remarkable functional diversification and refined classification of motion-sensitive visual areas elaborated in the monkey temporal cortex (Sean et al, 2001), our knowledge of the human visual cortex is still clearly lacking and prone to oversimplification.

ACKNOWLEDGMENT

This study was partially supported by the JSPS AA Science Platform Program and the JSPS Grant-in-Aid for Scientific Research (B) (21404002).

REFERENCES

Albright, T. D., & Desimone, R. (1987). Local precision of visuotopic organization in the middle temporal area (MT) of the macaque. *Experimental Brain Research, 65*, 582–592. doi:10.1007/BF00235981

Boussaoud, D., Desimone, R., & Ungerleider, L. G. (1992). Subcortical connections of visual areas MST and FST in macaques. *Visual Neuroscience, 9*, 291–302. doi:10.1017/S0952523800010701

Dubowitz, D. J., Chen, D. Y., Atkinson, D. J., Grieve, K. L., Gillikin, B., Bradley, W. G. Jr, & Andersen, R. A. (1998). Functional magnetic resonance imaging in macaque cortex. *Neuroreport, 9*, 2213–2218. doi:10.1097/00001756-199807130-00012

Duffy, C. J., & Wurtz, R. H. (1991b). Sensitivity of MST neurons to optic flow stimuli. I. A continuum of response selectivity to large-field stimuli. *Journal of Neurophysiology, 65*, 1329–1345.

Dukelow, S. P., DeSouza, J. F. X., Culham, J. C., van den Berg, A. V., Menon, R. S., & Vilis, T. (2001). Distinguishing subregions of the human MT+ complex using visual fields and pursuit eye movements. *Journal of Neurophysiology, 86*, 1991–2000.

Handel, B., Lutzenberger, W., Thier, P., & Haarmeier, T. (2007). Opposite dependencies on visual motion coherence in human area MT+ and early visual cortex. *Cerebral Cortex, 17*, 1542–1549. doi:10.1093/cercor/bhl063

Huk, A. C., Dougherty, R. F., & Heeger, D. J. (2002). Retinotopy and functional subdivision of human areas MT and MST. *The Journal of Neuroscience, 22*, 7195–7205.

Smith, A. T., Wall, M. B., Williams, A. L., & Singh, K. D. (2006). Sensitivity to optic flow in human cortical areas MT and MST. *The European Journal of Neuroscience, 23*, 561–569. doi:10.1111/j.1460-9568.2005.04526.x

Tootell, R. B., Reppas, J. B., Kwong, K. K., Malach, R., Born, R. T., & Brady, T. J. (1995). Functional analysis of human MT and related visual cortical areas using magnetic resonance imaging. *The Journal of Neuroscience, 15*, 3215–3230.

Yan, Y., Jin, F., & Wu, J. (2009). *Correlated size variations measured in human visual cortex V1/V2/V3 with functional MRI. (LNAI 5819)* (pp. 36–44). Berlin/ Heidelberg, Germany: Brain Informatics/ Springer-Verlag.

KEY TERMS AND DEFINITIONS

Functional MRI or Functional Magnetic Resonance Imaging (fMRI): Is a type of specialized MRI scan. It measures the hemodynamic response (change in blood flow) related to neural activity in the brain or spinal cord of humans and other animals. It is one of the most recently developed forms of neuroimaging. Since the early 1990s, fMRI has come to dominate the brain mapping field due to its relatively low invasiveness, lack of radiation exposure, and relatively wide availability.

Lateral Geniculate Nucleus (LGN): Is the primary processing center for visual information received from the retina. The LGN is found inside the thalamus of the brain and is part of the central nervous system. The LGN receives information directly from the ascending retinal ganglion cells via the optic tract and from the reticular activating system. LGN neurons send their axons through the optic radiation, a pathway leading directly to the primary visual cortex (V1), also known as the striate cortex. The primary visual cortex surrounds the calcarine fissure, a horizontal fissure in the medial and posterior occipital lobes. In addition, the LGN receives many strong feedback connections from the primary visual cortex. In mammals and humans, the two strongest pathways linking the eye to the brain are those projecting to the LGNd (the dorsal part of the LGN in the thalamus) and the superior colliculus.

Neuroimaging: This term includes the use of various techniques to directly or indirectly image the structure, function and pharmacology of the brain. It is a relatively new discipline within medicine and neuroscience/psychology.

Positron Emission Tomography (PET): Is a nuclear medicine imaging technique that produces a three-dimensional image or picture of functional processes in the body. The system detects pairs of gamma rays emitted indirectly by a positron-emitting radionuclide (tracer), which is introduced into the body on a biologically active molecule. Images of tracer concentration in three-dimensional or four-dimensional space (the fourth dimension being time) within the body are then reconstructed by computer analysis. In modern scanners, this reconstruction is often accomplished with the aid of a CT X-ray scan performed on the patient in the same machine during the same session.

Retinotopic: This term describes the spatial organization of neuronal responses to visual stimuli. In many locations within the brain, adjacent neurons have receptive fields that include slightly different but overlapping portions of the visual field. The position of the center of these receptive fields forms an orderly sampling mosaic that covers a portion of the visual field. Because of this orderly arrangement, which emerges from the spatial specificity of connections between neurons in different parts of the visual system, cells in each structure can be seen as forming a map of the visual field (also called a retinotopic or visuotopic map). Retinotopic maps are a particular case of topographic organization. Many brain structures that are responsive to visual input, including much of the visual cortex and visual nuclei of the brain stem (such as the superior colliculus) and thalamus (such as the lateral geniculate nucleus and pulvinar), are organized into retinotopic maps, also called visual field maps.

V1: (BA17): The primary visual cortex is the best-studied visual area in the brain. In all mammals studied, it is located in the posterior pole of the occipital cortex, which is responsible for processing visual stimuli. It is the simplest, earliest cortical visual area. It is highly specialized for processing information about static and moving objects and is excellent at pattern recognition. The functionally defined primary visual cortex is approximately equivalent to the anatomically defined striate cortex. The name "striate cortex" is derived from the stria of Gennari, a distinctive stripe visible to the naked eye that represents myelinated axons from the lateral geniculate body that terminate in layer 4 of the gray matter.

V2 (BA18): The visual area V2, also called the prestriate cortex, is the second major area in the visual cortex and the first region within the visual association area. It receives strong feedforward connections from V1 and sends strong connections to V3, V4 and V5. It also sends strong feedback connections to V1. Anatomically, V2 is split into four quadrants, with dorsal and ventral representations in the left and right hemispheres. Together, these four regions provide a complete map of the visual world. Functionally, V2 has many properties in common with V1. Cells are tuned to simple properties such as orientation, spatial frequency, and color. The responses of many V2 neurons are also modulated by more complex properties, such as the orientation of illusory contours and whether the stimulus is part of the figure or the ground.

V3 (BA19): The term third visual complex refers to the region of the cortex located immediately in front of V2, which includes the region called visual area V3 in humans. The "complex" nomenclature is justified by the fact that some controversy still exists regarding the exact extent of area V3, with some researchers proposing that the cortex located in front of V2 may include two or three functional subdivisions. For example, David Van Essen et al. (1986) have proposed the existence of a "dorsal V3" in the upper part of the cerebral hemisphere that is distinct from the "ventral V3" (or ventral posterior area, VP), which is located in the lower part of the brain. Dorsal and ventral V3 have distinct connections with other parts of the brain, different appearances in sections stained with a variety of methods and contain neurons that respond to different combinations of visual stimuli (e.g., color-selective neurons are more common in the ventral V3). Additional subdivisions, including V3A and V3B, have also been reported in humans. These subdivisions are located near dorsal V3 but do not adjoin V2.

V5/MT: Visual area V5, also known as visual area MT (middle temporal), is a region of extrastriate visual cortex that is thought to play a major role in motion perception, the integration of local motion signals into global percepts and the guidance of some eye movements.

Visual Cortex: This term refers to the primary visual cortex (also known as the striate cortex or V1) and extrastriate visual cortical areas such as V2, V3, V4 and V5. The primary visual cortex is anatomically equivalent to the Brodmann area 17 (or BA17). The extrastriate cortical areas consist of Brodmann areas 18 and 19. There is a visual cortex for each hemisphere of the brain. The left hemisphere visual cortex receives signals from the right visual field and the right visual cortex from the left visual field.

Chapter 4
Visual Attention with Auditory Stimulus

Shuo Zhao
Graduate School of Natural Science and Technology, Okayama University, Japan

Chunlin Li
Graduate School of Natural Science and Technology, Okayama University, Japan

Jinglong Wu
Graduate School of Natural Science and Technology, Okayama University, Japan

Hongbin Han
Peking University, China

Dehua Chui
Neuroscience Research Institute / Third Hospital of Peking University, China

ABSTRACT

Visual orienting attention is best studied using visual cues. Spatial and temporal attention have been compared using brain-imaging data. This chapter's authors developed a visual orienting attention tool to compare auditory when a visual target was presented. They also designed a control task in which subjects had to click on the response key consistent with a simultaneous spatial task. The effect of clicking the response key was removed by subtracting the brain activations elicited by clicking the response key from the results of the visual voluntary attention task. The authors then measured brain activity in sixteen healthy volunteers using functional magnetic resonance imaging (Coull, Frith, Büchel & Nobre, 2000). In the task, visual spatial attention was manipulated by a visual cue, and participants were told to ignore the auditory stimulus. A neutral task was also performed, in which a neutral cue was used. Symbolic central cues oriented subjects to spatial location only (Coull & Nobre, 1998) or gave no information about spatial location. Subjects were also scanned during a resting baseline condition in which they clicked the reaction key ten times. The reaction time for spatial location attention was faster than that without an auditory stimulus. Brain-imaging data showed that the inferior parietal lobe (IPL) and anterior cingulated cortex (ACC) were activated in the visual-spatial attention task and that the activation was enhanced during the task with the auditory stimulus.

DOI: 10.4018/978-1-60960-559-9.ch004

INTRODUCTION

Given the rapid increase in the elderly population, dementia has become a major social problem. Alzheimer's disease is thought to be the most common cause of dementia.

Previous studies of spatial attention in patients with mild cognitive impairment suggest that there is a reorganization of the relationships between the limbic system and the spatial attention network during healthy aging with mild cognitive impairment. We therefore thought that the spatial attention system would be altered in early-stage Alzheimer's disease. Elucidation ofthe sophisticated mechanisms of spatial attention in the brain could in turn be useful in the diagnosis of early-stage Alzheimer's disease.

Previous studies on attention proposed various psychological models supported by a variety of psychological and physiological evidence. The neuronal substrate of the human attention system has also been investigated using positron emission tomography (Corbetta, Miezin, Shulman & Petersen, 1993) and functional magnetic resonance imaging (fMRI) as well as by examining visual and auditory attention in humans using audiovisual stimuli. The primary motor cortex (BA6), prefrontal cortex (BA46), parietal lobe (BA7), and middle frontal gyrus (BA40) are activated with top-down control of visual-spatial attention (Coull & Nobre, 1998; Coull, Frith et al., 2000; Nobre, Gitelman, Dias & Mesulam, 2000). The primary motor cortex (BA6/4), prefrontal cortex (BA46/9), parietal lobe (BA7), and middle frontal gyrus (BA40) are also activated with top-down control of auditory-spatial attention (Zatorre, Mondor & Evans, 1999; Schubotz, von Cramon & Lohmann, 2003; Degerman, Rinne, Salmi, Salonen & Alho, 2006).

However, we still lack a good understanding of the common and varying networks used by visual-spatial and auditory attention systems. Moreover, attention to distraction has not been sufficiently researched in terms of visual space, and few studies have compared the differences between visual-spatial attention with and without auditory distractions.

In this study, we analyzed visual-spatial attention using both visual and auditory stimuli. To evaluate these processes behaviorally, we conducted psychological experiments in which we measured the reaction times (RTs) for each task. To reveal the neuronal networks related to these attention systems, we measured hemodynamic changes using fMRI.

ATTENTION

Attention is defined as the ability to attend to some things while ignoring others (Michael S. Gazzaniga 2008). Attention is very important in cognitive neuroscience, in part because this cognitive ability supports our awareness and influences our ability to encode information in long-term memory. There is no better definition of attention than that of William James, who stated a century ago, "Everyone knows what attention is. It is the taking possessing of the mind in clear and vivid form of what seem several simultaneous objects of trains of thought" (James, 1890).

We often divide attention into two broad categories: involuntary attention and voluntary attention (Figure 1). Involuntary attention, a bottom-up stimulus-driven process, describes attention captured by a sensory event. Voluntary attention, a top-down goal-directed process, represents our plan to attend to something. In this study, we focus on the mechanisms of voluntary attention.

In human information-processing systems, voluntary attention plays an important role in selecting and integrating information (Figure 1). Selective attention suggests that individuals have a tendency to process information from only one part of the environment to the exclusion of other parts. For example, the cocktail party effect is typical of selective attention. A British psycholo-

Figure 1.Category of attention

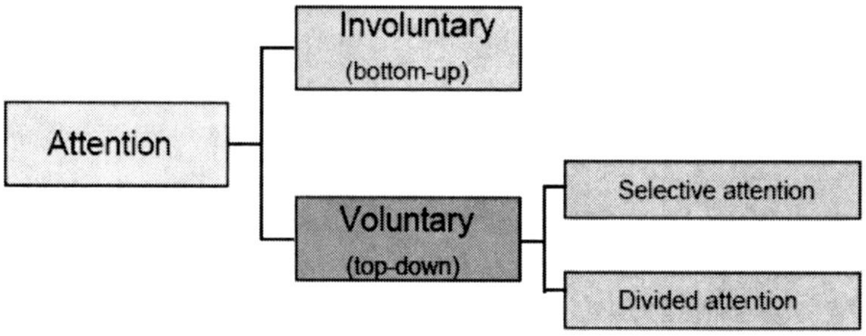

gist examined the so-called cocktail party effect: in the noisy, confusing environment of a cocktail party, we can still focus on a single conversation.

Multi-modal spatial integration is a common phenomenon in spatial perception. For example, we can make a phone call while driving a car. A previous study (Strayer, Drews and Crouch 2006) compared making a phone call while driving a car to making a phone call using one hand. They reported that making a phone call while driving a car was slower than making the call using one hand. In this study, we compared selective attention to integrated attention to reveal the neuronal networks related to these attention systems.

EXPERIMENT

Subjects

The subjects were 16 healthy right-handed college students aged 21–32 years. Informed consent was obtained from each participant following a detailed explanation of the study.

Experimental System

During fMRI scanning, visual stimuli were generated by a personal computer and presented to the subjects via a projector-screen–mirror system.

Experimental Stimuli

The visual stimulus consisted of a target ("X") with a diameter of 1° that was shown for 50 ms, 7° to the right or left of the central point on a screen located 130 cm in front of the subjects. Visual experiments included spatial tasks (S) and control tasks (N). The tasks were designed in a factorial format and are shown in Table 1.

Cue stimuli were used to direct the subjects' attention to a particular target location or onset time. The neutral cue provided spatial information, and the spatial (space) cue directed the subjects' attention to the left or right (Figure 3). The time from the end of stimulus presentation to the onset of the next stimulus was defined as the interval of the stimuli (IOS) and lasted 3000 ms (Figure 4). We recorded the RT, the time from the presentation of a stimulus to an indicated response, by a reaction key. The subjects responded to a right stimulus using the middle finger of their right hand and to a left stimulus with the forefinger of their right hand. The subjects performed 30 trials under each condition. There were two sessions, one with only visual stimuli and another to test

Table 1. Experimental tasks

	Visual	Visual with auditory distraction
Spatial	VS	VaS
Neutral	VN	VaN

Figure 2.fMRI experimental setup

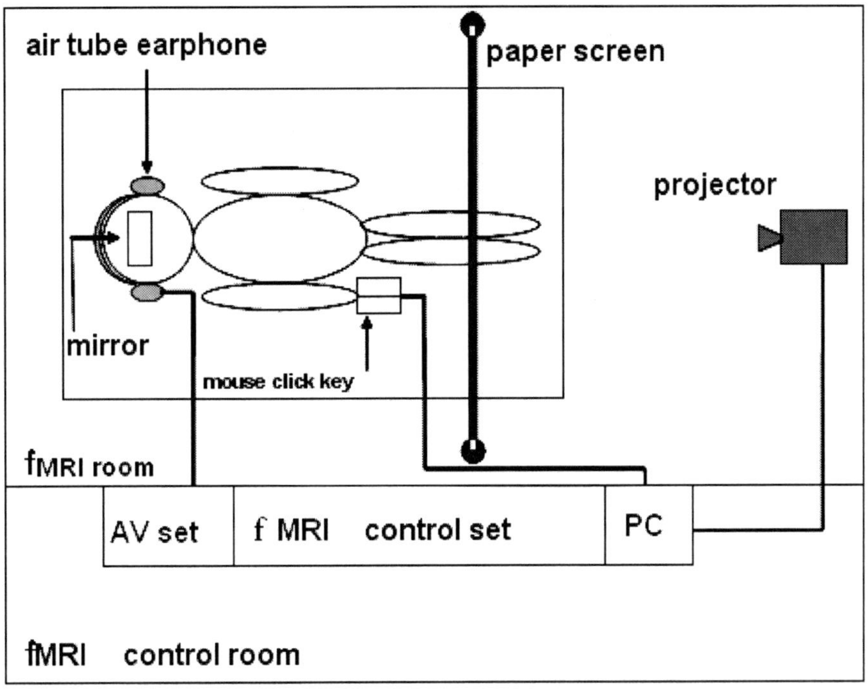

visual attention with auditory distraction. The visual and auditory stimuli were presented using a projector, as shown in Figure 2. The subject lay on MRI equipment and viewed the visual stimuli through the half mirror while the auditory stimuli were applied though the air tube earphone.

Methods

fMRI Scanning

We used a Philips 3.0 Tesla Magnetom Vision whole-body MRI system to measure brain activation using a head coil. The imaging area consisted of 32 functional gradient-echo planar imaging (EPI) axial slices (voxel size 3×3×4 mm, TR=4000 ms, TE=50 ms, FA=90°, 128×128 matrix) that were used to obtain T2-weighted fMRI images in the axial plane. The EPI images contained the entire cortex. For each task, we obtained 124 functional volumes. Before the EPI scan, a T2-weighted volume was acquired for anatomical alignment (TR=3500 ms, TE=100 ms, FA=90°, 256×256 matrix, voxel size=0.75×0.75×4 mm). The T2 image acquisition used the same slices as the functional image acquisition.

The spatial cue was used in the spatial attention tasks. The stimulus consisted of lighting either the right or left half of a cube to give the subjects information on the target location (right or left).

Figure 3.Central cues used in the experimental task

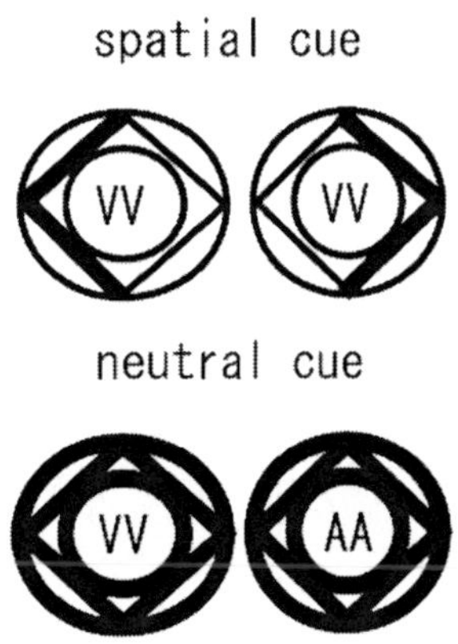

Figure 4. Task flow for each trial

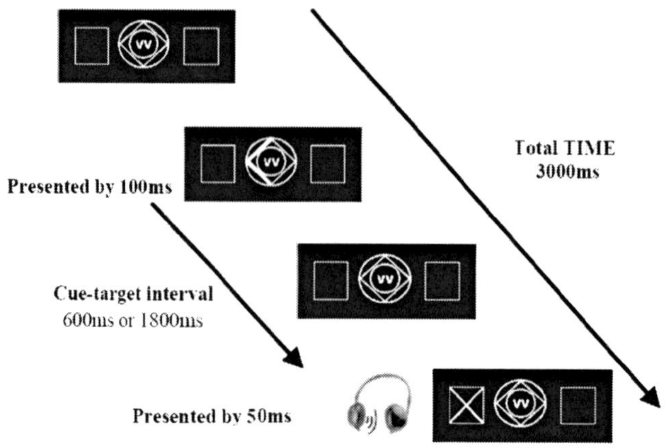

The neutral cue was used in the control task and gave neither spatial nor temporal information. A double 'V' in the center of the cue indicated a visual experiment.

In this example, the visual-spatial cue indicated spatial information but gave no information about the cue-target interval. The cue was lit for 100 ms, and the target was illuminated for 50 ms after the cue–target interval (600 or 1800 ms).

Data Analysis

Reaction times were used as behavioral data. The RT data during the fMRI experiment were analyzed using repeated measures analysis of variance (ANOVA; SPSS 12.0j for Windows). For each task, 60 RTs were acquired from each subject. We used the average of the RT data for the ANOVA, except for error trials (all subjects reacted with accuracy above 90%). Therefore, we had 16 RT values for each task. Four tasks were presented in this experiment, and we compared the visual and auditory tasks separately. Between the spatial and neutral conditions, we compared VS and VN as well as VaS and VaN.

For the functional images, we used MRIcro to change the DICOM files into MRIimg and MRIhdr files.

In each task, the functional images of the first four volumes were not used for the data analysis. The DICOM files were exported as MRIimg and MRIhdr files. In addition, the DICOM files for the T2 images were exported as MRIimg and MRIhdr files.

The functional images were analyzed using statistical parametric mapping (SPM5, Wellcome Department of Cognitive Neurology, London, UK). The functional images from each task were realigned using the first scan as a reference. T2-weighted anatomical images were co-registered to the first scan in the functional images. The co-registered T2-weighted anatomical images were then normalized to standard T2 template images as defined by the Montreal Neurological Institute. Finally, these spatially normalized functional images were smoothed using an isotopic Gaussian kernel of 8 mm.

Statistical analyses sought to identify the brain areas shared by visual-spatial attention with (VaS-VaN) and without (VS-VN) auditory distraction, as well as the brain areas selectively engaged in each task. To eliminate the brain activation caused by finger motion, we told the subjects to click the reaction key ten times during every rest. As a control task, we used VN for the visual attention task.

Table 2. Reaction time during each task (±SE)

Task	Mean reaction time (ms)
VS	409 (66.1)
VaS	398 (77.4)

RESULTS

Behavioral data were derived from the subject's performance during the fMRI experiment. The reaction time for each task (shown in Table 2) was computed from the data for the 16 subjects (the average of 16×27=432 trials).

We performed the paired *t*-test using SPSS. The comparison of RTs across visual tasks showed a significant difference between VS and VaS ($t_{(15)} = 2.53, p < 0.001$).

fMRIdata

Figure 5 shows the main results that contrast VaS-VaN (Figure 5A) and VS-VN (Figure 5B). The rendered results were made with a threshold of p<0.001 and a cluster size of 30. Figure 6 shows the activation area corresponding to Figure 5. This study focused on visual-spatial attention and visual-spatial attention with auditory distraction. Figure 5 compares the activation in VaS–VaN and VS–VN. The significant activations in the two attentional conditions are presented in Figure 6.

VaS vs. VaN

The areas of significant activation are shown in Figure 6A; the right frontal cortex showed more activation than the left. In the parietal cortex, BA7/40 was activated bilaterally. and the visual cortex showed greater activation on the left.

VS vs. VN

In this comparison, significant activation occurred only in the bilateral parietal cortex (Figure 6A). In a previous study (Coull and Nobre 1998), the medial premotor cortex (BA6) showed significant bilateral activation when the visual-spatial task was compared with baseline.

DISCUSSION

The current experiment contrasted performance on four pointing tasks with varying degrees of restriction of visual feedback. The results indicate that Fitts' law holds for pointing movements under different conditions of restricted visual feedback.

Baseline: At Rest or During the Neutral Task

The resting state has been used as the baseline in previous studies, so comparisons using visual fixa-

Figure 5.Activation during visual attention (p<0.001, cluster size=0)

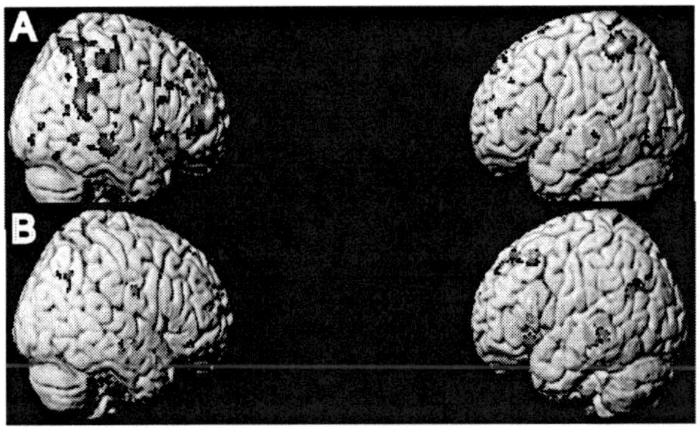

Figure 6.Areas of activation for each attentional condition in the cortex

VaS-VaN

Cluster (voxels)	Hemisphere	Location	Brodmann Area	Coordinate(mm) x	y	z	Z-score
585	Left	Lpi	BA40/ 7	-50	-44	58	5
524	Right	GFs	BA8	8	42	52	4.95
		GFd	BA9	14	40	34	4.94
		GC	BA32	2	36	26	3.81
	Left	GFd	BA9	-2	48	40	4.33
724	Right	LPi	BA40	56	-50	24	4.78
		LPs	BA7	34	-62	62	3.89
		GTs	BA22	44	-50	18	3.62
293	Left	GL	BA18	-24	-84	-2	4.64
230	Right	GPoC	BA1	62	-30	52	4.61
104	Right	Basal Ganglia		24	-24	10	4.46
299	Right	GTs	BA38/ 22	58	18	-8	4.26
		F i	BA47	54	28	-6	3.7
327	Left	CC		-6	-34	-6	4.18
	Right	CC		6	-40	10	4.06
579	Right	GFm	BA10	32	46	14	4.06
61	Right	GFs	BA6	4	14	72	3.99
148	Right	NL		18	2	8	3.97
144	Right	GFm	BA8	54	12	40	3.93
194	Right	Pcu	BA7	6	-54	50	3.87
67	Right	GFd	BA8	8	22	52	3.8
144	Right	GTm	BA21	62	-20	-12	3.8
41	Right	Gom	BA19	28	-74	2	3.55
32	Right	GFm	BA46	42	22	32	3.46
38	Right	GTm	BA37	54	-54	-4	4.27

b. VS-VN

Cluster (voexl)	Hemisphere	Location	Brodmann Area	Coordinate(mm) x	y	z	Z-score
645	Left	GFd	BA9	-6	48	40	4.66
		GFs	BA8	-2	20	58	4.54
	Right	GFd	BA9	6	42	26	4.33
57	Left	GFi	BA45	-54	-36	-2	3.85
		GTs	BA22	-60	-34	10	3.39
34	Right	GprC	BA4	54	-8	28	3.74
38	Left	GFi	BA45	-52	26	8	3.74
50	Left	GFi	BA47	-46	26	-8	3.71
63	Left	GFm	BA39	-44	-60	26	3.56
40	Right	GTs	BA39	54	-62	36	3.44

All areas are significant at an uncorrected threshold of $p<0.001$. K=30 voxels.
The approximate Brodmann areas are from MRIcro and the x, y and z coordinates are from SPM5.

tion controls are most compatible with previous reports (Corbetta, Miezin et al. 1993). In addition, the neutral condition itself engaged subjects' attention and oriented it between two spatial locations and two temporal intervals.

In this study, we focused on activation without finger movement, so subjects were asked to click the reaction key ten times during each rest period. We compared the activation during each task with that during rest. As a result, with the exception of the visual cortices, significant activation occurred in the somatosensory area and a small part of the motor area in the N task. Therefore, we used the N task as the baseline to reveal the activation resulting from spatial attention. The activation in VS–VN in the frontal (BA4/8) and parietal (BA39) cortices was similar to that identified in previous studies (Coull and Nobre 1998; Nobre, Gitelman et al. 2000). VaS–VN revealed bilateral activation in the parietal cortex (BA7/40) and in the right hemisphere of the frontal cortex (BA6/8) (Coull, Frith et al. 2000). The right hemisphere bias for spatial orientation in the VaS task in this study is consistent with a previous report (Coull and Nobre 1998). Therefore, we conclude that visual-orienting attention uses a frontal–parietal neural network for visual-spatial orienting attention both with and without auditory distraction.

Similarity between Visual VaS and VS Orienting Attention

A previous study (Badgaiyan & Posner, 1998) reported activation of BA6/8/32 when the frontal cortex was activated in spatial attention tasks.In this study, activation of BA6/8/32 wasrevealed inboth VaS and VS attention tasks. In some studies (Badgaiyan & Posner, 1998; Mesulam, 1999; Hahn, Ross et al., 2006), a contribution of BA6/8/32 was also reported for visual-spatial attention. As a result, we believe that the frontal cortex (BA6/8/32) is associated with both the VaS and VS neural networks.

The Activations of DLPFC (Dorsolateral Prefrontal Cortex)

Working memory within the rDLPFC as a function of executive and storage of information[8]. In the present study, we found that the rDLPFC was activated during the VaS tasks to a significantly different magnitude than in the VS task. A behavioral study (VROOMEN, Jean, GELDER and Beatrice 2000) found that auditory stimuli could enhance visual cognitive performance. An fMRI experiment (Kawashima, Imaizumi, Mori, Okada, Goto, Kiritani, Ogawa & Fukuda, 1999) found that the working memory within the rDLPFC was activated during visual cognition with synchronous auditory stimuli. In the present study, we found the same phenomenon, namely, that the auditory distraction enhanced the visual-spatial attention performance, although the subjects were told to ignore the auditory stimulus. We considered this to be an integration between visual and auditory stimuli that was completed subliminally.

CONCLUSION

In this study, we measured the CBF (Cerebral Blood Flow) during voluntary visual-spatial attention tasks using a 3Tesla fMRI machine. Our results revealed that the frontal-parietal neural network functioned for spatial attention and that brain activation was enhanced during an auditory distraction. The right DCPFC had a significantly higher activation in spatial attention tasks with VaS compared to the VS alone.

ACKNOWLEDGMENT

A part of this study was financially supported by JSPS AA Science Platform Program and JSPS Grant-in-Aid for Scientific Research (B) (21404002)

REFERENCES

Corbetta, M., Miezin, F. M., Shulman, G. L., & Petersen, S. E. (1993). A PET study of visuospatial attention. *The Journal of Neuroscience*, *13*(3), 1202–1226.

Coull, J. T., & Frith, C. D. (2000). Orienting attention in time: Behavioural and neuroanatomical distinction between exogenous and endogenous shifts. *Neuropsychologia*, *38*(6), 808–819. doi:10.1016/S0028-3932(99)00132-3

Coull, J. T., & Nobre, A. C. (1998). Where and when to pay attention: The neural systems for directing attention to spatial locations and to time intervals as revealed by both PET and fMRI. *The Journal of Neuroscience*, *18*(18), 7426–7435.

Degerman, A., & Rinne, T. (2006). Selective attention to sound location or pitch studied with fMRI. *Brain Research*, *1077*(1), 123–134. doi:10.1016/j.brainres.2006.01.025

Gazzaniga, M. S., Ivry, R. B., & Mangun, G. T. (2008). *Cognitive neuroscience*.

James, W. (1890). *Principles of psychology*. New York, NY: Holt. doi:10.1037/10538-000

Kawashima, R., & Imaizumi, S. (1999). Selective visual and auditory attention toward utterances-a PET study. *NeuroImage*, *10*(2), 209–215. doi:10.1006/nimg.1999.0452

Nobre, A. C., & Gitelman, D. R. (2000). Covert visual spatial orienting and saccades: Overlapping neural systems. *NeuroImage*, *11*(3), 210–216. doi:10.1006/nimg.2000.0539

Schubotz, R. I., & von Cramon, D. Y. (2003). Auditory what, where, and when: A sensory somatotopy in lateral premotor cortex. *NeuroImage*, *20*(1), 173–185. doi:10.1016/S1053-8119(03)00218-0

Strayer, D. L., & Drews, F. A. (2006). A comparison of the cell phone driver and the drunk driver. *Human Factors: The Journal of the Human Factors and Ergonomics Society*, *48*(2), 381–391. doi:10.1518/001872006777724471

Vroomen, J., & de Gelder, B. (2000). *Sound enhances visual perception: Cross-modal effects of auditory organization on vision*. Washington, DC: ETATS-UNIS, American Psychological Association.

Zatorre, R. J., & Mondor, T. A. (1999). Auditory attention to space and frequency activates similar cerebral systems. *NeuroImage*, *10*(5), 544–554. doi:10.1006/nimg.1999.0491

KEY TERMS AND DEFINITIONS

Attention: The ability to attend to some things while ignoring others.

DLPFC: The dorsolateral prefrontal cortex is the last area to develop in the human cerebrum. This area was defined as roughly equivalent to BA9 and BA46.

Functional MRI: A type of specialized MRI scan that measures the hemodynamic response correlated with neural activity in the brain or spinal cord of humans or animals.

Involuntary Attention: A bottom-up stimulus-driven process in which attention is captured by a sensory event.

Selective Attention: Individuals have a tendency to process information from only one part of the environment to the exclusion of other parts.

Spatial Integration: Among multi-modal task, this is a common phenomenon in space perception.

Voluntary Attention: A top-down, goal-directed process involving a plan to attend to something.

Chapter 5
Cerebral Network for Implicit Chinese Character Processing:
An fMRI Study

Xiujun Li
Graduate School of Natural Science and Technology, Okayama University, Japan

Chunlin Li
Graduate School of Natural Science and Technology, Okayama University, Japan

Jinglong Wu
Graduate School of Natural Science and Technology, Okayama University, Japan

Qiyong Guo
Department of Radiology, Shengjing Hospital of China Medical University, China

ABSTRACT

Recent event-related fMRI studies suggest that a left-lateralized network exists for reading Chinese words (to contrast two-character Chinese words and figures). In this study, the authors used a 3T fMRI to investigate brain activation when processing characters and figures in a visual discrimination task. Thirteen Chinese individuals were shown two Chinese characters (36 pairs) or two figures (36 pairs). The control task (two figures) was used to eliminate non-linguistic visual and motor confounds. The results showed that discrimination of Chinese characters is performed by a bilateral network that processes orthographic, phonological, and semantic features. Significant activation patterns were observed in the occipital region (BA17, 18, 19, and 37), temporal region (BA22 and 38), parietal region (BA7, 39, and 40), and frontal region (BA4, 6, 10, and 46) of the brain and in the cerebellum. The study concludes that a constellation of neural substrates provides a bilateral network that processes Chinese subjects.

DOI: 10.4018/978-1-60960-559-9.ch005

INTRODUCTION

Recent event-related fMRI studies have indicated that a left-lateralized network exists for processing Chinese logographs (Kuo, Yeh, Duann, Wu, Ho, Huang, Tzeng, Hsieh 2001). Written or spoken language activates certain parts of the brain. Previous neuroimaging studies using functional magnetic resonance imaging (fMRI) or positron emission tomography (PET) showed different activation patterns during alphabetic language processing (e.g., English) and logographic language processing (e.g., Chinese characters) (Kuo et al., 2001, Kuo, Yeh, Lee, Chen, Lee, Chen, Ho, Hung, Tzeng, Hsieh 2004, Petersson, Reis, Askelof, Castro-Caldas, Ingvar 2000, Petersson, Reis, Ingvar 2001, Tan, Liu, Perfetti, Spinks, Fox, Gao 2001, Tan, Spinks, Feng, Siok, Perfetti, Xiong, Fox, Gao 2003). Alphabetic language processing preferentially involves the left inferior frontal cortex (IFC), the left medial temporal lobe (MTL), and the left temporal occipital area (Booth, Burman, Meyer, Gitelman, & Parrish, 2002; Jobard, Crivello, & Tzourio-Mazoyer, 2003). Chinese logographic characters have different square configurations of a similar size that are packed by numerous stokes and map onto morphemes rather than direct phonemes (Tan et al., 2003). Accordingly elaborate visuospatial processing is pecessary to process the Chinese logographic system (Tan, Spinks, Gao, Liu, Perfetti, Xiong, Stofer, Pu, Liu, & Fox, 2000; Tan, Chan, Ka, Khong, Yip, & Luke, 2008).

Language, as an important part of cognitive neuroscience, is influenced by the socio-cultural background. Previous studies have elucidated a left-lateralized network for processing Chinese words (two-character Chinese words and two figures) (Kuo et al., 2001). Therefore, the pattern of interactions between large-scale functional-anatomical networks for language processing may differ during certain language tasks. Different regions of the brain are activated in behavioral and functional neuroimaging studies. To process alphabetic subjects, the functional architecture of the brain is adjusted by literacy and education. Kuo et al. reported that a left-lateralized network exists for reading Chinese words and figures (Kuo WJ et al., 2001). Whereas Tan et al. reported an extensive activation of bilateral hemispheric structures during Chinese character processing in semantic and a homophone tasks (Tan LH et al., 2003).

Moreover, our previous study found activation differences when processing Chinese characters by a visual modality in the left superior temporal gyrus (BA39/40), right inferior parietal lobule (BA40) and right middle frontal gyrus (BA10). Such differences are more obvious and easier to determine visually because lexical processing is nearly non-existent. Individuals receive information by through visual or auditory routes. Thus, we performed a visual fMRI study to investigate character processing by Chinese individuals. We hypothesized that there is a bilateral cortical network for Chinese character processing during judgment tasks through a visual modality.

In our study, we used whole-brain 3T fMRI to observe brain responses during the judgment of Chinese characters and figures. The goals of the current study are threefold: (1) to inspect the commonality and particularity of brain organization used for processing Chinese characters relative to that used for alphabetic languages. (2) to use a control task to eliminate non-linguistic visual and motor confounds. (3) to propose that Chinese word recognition might mandate perceptual and attention mechanisms that target the bilateral hemisphere. These provide advantageous sensitive analysis of the spatial properties of Chinese characters.

LANGUAGE

Language is succinctly defined in our Glossary as a "human system of communication that uses arbitrary signals, such as voice sounds, gestures, or written symbols." However, in practical terms, language is far too complicated, intriguing, and mysterious to be adequately explained by this definition. Language is a particular kind of system used for encoding and decoding information. Ever Since language (logos) and languages (logogn) were studied by the ancient grammarians, the term has had many definitions. The English word derives from the Latin word lingua meaning, "language, tongue," with a reconstructed Proto-Indo-European root of "tongue," a metaphor based on the use of this organ to generate speech.

Language processing has been classified as orthographic, phonological and semantic. However, one of the central concepts in word representation is that of the mental lexicon-a mental store of information about words that includes semantic information, syntactic information, and the details of word forms. Most psycholinguistic theories agree on the central role for a mental lexicon for both language comprehension and production, while other models distinguish between input and output lexica. The representation of orthographic and phonological forms must be considered in a given model. However, the principal concept is that a store of information about words exists in the brain. We have some albeit limited, ideas about how language is conceptually organized (Michael, Richard & George, 2002).

A key property of language is that its symbols are arbitrary. Any concept or grammatical rule can be mapped onto a symbol. In other words, most languages make use of sound, but a combination of sounds does not have any necessary and inherent meaning. Words are merely a common convention used to represent a certain thing by users of that language. For instance, the sound combination nada carries the meaning of "nothing" in the Spanish language and the meaning "thread" in the Hindi language. There is nothing about the word nada itself that forces Hindi speakers to convey the idea of "thread", or the idea of "nothing" for Spanish speakers. Other sets of sounds (for example, the English words nothing and thread) could also be used to represent the same concepts; however, Spanish and Hindi speakers have acquired or learned to correlate their own meanings for this particular sound pattern. Indeed, for speakers of Slovene and some other South Slavic languages, this sound combination carries the meaning of "hope", whereas in Indonesian, it means "tone" (http://en.wikipedia.org/wiki/Language).

EXPERIMENT

Subjects

Healthy subjects from North China were used in this study. All subjects were college teachers in Shenyang city and were comprised of thirteen right-handed participants. The average age of these subjects was 44.38 years (7 males, 6 females). They participated in the fMRI study after providing informed written consent. We explained the details of the information form and the consent form to them before we obtained their fingerprints and signature. Protocols were approved by the Ethics Committee of the Shengjing Hospital at the China Medical University.

Method

Seventy-two pairs of characters (36 pairs) and control stimuli (36 pairs of simple figures) were adopted during the fMRI experiments (Figure 2). All subjects were asked to perform the experimental tasks as quickly and accurately as possible.

All MRI studies were performed on a 3T Philips signal scanner at the Shengjing Hospital at the China Medical University (Figure 1). Two hundred and eighty-nine fMRI images were collected during each run, and each fMRI run consisted of one task. An event-related design was used. The subjects were asked to focus on a small crosshair during the resting period. Each pair of Chinese characters or figures was shown through a projector for 4000ms, with an interpair interval

Figure 1. fMRI experiment device

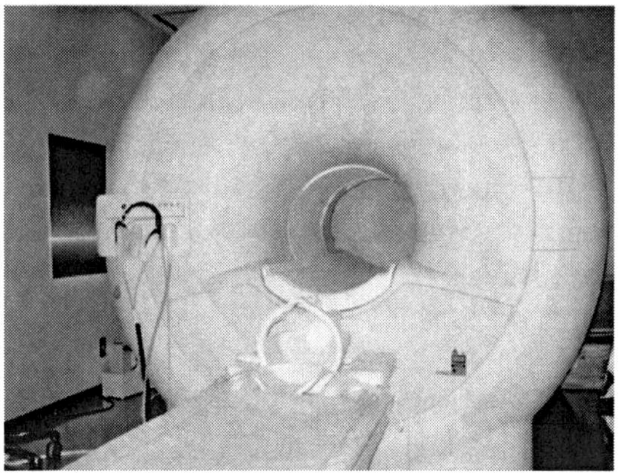

of 2000ms, 4000ms or 6000ms between the stimuli. Each task consisted of an equal number of Chinese characters and figures. The subjects were asked to press the right key with their right thumbs when they thought the two characters or figures were the same and press the left key with their left thumbs when they thought they were different.

Statistical Parametric Mapping 2 (SPM2) software and Matlab7.0 software were used for the image and statistical analysis. Initially, each of the 289 fMRI images was automatically re-aligned to the first image in the time series to correct for head movements during fMRI acquisition. Afterward, T1-weighted anatomical images were co-registered to the first scan in the functional images. Next, the co-registered T1-weighted anatomical images were normalized to a standard T1 template image, as defined by the Montreal Neurological Institute. Finally, these spatially normalized functional images were smoothed with an isotopic 8-mm Gaussian kernel. As analyzed by a one-sample t-test, activations that fell within clusters of 0 or more contiguous voxels that exceeded the false discovery rate (FDR)-corrected statistical threshold (P<0.05) were considered to be significant.

RESULTS

The average reaction time and response accuracy in the behavioral experiment are shown in Figure 3. The average reaction time of the control task was shorter than that of the language task; however, the average response accuracy of the control task was higher than that of the language task.

In the fMRI experiment significant activation was detected during presentation of language and control stimuli. Figure 4 shows the maps of average activation (n=13) for the Chinese character task and the figure task. Regions with significant activation during the two tasks relative to the respective resting state are shown in Table 1.

The results are briefly summarized below. The language and control stimuli produced significant activation of in the occipital region (BA17, 18, 19, and 37), temporal region (BA22 and 38), parietal region (BA7, 39, and 40), frontal region (BA4, 6, 10, and 46) and the cerebellum (Figure 4 and Table 1). (*P*<0.05 corrected cluster size>0 voxels).

Figure 2. Examples of experimental stimuli used in the fMRI behavioral experiment. The subject judged whether the two Chinese characters or the two figures were the same.

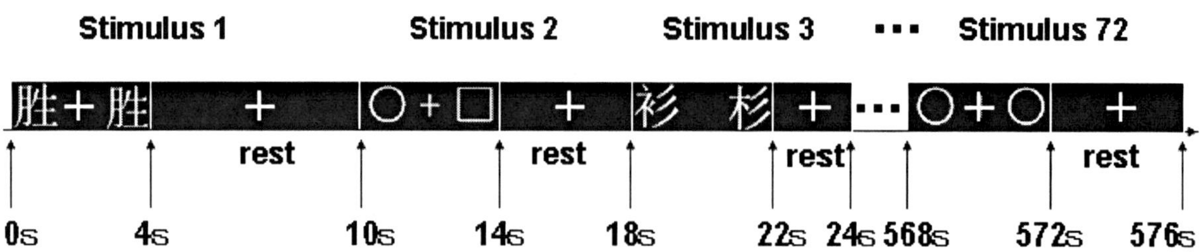

Figure 3. Average reaction time and response accuracy in the behavioral experiments. Language: Chinese character stimulus; Control: figure stimulus.

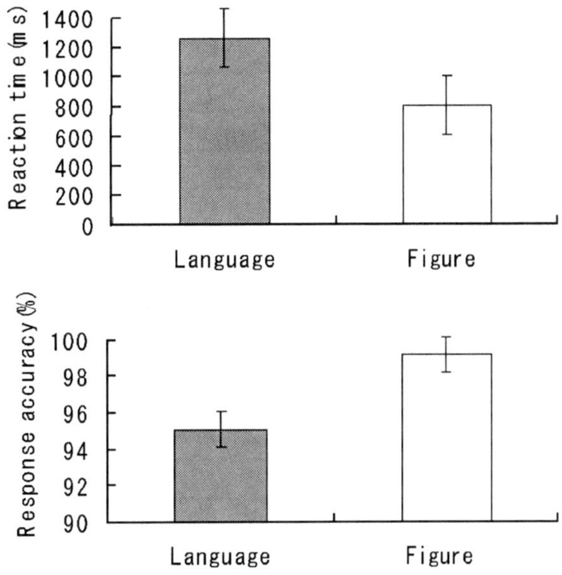

Figure 4. Functional brain maps during presentation of language stimuli and control stimuli. Mean normalized brain maps were overlaid on the corresponding T1-weighted images that showed significant activation (in color; p<0.05, corrected, FDR cluster size>0 voxels).

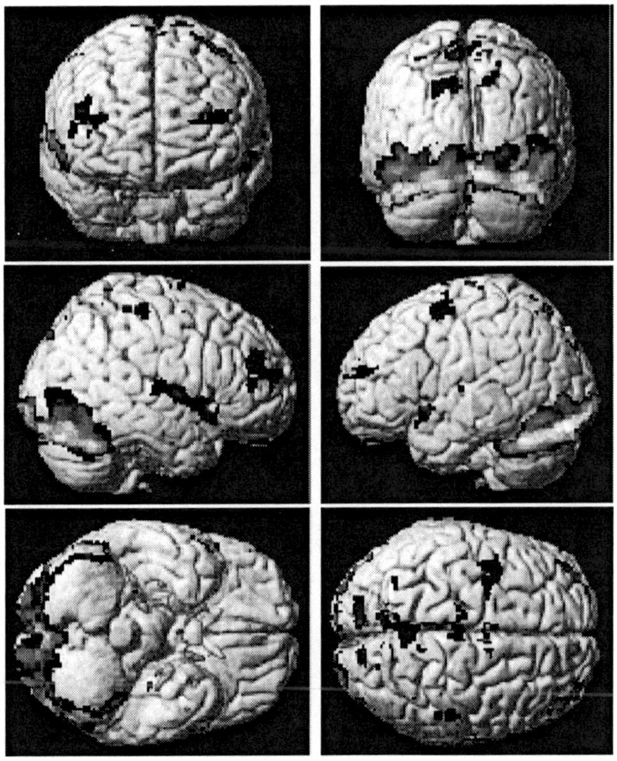

Table 1. Stereotactic coordinates, Z values, and corresponding Brodmann Areas (BAs) for significantly activated regions (brain activation in literate subjects).

Brain areas	Coordinates					
	BA	x	y	z	Ke	Z
Right middle occipital gyrus	17/18	3	-91	-19	6237	5.84
Cerebellum		43	-60	-30		5.4
Left fusiform gyrus	37	-43	-60	-26		5.07
Right middle occipital gyrus	18	29	-91	-21		4.78
Left middle occipital gyrus	19	-47	-71	-16		4.73
Right middle occipital gyrus	19	41	-73	-22		4.6
Cerebellum		-38	-50	-33		4.54
Left middle occipital gyrus	17/18	-3	-89	-21		4.5
Left middle occipital gyrus	18	-22	-93	-21		4.41
Right fusiform gyrus	37	48	-62	-19		4.36
Superior longitudinal gyrus	4	-40	-1	49	87	4.31
Left middle frontal gyrus	6	-29	-7	57		3.51
Right superior temporal gyrus	22	57	-7	5	248	4.09
Right superior temporal gyrus	38	48	14	-10		3.75
Left superior parietal gyrus	7	-6	-73	49	124	4.07
Cerebellum		3	-50	-6	123	4.02
Right middle frontal gyrus	10	41	39	23	155	3.75
Right middle frontal gyrus	46	40	45	16		3.6
Right superior parietal gyrus	39	45	-29	49	25	5.07
Superior longitudinal gyrus	4	-13	-21	67	58	4.91
Superior longitudinal gyrus	4	3	-27	63		4.35
Left superior temporal gyrus	38	-48	6	-7	75	4.83
Left middle frontal gyrus	10	-31	55	17		4.74
Left middle frontal gyrus	46	-20	61	17		4.06

DISCUSSION

We investigated the commonality and particularity of brain organization when reading two-character words and other alphabetic languages. The results of this study, in contrast to those of visuo-motor control, support the existence of a bilateral cortical network that orchestrates orthographic, phonological, and semantic processing when observing Chinese words and figures. Language processing corresponds to certain areas of brain in which activation is related to changes in the regional cerebral blood flow, as recorded by fMRI. Chinese is a logographic, albeit complex, system in which characters not only symbolize whole morphemes, but also represent phonemes. We wanted to clarify brain activation patterns that are related to Chinese character processing during visual recognition.

We administered a Chinese character and figure task to Chinese subjects to determine network interactions of character processing. We used an SPM analysis of the fMRI data to show the different activation patterns. After comparison of character and control stimuli, we found significant activations during Chinese character processing.

As expected activation of superior temporal gyri (BA22, and38) indicated the involvement of the auditory cortex. BA47 is part of the frontal cortex in the human brain. Recent fMRI data indicate that PFC (BA47) activity may be sensitive to the material being encoded or retrieved from long-term memory (Kelley, Miezin, McDermott, Buckner, Raichle, Chohen, Ollinger, Akbudak, Conturo, Snyder, & Petersen, 1998: Tan et al., 2001; Tan et al., 2003; Tan et al., 2008). It is also possible that PFC activity is modulated by the encoding strategy. Human language processing ability may be enhanced by literacy, as indicated by our previous visual fMRI study on character processing. Activation of BA17, 18, 19, and 37 may depend on the visual stimulus.

Moreover, the middle frontal gyrus (BA4, 6, 10, and 46) is uniquely activated in subjects. Activation of left middle frontal gyrus (BA9) is associated with word encoding, especially with Chinese character processing (Gabrieli, Poldrack, & Desmond, 1998; Tan et al., 2001; Tan et al., 2000). Activation of the bilateral precentral gyrus (BA6, the premortor and supplementary motor area) may be the result of quicker finger tapping: this is in agreement with the results of the behavioral experiments. Activation of the left superior temporal gyrus (BA39/40) and right inferior parietal lobule (BA40) as well as portions of Wernicke's area is strongly associated with orthographic and phonological processing and working memory. This is probably due to the unique square spatial configuration of Chinese characters, as the routine activation these areas was shown in some other verbal working memory tasks (Kuo et al., 2004). Based on this analysis, our hypothesis that certain brain regions are activated during character processing was confirmed. This phenomenon may be acquired during education.

In conclusion, a bilateral cortical network for Chinese character processing exists, and this type of brain plasticity may be acquired during education.

ACKNOWLEDGMENT

The authors would like to thank Hongzan Sun of the Shengjing Hospital at the China Medical University, for providing valuable instruction during the functional MRI experiment. We thank the subjects who participated in this study and the staff of the Shengjing Hospital at the Shenyang Medical College for their assistance with data collection. A portion of this study was financially supported by the JSPS AA Science Platform Program and a JSPS Grant-in-Aid for Scientific Research (B) (21404002). This research was supported by the 2009 Kagawa University Characteristic Prior Research Fund.

REFERENCES

Booth, J. R., Burman, D. D., Meyer, J. R., Gitelman, D. R., Parrish, T. B., & Mesulam, M. M. (2002). Functional anatomy of intra- and cross-modal lexical tasks. *NeuroImage*, *16*, 7–22. doi:10.1006/nimg.2002.1081

Gabrieli, J. D., Poldrack, R. A., & Desmond, J. E. (1998). The role of left prefrontal cortex in language and memory. *Proceedings of the National Academy of Sciences of the United States of America*, *95*, 906–913. doi:10.1073/pnas.95.3.906

Gazzaniga, M. S., Ivry, R. B., & Mangun, G. R. (2002). *Cognitive neuroscience*.

Jobard, G., Crivello, F., & Tzourio-Mazoyer, N. (2003). Evaluation of the dual route theory of reading: A metanalysis of 35 neuroimaging studies. *NeuroImage*, *20*, 693–712. doi:10.1016/S1053-8119(03)00343-4

Kelley, W. M., Miezin, F. M., McDermott, K. B., Buckner, R. L., Raichle, M. E., & Chohen, N. J. (1998). Hemispheric specialization in human dorsal frontal cortex and medial temporal lobe for verbal and nonverbal memory encoding. *Neuron*, *20*, 927–936. doi:10.1016/S0896-6273(00)80474-2

Kuo, W. J., Yeh, T. C., Duann, J. R., Wu, Y. T., Ho, L. T., & Huang, D. (2001). A left-lateralized network for reading Chinese words: A 3T fMRI study. *Neuroreport*, *12*, 3997–4001. doi:10.1097/00001756-200112210-00029

Kuo, W. J., Yeh, T. C., Lee, J. R., Chen, L. F., Lee, P. L., & Chen, S. S. (2004). Orthographic and phonological processing of Chinese characters: An fMRI study. *NeuroImage*, *21*, 1721–1731. doi:10.1016/j.neuroimage.2003.12.007

Petersson, K. M., Reis, A., Askelof, S., Castro-Caldas, A., & Ingvar, M. (2000). Language processing modulated by literacy: A network analysis of verbal repetition in literate and illiterate subjects. *Journal of Cognitive Neuroscience*, *12*, 364–382. doi:10.1162/089892900562147

Petersson, K. M., Reis, A., & Ingvar, M. (2001). Cognitive processing in literate and illiterate subjects: A review of some recent behavioral and functional neuroimaging data. *Scandinavian Journal of Psychology*, *42*, 251–267. doi:10.1111/1467-9450.00235

Tan, L. H., Chan, A. H. D., Kay, P., Khong, P. L., Yip, L. K. C., & Luke, K. K. (2008). Language affects patterns of brain activation associated with perceptual decision. *Proceedings of the National Academy of Sciences of the United States of America*, *105*, 4004–4009. doi:10.1073/pnas.0800055105

Tan, L. H., Liu, H. L., Perfetti, C. A., Spinks, J. A., Fox, P. T., & Gao, J. H. (2001). The neural system underlying Chinese logograph reading. *NeuroImage*, *12*, 836–846. doi:10.1006/nimg.2001.0749

Tan, L. H., Spinks, J. A., Feng, C. M., Siok, W. T., Perfetti, C. A., & Xiong, J. (2003). Neural systems of second language reading are shaped by native language. *Human Brain Mapping*, *18*, 158–166. doi:10.1002/hbm.10089

Tan, L. H., Spinks, J. A., Gao, J. H., Liu, H. L., Perfetti, C. A., & Xiong, J. H. (2000). Brain activation in the processing of Chinese characters and words: A functional MRI study. *Human Brain Mapping*, *10*, 16–27. doi:10.1002/(SICI)1097-0193(200005)10:1<16::AID-HBM30>3.0.CO;2-M

Wikipedia. (2010). *Language*. http://en.wikipedia.org/wiki/Language.

KEY TERMS AND DEFINITIONS

Chinese Character (also known as a Han Character): A logogram used in the written Chinese language.

Figure: A particular shape formed by lines or surfaces.

Functional Magnetic Resonance Imaging (fMRI): A type of specialized MRI scan. It measures the hemodynamic response (change in blood flow) related to neural activity in the brain or spinal cord of humans or other animals.

Judgment: The ability to recognize and understand the difference between two items.

Network: A system of items that are connected and operate together.

Neuroimaging: Includes the use of various techniques to either directly or indirectly image the structure and function/pharmacology of the brain. It is a relatively new discipline within the medicine and neuroscience/psychology community.

Visual: If or connected with seeing or sight.

Chapter 6
Neuronal Substrates for Language Processing and Word Priming

Chunlin Li
Graduate School of Natural Science and Technology, Okayama University, Japan

Xiujun Li
Graduate School of Natural Science and Technology, Okayama University, Japan

Jinglong Wu
Graduate School of Natural Science and Technology, Okayama University, Japan

Hiroshi Kusahara
Toshiba Medical Systems Corporation, Japan

ABSTRACT

The authors of this chapter studied behavioral performance and brain activities associated with word priming using a Japanese Word Stem Completion (WSC) task. They compared the results of this task with the results of a Korean character cognitive task. Their results showed facilitatory effects on subject performance. The percentage of correct answers in the non-priming (P/N) word condition was 94%, whereas the priming (P/Y) condition yielded 100% correct answers. The average reaction time during the P/N word condition was 1501 ms, whereas it was 978 ms and 3106 ms for the P/N non-word and word P/Y word conditions, respectively. In the fMRI experiment, the same tasks were performed using a block-design experimental paradigm without any overt response from the MRI scanner. As seen in the fMRI results, the bilateral middle and inferior frontal gyrus were active with a right hemispheric prevalence. In addition, the superior and inferior parietal gyrus and the supplementary motor area were activated. The prefrontal-parietal network observed in this study is consistent with the areas that were activated during an English word stem task. These results suggest that the facilitatory effects observed in the WSC test were successful for implicit memory retrieval.

DOI: 10.4018/978-1-60960-559-9.ch006

INTRODUCTION

Serious diseases, such as dementia, result from dysfunctional memory formation. To improve the quality of life of the patients and their families, it is important to detect disease symptoms in the early stages and administer treatment immediately. To provide early screening, we have to understand how the human memory system works. Despite much research in the memory field, the fundamental mechanisms of memory formation remain unclear. In this study, we focused on priming, which is a specialized form of implicit memory.

Priming is measured as the ability to identify a word as a result of a specific previous encounter with the item that the word describes. To investigate the neuronal substrates that control priming, we conducted functional magnetic resonance imaging (fMRI) while patients performed a word stem completion (WSC) test in Japanese (e.g., ホ○レン○ウ). In the WSC paradigm, a word is used as the pre-stimulus and then a portion of the word is used as the experimental stimulus (Figure 1).

The response time and the percentage of correct answers on the WSC test were measured. Based on the behavioral experiment, we deigned an fMRI experiment and evaluated brain activity by measuring the blood oxygenation level.

WORD PROCESSING

Language processing is classified as orthographic, phonological and semantic. One of the central concepts in word representation is the existence of a lexicon, i.e., a mental store of information about words that includes semantic information, syntactic information, and the details of word forms. Most psycholinguistic theories agree that a mental lexicon is central for the development of language comprehension and production, while other models distinguish between input and output lexica. The representation of orthographic and phonological forms must be considered in any model. The principal concept, though, is that a store of information about words exists in the brain, and we have some, albeit limited, theories about how information must be conceptually organized (Michael S. Gazzaniga, Richard B. Ivry & George R. Mangun, 2002).

PRIMING EFFECT

Priming provides a facilitatory and control effect that can facilitate the identification of successive stimuli that were previously subconsciously obtained. Priming is a form of implicit memory. Direct priming occurs when the precedent stimu-

Figure 1. Example of a priming test

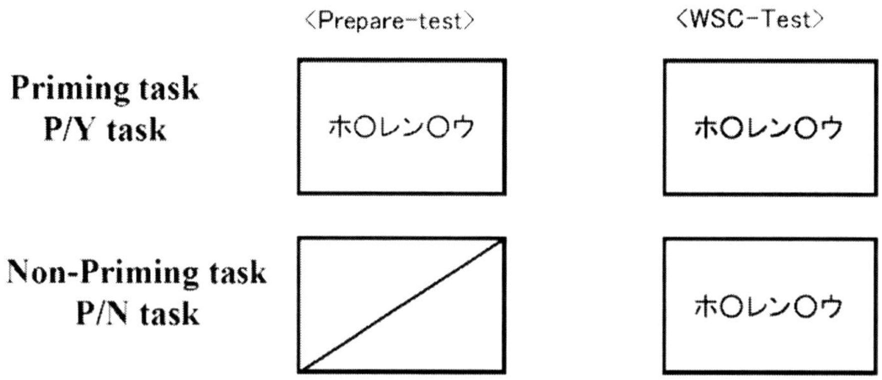

lus and successive stimulus are the same. Direct priming is further divided into perceptual priming and conceptual priming. The WSC test, which uses a word as a pre-stimulus and a portion of that word as the experimental stimulus, is often used to assess priming.

EXPERIMENT

Subjects and Tasks

Sixteen young healthy men (aged 21 to 24) participated in our experiments. All were native Japanese speakers. The words and categories used in our study were based on the frequency-of-appearance table that has been summarized in previous research (Akita, 1980; Ogawa, 1972). All the words were nouns composed of six letters. We examined the frequency at which the words were used in a preliminary study of fifty university students. In addition, we selected 120 words that are commonly used. Subjects performed both a PRE (prepare-test) and WSC test. In the PRE test, 120 words were visually presented and subjects were instructed to passively view the words. At this time, subjects were not given any information about the WSC test. After five days, the WSC test was conducted. During this test, subjects had to complete a word fragment, which was generated from previously presented words (primed words; P/Y-trial) or words that were not previously presented (non-primed words; P/N-trial). The word fragments in the P/Y and P/N trials were randomly presented to subjects. Subjects pressed a reaction key and orally completed the word as soon as they thought of the word. The reaction time and the percentage of correct answers were measured as the subject's performance score. The experiment was conducted in a quiet, dark room. To exclude sound from the outside, all subjects put on headphones. The stimulus was presented on a CRT, and the reaction of subjects was measured using a PC mouse. Answers were recorded (Figure 2). The figure form task was presented at the same time as the word.

Figure 2. Experimental setup

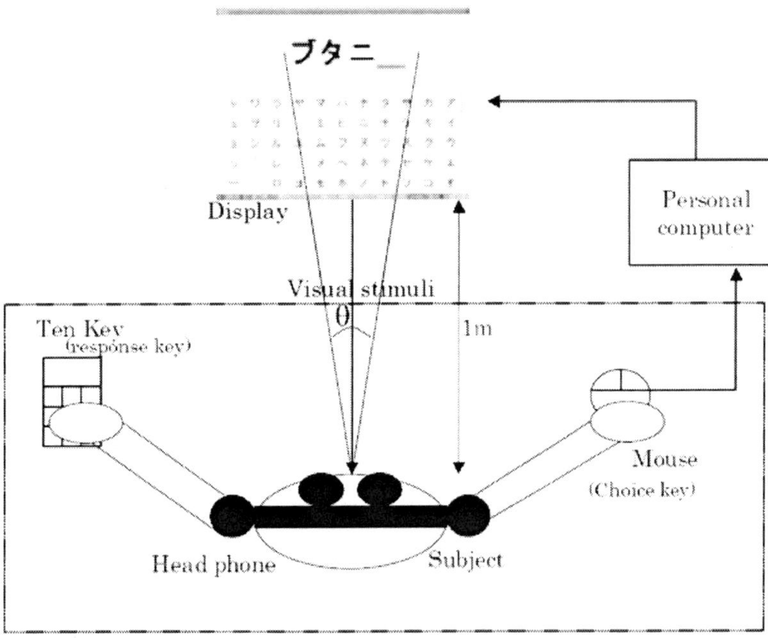

For the fMRI experiment, sixteen healthy men (aged 21 to 24) were used. The same behavioral tasks were performed in a block-design experimental paradigm without any overt response using the MRI scanner. The fMRI experiment began two hours after the pre-test. The task consisted of four conditions: word P/Y condition, word P/N condition, figure P/Y condition, and P/N condition. In the control task, subjects only observed nonsense KANA words. In the P/Y condition and the P/N condition, subjects were instructed to perform the WSC task (i.e. complete the word from a fragment) (Figure 4) without the use of speech. Each task condition lasted 30 sec and was alternated with a 30-sec control task (Figure 4). Every task session contained 5 questions that were presented for 5 seconds. To instruct the subjects at the beginning of the task or control condition, a fixation point was shown for 2.5 seconds. Each session lasted 360 seconds, and each subject performed four sessions. The word stimulus was presented using a projector, as shown in Figure 5. An MRI was performed while the stimuli were presented through a mirror. In the figure form task, four Korean words with one triangle in the head followed by another triangle and a blank at the end were shown.

Figure 3. Behavioral experiment apparatus. (a) Japanese word stimuli (b) Korean word stimuli

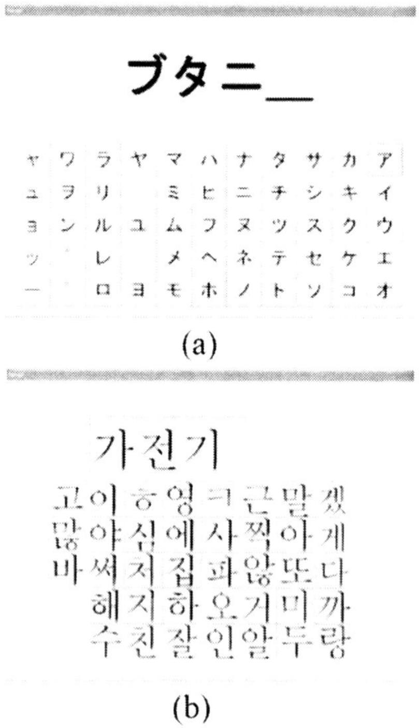

MRI Acquisition

Images were acquired using a 1.5-T scanning system (EchoSpeed 1.5T, GE) with a standard radio frequency head coil for signal transmission and reception. The functional images consisted of 20

Figure 4. Presentation sequence of fMRI experiment

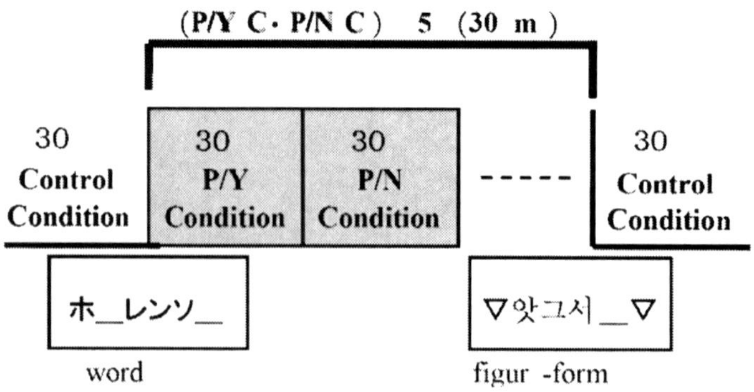

Figure 5. fMRI experimental setup

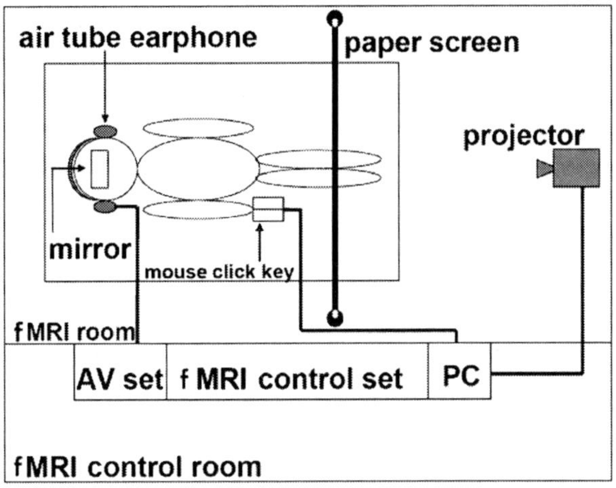

consecutive slices that covered the entire cerebral cortex. A T2*-weighted gradient echo-planar imaging sequence was used with the following parameters: TR/TE, 6000/50 msec; FA, 90°; matrix size, 64×64; voxel size, 4×4×5.5 mm. Before the acquisition of functional images, T2-weighted anatomical images were obtained in the same plane as the functional images using a spin echo sequence (voxel size, 1×1×5.5). High-resolution anatomical images were also acquired.

Image Analysis

Image analysis and statistical analysis were performed using the Statistical Parametric Mapping package SPM2 software (http://www.fil.ion.ucl.ac.uk/spm) implemented in MATLAB (Mathworks Inc., Sherborn MA, USA). Initially, to correct for head movements, functional images of each run were realigned using the first scan as a reference. Then the T2-weighted anatomical images, which were scanned in planes identical to that of the functional imaging slice, were co-registered to the first scan of the functional images. The co-registered T2-weighted anatomical images were then normalized to a standard T2 template image, as defined by the Montreal Neurological Institute (MNI), using linear and non-linear three-dimensional transformations. The parameters from this normalization process were applied to each functional image. Finally, the spatial-normalized functional images were re-sampled to a voxel size of 2 x 2 x 2 and smoothed with a 8-mm isotopic Gaussian kernel to compensate for anatomical variability amongst the subjects.

Significantly activated voxels of interest were found using a fixed effect analysis. The task-related neural activities for each condition were modeled using a boxcar function in combination with a canonical hemodynamic response function. In addition, we used a high-pass filter, which was composed of a discrete cosine function with a cut-off period of 128, to eliminate low-frequency trends and a low-pass filter to swamp serial autocorrelation across the scans. Least-square estimation was performed on data filtered through a band pass and the design matrix, which estimated the parameters of interest. Pre-planned comparisons were thereafter performed to test the main effects of the P/Y condition vs. control, P/N condition vs. control, and P/Y condition vs. P/N condition using the appropriate linear contrast. For these analyses, significantly activated voxels were identified if they reached the extent threshold ($p<0.05$) and were corrected for multiple comparison with a height threshold of $p<0.001$ (uncorrected).

RESULTS AND DISCUSSION

Results of Behavioral Experiments

Figure 6 shows the average reaction time and number of correct answers when subjects were presented with the P/Y and P/N conditions. The average reaction time of the P/Y word condition was 978 ms and 1501 ms. The difference in reaction time between the P/Y condition and the P/N condition was significant [$t(15)=2.26$, $p<0.001$]. The average reaction time in the P/Y task was 2873.06 ms and no reaction was observed during the P/N task.

The percentage of correct answers in the word P/N condition and P/Y condition was 94% and 100%, respectively. The percentage of correct answers in the P/N condition was unexpectedly high; however, subjects took a long time to recall correct answers, as shown in Figure 6. The percentage of correct answers in the figure form task (P/Y) and the P/N task was 20% and 0%, respectively.

Results of fMRI Experiments

We determined brain activity during the priming effect and non-priming effect. In the word task, the PY was greater than the PN and a contrast figure was made. The activation region within the two contrast images is shown in TABLE I. Each area was significant using an uncorrected threshold of $p<0.001$ (K=150 voxels).

Activated Area in Word PY>PN

Brain activation during the word PY>PN condition is shown in Figure 7. When the priming effect occurred during the word task, it caused significant activation of the parietal cortex and posterior angulate gyrus in comparison to the non-priming condition.

Activated Areas during Figure Presentation

Brian activations during presentation of the PY>PN figure are shown in Figure 8. The frontal cortex was primarily activated during the figure

Figure 6. Results of the behavioral experiment

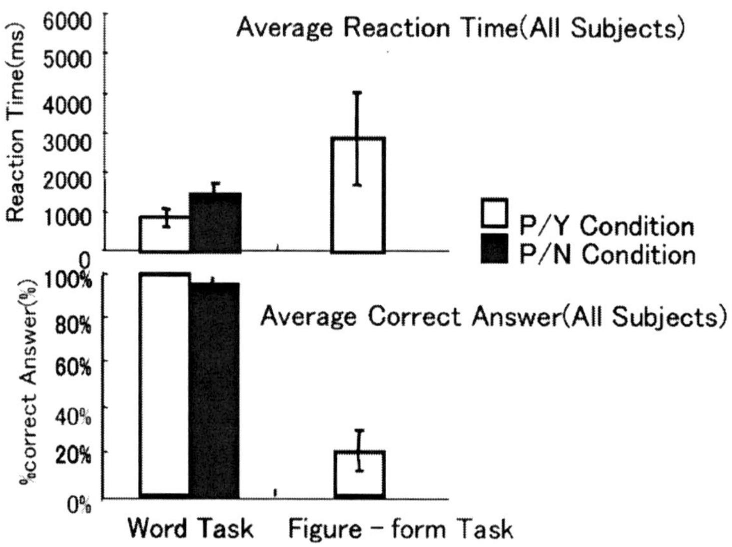

Table 1. Activation during tasks

Region		(x y z)mm	t-value
Word task			
1.	Left Precuneus (BA31)	(-12 -64 26)	5.65
2	Left Superior Temporal Gyrus (BA39)	(-38 -58 32)	5.55
3.	Right Middle Temporal Gyrus	(50 -70 26)	4.66
4.	Right Parietal Lobe, Postcentral Gyrus (BA2)	(60 -20 23)	4.31
5.	Cingulate Gyrus	(2 -72 26)	4.09
Figure-form task			
1.	Right Medial Frontal Gyrus	(6 24 44)	5.86
2.	Right Inferior Frontal Gyrus (BA9)	(40 8 22)	5.48
3.	Left Middle Occipital Gyrus	(-24 -82 24)	4.96
4.	Right Middle Frontal Gyrus (BA9)	(34 34 36)	4.55

Figure 7. Activated area in the word PY>PN condition. (a) Brain activation is shown on the surface in the left and right hemispheres. (b) Sections show brain activation. (c) The number of clusters is consistent with the activation shown in Table 1

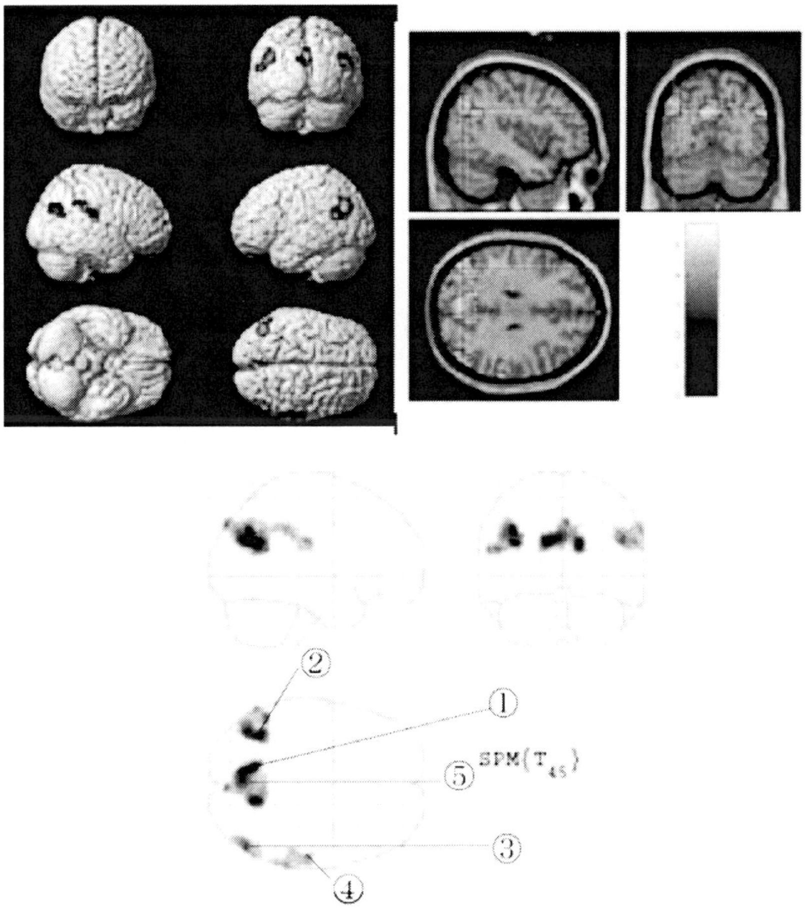

Figure 8. Activated area in figure form task. (a) Brain activations are shown in the surface rendering of left and right hemispheres. (b) Section results show brain activation. (c) The number of clusters is consistent with the activation shown in Table 1

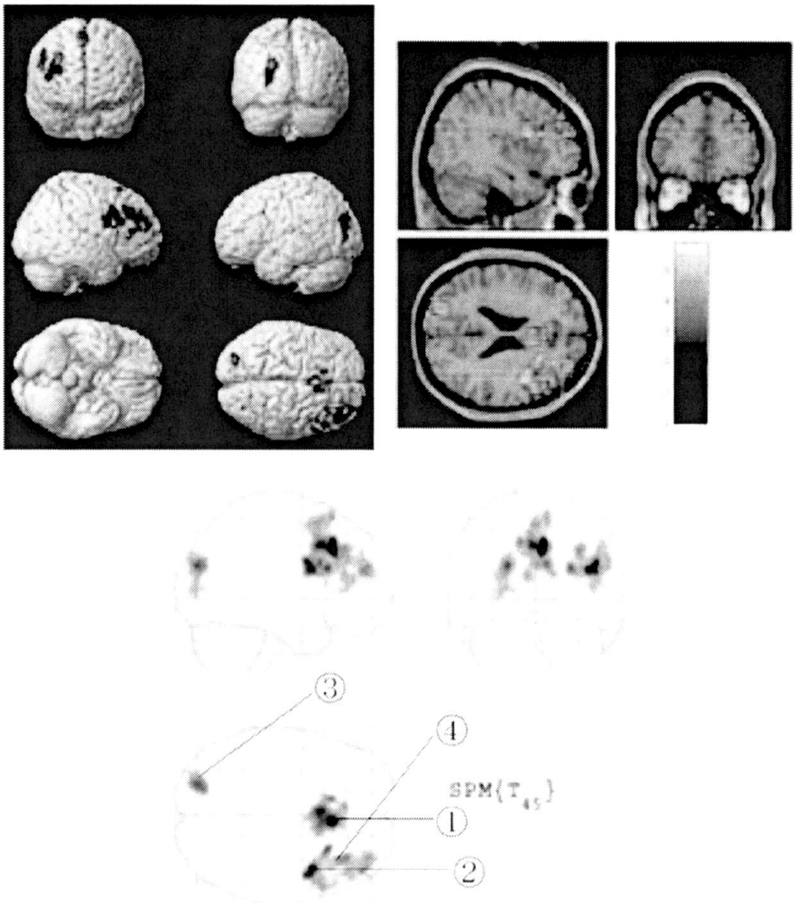

form task when priming occurred. In addition, the right frontal cortex and the visual cortex were significantly activated in the left hemisphere.

DISCUSSION

In the behavioral experiments, we found that the percentage of correct answers increased and the reaction time decreased during the P/Y trial. Because nearly every subject was unconscious, the difference between the P/Y trial and P/N trial indicated a successful priming effect. These results are consistent with many previous studies of word priming using various language and stimulus modalities. Schacter et al. (Schacter et al., 1999; Badgaiyan R. D., Schacter et al., 1999) performed a priming test within (e.g., visually/aurally encoded and visually/aurally retrieved) and across modalities (e.g., aurally encoded and visually retrieved) and reported that the percentage of correct answers was approximately 50% in P/Y conditions, whereas the percentage was less than 20% in a P/N condition across modalities. Cabeza and Ohta (Cabeza et al., 1993) performed the priming test using the Kanji fragment task and observed significant priming effects. In our study, the percentage of correct answers during the P/N condition was comparatively higher because we used common words.

The parietal cortex was activated in the P/Y condition in our study and another previous study (Palmer et al., 2001). However, this area was often activated during a visual attention task (Coull et al., 1998). The supplementary motor area was activated in our study and also displayed attention-related activation. Activation of this region may be related to the visual attention to word stimuli that was implicitly induced by priming.

During the figure form task, the right prefrontal cortex was significantly activated when the priming effect occurred. This is consistent with a previous study (Kuo et al., 2004) in which Chinese and Korean words were shown to Chinese participants. Furthermore, Henson et al. (Henson et al., 2004) performed a visual object cognition task and found that the left middle occipital gyrus was significantly activated, similar to the present study. Finally, we determined that the visual presentation of Korean characters had no meaning.

In this study, we investigated the priming effect in a word and figure form task. We concluded that the word task resulted in more priming than the figure form task. Using fMRI, significant activation of the parietal and frontal cortex was observed during the contrast of PY>PN but not in the figure form task.

ACKNOWLEDGMENT

The authors would like to thank the subjects who participated in this study. A portion of this study was financially supported by JSPS AA Science Platform Program and JSPS Grant-in-Aid for Scientific Research (B) (21404002). This research was supported by the 2009 Kagawa University Characteristic Prior Research Fund.

REFERENCES

Badgaiyan, R. D., Schacter, D. L., & Alpert, N. M. (1999). Auditory priming within and across modalities: Evidence from positron emission tomography. *Journal of Cognitive Neuroscience*, *11*(4), 337–348. doi:10.1162/089892999563463

Cabeza, R., & Ohta, N. (1993). Dissociating conceptual priming, perceptual priming and explicit memory. *The European Journal of Cognitive Psychology*, *5*(1), 35–53. doi:10.1080/09541449308406513

Coull, J. T., & Nobre, A. C. (1998). Where and when to pay attention: The neural systems for directing attention to spatial locations and to time intervals as revealed by both PET and fMRI. *The Journal of Neuroscience*, *18*(18), 7426–7435.

Gazzaniga, M. S., Ivry, R. B., & Mangun, G. R. (2002). *Cognitive neuroscience*.

Henson, R. N., Rylands, A., Ross, E., Vuilleumeir, P., & Rugg, M. D. (2004). The effect of repetition lag on electrophysiological and haemodynamic correlates of visual object priming. *NeuroImage*, *21*, 1674–1689. doi:10.1016/j.neuroimage.2003.12.020

Kiyo, A. (1980). *Appear frequency of Japanese words* (pp. 42–87). Doushisya University Press.

Kuo, W.-J., Yeh, T.-C., Lee, J.-R., Chen, L.-F., Lee, P.-L., & Chen, S.-S. (2004). Orthographic and phonological processing of Chinese characters: An fMRI study. *NeuroImage*, *21*, 1721–1731. doi:10.1016/j.neuroimage.2003.12.007

Palmer, E. D., Rosen, H. J., Ojemann, J. G., Buckner, R. L., Kelley, W. M., & Petersen, S. E. (2001). An event-related fMRI study of overt and covert word stem completion. *NeuroImage*, *14*, 182–193. doi:10.1006/nimg.2001.0779

Schacter, D. L., Badgaiyan, R. D., & Alpert, N. M. (1999). Visual word stem completion priming within and across modalities: A PET study. *Neuroreport, 10*, 2061–2065. doi:10.1097/00001756-199907130-00013

Tsuguo, O. (1972). *Appear frequency of Japanese words* (pp. 1–62). Doushisya University Press.

KEY TERMS AND DEFINITIONS

Attention: When people choose useful information and ignore other information in the environment.

Neuroanatomy: The study of the anatomy of nervous tissue and neural structures of the nervous system.

Neuroimaging: The use of various techniques to either directly or indirectly image the structure and function/pharmacology of the brain. It is a relatively new discipline within the medicine and neuroscience/psychology community.

Neuroscience: The scientific study of the nervous system.

Word Priming Effect: A facilitatory effect or a control effect that facilitates the identification of a successive stimulus that was previously subconsciously observed.

Word Processing: Orthographic, phonological and semantic cognitive processing.

Chapter 7
Visual Gnosis and Face Perception

Shozo Tobimatsu
Department of Clinical Neurophysiology, Neurological Institute, Graduate School of Medical Sciences, Kyushu University, Japan

ABSTRACT

There are two major parallel pathways in humans: the parvocellular (P) and magnocellular (M) pathways. The former has excellent spatial resolution with color selectivity, while the latter shows excellent temporal resolution with high contrast sensitivity. Visual stimuli should be tailored to answer specific clinical and/or research questions. This chapter examines the neural mechanisms of face perception using event-related potentials (ERPs). Face stimuli of different spatial frequencies were used to investigate how low-spatial-frequency (LSF) and high-spatial-frequency (HSF) components of the face contribute to the identification and recognition of the face and facial expressions. The P100 component in the occipital area (Oz), the N170 in the posterior temporal region (T5/T6) and late components peaking at 270-390 ms (T5/T6) were analyzed. LSF enhanced P100, while N170 was augmented by HSF irrespective of facial expressions. This suggested that LSF is important for global processing of facial expressions, whereas HSF handles featural processing. There were significant amplitude differences between positive and negative LSF facial expressions in the early time windows of 270-310 ms. Subsequently, the amplitudes among negative HSF facial expressions differed significantly in the later time windows of 330–390 ms. Discrimination between positive and negative facial expressions precedes discrimination among different negative expressions in a sequential manner based on parallel visual channels. Interestingly, patients with schizophrenia showed decreased spatial frequency sensitivities for face processing. Taken together, the spatially filtered face images are useful for exploring face perception and recognition.

DOI: 10.4018/978-1-60960-559-9.ch007

ANATOMY AND PHYSIOLOGY OF THE VISUAL PATHWAYS

The human visual system consists of multiple, parallel streams that process different information, and each stream constitutes a set of the sequential processes. They are sometimes referred to as *channels*. Light increments (ON) and decrements (OFF), motion, stereoscopic depth, color, shape, etc., are processed separately and simultaneously. There are two major parallel pathways in humans: the parvocellular (P) and magnocellular (M) pathways (Figure 1). The former is responsible for carrying information about the form and color of an object because of its ability to detect stimuli with high spatial frequencies and color, while the latter plays an important role in detecting motion due to its ability to respond to high temporal stimuli (Livingstone, & Hubel, 1998; Tobimatsu, & Celesia, 2006). There is considerable cross talk between the two systems and much evidence supporting that these systems are integrated in a distributed network.

We have been studying the functions of the P- and M-pathways with evoked potentials by manipulating the characteristics of the visual stimulus (Arakawa, Tobimatsu, Kato, & Kira, 1999; Tobimatsu, 2002; Tobimatsu, & Kato, 1998; Tobimatsu, Celesia, Haug, Onofrj, Sartucci, & Porciatti, 2000; Tobimatsu, Shigeto, Arakawa, & Kato, 1999; Tobimatsu, Tomoda, & Kato, 1995; Tobimatsu, Goto, Yamasaki, Tsurusawa, & Taniwaki, 2006). Information on the characteristics of a face is first processed in the fusiform gyrus (V4) and carried by the P-pathway (Vuilleumier, Armony, Driver, & Dolna, 2003). Information on the motion of an object is processed in the MT/V5, and the information is carried by the M-pathway (Rizzolatti, & Matelli, 2003).

FACE PERCEPTION

Event-related potentials (ERPs) elicited by facial stimuli were recorded at multiple scalp sites in normal subjects. As shown in Figure 2, visual stimuli are decomposed into several spatial frequencies

Figure 1. Recent concepts of the parallel pathways. Adopted from Tobimatsu, Goto, Yamasaki, Nakashima, Tomoda, & Mitsudome, 2008.

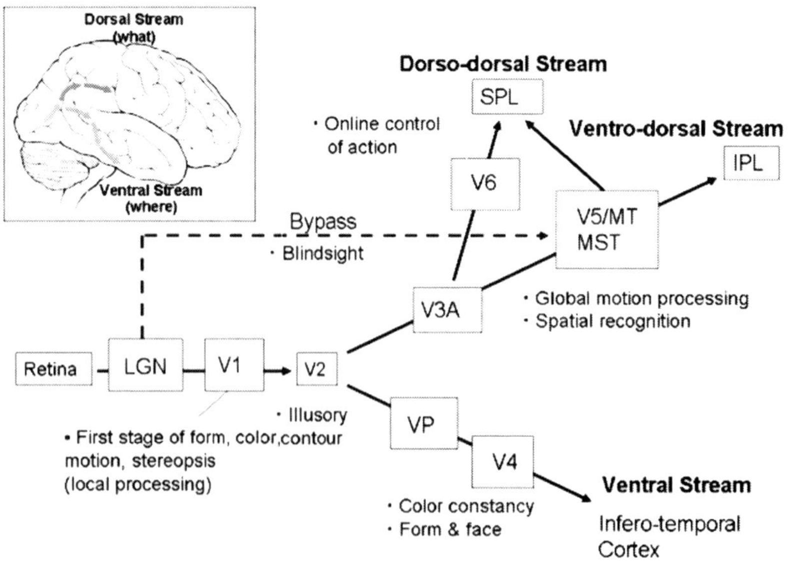

(SFs) (Tobimatsu, Goto, Yamasaki, Nakashima, Tomoda, & Mitsudome, 2008). The low-spatial-frequency (LSF) and high-spatial-frequency (HSF) information are processed by the M- and P-pathways, respectively. A photograph of a face was filtered to alter the SF components and used to investigate how the LSF and HSF components of the face contribute to its identification and recognition (Nakashima, Goto, Abe, Kaneko, Saito, Makinouchi, & Tobimatsu, 2008; Nakashima, Kaneko, Goto, Abe, Mitsudo, Ogata, Makinouchi, & Tobimatsu, 2008; Obayashi, Nakashima, Onitsuka, Maekawa, Hirano, Hirano, Oribe, Kaneko, Kanba, & Tobimatsu, 2009). The original stimuli were 256-level grayscale photographs of emotional (anger, fear and happiness) and neutral faces taken from Japanese and Caucasian Facial Expressions of Emotion (JACFEE) and Neutral Faces (JACNeuF), respectively (Matsumoto and Ekman, 1988). The object stimuli (houses) and target stimuli (shoes) were taken from our own 256-level grayscale photographs. Faces and houses for the LSF and HSF stimuli were created by image-engineering techniques with two-dimensional fast Fourier transformation (one-order Gaussian window methods for LSF; 35-order Hamming window methods for HSF) using our own program written in C language and MATLAB ver. 7 (The MathWorks Inc.). The BSF stimuli were original photographs and left unfiltered. The cutoff frequencies (< 2.5–4.0 cycles/face for LSF; > 30.0–50.0 cycles/face for HSF) were determined by measuring the psychophysical threshold for the recognition of facial expressions and houses using 30 other recruited subjects (10 females and 20 males; age range, 20-34 years; mean age, 25.7 years; unpublished data) prior to the ERP recordings. The mean luminance and contrast were controlled by normalizing the mean and standard deviation (SD) of the gray values of all stimuli using our own program written in C language (mean luminance, 48 cd/m^2; mean gray value ± SD, 128 ± 40). Representative examples of the stimuli (fearful expression) are shown in Figure 3.

Figure 2. Importance of the elementary components (luminance, contrast, color, spatial frequency and temporal frequency) of the visual images. Regarding spatial frequency, a checkerboard pattern is rather complex compared with sinusoidal gratings (left). A photograph of a face decomposed into several spatial frequencies (right). Adopted from Tobimatsu, Goto, Yamasaki, Nakashima, Tomoda, & Mitsudome, 2008.

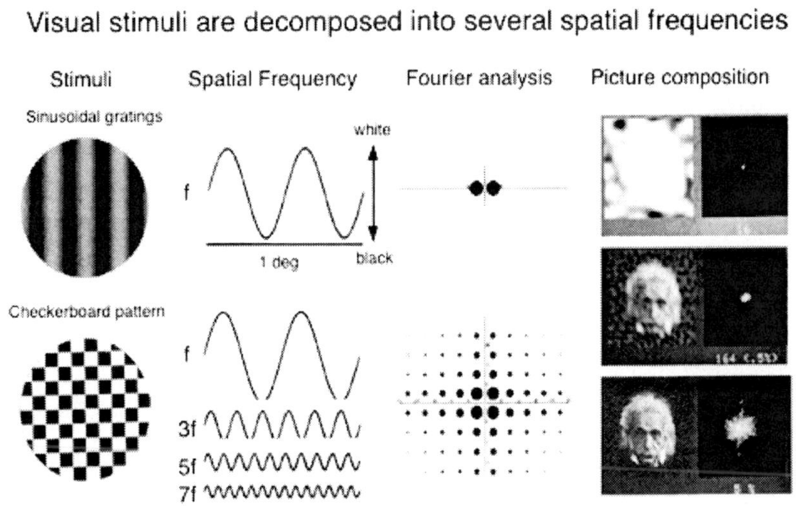

Figure 3. Representative examples of the stimuli used in this study. BSF is an original non-filtered image (left), which contains broad spatial frequency components. LSF and HSF faces are filtered by fast Fourier transformation. The LSF face consists of information with low spatial frequencies (<2.5-4 cycles/face width) and preserves the holistic facial image (right). The HSF face extracts information with high spatial frequencies (>30-50 cycles/face width) and emphasizes the detailed features of the facial components. Adopted from Tobimatsu, Goto, Yamasaki, Nakashima, Tomoda, & Mitsudome, 2008.

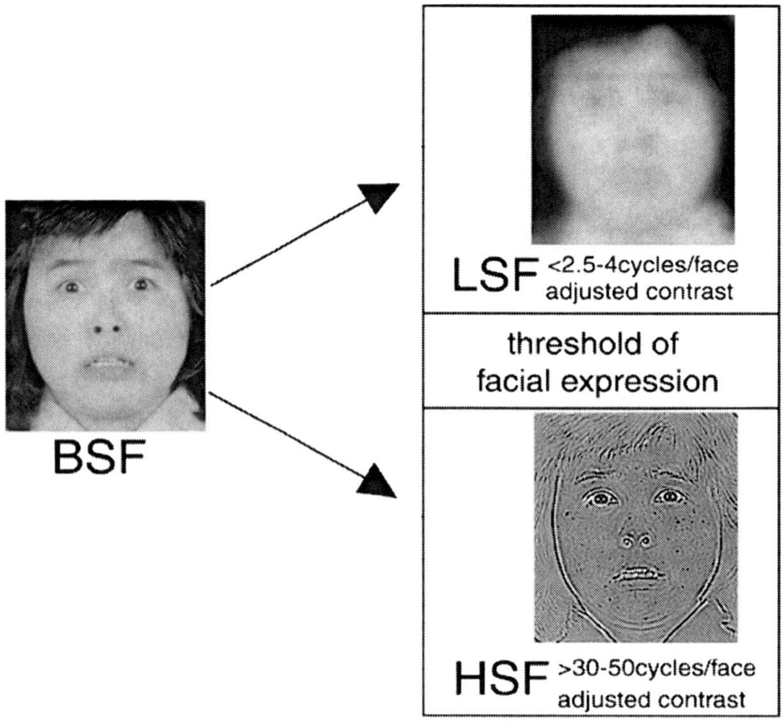

THE P100 COMPONENT

The grand-averaged P100 waveforms at Oz for each stimulus under the three conditions of spatial frequency are shown in Figure 4. The mean latency of P100 for faces was 110.2 ± 12.2 ms, while that of P100 for objects was 112.3 ± 16.6 ms. As shown in Figure 4 (upper panel), the P100 amplitudes for LSF faces tended to be greater than those for BSF faces. However, the P100 amplitudes for objects did not demonstrate this trend. ANOVA confirmed this tendency, showing a main effect of spatial frequency ($F(2, 24) = 25.743$, $p < 0.001$) and an interaction of spatial frequency (BSF, LSF and HSF) × stimuli (faces and objects) ($F(2, 24) = 6.619$, $p < 0.01$) for the P100 amplitudes. Moreover, an interaction contrast was found between LSF and BSF by post-hoc analysis ($F = 8.376$, $p < 0.05$). This interaction contrast suggested a clear difference in sensitivity to the spatial frequency between faces and objects for LSF in the early stage of perception. In other words, LSF faces activated the neural generators of P100, whereas LSF objects did not. In contrast, no significant difference was found for the P100 latency. Similarly, no significant interactions of spatial frequency (BSF, LSF and HSF) × facial expression (anger, fear, happiness and neutral) were observed for the P100 amplitudes and latency ($F(6, 72) = 1.799$, $p > 0.05$ and $F(6, 72) =$

Figure 4. P100 responses to each stimulus at the mid-occipital region (Oz) and N170 responses to each stimulus at the temporo-occipital electrodes (T5 and T6). The grand-averaged P100 is specifically larger for LSF faces (left) than for BSF (middle) and HSF (right) faces. The grand-averaged N170 for HSF faces is clearly larger than those for BSF and LSF faces with right hemisphere predominance. Adopted from Tobimatsu, Goto, Yamasaki, Nakashima, Tomoda, & Mitsudome, 2008.

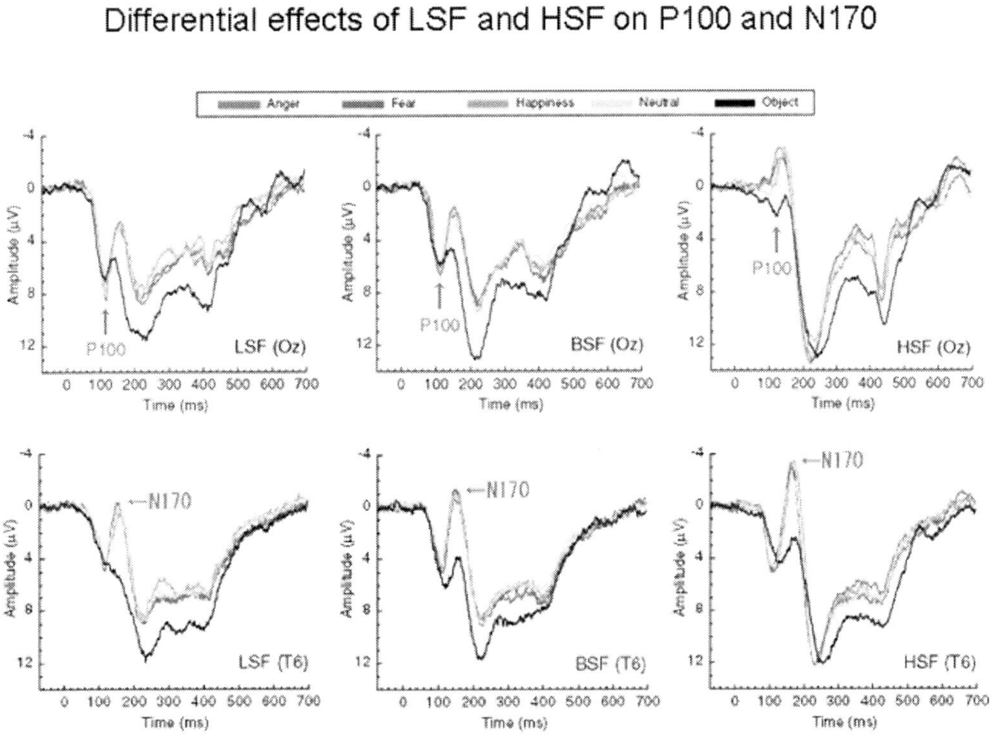

2.082, $p > 0.05$, respectively). Overall, the P100 amplitudes were significantly enhanced by LSF information of faces but not by that of objects, regardless of the facial expressions.

THE N170 COMPONENT

The grand-averaged N170 waveforms at the T5 and T6 electrodes are shown in Figure 4. The mean latency of N170 for faces was 158.4 ± 13.6 ms, while that of N170 for objects was 152.2 ± 21.4 ms. From Figure 4 (lower panel), it is apparent that the N170 amplitudes for faces increased to a much greater extent under the HSF condition than under the BSF condition with right hemisphere predominance. In contrast, the N170 amplitudes for objects did not increase under the HSF condition. Statistical analysis further confirmed a main effect of stimuli (T5: $F(1, 12) = 38.674$, $p < 0.001$; and T6: $F(1, 12) = 39.922$, $p < 0.001$) and spatial frequency (T5: $F(2, 24) = 7.222$, $p < 0.01$; and T6: $F(2, 24) = 12.618$, $p < 0.001$) regardless of the hemisphere. In addition, a significant interaction of stimuli × spatial frequency was only observed at T6 (T5: $F(2, 24) = 2.364$, $p > 0.10$; and T6: $F(2.24) = 4.461$, $p < 0.05$). A post hoc test revealed that a contrast interaction of BSF × HSF was only present at T6 ($F = 5.910$, $p < 0.05$). This interaction contrast indicated that HSF information of faces increased the N170 amplitudes in the right hemisphere, whereas the HSF components of objects had no effect. Thus, it is likely that N170 represents selective processing of HSF information for faces. A main effect of spatial frequency was found for the N170 latency, although it was only apparent at T6 ($F(2, 24) = 73.299$, $p < 0.001$). However, there was no interaction of faces × objects. Similarly, no significant interaction of spatial frequency (BSF, LSF and HSF) × facial expression (anger, fear, happiness and neutral) was found for the N170 amplitudes and latency. In summary, the N170 amplitudes in the right hemisphere were significantly augmented by HSF information of faces but not by that of objects, irrespective of the facial expressions.

LATE COMPONENTS IN THE TIME WINDOW OF 270-390 MS

Figure 5 shows enlarged waveforms of the late components for LSF, BSF and HSF faces at the T5 and T6 electrodes in Figure 4 for the time window of 200–450 ms. There was a significant difference in the amplitudes among the facial expressions for the LSF and HSF conditions. Under the LSF condition, happy facial images produced a negative potential compared with other expressions. Under the HSF condition, the fearful face induced a negative response, while the angry face evoked a positive potential. However, this difference was not significant under the BSF condition. The differences were statistically significant in the time windows of 270–290 and 290–310 ms for LSF ($F(3, 36) = 5.206$, $p < 0.01$ and $F(3, 36) = 4.847$, $p < 0.01$, respectively), and 330–350, 350–370 and 370–390 ms for the HSF condition ($F(3, 36) = 3.334$, $p < 0.05$, $F(3, 36) = 3.139$, $p < 0.05$ and $F(3, 36) = 3.057$, $p < 0.05$, respectively). A post-hoc paired comparison revealed that the differences in amplitudes for happiness vs. anger or happiness vs. fear (i.e., positive vs. negative) under the LSF condition were statistically significant ($p < 0.05$ and $p < 0.01$, respectively). In contrast, the difference in amplitudes for anger vs. fear (i.e., negative vs. negative) was only statistically significant for HSF faces ($p < 0.05$). These statistical results are summarized in Figure 5 as gray-scale boxes. Specifically, LSF images produced different responses between 'positive and negative' expressions in the relatively early phase of the late components, while HSF images induced different responses between 'negative and negative' expressions in the late phase of the late components.

GENERAL DISCUSSION

Information from the different components of the face is transmitted mainly by the P-pathway and processed in the fusiform gyrus (V4) (Vuilleumier, Armony, Driver, & Dolna, 2003). Direct recordings from the human V4 demonstrated that a surface-negative potential (N200) was evoked by faces but not by the other types of stimuli (Allison, Ginter, McCarthy, Nobre, Puce, Luby, & Spencer, 1994; Allison, Puce, Spencer, & McCarthy, 1999). Scalp-recorded ERPs showed that the N170 component was a face-specific potential, and it was predominant in the posterior temporal cortex (Bentin, Allison, Puce, Perez, & McCarthy, 1996). More specifically, it was most likely generated in the occipitotemporal sulcus lateral to the V4 (Bentin, Allison, Puce, Perez, & McCarthy, 1996). Our results suggest that P100 reflects holistic processing of faces, and face robustness further assures face-specific processing in the early component. Moreover, the N170 component analyzes fine facial features (Nakashima, Kaneko, Goto, Abe, Mitsudo, Ogata, Makinouchi, & Tobimatsu, 2008). Consequently, the N270–310 component is involved in the discrimination between positive and negative expressions, whereas the N330–390 component separates detailed information among

Figure 5. Waveforms of the late components for the facial expressions of each stimulus. The original waveforms in Fig. 3 in the time window of 200–450 ms are enlarged for comparison. The white square boxes on the abscissa indicate main effects of facial expressions, while the colored boxes show statistically significant differences revealed by paired comparisons (Bonferroni correction). Under the LSF condition, there were significant differences in amplitudes between positive (happiness) and negative (anger and fear) expressions during the time window of 270–310 ms, regardless of the hemisphere. In contrast, a significant difference was only found among negative expressions (anger vs. fear) during the time window of 330–390 ms under the HSF condition. Adopted from Tobimatsu, Goto, Yamasaki, Nakashima, Tomoda, & Mitsudome, 2008.

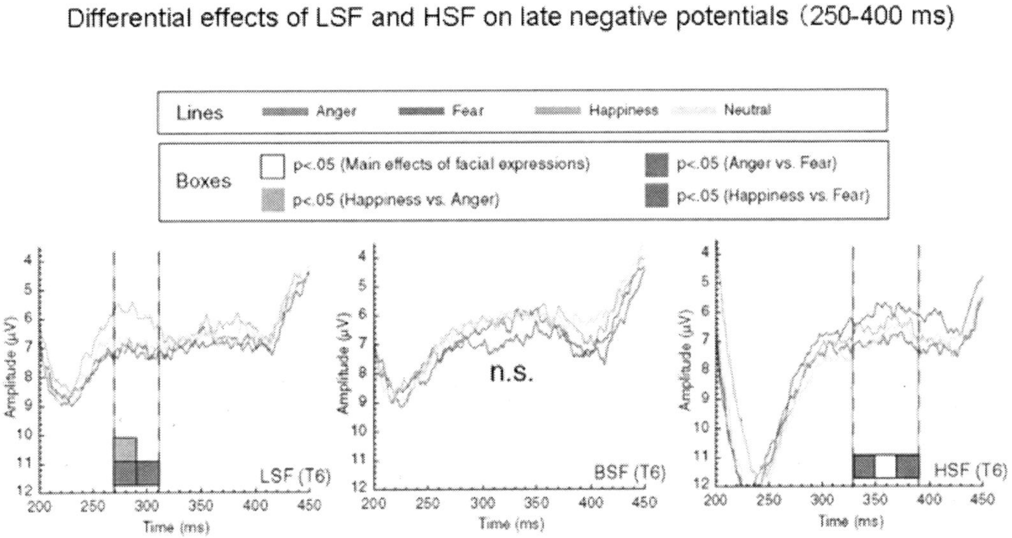

the negative expressions (Nakashima, Goto, Abe, Kaneko, Saito, Makinouchi, & Tobimatsu, 2008). Therefore, faces and facial expressions are sequentially processed in parallel based on the LSF and HSF information.

Recently, our laboratory demonstrated that schizophrenics showed abnormal P100 and N170 modulations in response to SF changes in faces (Figure 6), indicating decreased SF sensitivities for processing faces. These results further suggest that abnormal early visual processing may underlie at least some of the deficits associated with face recognition in schizophrenia (Obayashi, Nakashima, Onitsuka, Maekawa, Hirano, Hirano, Oribe, Kaneko, Kanba, & Tobimatsu, 2009).

In conclusion, our spatially filtered face images are useful for exploring face perception and recognition.

ACKNOWLEDGMENT

This study was supported by a Grant-in-Aid for Scientific Research on Innovative Areas, "Face perception and recognition", by the Ministry of Education, Culture, Sports, Science and Technology, Japan. I would also like to thank to my collaborators Drs. Y. Goto, K. Kaneko, T. Maekawa, T. Mitsudo, T. Nakashima, C. Obayashi, K. Ogata and T. Yamasaki.

*Figure 6. Response characteristics of P1 at O1/O2 and N170 at T5/T6 in normal controls and patients with schizophrenia. The data from P1s and N170s were averaged across three types of facial expressions (neutral, happy, and fearful faces) and across both hemispheres (O1 and O2, T5 and T6, respectively) with three spatial frequencies (LSF, BSF, and HSF). Error bars indicate the standard errors of the mean amplitude and latency. Asterisks indicate a significant difference between spatial frequencies (*p < 0.05, **p < 0.01, and ***p < 0.001). For P1 amplitudes, normal controls exhibited a significant LSF > BSF > HSF difference, while schizophrenics showed no significant LSF > BSF difference (A). For P1 latencies, normal controls showed significant LSF > BSF and LSF > HSF differences, whereas schizophrenics exhibited significant LSF > BSF and HSF > BSF differences (B). For N170 amplitudes, normal controls revealed a significant HSF > BSF > LSF difference, while schizophrenics showed no such HSF > BSF difference (C). For N170 latencies, both groups exhibited a significant HSF > LSF > BSF difference (D). Adopted from Obayashi, Nakashima, Onitsuka, Maekawa, Hirano, Hirano, Oribe, Kaneko, Kanba, & Tobimatsu, 2009.*

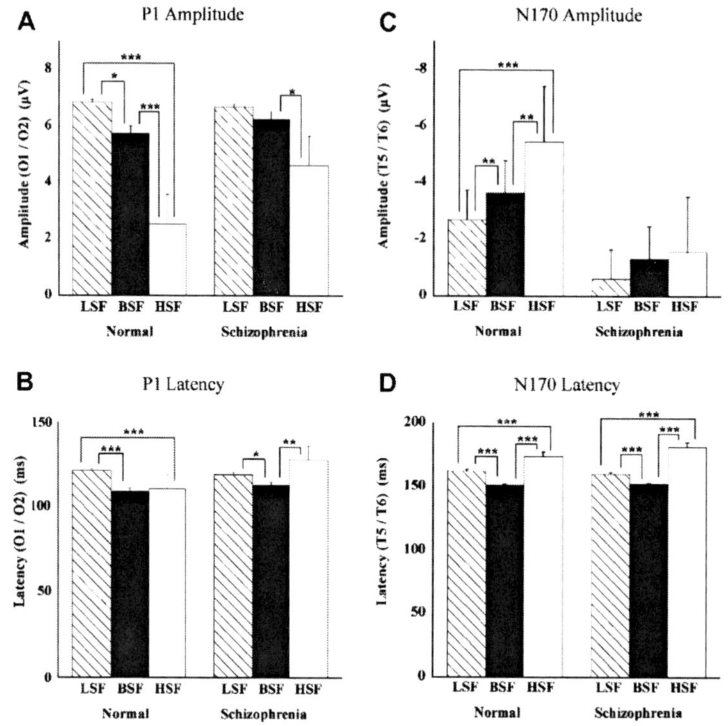

REFERENCES

Allison, T., Ginter, T. H., & McCarthy, H, G., Nobre, A. C., Puce, A., Luby, M., & Spencer, D. D. (1994). Face-recognition in human extrastriate cortex. *Journal of Neurophysiology*, *71*, 821–825.

Allison, T., Puce, A., Spencer, D. D., & McCarthy, G. (1999). Electrophysiological studies of human face perception. I: Potentials generated in occipitotemporal cortex by face and non-face stimuli. *Cerebral Cortex*, *9*, 415–430. doi:10.1093/cercor/9.5.415

Arakawa, K., Tobimatsu, S., Kato, M., & Kira, J. (1999). Parvocelluar and magnocellular visual processing in spinocerebellar degeneration and Parkinson's disease: An event-related potential study. *Clinical Neurophysiology*, *110*, 1048–1057. doi:10.1016/S1388-2457(99)00049-8

Bentin, S., Allison, T., Puce, A., Perez, E., & McCarthy, G. (1996). Electrophysiological studies of face perception in humans. *Journal of Cognitive Neuroscience*, *8*, 551–565. doi:10.1162/jocn.1996.8.6.551

Livingstone, M., & Hubel, D. (1998). Segregation of form, color, movement, and depth: Anatomy, physiology, and perception. *Science*, *240*, 740–749. doi:10.1126/science.3283936

Nakashima, T., Goto, Y., Abe, T., Kaneko, K., Saito, T., Makinouchi, A., & Tobimatsu, S. (2008). Electrophysiological evidence for sequential discrimination of positive and negative facial expressions. *Clinical Neurophysiology*, *119*, 1803–1811. doi:10.1016/j.clinph.2008.04.014

Nakashima, T., Kaneko, K., Goto, Y., Abe, T., Mitsudo, T., & Ogata, K. (2008). Early ERP components differentially extract facial features: Evidence for spatial frequency-and-contrast detectors. *Neuroscience Research*, *62*, 225–235. doi:10.1016/j.neures.2008.08.009

Obayashi, C., Nakashima, T., Onitsuka, T., Maekawa, T., Hirano, Y., & Hirano, S. (2009). Decreased spatial frequency sensitivities for processing faces in male patients with chronic schizophrenia. *Clinical Neurophysiology*, *120*, 1525–1533. doi:10.1016/j.clinph.2009.06.016

Rizzolatti, G., & Matelli, M. (2003). Two different streams from the dorsal visual system: Anatomy and functions. *Experimental Brain Research*, *153*, 146–157. doi:10.1007/s00221-003-1588-0

Tobimatsu, S. (2002). Neurophysiologic tools to explore visual cognition. *Electroencephalography and Clinical Neurophysiology*, *S54*, 261–265. doi:10.1016/S1567-424X(09)70459-3

Tobimatsu, S., & Celesia, G. G. (2006). Studies of human visual pathophysiology with visual evoked potentials. *Clinical Neurophysiology*, *117*, 1414–1433. doi:10.1016/j.clinph.2006.01.004

Tobimatsu, S., Celesia, G. G., Haug, B. A., Onofrj, M., Sartucci, F., & Porciatti, V. (2000). Recent advances in clinical neurophysiology of vision. *Electroencephalography and Clinical Neurophysiology*, *S53*, 312–322. doi:10.1016/S1567-424X(09)70174-6

Tobimatsu, S., Goto, Y., Yamasaki, T., Nakashima, T., Tomoda, Y., & Mitsudome, A. (2008). Visual ERPs and cortical function in Progress in epileptic disorders vol. 5, Event-related potentials in patients with epilepsy: From current state to future prospects. (A. Ikeda A and Y. Inoue, Eds). (pp. 37-48). Paris, France: John Libbey Eurotext.

Tobimatsu, S., Goto, Y., Yamasaki, T., Tsurusawa, R., & Taniwaki, T. (2006). An integrated approach to face and motion perception in humans. *Clinical Neurophysiology*, *S59*, 41–46.

Tobimatsu, S., & Kato, M. (1998). Multimodality visual evoked potentials in evaluating visual dysfunction in optic neuritis. *Neurology*, *50*, 715–718.

Tobimatsu, S., Shigeto, H., Arakawa, K., & Kato, M. (1999). Electrophysiological studies of parallel visual processing in humans. *Electroencephalography and Clinical Neurophysiology*, *S49*, 103–107.

Tobimatsu, S., Tomoda, H., & Kato, M. (1995). Parvocellular and magnocellular contributions to visual evoked potentials in humans: Stimulation with chromatic and achromatic gratings and apparent motion. *Journal of the Neurological Sciences*, *34*, 73–82. doi:10.1016/0022-510X(95)00222-X

Vuilleumier, P., Armony, J. L., Driver, J., & Dolna, R. J. (2003). Distinct spatial frequency sensitivities for processing faces and emotional expressions. *Nature Neuroscience*, *6*, 624–631. doi:10.1038/nn1057

KEY TERMS AND DEFINITIONS

Event-Related Potentials (ERPs): An event-related potential is any measured brain response that is directly the result of a thought or perception. More formally, it is any stereotyped electrophysiological response to an internal or external stimulus.

Face Perception: Face perception is the process by which the brain and mind understand and interpret the face, particularly the human face.

Late Components: Late components are ERP components peaking at 270-390 ms recorded from the posterior temporal area. These components probably reflect the visual processing of facial expressions.

N170: N170 is negative peak at around 170 ms recorded from the posterior temporal area. This component is considered to be a face-specific ERP component.

P100: P100 is a positive peak at around 100 ms and is an initial ERP response recorded from the occipital area. Hence, this peak is commonly called P100.

Parvocellular And Magnocellular Pathways: They contribute to the parallel visual processing. Parvocellular system has excellent spatial resolution with color selectivity while magnocellular stream shows excellent temporal resolution with high contrast sensitivity.

Spatial Frequencies: The spatial frequency is a measure of how often the structure repeats per unit of distance.

Chapter 8
Human Characteristics of Sound Localization under Masking for the Early Detection of Dementia

Kouji Nagashima
Graduate School of Natural Science and Technology, Okayama University, Japan

Jinglong Wu
Graduate School of Natural Science and Technology, Okayama University, Japan

Satoshi Takahashi
Graduate School of Natural Science and Technology, Okayama University, Japan

ABSTRACT

Sound localization ability differs among people, such as between a young person, a senior citizen, and a dementia patient. Therefore, it is possible to detect dementia at an early stage by measuring a difference in this ability. Experiments for sound source localization in the horizontal plane show that the ability is improved by separating the presented locations between the signal and a masker. However, there are few data regarding sound localization in the vertical plane. The threshold in the perpendicular plane has been measured, but only experiments in the median plane regarding sound localization have been reported, and its characterization in other aspects has not been clarified. Previous studies about localization ability in the vertical plane have reported contradictory results. One is that the sound source from an upper direction is perceptually superior for a subject, and the other is that a lower direction is superior. The purpose of this study in this chapter is to clarify sound localization ability in the vertical plane and to detect dementia in the early stage using the aging tendency of aural characteristics.

INTRODUCTION

The frequency of dementia (Alzheimer's disease, AD) increases drastically with an increase in the population of senior citizens. Because it is likely that dementia interferes with a patient's general life, it is desirable to discover symptoms at an early stage. MMSE is used for the early detection of dementia, but it is vague. Therefore, an effective method to diagnose dementia is necessary. We

DOI: 10.4018/978-1-60960-559-9.ch008

employ a human auditory characteristic for the early detection of the dementia.

A human being lives among various sounds in modern society and senses danger by understanding the direction of those sounds. If the sound source cannot be localized for various sounds, life in modern society becomes difficult. It may be said that sound source localization ability under sound masking is important.

A previous study has shown that there is a clear difference in sound localization ability between young people, senior citizens, and dementia patients. Therefore, it is thought that early detection of dementia is possible by examining the sound source localization ability of the subject. However, the sound source localization ability in the vertical plane between a physically unimpaired person and dementia patients was not elucidated in that study. The difference between subjects under the masking condition of daily, real-life noise is likewise unknown.

The difference between the horizontal plane and the vertical plane in sound source localization ability is the use of a head-related transfer function in the vertical plane but an interaural time difference or interaural level difference in the horizontal plane. Because the horizontal plane has many cues for localization, localization accuracy in the horizontal plane is higher than in the vertical plane. Sound source localization in the horizontal plane may be suitable for the early detection of dementia because it requires high localization ability. As for sound source localization in the vertical plane, it seems that a significant difference in ability exists between patients.

This study shows that sound source localization ability in the vertical plane is a means for the early detection of dementia. This is shown using a fundamental experiment about sound source localization ability in the vertical plane, and this study shows that the sound source localization ability is affected by a masking noise.

SOUND LOCALIZATION

Sound localization is an ability that allows a person to judge the direction of a sound source from the information of the sound. Figure 1 shows an example of masking. The cues for sound localization are interaural time and level differences and changes of the spectra. Interaural time and level differences are important in sound localization in the horizontal plane, and changes of the spectra are important in sound localization in the vertical plane.

MASKING

Masking refers to the inability to hear a signal because of a masker. There are various kinds of

Figure 1. Example of sound localization

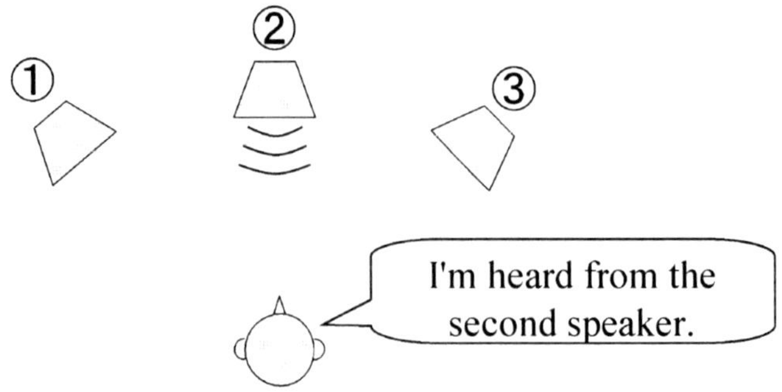

masking, but this study focuses on simultaneous masking. Figure 2 shows an example of masking.

EXPERIMENT

Subjects

Ten subjects ranging from 21 to 24 years in age were paid for their participation. All subjects had normal hearing as measured by pure-tone audiometry.

Stimuli

The experimental stimuli used were similar to a previous study. Table 1 shows the parameters of the signals and the maskers.

The signal was a 500-Hz or 4000-Hz pure tone. The signal was 1000 ms in duration. The signal that was measured at the position of the subject's head was constant at 60 dB. The masker was a 500-Hz pure tone, a 4000-Hz pure tone, or white noise (WN; 125–16000 Hz). The masker was always presented during an experiment. The pure-tone maskers of 500 Hz and 4000 Hz that were measured at the position of the subject's head were constant at 50 dB and 55 dB, and the white noise masker was constant at 50 dB.

Figure 2. Example of masking

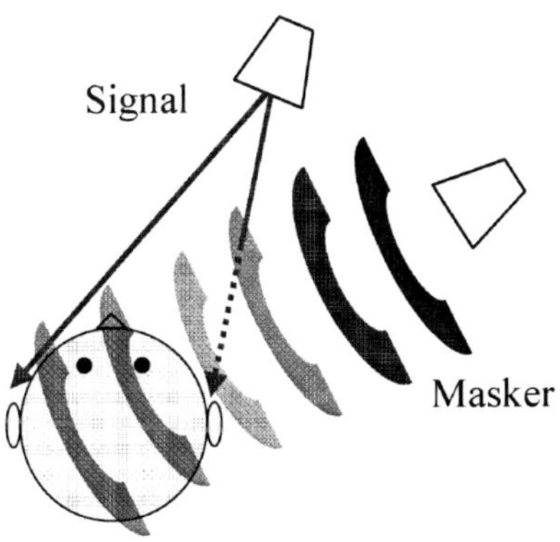

Apparatus

Figure 3 shows the arrangement of the seven speakers in this study. The speakers were arranged in an arc 1000 mm in radius centered at the subject's head. They were arranged in the vertical plane at a distance of 1000 mm from the head of the subject with a constant angle of 22.5 degrees between each other. The angle of the speaker facing the subject was defined to be 0 degrees in the vertical (φ) and horizontal (θ) directions. An experiment in the horizontal direction (θ = -90, 0, 90, 180 deg) is enabled by turning those speakers around the subject. The median plane was 0 to 180 deg, and the frontal plane was -90 to 90 deg.

Procedure

During the experiments, the subject was seated comfortably in a chair in the center of a completely dark, sound-attenuated room (H×W×L = 3.6×3.9×2.6 m). The subject responded with a response key to which of the speakers presented the signal. When a subject responded, the trial advanced to the next trial.

The first condition measured sound source localization ability without the masker. The signal was presented randomly from one of the seven speakers. This condition measured a response in θ = -90, 0, 90, 180 deg. The number of trials for this condition was 560.

The second condition measured sound source localization ability with the masker. The masker was presented by one of speakers at 67.5, 0, or -67.5 deg, and the signal was presented from one of the six remaining speakers randomly. This condition similarly measured a response in θ = -90, 0, 90, 180 deg. The trial was run 4,320 times in total (three presentational locations of the masker, three frequencies of the masker, six presentational locations of the signal, two frequencies of the signal, four θ directions, and trial numbers of 10 for each).

Figure 3. Speaker locations in the sound localization experiment

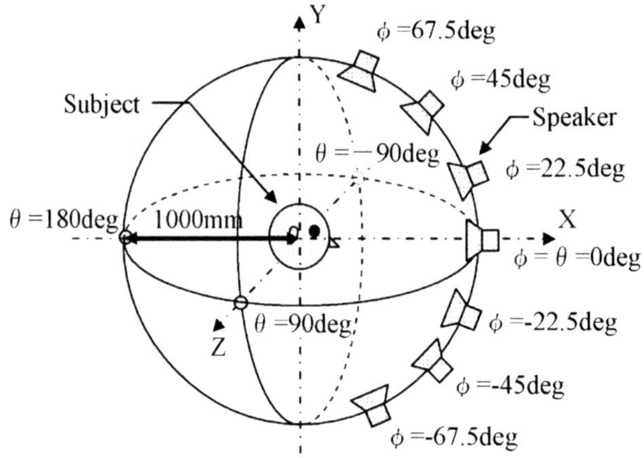

RESULTS AND DISCUSSION

Figure 4 shows the correct answer rate in the median and frontal planes versus the condition of the masker. The x-axis shows the condition of the masker (No-masker, 500 Hz, 4,000 Hz, WN (White Noise)), and the y-axis shows the correct answer rate. In the figure, gray bars show the median plane value, and white bars show the frontal plane value. The correct answer rate for the frontal plane was higher than that for the median plane in all conditions by approximately 10%. This result occurred from the difference in the cues that a subject uses for the sound localization in a median plane and a frontal plane. A previous study has indicated that a change of the spectrum

Figure 4. Relationship between the condition of the maskers and the condition of the median and frontal planes

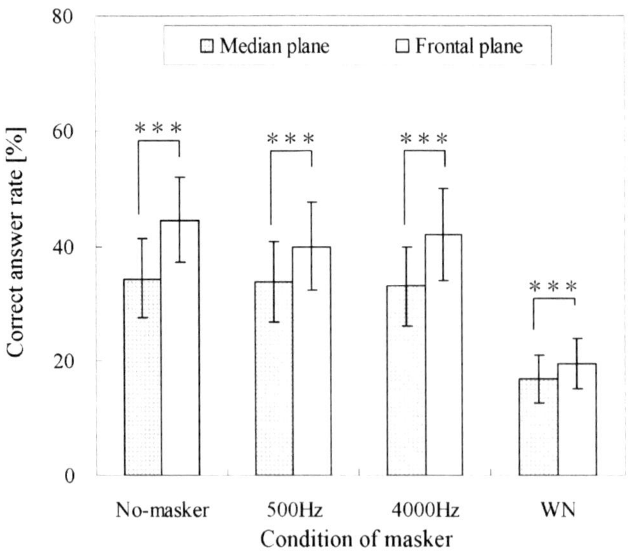

Figure 5. Relationship between the condition of the maskers and the condition of the signals

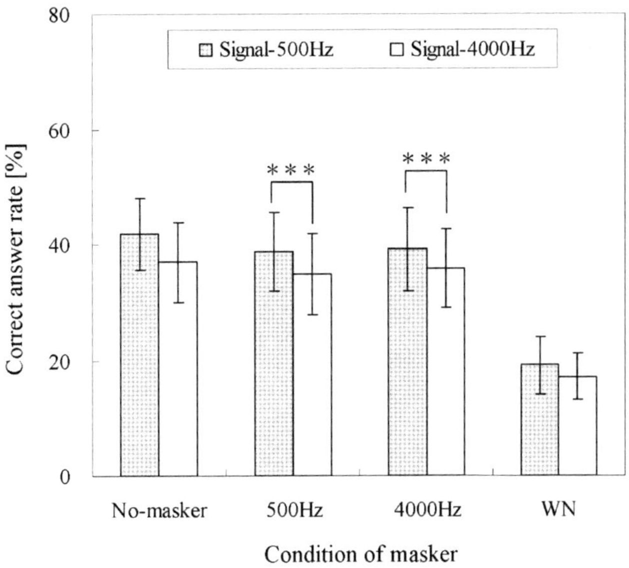

is the necessary cue for sound localization in the median plane. However, interaural time and level differences may raise localization precision in the frontal plane.

Figure 5 shows the correct answer rates for 500-Hz and 4000-Hz signals versus the condition of the masker. The x-axis shows the condition of the masker (No-masker, 500 Hz, 4000 Hz, WN), and the y-axis shows the correct answer rate. In the figure, gray bars show the 500-Hz signal value, and white bars show the 4000-Hz signal value. Under masker conditions the correct answer rate for the 500-Hz signal was higher than that for the 4000-Hz signal. A similar tendency was seen in the other conditions. We believe this result was caused by two factors. The first depends on the structure of the cochlea. In the structure of the cochlea, the high frequency is easily masked by the low frequency. The second depends on interaural time difference. High-frequency sound is localized by interaural level difference, and low-frequency sound is localized by interaural time difference. Therefore, perhaps the 4000-Hz signal was easier to mask.

Figure 6 shows the correct answer rate for the 500-Hz and 4000-Hz signals versus the presentation angle of the masker. The x-axis shows the presentation angle of the masker, and the y-axis shows the correct answer rate. In the figure, gray bars show the 500-Hz signal value, and white bars show the 4000-Hz signal value. The correct answer rate tended to increase in the order of no masker, -67.5 deg, 67.5 deg, and 0 deg. Perhaps the reason why a correct answer rate of 0 deg was high was that the answer of the subject was slanted around 0 deg generally. A correct answer rate at 67.5 deg was clearly higher than -67.5 deg. This result could have been caused by the different strength of the masking effect between the masker at -67.5 deg and the masker at 67.5 deg. Thus, our results indicate that the masking effect was stronger when the masker was at -67.5 deg.

This experiment was conducted in a young age group (21–24 years). It is likely that larger differences will be observed by comparing the data of senior citizens and dementia patients with the current findings.

Figure 6. Relationship between the presentation angle of the masker and the correct answer rate

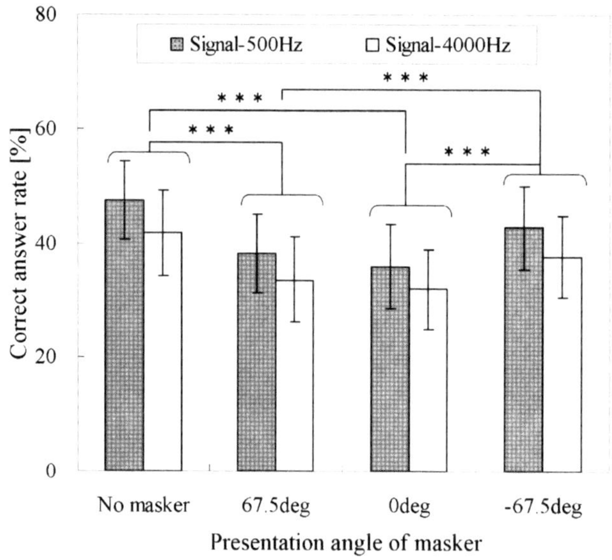

ACKNOWLEDGMENT

A part of this study was financially supported by JSPS AA Science Platform Program, JSPS Grant-in-Aid for Scientific Research (B) (21404002), and Kagawa University Characteristic Prior Research Fund 2009.

REFERENCES

Gilkey, R. H., & Good, M. D. (1996). Effects of frequency on free-field masking. *Human Factors*, *37*(4), 835–843. doi:10.1518/001872095778995580

Kurylo, D. D., Corkin, S., Allard, T., Zatorre, R. J., & Growdon, J. H. (1993). Auditory function in Alzheimer's disease. *Neurology*, *43*(10), 1893–1899.

Toshiyoki, K., Masashi, S., & Makoto, T. (2002). Sound localization with the speakers in the front vertical plane. (IEICE technical report). *ME and Bio Cybernetics*, *101*(733), 103–107.

KEY TERMS AND DEFINITIONS

Binaural Level and Time Difference: A difference occurs for the information of a sound signal due to the distance between the right and left ears.

Changes of the Spectra: The frequency characteristic of the signal changes due to the pinna and the body.

Dementia: Deterioration of developed intelligence due to diminished functioning of the brain.

Frontal Plane: The aspect that is perpendicular to the ground including the right and left ears.

Masking: The signal is interfered with by a masker.

Median Plane: The aspect that is perpendicular to the ground including the back of the head and the nose.

Sound Localization: Specifies the direction from which signals were presented.

Vertical Plane: The plane that is perpendicular to the ground.

Chapter 9
Kinetic Visual Field with Changing Contrast and Brightness

Hidenori Hiraki
Graduate School of Natural Science and Technology, Okayama University, Japan

Satoshi Takahashi
Graduate School of Natural Science and Technology, Okayama University, Japan

Jinglong Wu
Graduate School of Natural Science and Technology, Okayama University, Japan

ABSTRACT

Dynamic perimetry is the area in which a subject is able to recognize a moving target by eye. It is used in medical tests to diagnose glaucoma and cataracts. Evaluation of the kinetic visual field involves the use of an isopter. In a previous study, the area of the kinetic visual field was shown to become smaller with decreased target brightness and advancing age (Hashimoto, 2003). Moreover, the fields in the left and right eyes are the same. It is also known that dementia patients experience symptoms that lower their ability to recognize objects under conditions of weak contrast between the target object and the background (Trick, Trick, Morris, & Wolf, 1995). However, the exact relationship between this contrast and their visual fields is unknown. In this study, the areas of kinetic visual field were measured quantitatively on normal people as a fundamental study of the early detection of dementia in patients. These results were reported using an improved Goldmann perimeter, which has an electric slider to operate targets at constant speeds.

INTRODUCTION

Alzheimer's disease is a chronic, progressive, neurodegenerative disease that is characterized by clinical symptoms and pathological changes that are mainly characterized by signature disorders (senile plaques, nervous system fibril changes or nervous system cell death). With the progression of Alzheimer's disease, in addition to these signature disorders, cognitive functional disorders arise,

DOI: 10.4018/978-1-60960-559-9.ch009

including impairments in language faculty and visual space recognition. If Alzheimer's disease is detected early, the patient has the possibility of recovery through medical therapy and rehabilitation. However, with advancing disease, recovery becomes nearly impossible because the dead nerve cells caused by the disease cannot be restored (Kawakami & Fukushima, 2002). Therefore, regular checkups are very important for at-risk individuals to diagnose the disease early. Because cognitive function impairment in the initial stages of Alzheimer's disease is extremely slight and difficult to diagnose clinically, there is a limit to the symptoms that can be detected in early checkups. Thus, the development of a diagnosis that enables early disease detection is necessary. In this study, the decrease in contrast sensitivity and field of vision impairment (Andrew, 2004) that are known to occur in Alzheimer's patients were considered as possible early diagnosis tools. Specifically, we used the Goldman perimeter in this study; in this technique, the dynamic perimetry was measured with changing contrast and brightness (Figure 1) on ten people with normal sight abilities.

STATIC AND KINETIC VISUAL FIELDS

A. Static Visual Field

The static visual field is defined as the area in which targets do not move in static perimetry experiments. Measurement points were set to measure visual fields. The brightness of the measurement points was changed from dark to bright, and sensitivity thresholds were determined. Therefore, by determining the sensitivity thresholds at each measurement point, visual fields were evaluated. The normal extent of the static visual field for a bright stimulus is 60 degrees up, 75 degrees down, 100 degrees temporally and 60 degrees nasally. Figure 2 illustrates this extent of visual field. It is difficult for both disabled and normal people to recognize targets and focus on fixed points continuously in the experiment in whole area. However, it is known that the central visual field in 30 degrees tends to have a trouble during the first stage of glaucoma (Hashimoto, 2003; David, 1993). Thus, static perimetry is well suited for glaucoma diagnosis.

Figure 1. Target contrast and brightness in the Goldmann perimeter

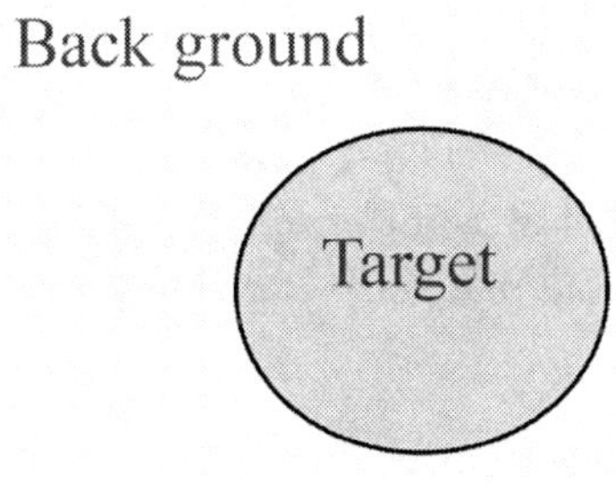

B. Kinetic Visual Field

Dynamic perimetry is defined as the way in which a subject finds a target that moves from outside the visual field to inside the visual field. The kinetic visual field is measured to determine the range in which the target can be seen. The range is shown by a curve known as an isopter (Figure 3). Abnormal characteristics of the visual field were inspected from the area and shape of the isopter. In a previous study involving a normal person, the area of the kinetic visual field becomes smaller with increasing target brightness and advancing age. Moreover, the fields in the left and right eyes are the same.

VISUAL FIELD AND ALZHEIMER'S DISEASE

Trick et al. performed automated perimetry (Humphrey) on 61 patients with AD and 61 age-matched controls. Differential luminance sensitivity was decreased (especially in the inferonasal and inferotemporal arcuate regions) in the AD group

Figure 2. Normal visual field. (A) shows a vertical visual field, and (B) shows a horizontal visual field

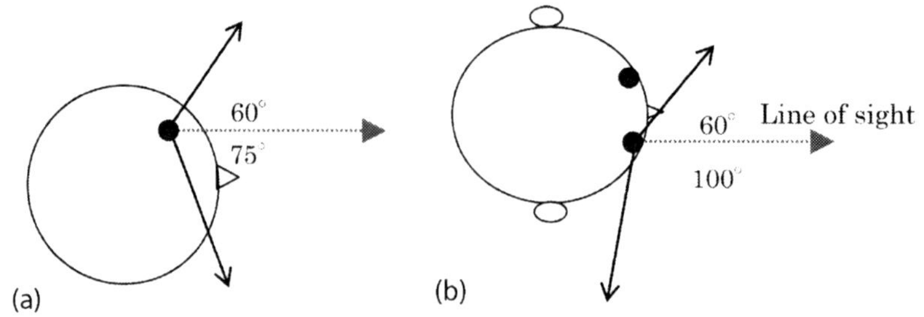

Figure 3. The isopter was measured for the right eye of a normal person with a target speed of 5 deg/s

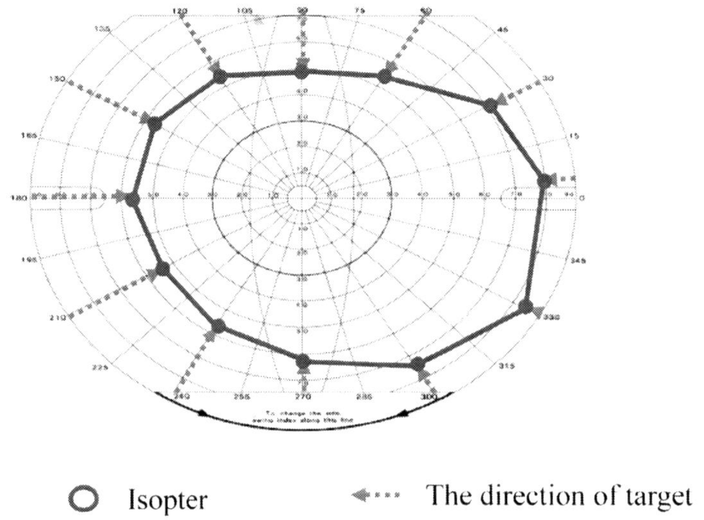

compared to the control group. Previous study described homonymous visual field defects in patients with no corresponding structural lesions on neuroimages. Previous study described six patients on whom they performed a formal (Goldmann) perimetry experiment; four patients demonstrated paracentral homonymous hemianopsias. Two patients could not perform a reliable or valid formal visual field assessment, and confrontation visual field testing showed nonspecific constriction in both eyes. The inability to perform an accurate visual field test is a major problem when testing patients with dementia (Andrew, 2004).

EXPERIMENT

A. Equipment

The Goldman perimeter that is used for dynamic perimetry moves a target by manual operation. Thus, quantitative measurements are difficult to perform (Nowomiejsk, 2005; Fischer, & Schmidt, 1998). Therefore, in this study, an electromotive slider that can be controlled by a controller was fixed to the Goldman perimeter to measure the kinetic visual field quantitatively. The target arm was moved at a uniform speed through the improved Goldman perimeter (Figure 4).

Figure 4. Improved Goldmann perimetry. (A) shows the front side of the equipment, and (B) shows the back side of the equipment

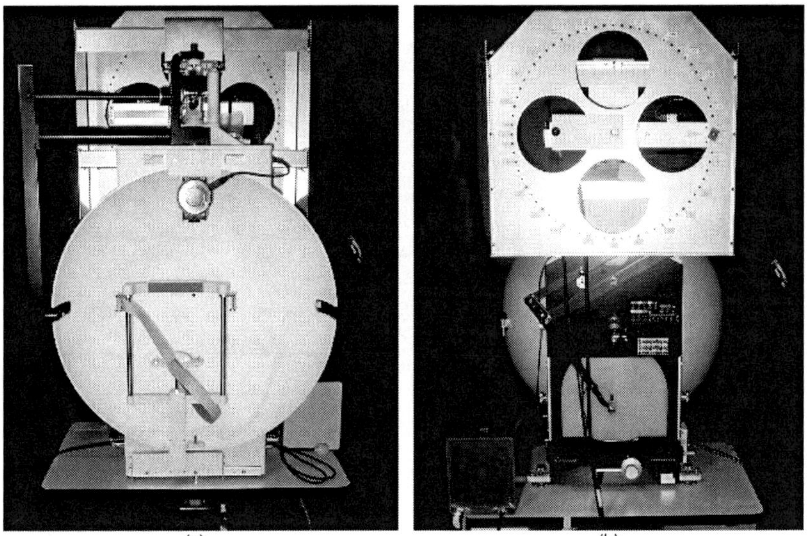

(a) (b)

B. Method

Dynamic perimetry was measured in a dark room with the only light being the background light of the perimeter in a hemisphere-type dome. The background brightness in the hemisphere-type dome assumes that there are three conditions occurring, including photopia (200 lx), mesopic vision (5 lx) and scotopic vision (0.01 lx). The background brightness was measured by a light meter attached to the perimeter. The target was oval shaped, and the brightness was adjusted with a neutral density filter. The contrast (brightness ratio) of the target for each background brightness level was chosen from three conditions, including 1.0-1.5 (very difficult to distinguish), 1.5-2.0 (difficult to distinguish) and 2.0-2.5 (easy to distinguish). The target speeds were 5 deg/s and 15 deg/s. The target size was 16 mm^2. Table 1 shows the experimental conditions. The perimetry was measured in 18 trials of right cyclopean eyes. Each subject's left eye was covered with an eye bandage. The dynamic perimetry was measured five times in each condition. The ten subjects had no vision corrections and their eyesights were over 1.0 by the naked eye. The subjects held their heads in the chin stand of the perimeter and focused on the target at the center of hemisphere-type dome throughout the experiment. They pushed a button at the moment when they saw the target that moved from outside the visual field to the center of the visual field. The target was moved 30 degrees in 12 directions. Degree zero was not measured to avoid the blind spot; five degrees were measured instead. The target position was recorded by a ● mark in Figure 2, and the isopter was constructed while considering the reaction time of each subject. The results were measured five times at each angle and then averaged. The area of the kinetic visual field was calculated from the coordinates of each reply point.

C. Kinetic Visual Field calculation Method

In a previous study, Hashimoto et al. divided the measured isopter to small triangle areas and calculated the area of the kinetic visual field by summing each area (Hashimoto, 2003). In this study, the isopter was divided into 12 sections, and

Table 1. Experimental conditions. (A) shows the conditions of background brightness at 0.01 lx. (B) shows the condition of background brightness at 5 lx. (C) shows the condition of background brightness at 200 lx.

(A)				
Target Size (mm²)		16		
Target Speed (mm²)		5.15		
Background Brightness	(lx)	$1.0*10^{-2}$		
	(cd/mm²)	$4.3*10^{-2}$		
Target Luminance (cd/mm²)		$6.2*10^{-2}$	$7.3*10^{-2}$	$9.2*10^{-2}$
Contrast Ratio		1.4	1.7	2.1
(B)				
Target Size (mm²)		16		
Target Speed (mm²)		5.15		
Background Brightness	(lx)	5		
	(cd/mm²)	1.2		
Target Luminance (cd/mm²)		1.5	1.9	2.5
Contrast Ratio		1.3	1.6	2.1
(C)				
Target Size (mm²)		16		
Target Speed (mm²)		5.15		
Background Brightness	(lx)	200		
	(cd/mm²)	4.3		
Target Luminance (cd/mm²)		5.6	6.9	9.8
Contrast Ratio		1.3	1.6	2.3

each inside area was calculated using Equation 1 (Figure 5). The total area A (deg²) was calculated by summing A_1 through A_{12} (Figure 6). From this value, the visual fields were evaluated.

$$1/2 \times a \times b \times \sin \theta = A_1 \qquad (1)$$

RESULTS

The areas of the kinetic visual fields differed between subjects. Representative results from one subject are shown in Figure 7. To analyze all ten subjects, a reference condition (background brightness 200 lx, contrast ratio 1.3, target speed 5 deg/s) was chosen. This reference condition was determined by identifying the conditions with the smallest coefficients of variation. The dimension-

Figure 5. Calculation of the divided areas

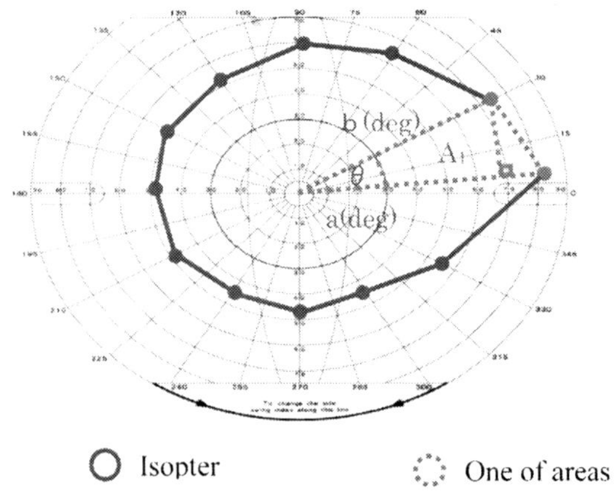

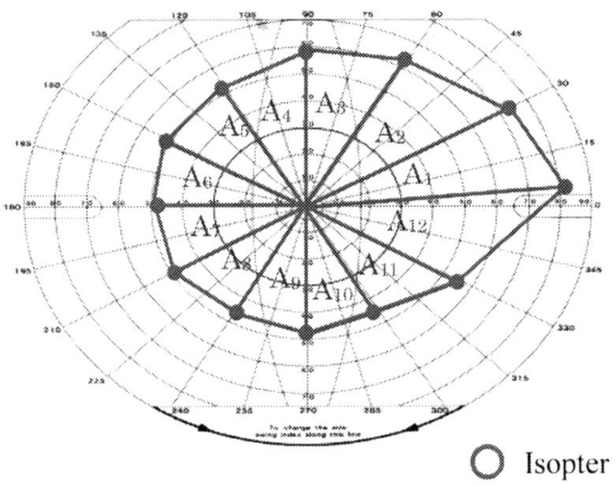

Figure 6. Calculation of the division of the kinetic visual field

less results from all subjects were averaged. The kinetic visual fields are shown in Figure 6; from this figure, it can be seen that as the contrast ratio decreased with constant background brightness, the kinetic visual field decreased at each background brightness level. As the background brightness decreased with a constant contrast ratio, the kinetic visual field area decreased with decreasing contrast. The variation of the kinetic visual field area compared to the variation of the contrast ratio increased as the background brightness level decreased.

DISCUSSION

As the background brightness decreased with constant contrast ratios, the area of the kinetic visual field was smaller at each contrast ratio. As the contrast ratio decreased with constant background brightness, the kinetic visual field decreased at each background brightness level.

Figure 7. Representative results from one subject. (A) shows the conditions of the target speed at 5 deg/s, and (B) shows the conditions of the target speed at 15 deg/s

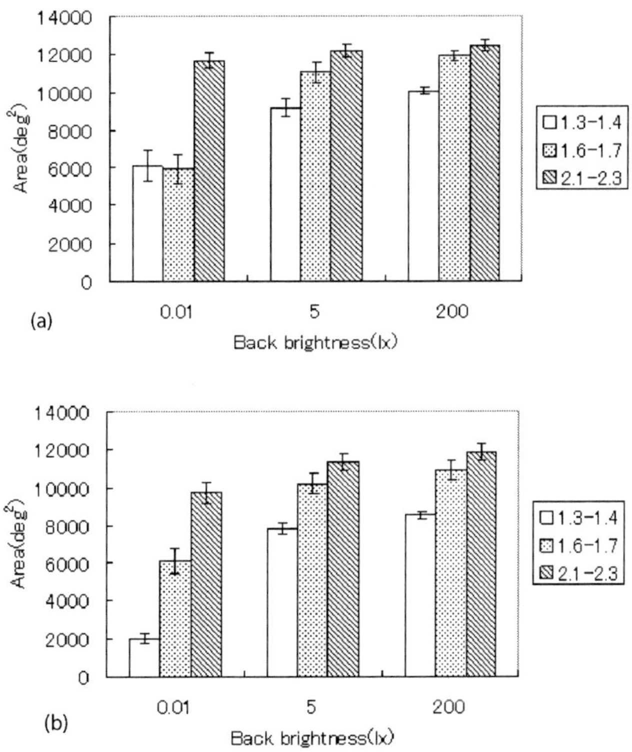

The reason underlying these results arises from the fact that when the background brightness is decreased, the quantity of light is also decreased, and the eye's sensitivity must be increased to sense the available light, decreasing the kinetic visual field (Figure 8). The variation in kinetic visual field area became larger compared to the variation in contrast ratio when the background brightness was lower. As the background brightness decreased, the quantity of light decreased, and the target brightness decreased. The eye's sensitivity was highly variable when viewing dark targets. Therefore, the variation in kinetic visual

Figure 8. The results of the dimensionless kinetic visual field area. (A) shows the conditions of the target speed at 5 deg/s, and (B) shows the conditions of the target speed at 15 deg/s

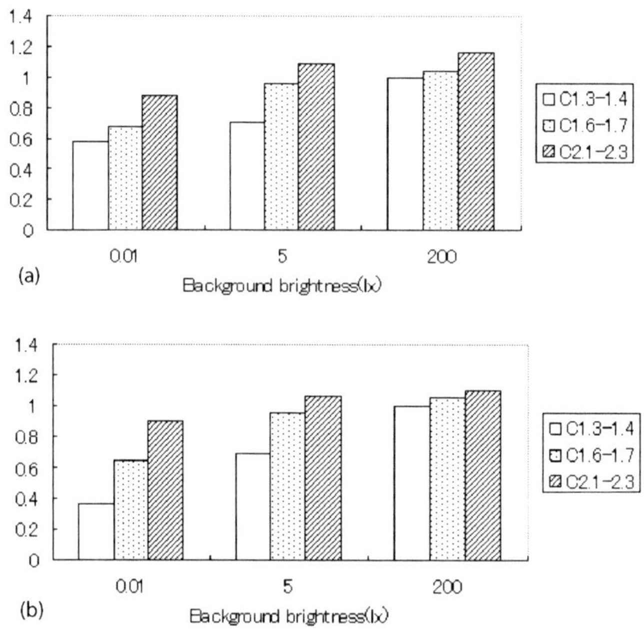

Figure 9. Stimulus intensity depended on the visual field

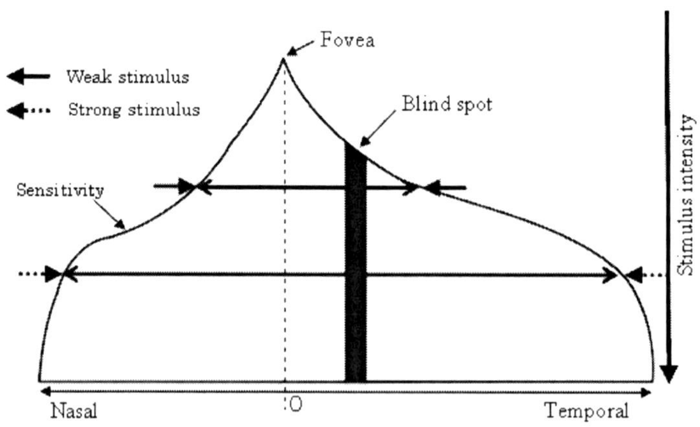

field area was large compared to the variation in contrast ratio (Figure 9).

ACKNOWLEDGMENT

This study was supported in part by a Grant-in-Aid for Scientific Research (B) 21404002 in Japan and AA Science Platform Program of the Japan Society for the Promotion Science.

REFERENCES

Andrew, G. L. (2004). Neuro-opthalmic findings in the visual variant of Alzheimer's disease. *Opthalmology, 111*, 376–380. doi:10.1016/S0161-6420(03)00732-2

David, B. H. (1993). *Visual fields* (p. 2). Oxford Medical Publishers.

Fischer, F. W., & Schmidt, Y. H. (1998). 40year's of the perimetry. *Klinische Monatsblatter fur Augenheilkunde, 193*, 237–242. doi:10.1055/s-2008-1050251

Hashimoto, S. (2003). The dynamic perimetry program by using an automatic perimeter. *Kinki University Medical Journal, 28*, 207–221.

Kawakami, Y., & Fukushima, S. (2002). *The development of the Alzheimer's disease diagnosis system by using ocular movement.* (pp. 63-67). (Technological University of Nagaoka Report 24).

Nowomiejsk, K. (2005). Comparison between semiautomated kinetic oerimetry and conventional Goldmann manual kinetic perimetry in advanced visual field loss. *Ophthalmology, 112*, 1343–1354. doi:10.1016/j.ophtha.2004.12.047

Trick, G. L., Trick, L. R., Morris, P., & Wolf, W. (1995). Visual field loss in senile dementia of the Alzheimer's type . *Neurology, 45*, 68–74.

KEY TERMS AND DEFINITIONS

Alzheimer's Disease: A chronic progressive neurodegenerative disease.

Background Brightness: The brightness on the surface of dome in the Goldmann perimeter.

Contrast Ratio: The ratio between target luminance and background luminance.

Goldmann Perimeter: The equipment used to measure the kinetic visual field.

Kinetic Visual Field: The area in which a subject is able to recognize a moving target by eye.

Static Visual Field: The area in which a subject is able to recognize a static target by eye.

Visual Field: The area in which a subject is able to recognize the target by eye.

Chapter 10
Effects of Stimulus Complexity on Bisensory Audiovisual Integration

Qi Li
Graduate School of Natural Science and Technology, Okayama University, Japan & School of Computer Science and Technology, Changchun University of Science and Technology, China

Naoya Nakamura
Graduate School of Natural Science and Technology, Okayama University, Japan

Jinglong Wu
Graduate School of Natural Science and Technology, Okayama University, Japan

Yasuyuki Ohta
Graduate School of Medicine, Dentistry, and Pharmacological Sciences Okayama University, Japan

Koji Abe
Graduate School of Medicine, Dentistry, and Pharmacological Sciences Okayama University, Japan

ABSTRACT

With the rapid increase in the number of elderly people, the number of people with dementia is also increasing. The most common form of dementia is Alzheimer's disease, which accounts for 50-70% of all dementia cases. Until the present time, however, there was no effective early detection method for Alzheimer's disease. A recent study showed that brain glucose metabolism in healthy volunteers was different than glucose metabolism in Alzheimer's patients during the response to passive audio-visual stimulation. This result suggested that the mechanism of audiovisual integration in patients with Alzheimer's disease was influenced by the disease. In the present study, the authors investigated the effects of modality-specific selective attention on audiovisual integration using simple visual and auditory stimuli in healthy human subjects. Three different attentional instructions were accessed: (1)

DOI: 10.4018/978-1-60960-559-9.ch010

visual selective attention, in which subjects were instructed to focus their attention on visual stimuli; (2) auditory selective attention, in which subjects were instructed to focus their attention on auditory stimuli; and (3) audiovisual divided attention, in which subjects were instructed to focus their attention on both visual and auditory stimuli. The results showed that significant bimodal enhancement was present only in the divided attention condition, which is similar to the results of a previous study using complex semantic stimuli. Therefore, the authors conclude that stimulus complexity does not influence the modality-specific selective attention effects of audiovisual integration. A future study will examine the mechanism of audiovisual integration in patients with Alzheimer's disease using the same experimental design (using simple stimuli), which will hopefully help find a new method for the early detection of Alzheimer's disease.

INTRODUCTION

Audiovisual Integration

Humans are constantly bombarded with information from multiple sensory organs. For instance, when driving a car, we are surrounded by visual (road, roadside billboards, signaling lamps, etc.), auditory (car engine, music from vehicle CD player, etc.), and somatosensory (feeling the steering wheel, etc.) information. Some of this information is task-relevant (road, signal lamp, car engine, feeling the steering wheel), while other information is task-irrelevant (roadside billboard, music from vehicle CD player). To focus on the relevant information and ignore the irrelevant information, the human brain is equipped with a selection mechanism known as attention. The attention system allows us to dynamically select and enhance the processing of objects and events that are the most relevant at each moment. The brain can then combine the task-relevant information from anatomically different sensory pathways to form unified percepts.

A typical example of the audiovisual interaction is the McGurk effect, which was first described in a paper by McGurk and MacDonald in 1976. When a video of one phoneme production is dubbed onto a sound recording of a different phoneme that is spoken, the perceived phoneme is a third, intermediate phoneme. For example, a visual /ga/ combined with an audio /ba/ is often heard as /da/. The McGurk effect demonstrates an interaction between hearing and vision in speech perception (McGurk & MacDonald, 1996).

Alzheimer's Disease and Audiovisual Integration

The population of elderly people is increasing rapidly, and the number of people with dementia is increasing accordingly. It is estimated that there are currently approximately 18 million people worldwide with Alzheimer's disease (AD). This number is expected to nearly double by 2025 to 34 million. Unfortunately, we currently have no effective early detection method for Alzheimer's disease. AD is a progressive, degenerative brain disorder, and a recent study showed that brain glucose metabolism in healthy volunteers differed from glucose metabolism in Alzheimer patients during their response to passive audiovisual stimulation (Pietrini et al., 2000). This result suggested that the mechanism of audiovisual integration was altered in AD patients. Therefore, it might be possible to detect Alzheimer's disease at an early stage by observing a patient's audiovisual integration.

Previous Studies Regarding Audiovisual Integration

Many studies have investigated the bimodal audiovisual integration in healthy individuals

(Fort, Delpuech, Pernier, & Giard, 2002; Sophie Molholm et al., 2002; Teder-Salejarvi, Di Russo, McDonald, & Hillyard, 2005; Teder-Salejarvi, McDonald, Di Russo, & Hillyard, 2002; Vidal, Giard, Roux, Barthelemy, & Bruneau, 2008) when visual and auditory information are presented synchronously as a bimodal object. Behavioral results showed that responses to audiovisual targets are more rapid and accurate than the responses to either unimodal visual or auditory targets in divided-attention tasks (Molholm et al., 2002; Teder-Salejarvi et al., 2005; Teder-Salejarvi et al., 2002).

In more recent studies, it was reported that attention could affect audiovisual integration when both visual and auditory modalities of bimodal audiovisual stimulus were sensed (Eimer & Schroger, 1998; Talsma & Woldorff, 2005). Using semantically complex stimuli, Jennifer et al. (2008) demonstrated that selective attention to a single sensory modality prevented the integration of semantic matching bimodal stimuli that are normally observed when attention is divided between sensory modalities (Mozolic, Hugenschmidt, Peiffer, & Laurienti, 2008). However, it is difficult to use these semantically complex stimuli with AD patients to explore the mechanism of audiovisual integration.

Study Aim

In the present study, we mainly discuss the effects of modality-specific selective attention on audiovisual integration using simple visual and auditory stimuli. We ascertain whether the effects depend on stimulus complexity by comparing the results of previous studies in which semantically complex stimuli were used. In a future study, we will observe the mechanism of audiovisual integration in patients with Alzheimer's disease using the same experimental design, and we hope to find a new method for the early detection of Alzheimer's disease by comparing these results with the audiovisual integration mechanisms of healthy individuals.

EXPERIMENT

Subjects

Fifteen healthy adults participated in this experiment (all subjects were males, aged 21-25 years, with a mean age of 22.4 years). All subjects had normal or corrected-to-normal vision and normal hearing capabilities. The experimental protocol was approved by the Ethics Committee of Okayama University. After receiving a full explanation regarding the purpose and risks of the study, subjects provided written informed consent as per the protocol approved by the institutional research review board.

Stimuli and Task

The experiment contained three stimulus types, including unimodal visual (V) stimuli, unimodal auditory (A) stimuli, and bimodal audiovisual (AV) stimuli. Unimodal V stimuli included a checkboard subtending at a 5-degree visual angle that was presented against a black background. These V stimuli were presented unilaterally to lateral locations on either the left or right of the display at a 12-degree visual angle that was below 5-degree in the vertical direction relative to the fixation point in the horizontal direction (Figure 1A). The duration of the stimulus was 150 ms. Unimodal A stimuli consisted of 1600 Hz tones with linear rise and fall times of 5 ms and intensities of 70 dB with durations of 150 ms. These A stimuli were presented through two speakers placed on either side of the display. Bimodal AV stimuli consisted of a combination of both unimodal auditory and visual stimuli. Presenting the visual and auditory stimuli simultaneously created the subjective impression of a single bimodal audiovisual object.

Figure 1. Stimulus and time sequence of the stimulus

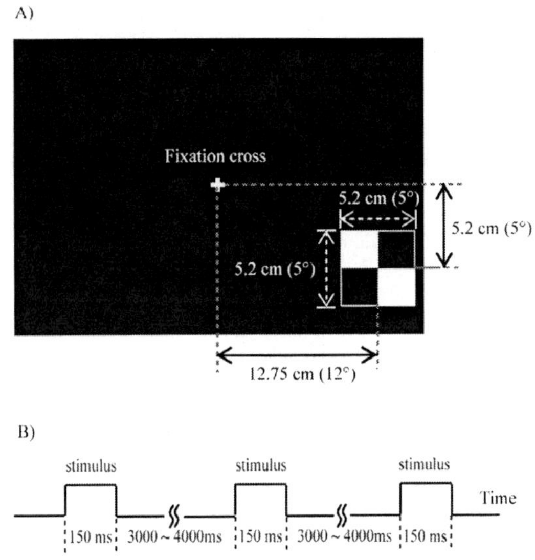

Subjects were given three types of attentional instructions, but in all cases, they were instructed to keep their eyes focused on the fixation cross and direct their attention covertly to a designated subset of presented objects. The first type of attention instruction probed the audiovisual divided attention condition; subjects were instructed to pay attention to all visual, auditory, and audiovisual stimuli. The second type of attention instruction probed the visual selective attention condition; subjects were instructed to pay attention to the unimodal visual stimuli and only the visual component of the bimodal stimuli. Finally, the third type of attention instruction probed the auditory selective attention condition; subjects were instructed to pay attention to unimodal auditory stimuli and only the auditory components of the bimodal stimuli. In all conditions, each subject was required to press a button with his left index finger when he identified a stimulus on his left side and to press a button with his right index finger when he identified a stimulus on his right side.

The interstimulus interval (ISI) of the stimuli varied randomly from 3000 to 4000 ms (mean ISI 3500 ms) (Figure 1B). For each condition (divided attention, visual attention or auditory attention), three sessions were executed. In each session, 72 unimodal V, 72 unimodal A, and 72 bimodal AV stimuli were presented. Of these 72 stimuli, 36 were presented on the left side, and the remaining 36 were presented on the right side. All stimuli were randomly presented.

Procedure

Each subject was seated in a comfortable chair in a dimly lit, sound-attenuated, electrically shielded room. The subject's head was fixed on a chin rest to keep head and eye movements to a minimum. At the beginning of the experiment, the subject performed a few practical trials to ensure that he understood the paradigm and became familiar with the stimuli. The subject was allowed to take short breaks of approximately one to five minutes between experimental sessions.

Data Analysis

The reaction times (RTs) for the correct detection of targets and the subject's accuracy were computed separately for the different attention conditions. These data were subjected to an analysis of variance (ANOVA) to determine whether mean RTs or accuracy differed by stimulus type (unimodal or bimodal) for each attention condition.

Although the ANOVA comparison of RTs could identify responses for bimodal targets that were faster than responses to either unimodal targets, this analysis did not take into account the fact that faster responses to bimodal targets were possibly due to the presence of two stimuli in the bimodal objects compared to a single stimulus. This potential effect was termed the "redundant signal effect." To control for the redundant nature of bimodal objects, an independent race model was adopted (Miller, 1982, 1986; Mozolic et al., 2008). In race models, each stimulus of a multimodal object competes independently for response initiation, and the faster of the two stimuli mediates the response for any trial. According to this model, the probability summation produces a redundant signal effect because the likelihood of either of the two stimuli yielding a faster reaction time is higher than that from one stimulus alone. To perform an analysis of this possibility, cumulative distribution functions (CDFs) for each trial type were generated for each subject using 2-ms time bins. Each subject's unimodal CDFs were then used to calculate the race distribution using the following formula at each time bin:

$$[P(A)+P(V)]-[P(A)\times P(V)] \quad (1)$$

In this formula, P(A) is the probability of responding by a given time with a unimodal auditory object stimulus, and P(V) is the probability of responding by a given time with a unimodal visual object stimulus. Two different race model predictions were generated for each subject in a manner that were in line with a previous study (Mozolic et al., 2008). The first race model used the selective attention race model, which was based on responses to unimodal targets when subjects were instructed to selectively attend to either vision or audition. The second race model was the divided attention race model, which was based on responses to unimodal targets when subjects were instructed to divide their attention between vision and audition.

After these individual CDFs were completed, group mean CDFs were generated for each stimulus type, and individual race models were averaged to obtain group predictions for responses made under selective attention and divided attention conditions.

RESULTS

Reaction Times

Table 1 presents the mean RTs for each target type. Under the divided attention condition, there were significant differences among the modalities ($F(2,13)=68.68$, $p<0.001$). Multiple comparison results showed that the RTs to audiovisual targets were significantly faster than the RTs to visual targets ($p<0.001$) and auditory targets ($p<0.001$). No significant RT difference could be found between visual and auditory targets ($p>0.07$). Under the visual selective attention condition, the RTs to audiovisual targets were significantly faster than the RTs to visual targets ($F(1,14)=36.79$, $p<0.001$). Under the auditory selective attention condition, the RTs to audiovisual targets were significantly faster than the RTs to auditory targets ($F(1,14) = 39.58$, $p<0.001$).

Accuracy

Table 2 presents the percentage correctly identified to each target type. Accuracy was very high, with subjects averaging 98.6% correct over all stimulus types. Under the divided attention condition, there

Table 1. Mean response times to attended stimuli

	Stimulus					
	Auditory		Visual		Audiovisual	
	M	SE	M	SE	M	SE
Audiovisual divided attention	384	18.6	364	12.5	319	11.4
Auditory selective attention	402	15.5			378	14.4
Visual selective attention			378	17.3	355	15.3
All times are given in milliseconds. M: mean response times; SE: standard error.						

was no statistically significant accuracy difference between modalities (F(2,13) = 1.81, p>0.2). Under the visual selective attention condition, no statistically significant accuracy differences could be found between audiovisual and visual targets (F(1,14) = 0.63, p>0.4). Under the auditory selective attention condition, the responses to audiovisual targets were no more accurate than those to auditory targets (F(1,14) = 1.35, p>0.26).

Cumulative Distribution Function

Due to the redundant nature of multimodal stimuli, it is possible that the increase in speed of RTs to multimodal stimuli found in this study was due to the availability of multiple pieces of information and not to the integration of these stimuli. To account for the increased probability of responding more quickly to multimodal stimuli, the distributions for multimodal responses were compared to the race model that was created from the summed probabilities of unimodal responses. Responses to multimodal targets under the divided attention condition were compared to the summed probabilities of responses to auditory and visual targets (race model distribution) under the divided attention condition (Figure 2a). The CDFs of the unimodal auditory targets are depicted with a blue dotted curve, the CDFs of unimodal visual targets are depicted with a red dashed curve, and the CDFs of multimodal targets are depicted with a green solid curve. The response probabilities predicted by summing the unimodal response probabilities (race modal) are depicted by the gray solid curve. It should be noted that fast response times were more likely to occur for multimodal targets than was predicted by the race model in several time bins. Two similar comparisons evaluated responses to multimodal targets under selective auditory attention and selective visual attention versus a selective attention race model distribution (Figure 2b). The CDFs of auditory targets are depicted with a blue dotted curve, and the CDFs of multimodal targets are depicted with a yellow solid curve during selective auditory attention. The CDFs of visual targets were depicted with a red dashed curve, and the CDFs of multimodal targets are depicted with a green solid curve during selective visual attention. The gray solid curve depicts race model predictions that are based on the summed probabilities of unimodal responses during the selective attention condition. Fast responses to multimodal targets under the selective attention condition were typically less likely to occur than was predicted by the race model.

Figure 2c shows that the difference in response probabilities between multimodal stimuli and the race model predictions under the divided attention (yellow solid curve), auditory selection attention (blue dotted curve), and visual selection attention (red dashed curve) conditions. In contrast to the mean RT comparisons that found similarly significant multimodal gains under all attention conditions, these comparisons indicated that

Table 2. Percentage correctly reported by attended stimuli

	Stimulus					
	Auditory		Visual		Audiovisual	
	Acc	SE	Acc	SE	Acc	SE
Audiovisual divided attention	97.7	0.75	99.2	0.18	99.1	0.29
Auditory selective attention	98.4	0.40			98.9	0.34
Visual selective attention			98.2	0.72	98.7	0.34
Acc: accuracy; SE: standard error.						

Figure 2. Cumulative distribution functions (CDFs) for responses to auditory, visual, and multimodal stimuli during divided and selective attention conditions. (a) CDFs are depicted during divided attention. (b) CDFs are depicted during selective attention. (c) Difference in response probabilities between multisensory trials and race model predictions under divided attention, auditory selection attention, and visual selection attention conditions.

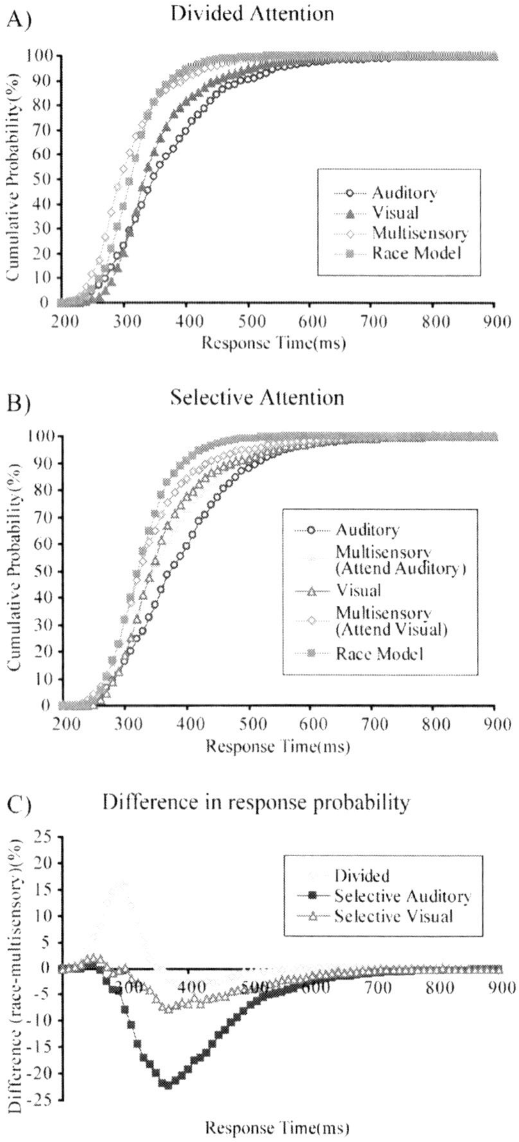

significant multimodal enhancements were present only under divided attention conditions.

DISCUSSION

The present study investigated the effects of modality-specific selective attention on the integration of bimodal audiovisual objects using simple visual and auditory stimuli. Comparisons between bimodal response distributions and a race model were used to identify whether the significant facilitation of RTs resulted from a true facilitation of processing due to bimodal integration or the simple probability summation of target information arriving over two independent channels. The data demonstrated that significant bimodal integration only occurred when subjects divided their attention between modalities. When selectively attending to either the auditory or visual modality, subjects obtained no significant performance enhancements compared to the race model.

The behavioral findings from this experiment are in accordance with results from an ERP study that suggested that the bimodal integration effects that can be detected when subjects attend to both visual and auditory modalities are absent when subjects attend to only one sensory modality at an early sensory processing stage (Talsma, Doty, & Woldorff, 2007). Moreover, other studies have shown that when attention is focused on a single sensory modality, activity is suppressed in the ignored cortex. This presumably results in less sensory information being available for integration (Johnson & Zatorre, 2005, 2006; Laurienti et al., 2002).

In the present study, we arrived at a similar conclusion as that of a previous study that used semantically complex semantically stimuli. Therefore, our data support the hypothesis that stimulus complexity did not influence the modality-specific selective attention effects on audiovisual integration. In a future study, we will compare the mechanism of audiovisual integration in AD patients with that of healthy subjects using the same experimental design. With these comparisons, we hope to find a new method for the early detection of AD.

REFERENCES

Eimer, M., & Schroger, E. (1998). ERP effects of intermodal attention and cross-modal links in spatial attention. *Psychophysiology*, *35*(3), 313–327. doi:10.1017/S004857729897086X

Fort, A., Delpuech, C., Pernier, J., & Giard, M.-H. (2002). Early auditory-visual interactions in human cortex during nonredundant target identification. *Brain Research. Cognitive Brain Research*, *14*(1), 20–30. doi:10.1016/S0926-6410(02)00058-7

Johnson, J. A., & Zatorre, R. J. (2005). Attention to simultaneous unrelated auditory and visual events: behavioral and neural correlates. *Cerebral Cortex*, *15*(10), 1609–1620. doi:10.1093/cercor/bhi039

Johnson, J. A., & Zatorre, R. J. (2006). Neural substrates for dividing and focusing attention between simultaneous auditory and visual events. *NeuroImage*, *31*(4), 1673–1681. doi:10.1016/j.neuroimage.2006.02.026

Laurienti, P. J., Burdette, J. H., Wallace, M. T., Yen, Y. F., Field, A. S., & Stein, B. E. (2002). Deactivation of sensory-specific cortex by cross-modal stimuli. *Journal of Cognitive Neuroscience*, *14*(3), 420–429. doi:10.1162/089892902317361930

McGurk, H., & MacDonald, J. (1976). Hearing lips and seeing voices. *Nature*, *264*(5588), 746–748. doi:10.1038/264746a0

Miller, J. (1982). Divided attention: Evidence for coactivation with redundant signals. *Cognitive Psychology*, *14*(2), 247–279. doi:10.1016/0010-0285(82)90010-X

Miller, J. (1986). Timecourse of coactivation in bimodal divided attention. *Perception & Psychophysics*, *40*(5), 331–343. doi:10.3758/BF03203025

Molholm, S., Ritter, W., Murray, M. M., Javitt, D. C., Schroeder, C. E., & Foxe, J. J. (2002). Multisensory auditory-visual interactions during early sensory processing in humans: a high-density electrical mapping study. *Brain Research. Cognitive Brain Research*, *14*(1), 115–128. doi:10.1016/S0926-6410(02)00066-6

Mozolic, J. L., Hugenschmidt, C. E., Peiffer, A. M., & Laurienti, P. J. (2008). Modality-specific selective attention attenuates multisensory integration. *Experimental Brain Research*, *184*(1), 39–52. doi:10.1007/s00221-007-1080-3

Pietrini, P., Alexander, G. E., Furey, M. L., Dani, A., Mentis, M. J., & Horwitz, B. (2000). Cerebral metabolic response to passive audiovisual stimulation in patients with Alzheimer's disease and healthy volunteers assessed by PET. *Journal of Nuclear Medicine*, *41*(4), 575–583.

Talsma, D., Doty, T. J., & Woldorff, M. G. (2007). Selective attention and audiovisual integration: Is attending to both modalities a prerequisite for early integration? *Cerebral Cortex*, *17*(3), 679–690. doi:10.1093/cercor/bhk016

Talsma, D., & Woldorff, M. G. (2005). Selective attention and multisensory integration: multiple phases of effects on the evoked brain activity. *Journal of Cognitive Neuroscience*, *17*(7), 1098–1114. doi:10.1162/0898929054475172

Teder-Salejarvi, W. A., Di Russo, F., McDonald, J. J., & Hillyard, S. A. (2005). Effects of spatial congruity on audio-visual multimodal integration. *Journal of Cognitive Neuroscience*, *17*(9), 1396–1409. doi:10.1162/0898929054985383

Teder-Salejarvi, W. A., McDonald, J. J., Di Russo, F., & Hillyard, S. A. (2002). An analysis of audio-visual crossmodal integration by means of event-related potential (ERP) recordings. *Brain Research. Cognitive Brain Research*, *14*(1), 106–114. doi:10.1016/S0926-6410(02)00065-4

Vidal, J., Giard, M. H., Roux, S., Barthelemy, C., & Bruneau, N. (2008). Cross-modal processing of auditory-visual stimuli in a no-task paradigm: a topographic event-related potential study. *Clinical Neurophysiology*, *119*(4), 763–771. doi:10.1016/j.clinph.2007.11.178

KEY TERMS AND DEFINITIONS

Audiovisual Integration: Audiovisual integration is the combination of individual visual and auditory information to form unified percepts.

Alzheimer's Disease: Alzheimer's disease (AD), also called Alzheimer disease, Senile Dementia of the Alzheimer Type (SDAT) or simply Alzheimer's, is the most common form of dementia. This incurable, degenerative, terminal disease was first described by German psychiatrist and neuropathologist Alois Alzheimer in 1906 and was named after him.

Attention: Attention is the cognitive process of selectively concentrating on one aspect of an environment while ignoring other aspects. Attention has also been referred to as the allocation of processing resources.

Cumulative Distribution Function (CDF): In probability theory and statistics, the cumulative distribution function or simply the distribution function, completely describes the probability distribution of a real-valued random variable X. Cumulative distribution functions are also used to specify the distribution of multivariate random variables.

Chapter 11
Tactile Pattern Delivery Device to Investigate Cognitive Mechanisms for Early Detection of Alzheimer's Disease

Jiajia Yang
Biomedical Engineering Laboratory, Graduate School of Natural Science and Technology, Okayama University, Japan

Takashi Ogasa
Biomedical Engineering Laboratory, Graduate School of Natural Science and Technology, Okayama University, Japan

Jinglong Wu
Biomedical Engineering Laboratory, Graduate School of Natural Science and Technology, Okayama University, Japan

Yasuyuki Ohta
Graduate School of Medicine, Dentistry and Pharmacological Sciences, Okayama University, Japan

Koji Abe
Graduate School of Medicine, Dentistry and Pharmacological Sciences, Okayama University, Japan

ABSTRACT

The cognitive symptoms in early Alzheimer's disease (AD) involve problems with learning, memory or planning. Currently, no medical tests are available to conclusively diagnose dementia pre-mortem. Previous studies have demonstrated that the cognitive deficits of AD can be detected during a preclinical period with neuropsychological tests. This chapter's hypothesis is that cognitive deficit symptoms of AD are detectable using a combination of tactile, kinetic, cognitive, and functional MRI tasks in the earliest stages of the disease. The authors of this chapter offer a novel approach to investigate the early detection of AD with tactile procedures. This chapter introduces the development of two tactile pattern delivery

DOI: 10.4018/978-1-60960-559-9.ch011

devices. The first delivery device is MRI-compatible and can serve to investigate the underlying neural mechanisms of active and passive tactile pattern discrimination. The second delivery device is designed to investigate the characteristics of passive shape discrimination for psychological experiments. These devices may contribute to the early detection of AD with neuropsychological approaches. The ultimate goal of this research was to confirm the human ability of tactile shape discrimination and determine the differences between age-matched healthy individuals and AD patients.

INTRODUCTION

Alzheimer's disease (AD) is one of the most devastating brain diseases in middle-aged and elderly humans in modern society. AD is an irreversible, progressive brain disease that slowly destroys memory, thinking skills and, eventually, the ability to carry out the simplest tasks of daily living. Worldwide, the number of AD patients was reported to be 24.3 million people in 2005, and it is estimated that the number of patients will increase to 42.3 million people in 2020. Currently, no medical tests are available to diagnose dementia conclusively pre-mortem.

The causes and progression of AD are not well understood. However, there are some hypotheses that exist about the cause of the disease. The oldest is the cholinergic hypothesis, which proposes that AD is caused by reduced synthesis of the neurotransmitter acetylcholine. This hypothesis has not maintained widespread support. Currently, the amyloid hypothesis postulates that amyloid β-peptide (Aβ) deposits are the fundamental cause of the disease, and this view is widely supported.

Usually, doctors at specialized centers use several cognitive tests (e.g., memory, problem solving, and attention tests) to diagnose "probable" AD. The Mini-Mental State Examination (MMSE) is one of the neuropsychological tests most commonly used to assess mental function. In addition, the Clinical Dementia Rating (CDR) is a widely used semi-objective instrument for staging dementia severity. These tests provide descriptive anchors that guide the clinician to make appropriate ratings based on interview data and clinical judgment.

The most commonly recognized symptom of AD patients is memory loss or cognitive deficits, such as difficulty in remembering recently learned facts. People with AD die an average of 4 to 6 years after diagnosis, but the duration of the disease can vary from 3 to 20 years. At a certain point, patients with AD display more rapid deterioration of cognitive function than healthy patients. At this point, it may be possible to detect AD with certain memory and planning tests. Some recent studies (Bäckman & Small, 1998, 2007) convincingly demonstrated that the cognitive deficits of AD can be detected by some simple cognitive tests during a preclinical period spanning several years. This theory was also supported by numerous neuropathological, electrophysiological and neuroimaging studies, as the cognitive deficits in AD are related to a possible disconnection between cortical areas (Delbeuck et al, 2003).

The somatosensory system is a diverse sensory system comprised of receptors and processing centers that produce the sensory modalities. Tactile object cognition, one of the major manual learning and memory skills of humans, requires many connections between cortical areas (Gardner & Kandel, 2002; Penelope et al, 2007). Thus, our hypothesis is that the tactile cognitive deficit symptoms of AD may be detectable using tactile cognitive tests.

In the present chapter, we introduced two tactile pattern delivery devices. The first device was designed to work under a Magnetic Resonance Imaging (MRI) environment for neuroimaging studies. The results of the evaluation experiment indicated that the performance of the device was unaffected by the magnetic field and that the device does not interfere with the magnetic field, making it usable for fMRI. The second device was designed to carry out tactile psychological experiments. This device consists of an electric slide to move the hand platelet along the horizontal axis in the transverse plane and a pattern stand to present a planar shape pattern. To evaluate the function of the second device, we performed two angle discrimination experiments with ten healthy young subjects. The results indicated that the device was operating correctly and can serve as an automated tactile delivery system for tactile behavioral experiments.

DEVELOPMENT OF AN MRI-COMPATIBLE DELIVERY DEVICE

Configuration of the Device

To eliminate the influence of the high magnetic field, plastic material was selected to build the device, and ultrasonic motors were used to drive the device. As shown in Figure 1, the system consists of a main device, a reaction key, a personal computer, a motor controller and an electronic amplifier unit connected to the output of the force sensors. To control and operate the system, we developed a program to achieve precise position control of the stimulus delivery, precise control of the subjects' finger movement orbits, accurate recording of real-time force data, reliable recording of reaction times, and monitoring of the systems operations and integrity.

Evaluation Experiments

We evaluated the function, precision and performance of the system in a magnetic field. Two healthy right-handed volunteers consented to participate in the experiment (male, 21- and 22-years-old). The experiment consisted of two tasks, each lasting 360 seconds. The tasks included finger tapping with the main device and finger tapping without the main device. The subjects were instructed to tap their fingers attentively during active blocks of the experiment and do nothing during baseline blocks.

As shown in Figure 2, the images of the subject show no geometric distortion in the presence of the main device. The brain activation related to the motor process found in both images should no longer be present in the resulting difference. The results suggest that the main device features allowed for controlled, reproducible and automated delivery of a variety of tactile stimuli that can be safely and compatibly delivered in an MRI environment.

Figure 1. MRI-compatible tactile delivery device

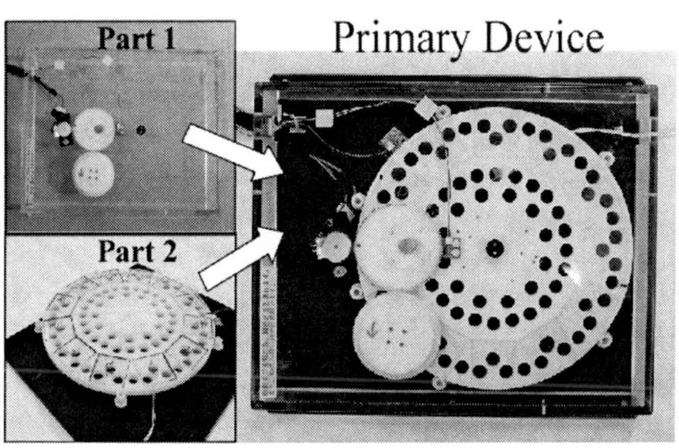

Figure 2. Evaluation results

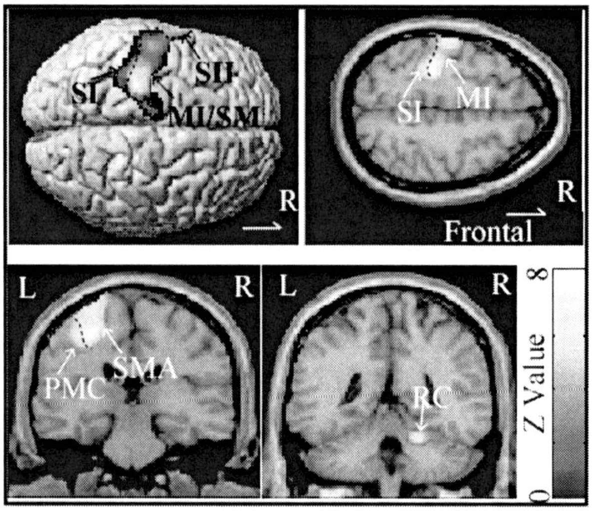

DEVELOPMENT OF A PASSIVELY TACTILE PATTERN DELIVERY DEVICE FOR PSYCHOLOGICAL EXPERIMENTS

Summary of an Experiment and the Device

Figure 3 shows a block diagram of the delivery device system. The control order is delivered by a computer via an exclusive controller, and it is conveyed by a presentation device. In the preliminary experiment, we used two kinds of raised angle patterns that consisted of 1 standard angle (SA) and fourteen comparison angles (CA). First, the experimenter clamped a pair of raised angle patterns, which consisted of a SA and a CA, onto the device. Then the angle pattern was moved by the device. The subjects' right index fingertips were moved between the edges of the angle following an imaginary bisector. The subjects were asked to verbally provide an answer whether the larger angle of each pair was the first or the second.

Figure 3. The block diagram of tactile pattern delivery device

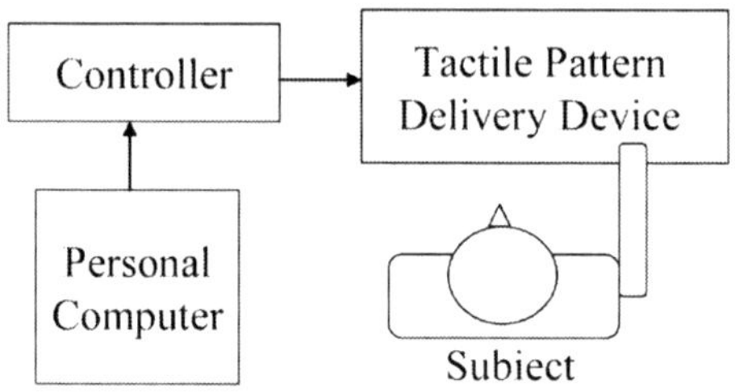

Tactile Pattern Delivery Device

Figure 4 shows the configuration of the main device of the tactile stimuli delivery system. The main device consists of an immovable hand plate, an angle pattern stand and an electric slide. The right index fingertips were allowed to contact the angle pattern from a gap in the immovable hand plate. The angle pattern stand was fixed on the electric slide (Oriental Motor Co., Ltd.), and the movement of the angle patterns was controlled at a constant speed. The electric slide moved the plate along a horizontal axis in a transverse plane within a maximum range of motion of 200.0 mm. The accuracy of the motion distance was 0.01 mm, and the range of motion speed was between

Figure 4. Passively tactile pattern delivery device

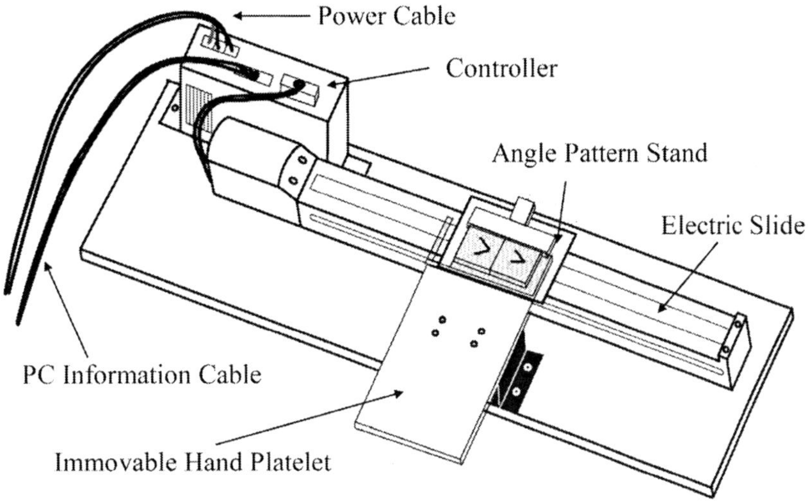

Figure 5. Hand position in present experiment

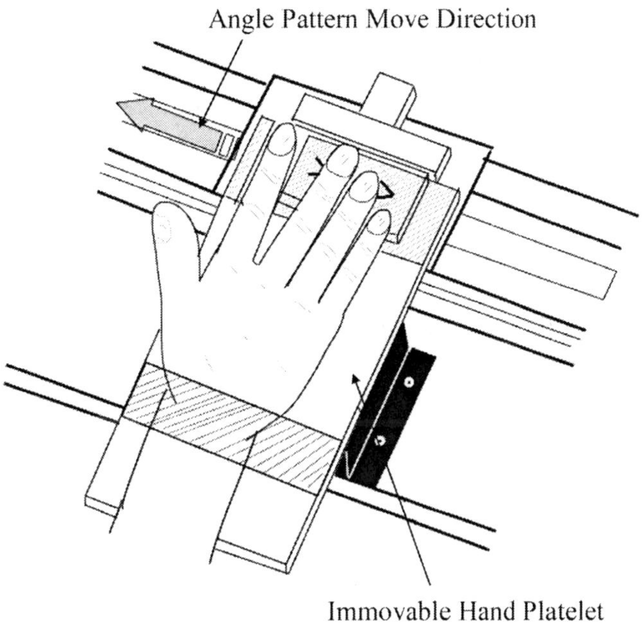

0.01 and 100.0 mm/s, which could be controlled by the computer. Figure 5 shows the hand position on the immovable hand plate. The direction of the arrow shows the direction of the angle pattern movement.

Configuration of the Tactile Pattern

Angle patterns consisted of a standard angle (SA) and a comparison angle (CA). The size of the standard angles was 60°. As shown in Figure 6, fourteen comparison angles that differed from

Figure 6. The configuration of tactile pattern

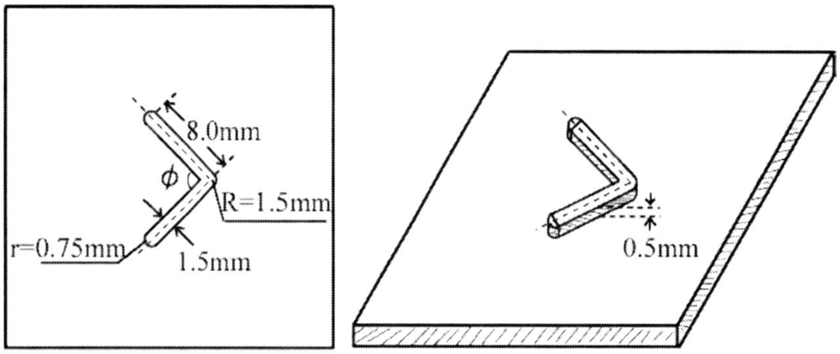

each standard angle by ±2°, 4°, 6°, 8°, 10°, 12°, or 14° were included in the study. The raised angle patterns were custom-built plastic shapes raised 0.5 mm from a 40-mm square base. Varying in two spatial dimensions, the angles were formed by two convex lines at the center of the 40-mm square base with an accuracy of ±0.1°. The length and width of the line were 8.0 mm and 1.5 mm, respectively.

EVALUATION EXPERIMENT

Subjects

Ten healthy, right-hand volunteers consented to participate in the experiment (all male, with a mean age of 24.3 years and an age range of 23-27 years). Before the start of the experiment, all subjects were included in a training test in which they were instructed about the protocol and had to perform all contractions.

Procedure

In this experiment, we measured angle discrimination thresholds based on the subjects' ability to judge whether an angle pattern is larger or smaller than the standard angle used as a reference size. The subjects were blindfolded and seated at a table. The experimenter instructed the subject to place their right index finger and arm in a vertical direction, and the right hand was affixed on the plate. Subjects performed the tests with their eyes closed and did not receive feedback throughout the experiment. First, the experimenter clamped a pair of raised angle patterns, which consisted of a standard angle and a comparison angle, on the apparatus. The subjects were then instructed to perceive each angle using the glabrous skin of the right index finger by passive angle pattern movement. The subjects also had to verbally provide an answer as to whether the larger angle of each pair was the first or the second angle. There were restrictions on contact force, and the passive scanning speed of the right index finger was maintained at 5.0 mm/s. One standard angle and ten comparison angles were presented ten times in a pseudorandom order for a total of 140 trials.

Results of the evaluation experiment

The mean accuracies of ten subjects during the experiment with the standard angle smaller than the comparison angle (SA<CA) and the standard angle larger than the comparison angle (SA>CA) are shown in Figure 5. Inspection of the results indicated that accuracies were not different between the SA<CA and the SA>CA conditions. Figure 6 shows the mean accuracy plotted as function of difference between SA and CA. The results indicate that accuracy improved as the difference between the SA and CA was increased.

Angle Discrimination Threshold

In this study, the 2AFC technique was used to measure threshold. Subjects were forced to make a choice (larger angle) between two angles, even if they could not detect a difference. Here we show the 2AFC results as a plot of percent correction averaged over all trials versus stimulus strength (Figure 6). The guess rate (chance level) for the 2AFC procedure was 50% for two alternatives, and the largest percentage was 100%. Therefore, the sigmoid psychometric function changed from 50 to 100%. The logistic curve is the most common sigmoid curve used extensively in cognitive psychological experiments for measuring threshold. Accordingly, the data were incorporated into a logistic function. The proportion of correct responses for a standard angle was computed (Figure 8). The accuracies were fitted to the following logistic function (1) (Voisin et al, 2002a,b):

$$Accuracy = \frac{1}{1 + e^{d \mid SA - CA \mid}} \qquad (1)$$

In this equation, d is the unique degree of freedom of the logistic curve that was adjusted to fit the raw data. The abbreviations SA and CA are the degree value of the standard angle and the comparison angle. The discrimination threshold is defined as the angle difference at an accuracy of 75%. The discrimination threshold is found at the cross point of the accuracy line and the 75% line. The discrimination thresholds (DT) were computed from the logistic function (2) as follows (X=75% accuracy):

$$DT = d^{-1} Ln(\frac{1 - X}{X}) \qquad (2)$$

Discrimination thresholds of all subjects are shown in Table 1. The mean discrimination threshold was estimated to be 6.0°.

Discussion

The present study used raised angle patterns to evaluate the ability of test subjects to discern different angles in a passive manner. The results indicate that accuracy improved as the difference between the SA and CA was increased. While similar results between test subjects were obtained, there were no significant differences between the SA<CA condition and SA>CA condition. These

Figure 7. The mean accuracy of all subjects in SA<CA and SA>CA condition

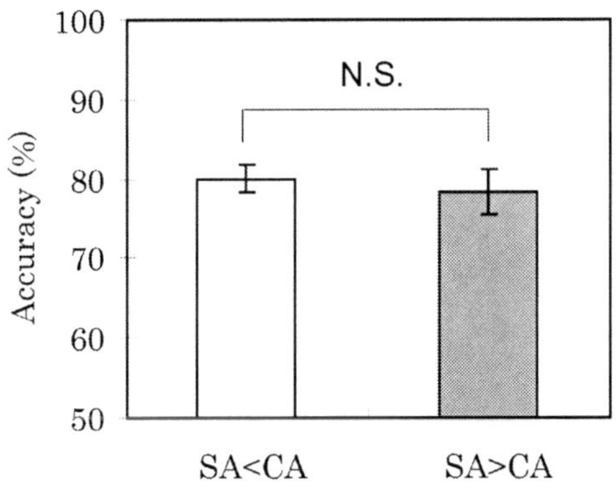

Figure 8. The relationship between accuracy and difference of the angle

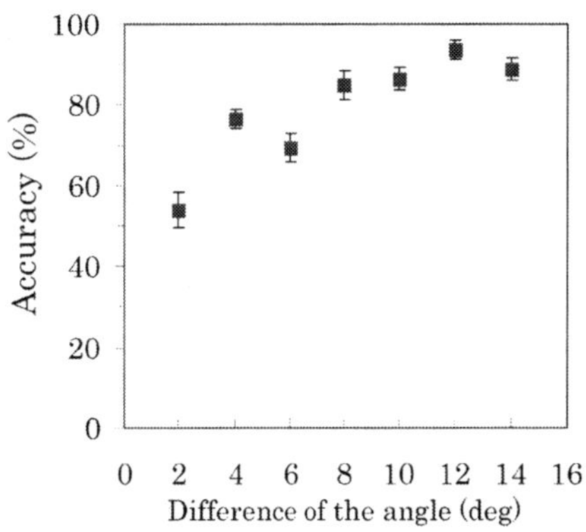

Table 1. Threshold values of all subjects

Subject	Threshold(°)
Sub1	4.18
Sub2	5.27
Sub3	4.57
Sub4	6.59
Sub5	5.23
Sub6	4.20
Sub7	5.02
Sub8	7.90
Sub9	7.79
Sub10	8.99
Mean	5.97(SE±0.5)

results suggested that the different conditions do not affect the difficulty of angle discrimination, and only the net difference between the SA and the CA affect the difficulty level of the experiment.

CONCLUSION

In the present chapter, we described the development of two tactile pattern delivery devices. To validate the compatibility of these devices, we performed an fMRI experiment and an angle discrimination experiment. The results indicated that the devices performed well under testing conditions. These devices can serve as automated tactile delivery systems for tactile behavior and fMRI experiments.

ACKNOWLEDGMENT

A part of this study was financially supported by JSPS AA Science Platform Program and JSPS Grant-in-Aid for Scientific Research (B) (21404002).

REFERENCES

Bäckman, L., & Small, B. J. (1998). Influences of cognitive support on episodic remembering: tracing the process of loss from normal aging to Alzheimer's disease. *Psychology and Aging*, *13*, 267–276. doi:10.1037/0882-7974.13.2.267

Bäckman, L., & Small, B. J. (2007). Cognitive deficits in preclinical Alzheimer's disease and vascular dementia: Patterns of findings from the Kungsholmen Project. *Physiology & Behavior*, *92*, 80–86. doi:10.1016/j.physbch.2007.05.014

Delbeuck, X., Van der Linden, M., & Collette, F. (2003). Alzheimer' disease as a disconnection syndrome? *Neuropsychology Review*, *13*, 79–92. doi:10.1023/A:1023832305702

Gardner, E. P., & Kandel, E. R. (2000). Touch. In Kandel, E. R. (Eds.), *Principles of neural science* (pp. 451–471). New York, NY: McGraw-Hill.

Kostopolous, P., Albanese, M. C., & Petrides, M. (2007). Ventrolateral prefrontal cortex and tactile memory disambiguation in the human brain. *Proceedings of the National Academy of Sciences of the United States of America*, *104*(24), 10223–10228. doi:10.1073/pnas.0700253104

Voisin, J., Benoit, G., & Chapman, C. E. (2002). Haptic discrimination of object shape in humans: Two-dimensional (2-D) angle discrimination. *Experimental Brain Research*, *145*, 239–250. doi:10.1007/s00221-002-1117-6

Voisin, J., Lamarre, Y., & Capman, C. E. (2002). Haptic discrimination of object shape in humans: Contribution of cutaneous and proprioceptive inputs. *Experimental Brain Research*, *145*, 251–260. doi:10.1007/s00221-002-1118-5

KEY TERMS AND DEFINITIONS

Active Touch: When both cutaneous and kinesthetic senses are activated during touch, it is referred to as active touch.

Alzheimer's Disease: A progressive neurodegenerative disease that is characterized by a loss of neurons and synapses in the cerebral cortex and certain subcortical regions. Which is named for German physician Alois Alzheimer, who first described it in 1906.

Amyloid β-Peptide: A peptide of 39–43 amino acids that appears to be the main constituent of amyloid plaques in the brains of Alzheimer's disease patients.

Cognitive Deficits: An inclusive term to describe any characteristic that acts as a barrier to cognitive performance.

Functional MRI: A type of specialized MRI scan. It measures the hemodynamic response (change in blood flow) related to neural activity in the brain or spinal cord of humans or other animals.

Passive Touch: When using the cutaneous sense alone during touch, it is referred to as passive touch.

Chapter 12
Prospective Memory Impairment in Remembering to Remember in Mild Cognitive Impairment and Healthy Subjects

Nobuko Ota
Graduate School of Health Science and Technology, Kawasaki University of Medical Welfare, Japan

Shinichiro Maeshima
Department of Rehabilitation Medicine, International Medical Center, Saitama Medical University, Japan

Aiko Osawa
Department of Rehabilitation Medicine, International Medical Center, Saitama Medical University, Japan

Miho Kawarada
Department of Rehabilitation Medicine, Kawasaki Medical School Kawasaki Hospital, Japan

Jun Tanemura
Department of Sensory Science, Kawasaki University of Medical Welfare, Japan

ABSTRACT

The authors of this chapter studied the prospective memory (PM) performance of 20 older people using the message task in delayed recall from the Rivermead Behavioral Memory Test (RBMT) (Wilson, Cockburn, & Baddeley, 1985; Watamori, Hara, Miyamori, & Eto, 2002). Nine of the subjects had mild cognitive impairment (MCI), while the remaining 11 were healthy subjects (HS). The retrievals in PM were divided into two components: remembering to remember and remembering the content (Umeda, & Koyazu, 1998). Cockburn (1995) suggested that four stages existed in the PM retrieval process: encoding, retention, recognition of the prospective memory cue (PM cue) and retrieval of the intended

DOI: 10.4018/978-1-60960-559-9.ch012

action. The authors administered neuropsychological tests corresponding to each of these stages to investigate the impairment process. Ten subjects showed impairment in remembering to remember and had low performance in encoding, recognition and retrieval in both the auditory verbal memory test and the fluency test, which requires divergent thinking and semantic memory. The other ten subjects were unimpaired, but they also showed low performance in the recognition process of the PM cue with the fluency test. Neither the MCI nor the HS showed impairment in remembering the content. The results suggest that PM impairment in remembering to remember for both MCI and HS results from impairments in frontal lobe function and retrospective memory in the auditory verbal task related to the cue accessibility of spontaneous retrieval.

INTRODUCTION

"Prospective memory (PM)" is a behavioral memory to do something in the future (Munsat, 1966), and the intended action is encoded as "intention." PM is an important part of daily life. PM is distinguishable from retrospective memory because spontaneous retrieval requires retrospective memory as well as frontal lobe function/ executive function (Shallice, & Burgess, 1991; Cockburn, 1995). Healthy older people and patients with amnestic syndrome or dementia caused by organic brain damage show PM impairment (Umeda, 2004). One report indicated that PM is not impaired in event-based prospective memory (PM) tasks, but it is impaired in time-based prospective memory (PM) tasks in normal older subjects (Einstein, & McDaniel, 1990). However, other reports suggest that PM is impaired in both tasks, because both require a procedural control process, and the processing resources of PM diminish with age (Craik, 1986). We investigated the PM impairment process in MCI and HS with an event-based PM task using the four stages in the PM retrieval process (Cockburn, 1995).

METHOD

Subjects

Twenty subjects who consulted with our memory clinic were studied. Nine of the subjects (6 men, 3 women) were diagnosed as MCI according to conventional criteria (Petersen, et al., 1999), while 11 of them (3 men, 8 women) were diagnosed as HS. The mean age was 72.9±10.5 years old. The average years of education were 11.7±10.5 years, and the duration of forgetfulness was 28.7±27.3 months

Neuropsychological Tests

Prospective Memory Task

PM performance was measured with the message task in delayed recall in the RBMT. This is an event-based PM task. When the tester gives a cue, the subject recognizes the event as a PM cue and spontaneously picks up an envelope. Then (s) he walks around the room via a route previously learned (e.g. in version A: to a chair, a door, a window, a desk, and then the chair) and puts the envelope down at a certain place (e.g. in version A: on the desk). According to the PM components, the PM retrievals were divided into two components (Umeda, et al., 1998). The first is remembering to remember, which corresponds to picking up the envelope spontaneously. The other is remembering the content, which corresponds to placing the envelope in the correct location, irrespective of the prompt from the tester when the subject shows no response to the PM cue. The PM performances were judged according to these components.

Four Stages in the PM Retrieval Process and Neuropsychological Tests

Cockburn (1995) suggested that four stages exist in the PM retrieval process and that an impairment in any stage led to overall PM impairment. We administered neuropsychological tests for each of these stages (see Table 1).

We investigated the impairment process by judging each mean score in each stage to determine if it was or was not lower than the cut-off score or 2 SD lower than the criteria. The four stages in the PM retrieval process and the corresponding neuropsychological tests were as follows:

Stage 1 was encoding the PM task when instructed orally. The Rey's auditory verbal learning test (RAVLT) is an auditory verbal memory test in which 15 words are presented orally, and the subject recalls as many words as possible immediately after the presentation (Rey, 1964; Wakamatsu, Anamizu, & Kato, 2003). The total number of words remembered after five trials constituted the score on this test.

Stage 2 was switching attention between an ongoing task and monitoring for the target context, such as PM intention, which requires divided attention. The Kana-hiroi test (Kaneko, 1990), which is the assessment of attention divided between checking five Kana-letters, "a", "i", "u", "e", and "o", in sentences and grasping the meaning of the sentences in two minutes, was used.

Stage 3 was activation of the target context to recognize the PM cue. Divergent thinking to relate the event, represented by the instruction from the tester, to the target PM cue is necessary. Verbal fluency tests assess divergent thinking, so the Category Fluency Test (CFT) and the Letter Fluency Test (LFT) (Saito, Kato, Kashima, Asai, & Hosaki, 1992) were used. In the CFT, subjects are asked to generate as many words as possible in the categories of "animal", "fruit" and "vehicle" with one minute for each category. The LFT requires the subject to generate words that begin with the sound of "shi", "i" and "re" with one minute for each sound. The total number of generated words constitutes the scores of the LFT and the CFT. Recognition of the PM cue is the ability to judge the event as a cue. Recognition in the RAVLT, which assesses the recognition of 15 words encoded in the RAVLT from a group of distracters, was used.

Stage 4 was retrieval of the content of the intended action by delayed recall. The PM content is stored in visual images as well as in auditory memory (Koriat, Ben-Zur, & Nussbaum, 1990). Delayed recall in the RAVLT, which assesses auditory verbal memory from the 15 encoded words, and Raven's Colored Progressive Matrices (RCPM) (Raven, 1976; Sugishita, & Yamazaki, 1993), which assesses the visual process, were used. We also administered the mini-mental state examination (MMSE) to assess general cognitive

Table 1. Four stages in the PM retrieval process and neuropsychological process

Four stages in PM retrieval	Neuropsychological process	Neuropsychological tests
1. Map the target action onto the target context at encoding	Memory: Encoding the event as the PM cue and the content of the intended action	Immediate recall in the Rey's auditory verbal learning test (RAVLT)
2. Divide attention between an ongoing task and monitoring for the target context	Attentional switching: divided attention between the ongoing task and the intention	Kana-hiroi test
3. Activate the target context as a trigger for activation of the intended action	Recognition of the PM cue	Letter fluency test (LFT) Category fluency test (CFT) Recognition in the RAVLT
4. Retrieve the content of the intended action to perform	Retrieval of the content of the intended action with auditory verbal memory and visual process	Delayed recall in the RAVLT Raven's Colored Progressive Matrices (RCPM)

function (Folstein, Folstein, & McHugh, 1975; Mori, Mitani, & Yamadori, 1985).

RESULTS

PM Performance

Ten subjects (MCI: 6, HS: 4) showed impairments in remembering to remember, while the remaining 10 subjects (MCI: 3, HS: 7) showed no impairment (see Figure 1). There was no significant difference between the impairment rates in remembering to remember between MCI and HS (χ^2 test). None of the subjects showed any impairment in remembering the content. There is no significant difference between the two groups with regard to age or the duration of forgetfulness, but the years of education were significantly greater in the unimpaired group than in the impaired group (see Table 2).

Performance on Neuropsychological Tests

The scores of immediate recall in the RAVLT, the Kana-hiroi test, and the CFT of the impaired group were significantly lower than those in the unimpaired group. There was no significant difference between the two groups in the scores of the MMSE, recognition in the RAVLT, the LFT or the RCPM (see Table 3).

Four Stages in the PM Retrieval Process and Neuropsychological Test Performance

The four stages of the PM retrieval process and results of the neuropsychological tests are shown in Table 4. The performances on the LFT in both groups were low. For the impaired group, the performances on the immediate recall in the

Figure 1. Comparison of prospective memory impairments rates by diagnosis

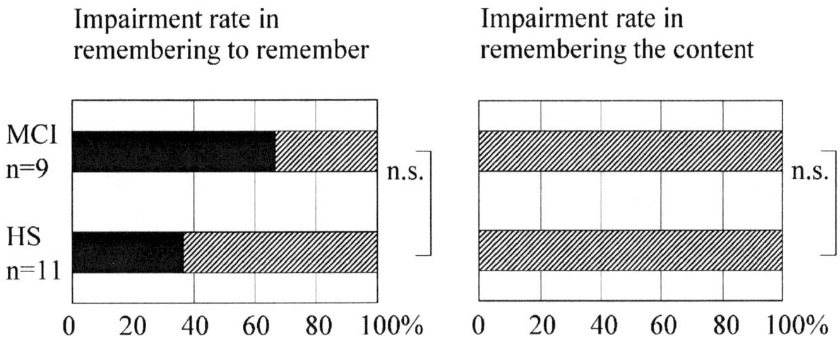

The impairment rates show no significant difference by diagnosis, ■ : impaired, ▨ : unimpaired, n. s. : not significant, χ^2 test.

Table 2. Subjects in the two groups

PM performance in remembering to remember	Impaired n=10	Unimpaired n=10
Age: Mean ± SD (years old)	74.0± 7.7	71.8±13.3
Duration of forgetfulness (months)	31.4±19.5	26.3±33.8
Education period (years)	10.6± 1.6	12.8± 1.5**

**Significant at p <.01, t-test.

Table 3. Comparison in performance of neuropsychological tests

Cognitive functions	Neuropsychological tests	Impaired n=10	Unimpaired n=10
General cognitive function	MMSE	27.1± 2.6	27.9±2.2
Auditory verbal Memory	RAVLT Immediate recall: IR Recognition Delayed recall: DR	26.5± 8.1 9.4± 2.6 4.5± 3.0	36.1±11.2* 11.4± 2.6 6.2± 3.8
Frontal lobes function	Kana-hiroi test Fluency: Category FT : Letter FT	14.6± 6.0 24.4± 9.2 14.4± 5.2	23.7± 9.3* 32.5± 7.0* 14.5± 6.9
Visual process	RCPM	26.8± 3.0	29.0± 4.3

* Significant at $p<.05$, t-test.

RAVLT, as well as delayed recall in the RAVLT and the CFT, were low. Neither group showed low performance on the MMSE, the Kana-hiroi test, recognition in the RAVLT or the RCPM.

DISCUSSION

In our study, groups that demonstrated impairments in remembering to remember also had low performances in Stage 1, Stage 3 and Stage 4 of the PM process (Cockburn, 1995). The unimpaired group showed low performance in Stage 3 only. Stage 1 reflects encoding and Stage 4 reflects retrieval, so both stages are related to memory. On the other hand, there was a difference between the two groups in their performance on Stage 3. Neither group showed any decline in recognition in the RAVLT. While both groups had low scores in fluency on the LFT, there was no significant difference between the two groups. Scores in the CFT were significantly lower in the impaired group. This suggests that this stage is primarily responsible for the spontaneous prospective remembering in remembering to remember that activates the target context as a trigger. It is possible that the impaired group could retrieve the previously present words, because they showed no decline in recognition when the subjects did not have to retrieve the contents spontaneously. In other words, they might have cue accessibility with the previous retrieval cue in retrospective memory. On the other hand, they were unable to recognize the prospective cue unless an apparent

Table 4. Comparison in performances in the four retrieval stages between the groups

Four retrieval stages (Cockburn, 1995)	Neuropsychological Tests	Impaired n=10	Unimpaired n=10
1. Map the target action onto the target context at encoding	RAVLT: IR	*	
2. Divide attention between an ongoing task and monitoring for the target context	Kana-hiroi test		
3. Activate the target context as a trigger for activation of the intended action	LFT CFT RAVLT: Recognition	* *	*
4. Retrieve the content of the intended action	RAVLT: DR RCPM	*	

*Low performance: the mean score is lower than the cut-off score or 2 SD lower than the criteria.

cue for the retrieval cue was presented, as reflected by the low scores in both in the CFT and the LFT. By collecting certain words by category or sound, the verbal fluency tests assess executive function and engage working memory to monitor the words that have already been collected and to retrieve other words (Lezak, 1995). Past 50 years of age, frontal lobe functions, including fluency, decline with age (Troyer, 2000). In studies of regional cerebral blood flow, the LFT is correlated with activity in the left dorsolateral prefrontal cortex and cingulated gyrus, while the CFT is associated with activity in the left medial temporal lobe (Warkentin, Risberg, & Nilsson, 1991). In our study, the only low performance that did not indicate PM impairment in remembering to remember was in the LFT. Activation areas differ between CFT and the LFT (Warkentin et al., 1991). The LFT reflects the retrieval process with a phonological cue, and we assume that low scores in the LFT are sensitive to a decline in frontal lobe function as a result of reduced processing resources due to aging. However, this decline alone does not lead to impairment in remembering to remember. The impaired group showed low performance in both the CFT and the LFT. The CFT reflects retrieval from semantic memory (Warkentin et al., 1991). In the PM retrieval, cue accessibility and cue sensitivity are important, and cue accessibility declines with age (Craik, 1986). We suggest that an impairment in remembering to remember results from an impairment in divergent thinking and poor retrieval from both semantic memory and episodic memory. This results in a lack of cue accessibility in retrospective memory, which leads to an impairment in remembering to remember. Neither group showed impairment in remembering the content in Stage 2 or Stage 4. Stage 2 involves retaining the intention with attentional switching between the ongoing task and the target context. The content of the action to be executed is stored in visual images (Koriat, et al., 1990). We suggest that remembering the content is not impaired because there was no impairment in the retention of content with the visual process in the RCPM.

In our study, both subjects who were diagnosed as MCI and HS showed impairment in remembering to remember in PM. The impaired group had fewer years of education, and in the RBMT message task of delayed recall, received lower scores on immediate recall in RAVLT, the Kana-hiroi test, and the CFT than those in the unimpaired group. The number of years of education has been shown to effect performance on fluency tests (Ito, Hatta, Yasuhiro, Kosuge, & Watanabe, 2004) and RAVLT (Ponton et al., 1996). Based on our data, we propose that the poor performance of the impaired subjects can be attributed to the strategic process in encoding and divergent thinking in fluency. The message task in the RBMT is an event-based PM task. Non-dementia subjects were impaired in the event-based PM task with the procedural control process (Craik, 1986). We suggest that the performance on the event-based PM task in our subjects was impaired because the message task in the RBMT requires a procedural control process to pick up the envelope and to put it in the correct location after following the previously learned route. Due to a reduction in processing resources for memory and divergent thinking in frontal lobe function, the impaired group was unable to complete the task. Older people who have reached a stage of Age-associated Memory Impairment, Aging-associated Cognitive Decline (Levy, 1994) or MCI show various cognitive impairments, and they are at increased risk to progress to a state of dementia (Richie, Artero, & Touchon, 2001). Other studies have reported that older subjects with MCI showed greater PM impairments relative to non-dementia subjects (Maeshima, Tanemura, Osawa, Kawarada, & Yamada, 2006; Troyer, & Murphy, 2007), but our results are not consistent with those conclusions. It is possible that the total number of subjects in our study was too small to show a significant difference between MCI and HS, and that further investigation is needed to determine if PM impairment in the message task in delayed recall in the RBMT could be used distinguish MCI from HS. In the early stage of dementia, patients show slight failures in daily activities related to a mild decline in judgment and planning, which are necessary for executive functions/frontal lobe functions as well as memory (Takayama, 2003). PM impairment is an indicator of the early stage of dementia (Huppert, & Beardsall, 1993). In our study, PM impairment resulted in reduced frontal lobe function and retrospective memory in an auditory verbal task, so we conclude that PM impairment could offer important information regarding the behavior of older people prior to dementia onset. Follow-up work is necessary for the PM-impaired older.

ACKNOWLEDGMENT

We wish to give special thanks to the patients and their families who were tested and underwent rehabilitation at Kawasaki Medical School Kawasaki Hospital.

REFERENCES

Cockburn, J. (1995). Task interruption in prospective memory: A frontal lobe function? *Cortex*, *31*, 87–97.

Craik, F. I. M. (1986). A functional account of age differences in memory. In Clix, F., & Hangendorf, H. (Eds.), *Human memory and cognitive capabilities: Mechanisms and performances* (pp. 409–422). Amsterdam, The Netherlands: Elsevier.

Einstein, G. O., & McDaniel, M. A. (1990). Normal aging and prospective memory. *Journal of Experimental Psychology. Learning, Memory, and Cognition*, *16*, 717–726. doi:10.1037/0278-7393.16.4.717

Folstein, M. F., Folstein, S. E., & McHugh, P. R. (1975). Mini-mental state examination: A practical method for grading the cognitive state of patients for clinician. *Journal of Psychiatric Research*, *12*, 182–198. doi:10.1016/0022-3956(75)90026-6

Huppert, F. A., & Beardsall, L. (1993). Prospective memory impairment as an early indicator of dementia. *Journal of Clinical and Experimental Neuropsychology*, *15*, 805–821. doi:10.1080/01688639308402597

Ito, E., Hatta, T., Yasuhiro, I., Kosuge, T., & Watanabe, H. (2004). Performance of verbal fluency tasks in Japanese healthy adults: Effect of gender, age and education on the performance. *Japanese Journal of Neuropsychology*, *20*, 254–263.

Kaneko, M. (1990). Dementia and frontal lobe function. *Higher Brain Function Research*, *10*, 127–131. doi:10.2496/apr.10.127

Koriat, A., Ben-Zur, H., & Nussbaum, A. (1990). Encoding information for future action; Memory for to-be-performed tasks versus memory for to-be-recalled tasks. *Memory & Cognition*, *18*, 568–578. doi:10.3758/BF03197099

Levy, R. (1994). Aging -associated cognitive decline. *International Psychogeriatrics*, *6*, 63–68. doi:10.1017/S1041610294001626

Lezak, M. D. (1995). *Neuropsychological assessment* (3rd ed.). New York, NY: Oxford University Press.

Maeshima, S., Tanemura, J., Osawa, A., Kawarada, M., & Yamada, Y. (2006). Prospective memory in the Elderly: The difference between presence and contents of intentions to remember. *Japanese Journal of Rehabilitation Medicine*, *43*, 446–453. doi:10.2490/jjrm1963.43.446

Mori, E., Mitani, Y., & Yamadori, A. (1985). Usefulness of a Japanese version of the mini-mental state test in neurological patients. *Japanese Journal of Neuropsychology*, *1*, 82–90.

Munsat, S. (1966). *The concept of memory*. New York, NY: Random House.

Petersen, R. C., Smith, G. E., Waring, S. C., Ivnik, R. J., Tangalos, E. G., & Kokmen, E. (1999). Mild cognitive impairment; clinical characterization and outcome. *Archives of Neurology*, *56*, 303–308. doi:10.1001/archneur.56.3.303

Ponton, M. O., Satz, P., Herrera, L., Ortiz, F., Urrutia, C. P., & Young, R. (1996). Normative data stratified by age and education for the Neuropsychological Screening Battery for Hispanics (NeSBHIS): Initial report. *Journal of the International Neuropsychological Society*, *2*, 96–104. doi:10.1017/S1355617700000941

Raven, J. C. (1976). *Colored progressive matrices. London, UK.* Lewis: Oxford Psychologists Press.

Rey, A. (1964). *L'examen clinique en psychogie*. Paris, France: Presses Universitaires de France.

Richie, K., Artero, S., & Touchon, J. (2001). Classification criteria for mild cognitive impairment: A population based validation study. *Neurology*, *56*, 37–42.

Saito, H., Kato, M., Kashima, H., Asai, M., & Hosaki, H. (1992). Effects of disinhibition on performance of the Word Fluency Test in patients with frontal lesions. *Higher Brain Function Research*, *12*, 223–231. doi:10.2496/apr.12.223

Shallice, T., & Burgress, P. W. (1991). Higher order cognitive impairments and frontal lobe lesions in man. In Levin, H. S., Eisenberg, H. M., & Benton, A. L. (Eds.), *Frontal lobe function and dysfunction* (pp. 125–138). New York, NY: Oxford University Press.

Sugishita, M., & Yamazaki, K. (1993). *Japanese raven's coloured progressive matrices*. Tokyo, Japan: Nihon-bunnkakagakusya.

Takayama, Y. (2003). Conditions necessary for the screening tests to detect early stage of dementia. *Japanese Journal of Geriatric Psychiatry*, *14*, 13–19.

Troyer, A. K. (2000). Normative data for clustering and switching on verbal fluency tasks. *Journal of Clinical and Experimental Neuropsychology*, *22*, 370–378. doi:10.1076/1380-3395(200006)22:3;1-V;FT370

Troyer, A. K., & Murphy, J. K. (2007). Memory for intentions in amnestic mild cognitive impairment; Time- and event-based prospective memory. *Journal of the International Neuropsychological Society*, *13*, 365–369. doi:10.1017/S1355617707070452

Umeda, S. (2004). Prospective memory impairment in elderly. *Japanese Journal of Geriatric Psychiatry*, *15*, 725–730.

Umeda, S., & Koyazu, T. (1998). Prospective memory and its theoretical consideration. *Shinrigaku Kenkyu*, *69*, 317–333.

Wakamatsu, N., Anamizu, S., & Kato, M. (2003). Rey Auditory Verbal Learning Test (RAVLT). *Japanese Journal of Clinical Medicine*, *61*(9), 279–284.

Warkentin, S., Risberg, J., & Nilsson, A. (1991). Cortical activity during speech production; A study of regional blood flow in normal subjects performing a word fluency task. *Neuropsychiatry, Neuropsychology, and Behavioral Neurology*, *4*, 305–316.

Watamori, T., Hara, H., Miyamori, T., & Eto, F. (2002). *The Japanese version of the Rivermead Behavioural Memory Test*. Tokyo, Japan: Chiba Test Center.

Wilson, B. A., Cockburn, J. M., & Baddeley, A. D. (1985). *The Rivermead Behavioral Memory Test. Bury St.* Edmunds, England: Thames Valley Test Company.

KEY TERMS AND DEFINITIONS

Event-Based Prospective Memory (PM) Task: A prospective memory task with an external prospective cue (e.g. alarm, verbal cue from the tester, etc.).

Executive Function: Necessary to perform a series of goal-oriented actions and includes four components: goal formulation, planning, carrying-out activities and effective performance.

Frontal Lobe Function: Cognitive and behavioral functions related to the frontal lobes.

Mild Cognitive Impairment (MCI): Generally used to refer to a transitional zone between normal cognitive function and clinical dementia. In our study, it refers to amnestic MCI diagnosed according to Petersen's criteria.

Prospective Memory (PM): The ability to spontaneously remember to do previously planned actions.

Remembering the Content: Demembering the content of the action to be performed with the prospective intention.

Remembering to Remember: Spontaneously remembering the prospective intention to do something when the prospective memory cue is given.

Retrospective Memory: Memory with content about past events; this is in contrast to prospective memory.

Time-Based Prospective Memory (PM) Task: A prospective memory task with an internal prospective cue (e.g. a clock or a timer monitoring).

Chapter 13
Cognitive Decline in Patients with Alzheimer's Disease:
A Six-Year Longitudinal Study of Mini-Mental State Examination Scores

Hikaru Nakamura
Department of Welfare System and Health Science, Okayama Prefectural University, Japan

ABSTRACT

The authorof this chapter present six years of longitudinal data on Mini-Mental State Examination (MMSE) scores in Japanese patients with Alzheimer's disease (AD). Fifty-eight subjects were treated with donepezil, and nineteen served as controls. The MMSE scores recorded at the first medical examination and at the one-, three- and six-year follow-up examinations were analyzed. Over six years, the mean MMSE scores fell from 21.9 to 15.0 in the medication group and from 21.6 to 10.2 in the control group. The difference in the rate of decline between the two groups was significant. In the medication group, subjects' sex, age and severity of cognitive impairment at entry did not affect the rate of MMSE score decline. Thirty-two patients in the medication group remained residents during the six-year period (resident group), twenty-one began as residents but were subsequently institutionalized, and five were institutionalized from the outset. The rate of decline in MMSE scores was significantly smaller in the resident group than in the other two groups. These data suggest that donepezil contributes to long-term maintenance of cognitive ability in AD patients and that a residential community setting, which is rich in stimuli, suppresses cognitive decline.

INTRODUCTION

Cognitive impairment is the key clinical feature of Alzheimer's disease (AD). Researchers are greatly interested in how impairment progresses and the most effective preventative measures. The Mini-Mental State Examination (MMSE) (Folstein, Folstein, & McHugh, 1975) is the most widely used tool for measuring cognitive ability in brain-damaged patients. It is a paper and pencil test with a maximum total score of 30. The MMSE

DOI: 10.4018/978-1-60960-559-9.ch013

is easy to administer and has high reliability and validity. It is comprised of subtests in five cognitive domains: orientation, registration (short-term memory), attention, recall (long-term memory) and language.

In 1998, Bracco, Piccini, and Amaducci reviewed longitudinal studies on cognitive decline measured by the MMSE in AD patients. They reported that the rate of MMSE score decline in AD patients differed considerably among studies, ranging from 1.8 to 4.5 points per year. In 2000, Han, Cole, Belavance, Cusker, and Primeau executed a meta-analysis to estimate the annual rate of MMSE score decline. They analyzed 37 longitudinal studies involving 3,492 AD patients followed over an average of two years. They concluded that the pooled average of the annual rate of MMSE decline was 3.3 (95% confidence interval 2.9-3.7). In addition, the above two reports indicated some possibility that the patients' sex, age at entry (at the first examination), or severity of cognitive impairment (MMSE scores) at entry affected the progression of cognitive decline.

These reports are not up to date. In addition, they only presented studies performed in Western countries. Here, we present longitudinal data comprised of MMSE scores in recently treated Japanese patients with AD.

METHODS

Subjects

The subjects were patients examined as outpatients at a general hospital in Okayama between 1999 and 2008. The inclusion criteria included the following: (1) a diagnosis of dementia of the Alzheimer's type according to DSM-IV criteria, early in their course of treatment; (2) the availability of more than six years of follow-up data. Patients were excluded if they had other obvious neurological or psychiatric diseases such as cerebrovascular disease or major depression. Seventy-seven patients fulfilled the above criteria.

Procedure

The MMSE scores recorded at the first medical examination (T0) and at the one-year (T1), three-year (T2), and six-year (T3) follow-up examinations were analyzed retrospectively. A two-way analysis of variance (ANOVA) was conducted to test whether time (T0-T3), medication, sex, age at T0, severity of cognitive impairment at T0, or residential state affected the MMSE scores.

RESULTS

Medication

Fifty-eight of the subjects (19 men and 39 women; mean age, 75.5 years) were continuously treated with donepezil, whereas nineteen (4 men and 15 women; mean age, 80.6 years) were not. The most frequent reason for non-medication was gastrointestinal side effects. Table 1 shows the patients' MMSE scores. In the medication group, the mean MMSE score fell 6.9 points during the six-year period (annual rate of decline was 1.2). In the non-medication (control) group, the cor-

Table 1. Means and SDs of MMSE scores in the subjects

Group	Test Period							
	T0		T1		T2		T3	
	M	SD	M	SD	M	SD	M	SD
Medication	21.9	5.2	21.8	5.3	18.1	6.5	15.0	8.0
Non-medication	21.6	4.6	18.2	4.8	16.7	5.6	10.2	7.0

responding value was 11.4 points (annual rate of decline was 1.9). An ANOVA revealed significant main effects for both time and medication. The interaction between time and medication was also significant, indicating that the medication group exhibited a slower rate of decline.

Sex, Age, and Severity

The following analyses were conducted only in the medication group. Table 2 shows their MMSE scores.

Sex: An ANOVA revealed a significant main effect for time. However, the main effect for sex and the interaction between time and sex were not significant.

Age: The subjects were divided into three subgroups based on their age at T0. Of these, 9 were under 70 years old, 33 were 70-79 years old, and 16 were over 79 years old. An ANOVA failed to reveal a significant main effect for age or an interaction between time and age.

Severity: The subjects were divided into three groups based on the severity of cognitive impairment as determined by MMSE scores (Hodges & Patterson, 1995) at T0. Twenty-five of the subjects had very mild cognitive impairment (MMSE > 23), 25 had mild impairment (23-17), and 8 had moderate to severe impairment (< 17). An ANOVA failed to revealed a significant main effect for severity. However, or the interaction between time and severity were not significant.

Residential State

In the medication group, the subjects were divided into three subgroups based on their residential state. Thirty-two were community residents at both T0 and T3 (resident group); twenty-one were residents at T0 but were institutionalized at T3 (resident-institutionalized group); and five were institutionalized at both T0 and T3 (institutionalized group). In the resident group, the mean MMSE score fell 5.1 points over the six-year period. In the resident-institutionalized and institutionalized groups, the mean scores fell 9.2 and 9.6 points, respectively. An ANOVA revealed a significant main effect for residential state. It also revealed a significant interaction between time and residential state, with the residential group exhibiting a slower rate of decline than the other groups.

Table 2. Means and SDs of MMSE scores in the medication group subjects

Subgroup	Test Period							
	T0		T1		T2		T3	
	M	SD	M	SD	M	SD	M	SD
Sex								
Male	22.7	4.5	22.5	3.0	20.5	3.4	17.6	6.3
Female	21.5	5.4	21.5	6.0	17.0	7.3	13.7	8.3
Age								
< 70	20.9	6.9	20.6	7.3	17.0	6.9	15.1	7.1
70-79	22.7	4.7	22.8	3.6	19.7	5.6	16.2	8.1
> 79	20.7	5.3	20.4	6.8	15.5	7.6	12.3	8.0
Initial severity								
Very mild	26.1	1.7	24.7	3.3	21.5	5.8	19.2	5.5
Mild	21.0	1.8	21.4	3.5	17.4	3.5	14.0	7.5
Moderate-severe	11.5	3.1	14.0	6.2	10.4	6.2	5.9	6.5
Residential State								
Resident	22.3	5.6	22.7	5.1	19.5	6.2	17.2	6.6
Resident-institutionalized	22.3	4.2	21.1	5.8	16.7	6.9	13.1	8.7
Institutionalized	17.6	6.1	19.2	3.9	14.8	5.7	8.0	8.3

DISCUSSION

The annual rate of MMSE score decline in this group of AD patients, especially those who were treated with donepezil, was much smaller than the declines reported in the studies reviewed by Bracco et al. (1998) and Han et al. (2000). Two factors that were not commonly applied to AD patients more than ten years ago likely contributed to the preservation of cognitive ability in these patients. The first factor is donepezil. No obvious decline in the MMSE score was observed in the medication group during the first year of treatment. Donepezil is known to prevent the progression of AD by several months at a minimum (American Psychiatric Association, 2007; Farlow & Cummings, 2007; Nakamura, 2004), consistent with the data presented here. The second factor is rehabilitation. Most of the patients in the medication group participated in rehabilitation programs such as physical exercise, music therapy, reminiscence therapy, and/or memory training. Some researchers have reported that such programs are effective for the cognitive and/or mental domains in patients with dementia (American Psychiatric Association, 2007; Nakamura, 2004).

Some studies have pointed out that the patients' sex, age at entry, or cognitive state at entry affected the rate of MMSE score decline. The effects of these factors, however, could not be confirmed in the present study. If the influence of these factors is indeed significant, it might be rather weak. In addition, most of the subjects in the present study were relatively old. Studies that include subjects with a wider age range should be analyzed.

The rate of MMSE score decline among the patients who were continuous residents in a community setting was slower than that of the other patients. A community setting, which is rich in stimuli, might slow cognitive decline. However, the reverse causal relationship should also be considered. More specifically, patients who did not exhibit cognitive deterioration were able to continue residing in their homes, whereas patients who exhibited prominent decline were forced to move into institutions. Further investigations are needed.

REFERENCES

American Psychiatric Association. (2007). *Practice guideline for the treatment of patients with Alzheimer's disease and other dementias, 2nd ed.* American Psychiatric Association, Inc. Retrieved from http://www.psychiatryonline.com/pracguide/pracguidetopic_3.aspx

Bracco, L., Piccini, C., & Amaducci, L. (1998). Rate of progression of mental decline in Alzheimer disease: Summary of European studies. *Alzheimer Disease and Associated Disorders*, *12*, 347–355. doi:10.1097/00002093-199812000-00016

Farlow, M. R., & Cummings, J. L. (2007). Effective pharmacologic management of Alzheimer's disease. *The American Journal of Medicine*, *120*, 388–397. doi:10.1016/j.amjmed.2006.08.036

Folstein, M. F., Folstein, S. E., & Mchugh, P. R. (1975). Mini-mental state: A practical method for grading the cognitive state of patients for the clinician. *Journal of Psychiatric Research*, *12*, 189–198. doi:10.1016/0022-3956(75)90026-6

Han, L., Cole, M., Bellavance, F., McCusker, J., & Primeau, F. (2000). Tracking cognitive decline in Alzheimer's disease using the miniMini-mentalMental stateState examinationExamination: A meta-analysis. *International Psychogeriatrics*, *12*, 231–247. doi:10.1017/S1041610200006359

Hodges, J. R., & Patterson, K. (1995). Is semantic memory consistently impaired early in the course of Alzheimer's disease? Neuroanatomical and diagnostic implications. *Neuropsychologia*, *33*, 441–459. doi:10.1016/0028-3932(94)00127-B

Nakamura, S. (2004). A guideline for the treatment of dementia in Japan. *Internal Medicine (Tokyo, Japan)*, *43*, 18–29. doi:10.2169/internalmedicine.43.18

KEY TERMS AND DEFINITIONS

Alzheimer's Disease: The most common form of dementia in both Western countries and Japan. Neuropathologically, this disease is characterized by amyloid plaques, neurofibrillary tangles, and loss of neurons in the brain.

Donepezil: A drug used to treat Alzheimer's disease. Donepezil was approved in the USA in 1996 and in Japan in 1999. It acts as a reversible acetylcholinesterase inhibitor that increases acetylcholine in the brains of patients with Alzheimer's disease.

DSM-IV: The abbreviation for the Diagnostic and Statistical Manual of Mental Disease, Fourth Edition, determined by American Psychiatric Association. This manual provides the most authoritative criteria on mental illness.

Meta-Analysis: A statistical analysis that combines the results of several studies having similar research questions and methods with the aim of gaining more reliable results.

Mini-Mental State Examination (MMSE): A paper and pencil test developed by Folstein et al. in 1975. The MMSE is currently the most widely used tool in the world to rapidly measure cognitive ability in brain-damaged patients.

Music therapy: An interventional technique for people with disabilities. In this therapy, music is used intentionally to recover or maintain patients' physical and mental health.

Reminiscence Therapy: An intervention technique for people of advanced age and/or dementia. In this therapy, the participants are required to review their life and are expected to recover their identity and good mental health.

Chapter 14
The Clinical Analysis of Combined Effects of Huperzine A and Memantine for Alzheimer's Disease

Shouzi Zhang
Beijing Geriatric Hospital, China

Qinyun Li
Beijing Geriatric Hospital, China

Maolong Gao
Beijing Geriatric Hospital, China

ABSTRACT

The purpose of this study was to evaluate the clinical effects of a combination of Huperzine A and memantine for the treatment of Alzheimer's disease (AD). Sixty patients (aged 69 ± 4.5), treated in both outpatient and hospital settings, were divided into two groups, the treated group and the control group. Over 24 weeks of clinical therapy, 30 patients received treatment with Huperzine A (0.2 mg/d), and the other 30 patients received a combination of Huperzine A (0.2 mg/d) and memantine (20 mg/d). Mini-mental State Examination (MMSE) was taken as the main value target. Activity of Daily Living Scale (ADL) and Neuropsychiatric Inventory (NPI) were secondary targets. Results: After 24 weeks, the scores from the MMSE, ADL, and NPI of the treatment group were more improved than those of the control group (P≤0.05). Combination treatment with Huperzine A and memantine will be more effective for treating AD than treatment with Huperzine A alone.

INTRODUCTION

Alzheimer's disease (AD) is a neurodegenerative disorder affecting higher cognitive functions such as memory, orientation and attention, and is the most common cause of dementia. Cholinesterase inhibitors such as donepezil have shown the best efficacy and are approved for use in mild to moderate cases of AD. Another cholinesterase inhibitor, Huperzine A (from Huperziaserrata) is

DOI: 10.4018/978-1-60960-559-9.ch014

widely used to treat AD in China. The glutamate antagonist memantine is a low- to moderate-affinity, uncompetitive N-methyl-D-aspartate receptor antagonist. Controlled trials have demonstrated the safety and efficacy of memantine monotherapy for patients with moderate to severe AD. While memantine has been widely prescribed, often in the later stages of AD, there is little evidence to guide clinicians as to the treatment options to use as AD advances, particularly as the condition progresses from moderate to severe. Options include continuing treatment with cholinesterase inhibitors irrespective of decline, adding memantine to the cholinesterase inhibitors, or prescribing memantine instead of cholinesterase inhibitors. The aim of this trial is to establish the combinative value of Huperzine A and memantine for AD patients who are progressing from moderate to severe dementia.

EXPERIMENT

Subjects

Sixty AD patients (29 males, 31 females; age range 69 ± 4.5 years) treated in both outpatient and hospital settings were selected. All patients were required to have had stable physical health for the previous year and meet the National Institute of Neurological and Communicative Diseases and Stroke -Alzheimer's Disease and Related Disorders Association (NINCDS-ADRDA) and the Diagnostic and Statistical Manual of Mental Disorders, 4th Edition (DSM-IV) criteria for probable Alzheimer's disease (AD), have a Global Deterioration Scale (GDS) score of 4 to 5 at the time of enrollment, have no contraindication to taking Huperzine A, remained stable regarding other medications, and be able to give informed consent (or not object to participating).

Method

Patients were randomly assigned by lottery to the control (Huperzine A alone) or treatment group (Huperzine A and memantine) and given treatment for one year. Both groups received Huperzine A. The treatment group patients started taking memantine at the time of enrollment, beginning with a dose of 5 mg per day, which was increased to 20 mg per day by the end of the study. All follow-up assessments included baseline measurements. Patient assessment included the Mini-Mental State Examination (MMSE), Alzheimer's Disease Cooperative Study – Activities of Daily Living (ADCS-ADL) and Neuropsychiatric Inventory (NPI). The MMSE, ADCS-ADL, and NPI results were evaluated, as well as cognition, the activities of daily living and behavioral and psychological symptoms. These outcomes were assessed at baseline and 24 weeks, and all participants will be subsequently followed for one year by telephone interview to record institutionalization.

RESULTS

The baseline characteristics of the patients are summarized in Table 1. Treatment and control group subjects did not differ significantly at enrollment with respect to MMSE, ADCS-ADL, NPI, gender or age. After 24 weeks, the scores of the MMSE, ADL and NPI tests for the control and treatment group subjects were statistically analyzed using SAS9.1.3 software. Data were expressed as Mean±SD. There were significant differences between the control and treatment groups.

DISCUSSION

Alzheimer's disease (AD), the most common form of dementia, is a neurodegenerative disorder characterized by a gradual progression of cognitive, functional, and behavioral deficits. The effect of

Table 1. Comparison of the baseline characteristics for control and treatment groups ($\overline{x} \pm S$)

	Age	MMSE	ADL	NPI
Control group	70.5±5.9	8.5±0.8	60±2.6	25±3.1
Treatment group	71.2±6.1	7.6±0.6	45±4.2	24±4.3
t test	0.435	1.564	0.370	0.249
p test	0.562	0.741	0.538	0.783

α=0.05

Table 2. Comparison of the scores of control and treatment groups after 24 weeks of treatment ($\overline{x} \pm S$)

	MMSE	ADL	NPI
Control group	10.8±1.3	56±3.4	23±2.5
Treatment group	12±1.4	33±2.3	15±1.2
t test	2.28	2.45	2.12
p test	0.034	0.010	0.030

α=0.05

cholinesterase inhibitors in delaying the progression of AD has been established (Evans et al., 2004). There is a significant body of evidence to support the use of the cholinesterase inhibitors such as donepezil in people with mild to moderate AD (Birks et al., 2003; Ritchie, 2004). To explain the neuroprotective effect of cholinesterase inhibitors, mechanisms based on beta-amyloid metabolism have been postulated. Accumulation of amyloid is one of the earliest changes in Alzheimer's disease pathology (Hardy & Allsop, 1991; Hardy & Higgins, 1992) and may cause neuronal death in the CNS. In vitro studies have demonstrated a link between cholinergic activation and beta-amyloid precursor protein metabolism.

We postulate that the combination of cholinesterase inhibitors and a glutamate antagonist for the treatment of AD will reduce the symptoms of dementia. The results of our experiment support this hypothesis. Donepezil can delay the progression of AD. Previous studies report that the annual decline of MMSE scores in AD patients was about 1.8–2.3 (Jones et al, 2002). Although the exact pathophysiology of AD has not been fully established, the cognitive deficits associated with the disease are primarily related to cholinergic deficits. A longitudinal neuroimaging study using single photon emission computed tomography (SPECT) demonstrated that treatment of patients with Alzheimer's disease with donepezil for one year reduced the decline in regional cerebral blood flow (rCBF) (Nakano et al., 2001). The development of potential therapies has, therefore, focused on enhancing cholinergic neurotransmission. Cholinesterase inhibitors, which enhance cholinergic function, are the standard pharmacologic treatment for mild-to-moderate AD. Analysis of the effects of donepezil for patients with relatively severe behavioral disturbances indicates that donepezil has a significant behavioral effect, reducing mood disturbances and psychotic symptoms (Suh et al., 2004). The glutamate antagonist memantine has been widely prescribed, often in the later stages of AD.

One dilemma in the treatment of AD is what to do as the condition progresses from the moderate to severe stage. Options include continuing cholinesterase inhibitors irrespective of decline, adding memantine to cholinesterase inhibitors, or prescribing memantine instead of cholinesterase inhibitors. Randomized double-blind placebo-controlled trials of cholinesterase inhibitors that have included moderately to severely affected patients have shown significant benefits over 24 weeks in cognitive, behavioral, and functional outcomes (Cummings et al, 2006). In accordance with the results of our trial, Raina P,et al reported both cholinesterase inhibitors and memantine had consistent effects in the domains of cognition and global assessment. The treatment of dementia with cholinesterase inhibitors and memantine can result in statistically significant, but clinically marginal, improvement in the measures of cognition and global assessment of dementia (Raina et al., 2008).

ACKNOWLEDGMENT

This study was supported by Capital Medicine Development Scientific Research Foundation.

REFERENCES

Birks, J. S., Melzer, D., & Beppu, H. (2003). Donepezil for mild and moderate Alzheimer's disease. *Cochrane Database of Systematic Reviews*, 3.

Cummings, J. L., McRae, T., & Zhang, R. (2006). Effects of donepezil on neuropsychiatric symptoms in patients with dementia and severe behavioral disorders. *The American Journal of Geriatric Psychiatry*, *14*(7), 605–612. doi:10.1097/01.JGP.0000221293.91312.d3

Evans, J. G., Wilcock, G., & Birks, J. (2004). Evidence-based pharmacotherapy of Alzheimer's disease. *The International Journal of Neuropsychopharmacology*, *7*, 351–369. doi:10.1017/S1461145704004444

Hardy, J. A., & Allsop, D. (1991). Amyloid deposition as the central event in the aetiology of Alzheimer's disease. *Trends in Pharmacological Sciences*, *12*, 383–388. doi:10.1016/0165-6147(91)90609-V

Hardy, J. A., & Higgins, G. A. (1992). Alzheimer's disease: The amyloid cascade hypothesis. *Science*, *256*, 184–185. doi:10.1126/science.1566067

Jones, S., Small, B. J., Fratiglioni, L., & Backman, L. (2002). Predictors of cognitive change from preclinical to clinical Alzheimer's disease. *Brain and Cognition*, *49*(2), 210–213.

Nakano, S., Asada, T., Matsuda, H., Uno, M., & Takasaki, M. (2001). Donepezil hydrochloride preserves regional cerebral blood flow in patients with Alzheimer's disease. *Journal of Nuclear Medicine*, *42*, 1441–1445.

Raina, P., Santaguida, P., Ismaila, A., Patterson, C., Cowan, D., & Levine, M. (2008). Effectiveness of cholinesterase inhibitors and memantine for treating dementia: Evidence review for a clinical practice guideline. *Annals of Internal Medicine*, *148*(5), 379–397.

Ritchie, C. W. (2004). Meta-analysis of randomised trials of the efficacy and safety of donepezil, galantamine and rivastigmine for the treatment of Alzheimer's disease. *The American Journal of Geriatric Psychiatry*, *12*, 358–369.

Suh, G. H., Ju, Y. S., Yeon, B. K., & Shah, A. (2004). A longitudinal study of Alzheimer's disease: Rates of cognitive and functional decline. *International Journal of Geriatric Psychiatry*, *19*(9), 817–824. doi:10.1002/gps.1168

KEY TERMS AND DEFINITIONS

Alzheimer's Disease (AD): A neurodegenerative disorder,including higher cognitive functions like memory, orientation and attention.

Huperzine A: A Cholinesterase inhibitor, which is from Huperziaserrata, widely used to treat AD.

Memantine: A low- to moderate-affinity, uncompetitive N-methyl-D-aspartate receptor antagonist,used to treat AD.

Section 2

Chapter 15
From Bench to Bedside: BACE1, Beta-Site Amyloid Precursor Protein Cleaving Enzyme 1, From Basic Science to Clinical Investigation

Yong Shen
Center for Advanced Therapeutic Strategies for Brain Disorders(CATSBD), Raskamp Institute, USA

I. ABSTRACT

Alzheimer's disease (AD) is a constantly progressive and highly complex neurodegenerative disease, and there are many ways to molecularly characterize the various stages. Morphologically, AD patients are characterized by neurofibrillar abnormalities associated with pathological hyperphosphorylation of tau protein, and deposits of β– amyloid peptides (Aβ). There is an overwhelming amount of information to support the hypothesis that generation, formation, and β-amyloid deposits play key mechanistic roles in the early development of AD. It is known that the cause of early-onset familial AD (FAD) is due to mutations in three genes which cause an increase in the production of the toxic peptide, Aβ42. The molecules that cause the proteolytic activities of beta and gamma secretase, two proteases that free the Aβ-peptide by endoproteolyzing APP, have recently been discovered. Homologous to BACE1, BACE2 was also a recent discovery (Lin et al, 2000; Vassar et al, 1999; Yan et al, 1999), and together these two enzymes make up a new family of transmembrane aspartic proteases. The key enzyme, BACE1, initiates the formation of Aβ, represents a candidate biomarker, as well as a drug target for AD, exhibit all the functional properties of β–secretase. This chapter will review the biology of BACE1 and focus attention to BACE1 as a candidate biomarker for the early detection, prediction, and biological activity in AD.

II. DISCOVERY AND CLONING OF BACE1

Several groups have independently cloned and characterized BACE1 as a transmembrane aspartyl protease with all the known characteristics of APP β-secretase (Lin et al, 2000; Vassar et al, 1999; Yan et al, 1999; Sinha et al, 1999). The activity of BACE1 in the human brain, both, in vitro and in vivo, is highly specific for the β-cleavage site; however, over-expression of this enzyme increases the amount of the BACE1 cleavage products which are C99 and C89. The enzyme shows enhanced cleavage of the substrate carrying

DOI: 10.4018/978-1-60960-559-9.ch015

the Swedish mutation as compared to wild type substrate, which is in agreement with the results obtained from other cellular studies (Yan et al, 1999; Sinha et al, 1999). The role of BACE1 in Aβ production in vitro might explain the higher production of Aβ peptide in sporadic AD and the early onset of Swedish familial Alzheimer's disease. The highest levels of enzymatic activity are found in cells and tissues of the central nervous system, therefore supporting its role as human brain β-secretase. BACE1 cleavage occurs at the known β-cleavage sites of APP, Asp 1 and Glu 11 (Vassar et al, 1999; Lee et al, 2003).

Studies indicate that over-expression of BACE1 in vitro results in increased β-cleavage products; although expression of an antisense oligonucleotide against BACE1 reduces the generation of β-cleavage products (Vassar et al, 1999; Yan et al, 1999). Consistent with the site for Aβ generation, BACE1 is intracellularly localized to the Golgi apparatus, secretory vesicles, endosomes and the cell surface. Tunicamycin or Nglycosidase F treatment in vitro abolishes the Nglycosylation of BACE1 in cells (Haniu et al, 2000), suggesting that posttranslational modification of BACE1 occurs during transport from ER to the cell surface. Trafficking of BACE1 through the Golgi apparatus requires the cytoplasmic tail of BACE1, and deletion of the C-terminal region of BACE1 prevents maturation. However, a soluble BACE1 molecule, without the transmembrane domain and the cytoplasmic tail, matures at an enhanced rate as compared to full length BACE1 (Capell et al, 2000). Although there is a cytoplasmic di-Leucine motif that may direct BACE1 to endosomes, there is no co-localization of BACE1 with lysosomal markers, and the half-life of BACE1 is over 16 hrs. (Huse et al, 2000) β-secretase activity is the highest in compartments of the secretary pathway, including the Golgi apparatus, secretory vesicles, and endosomes. It is possible that even a small increase in the amount of BACE1 protein in the brain would have a significant impact on Aβ production.

III. PATHOLOGY OF BACE1 IN AD BRAINS

Because BACE1 has been localized to the neurons in the brain, we can assume that they are the main source for β- amyloid peptides. Adversely, astrocytes, have been known to provide trophic support to neurons, form protective barriers between β-amyloid deposits and neurons, as well as their importance in the clearance and degradation of β- amyloid. Recently, we and two other independent research groups demonstrated an elevation of BACE1 activity in brain tissue of sporadic AD cases particularly, temporal cortex, hippocampus (Yang et al, 2003; Holsinger et al, 2002; Fukumoto et al, 2002). BACE1 mRNA is distributed in entire brain regions at moderate levels (Vassar et al, 1999; Sinha et al, 1999). Moreover, we have found that BACE1 mRNA expression levels are increased in AD brains although two recent studies (Holsinger et al, 2002; Gatta et al, 2002) failed to detect the difference in BACE1 mRNA in tissues from AD and non-demented brains. We noticed that both studies used tissues had long PMIs (> than 8 hrs). Northern blot analysis demonstrated non-differentiable or non- detectable BACE1 expression in the tissues with long PMIs. Furthermore, both studies lacked age-matched control tissues, and included a wide range of ages (from 53-86 years), as well as a wide range of MMSE scores, which might increase variability. Our laboratory has access to tissues with short PMI (< 3hrs), preserving intact RNA, and a large brain bank from which to select age-matched tissue samples. Therefore, it is important to rigorously examine BACE1 mRNA in the AD and non-demented (ND) brain tissue using our technologies.

Increases of BACE1 levels in sporadic AD brains may suggest that either BACE1 promotes Aβ production and AD, or it is just an epiphenomenon of late stage AD. BACE1 knockout mice did not show any production of β-amyloid, and did not have neuronal loss or specific memory deficits which are characteristic of AD associated pathologies. The fact that BACE1 directly initiates the generation of β- amyloid, and the observation that BACE1 levels are elevated in this disease provide direct and compelling reasons to develop mechanistic therapies directed at BACE1 inhibition thus reducing β-amyloid and its associated toxicities. However, new data indicates that complete abolishment of BACE1 may be associated with specific behavioral and physiological alterations.

IV. CLINICAL CSF STUDIES WITH BACE1 IN ALZHEIMER'S DISEASE

Since the CSF is in direct contact with the extracellular space of the central nervous system, biochemical changes in the brain can potentially be reflected in CSF. Recently, first studies have demonstrated measurement of BACE1 activity in CSF (Holsinger et al, 2006; Verheijen et al, 2006), of which one was a small pilot study indicating that BACE1 is slightly increased in AD and CJD compared with other dementia disorders and controls (Holsinger et al, 2006).

Our group was particularly interested in whether BACE1 could be identified in the CSF of subjects with MCI due to the high risk for AD in this population (Zhong et al, 2007). We used 2 sandwich enzyme-linked immunosorbent assays, for BACE1 enzymatic activities by means of synthetic fluorescence substrate, and total amyloid-beta peptide.

To discover the CSF levels of the BACE1 protein and their correlation to AD or MCI risk factors, we must first establish two BACE1 protein sandwich-ELISAs. The first used a combination of anti-BACE1 polyclonal antibody SECB2 as a capture antibody and biotinylated anti-BACE1 polyclonal antibody SECB1 as a detecting body. The second ELISA used anti-BACE1 polyclonal antibody B280 as a capture antibody, and anti-BACE1 monoclonal antibody (R&D) as a detection antibody. To compare our results, we used recombinant BACE1 from Amgen as the standard, and of course, assayed under the same conditions. The concentration of BACE1 was then calculated from the standard curve and expressed as μg/ml. BACE1 antibodies (R&D systems) were used to immunoprecipitate 200 of CSF from MCI, AD, and HC patients and incubated with Protein G-agarose (Sigma). For accuracy, the beads were washed four times with washing buffer and immunoprecipitates were eluted by boiling β-mercaptoethanol. We found increased CSF-levels of BACE1 protein which were associated with an increased risk ratio for MCI subjects when compared to HC (risk ratio = 2.08, 95% CI = 1.58 – 2.58) and AD (1.65, 95% CI = 1.19 – 2.03). Activity assays of BACE1 were performed by using synthetic peptide substrates containing the BACE1 cleavage site (Zhong et al, 2007) at a 50 mM concentration in reaction buffer. To examine BACE1 activity, 10μl of CSF from each sample was used, and to observe fluorescence, a fluorescent microplate reader with excitation wavelength at 320nm and emission wavelength at 383 was used. Similarly, MCI subjects showed increased levels of BACE1 activity when compared to HC (risk ratio = 2.17; 95% CI = 1.66 – 2.71) and AD (3.71, 95% CI = 2.74 – 4.36). CSF total tau (T-tau) was determined by using a sandwich ELISA that measured total tau: normal and hyperphosphorylated. For total Aβ and tau, increased CSF levels were associated with a higher risk of MCI when compared to HC. Due to these results, we were curious to see if there was a correlation between BACE1 activity and BACE1 protein level. Therefore, BACE1 cDNA was subcloned into pcDNA and Kozak sequence was added in front of the translation start codon. Next, 293T cells were split into two groups: one group was maintained in DMEM, and the other was transfected with 0.1μg and 0.5μg BACE1 expression plasmid by lipofectamine. Cells were then harvested after 48 hours of transfection, and both cells and brain tissue were homogenized in lysis buffer with PMSF and protease inhibitor mix. Western blot was then performed and BACE1 enzymatic activity assay and Deglycosylation were performed. BACE1 activity was significantly correlated with BACE1 protein level (Rho=0.23, P<0.001) and Aβ level (Rho=0.39, P<0.001), with Aβ being itself correlated with the BACE1 protein level (Rho=0.30, P<0.001) (Zhong et al, 2007).

BACE1 activities have been reported to be detectable in human CSF (Yan et al, 1999; Sinha et al, 1999; Yang et al, 2003). Our study demonstrated that we detected BACE1 levels and activities in CSF of AD and MCI subjects, as well as in healthy elderly controls and we found that CSF BACE1 levels and activity were significantly altered in MCI subjects but not in AD patients when compared to HC. Importantly, CSF BACE1 levels were statistically correlated with its activity. However, we noticed that the correlation was not very strong, this could be because: 1) of the possibility that other gamma-secretaselike enzymes could exist in the CSF, which could affect the BACE1 activity assay; 2) glycosylation interferes with the biological activity of proteins and affects their folding as well as stability (Andreasen et al, 2003). Recent proteomic studies showed glycosylation changes in AD (Hampel et al, 2004). BACE1 has been identified as 54kDa transmembrane protein with 4 potential glycolsylation sites (Herukka et al, 2005; Solfrizzi et al, 2004); three of four potential sites were found to be glycosylated in the ER16 and further processed in the Golgi, giving rise to a glycoprotein with heterogeneous oligosaccharides contributing to an apparent molecular weight of approximately 70KDa of the mature Endo-H-resistant form of BACE1 (Herukka et al, 2005; Jack et al, 1999). Glycosylation has been reported to play an important role in BACE1 enzymatic activity (Maruyama et al, 2004). Increased BACE1 maturation contributes to increased BACE1 enzymatic activity and increased Aβ production. When treated with the drug Tunicamycin, which inhibits N-glycosylation, BACE1 activity was reduced (Maruyama et al, 2004), which is consistent with our results that showed that immature BACE1 protein exhibited much lower enzyme activity than the mature BACE1 protein. Glycosylation can also affect protein folding. This reminded us that in our experiment and previous studies (Farrer et al, 1997; Skoog et al, 2003) nonglycosylated BACE1 protein expressed in E. coli system could easily form insoluble inclusion bodies, suggesting that full glycosylation in mammalian cells could be critical for solubility and stability of BACE1 protein. In our study, BACE1 ELISA assays detected total BACE1 levels. On the other hand, our study showed BACE1 enzymatic activity correlated with mature BACE1 level instead of total BACE1 level; this might be the reason why the correlation between BACE1 levels and activity was low in our assay.

V. PERSPECTIVES OF NEUROCHEMICAL BIOMARKER DEVELOPMENT IN ALZHEIMER'S DISEASE

A number of in vivo neurochemistry and neuroimaging techniques, which can reliably assess aspects of physiology, pathology, chemistry, and neuroanatomy, hold promise as biological markers. These neurobiological measures appear to relate closely to pathophysiological, neuropathological and clinical data, such as hyperphosphorylation of tau, abeta metabolism (such as BACE1), lipid peroxidation, pattern and rate of atrophy, loss of neuronal integrity, functional and cognitive decline, as well as risk of future decline. CSF levels of Aβ42, total tau (Hampel et al, 2004) and phosphorylated-tau (p-tau), as single markers and even more pronounced in combination (Hanson et al, 2006) can distinguish subjects with MCI who are likely to progress to AD. They also show preclinical alterations that predict later development of early AD symptoms. Studies on plasma Aβ are not entirely consistent, but recent findings suggest that decreased plasma Aβ42 relative to Aβ40 may increase the risk of AD (Graff-Radford et al, 2007). Increased production of Aβ in aging is suggested by elevation of BACE-1 protein and enzyme activity in the brain and CSF of subjects with MCI. CSF tau and p-tau are increased in MCI subjects, as well and show promising predictive value (Buerger et al, 2005; Buerger et al, 2002; Ewers et al, 2007). Other biomarkers may indicate components of a cascade initiated by Aβ, such as oxidative stress or inflammation, merit further study in MCI and subjects in early stages. Other interesting novel marker candidates derived from blood are being currently proposed (phase I stage of development). Biomarker discovery through proteomic approaches requires further research. Large-scale international controlled multicenter trials (such as the US-, European-, Australian- and Japanese ADNI and the German Dementia Network) are engaged in phase III stage of development of the proposed core feasible imaging and CSF biomarker candidates in AD (Frank et al, 2003).

Core feasible biological marker candidates of mechanisms related to AD pathology are in an ever maturing process leading to implementation as secondary and even primary outcome variables into regulatory guideline documents regarding study design and approval for novel compounds claiming disease modification.

REFERENCES

Andreasen, N., Vanmechelen, E., Vanderstichele, H., Davidsson, P., & Blennow, K. (2003). Cerebrospinal fluid levels of total-tau, phospho-tau and A beta 42 predicts development of Alzheimer's disease in patients with mild cognitive impairment. *Acta Neurologica Scandinavica*, *179*, 47–51. doi:10.1034/j.1600-0404.107.s179.9.x

Buerger, K., Ewers, M., Andreasen, N., Zinkowski, R., Ishiguro, K., & Vanmechelen, E. (1502-1503). … Hampel, H. (2005). Phosphorylated tau predicts rate of cognitive decline in MCI subjects: A comparative CSF study. *Neurology*, *65*(9).

Buerger, K., Zinkowski, R., Teipel, S. J., Tapiola, T., Arai, H., & Blennow, K. (2002). Differential diagnosis of Alzheimer disease with cerebrospinal fluid levels of tau protein phosphorylated at threonine. *Archives of Neurology*, *59*(8), 1267–1272. doi:10.1001/archneur.59.8.1267

Capell, A., Steiner, H., Willem, M., Kaiser, H., Meyer, C., & Walter, J. (2000). Maturation and propeptide cleavage of beta-secretase. *The Journal of Biological Chemistry*, *275*(40), 30849–30854. doi:10.1074/jbc.M003202200

Ewers, M., Buerger, K., Teipel, S. J., Scheltens, P., Schroeder, J., Zinkowski, R., … Hampel, H. (2007). *Multicenter assessment of CSF-phosphorylated tau for the prediction of conversion of MCI.*

Farrer, L. A., Cupples, L. A., Haines, J. L., Hyman, B., Kukull, W. A., & Mayeux, R. (1997). Effects of age, sex, and ethnicity on the association between apolipoprotein E genotype and Alzheimer disease. A meta-analysis. [APOE and Alzheimer Disease Meta Analysis Consortium]. *Journal of the American Medical Association*, *278*(16), 1349–1356. doi:10.1001/jama.278.16.1349

Frank, R. A., Galasko, D., Hampel, H., Hardy, J., de Leon, M. J., & Mehta, P. D. (2003). Biological markers for therapeutic trials in Alzheimer's disease. *Neurobiology of Aging*, *24*(4), 521–536. doi:10.1016/S0197-4580(03)00002-2

Fukumoto, H., Cheung, B. S., Hyman, B. T., & Irizarry, M. C. (2002). Beta-secretase protein and activity are increased in the neocortex in Alzheimer disease. *Archives of Neurology*, *59*(9), 1381–1389. doi:10.1001/archneur.59.9.1381

Gatta, L. B., Albertini, A., Ravid, R., & Finazzi, D. (2002). Levels of beta-secretase BACE and alpha-secretase ADAM10 mRNAs in Alzheimer hippocampus. *Neuroreport*, *13*(16), 2031–2033. doi:10.1097/00001756-200211150-00008

Graff-Radford, N. R., Crook, J. E., Lucas, J., Boeve, B. F., Knopman, D. S., & Ivnik, R. J. (2007). Association of low plasma Abeta42/Abeta40 ratios with increased imminent risk for mild cognitive impairment and Alzheimer disease. *Archives of Neurology*, *64*(3), 354–362. doi:10.1001/archneur.64.3.354

Hampel, H., Teipel, S. J., Fuchsberger, T., Andreasen, N., Wiltfang, J., & Otto, M. (2004, Jul). Value of CSF beta-amyloid1-42 and tau as predictors of Alzheimer's disease in patients with mild cognitive impairment. *Molecular Psychiatry*, *9*(7), 705–710.

Haniu, M., Denis, P., Young, Y., Mendiaz, E. A., Fuller, J., & Hui, J. O. (2000). Characterization of Alzheimer's beta -secretase protein BACE. A pepsin family member with unusual properties. *The Journal of Biological Chemistry*, *275*(28), 21099–21106. doi:10.1074/jbc.M002095200

Hanson, R. L., Looker, H. C., Ma, L., Muller, Y. L., Baier, L. J., & Knowler, W. C. (2006). Design and analysis of genetic association studies to finely map a locus identified by linkage analysis: Sample size and power calculations. *Annals of Human Genetics*, *70*(3), 332–349. doi:10.1111/j.1529-8817.2005.00230.x

Herukka, S. K., Hallikainen, M., Soininen, H., & Pirttila, T. (2005). CSF Abeta42 and tau or phosphorylated tau and prediction of progressive mild cognitive impairment. *Neurology*, *64*(7), 1294–1297.

Holsinger, R. M., Lee, J. S., Boyd, A., Masters, C. L., & Collins, S. J. (2006). CSF BACE1 activity is increased in CJD and Alzheimer disease versus other dementias. *Neurology*, *67*(4), 710–712. doi:10.1212/01.wnl.0000229925.52203.4c

Holsinger, R. M., McLean, C. A., Beyreuther, K., Masters, C. L., & Evin, G. (2002). Increased expression of the amyloid precursor beta-secretase in Alzheimer's disease. *Annals of Neurology*, *51*(6), 783–786. doi:10.1002/ana.10208

Huse, J. T., & Doms, R. W. (2000). Closing in on the amyloid cascade: recent insights into the cell biology of Alzheimer's disease. *Molecular Neurobiology*, *22*(1-3), 81–98.

Jack, C. R. Jr, Petersen, R. C., Xu, Y. C., O'Brien, P. C., Smith, G. E., & Ivnik, R. J. (1999). Prediction of AD with MRI-based hippocampal volume in mild cognitive impairment. *Neurology*, *52*(7), 1397–1403.

Lee, M. S., Kao, S. C., Lemere, C. A., Xia, W., Tseng, H. C., & Zhou, Y. (2003). APP processing is regulated by cytoplasmic phosphorylation. *The Journal of Cell Biology*, *163*(1), 83–95. doi:10.1083/jcb.200301115

Lin, X., Koelsch, G., Wu, S., Downs, D., Dashti, A., & Tang, J. (2000). Human aspartic protease memapsin 2 cleaves the beta-secretase site of betaamyloid precursor protein. *Proceedings of the National Academy of Sciences of the United States of America*, *97*(4), 1456–1460. doi:10.1073/pnas.97.4.1456

Maruyama, M., Matsui, T., Tanji, H., Nemoto, M., Tomita, N., & Ootsuki, M. (2004). Cerebrospinal fluid tau protein and periventricular white matter lesions in patients with mild cognitive impairment: Implications for 2 major pathways. *Archives of Neurology*, *61*(5), 716–720. doi:10.1001/archneur.61.5.716

Sinha, S., Anderson, J. P., Barbour, R., Basi, G. S., Caccavello, R., & Davis, D. (1999). Purification and cloning of amyloid precursor protein beta-secretase from human brain. *Nature*, *402*(6761), 537–540. doi:10.1038/990114

Skoog, I., Davidsson, P., Aevarsson, O., Vanderstichele, H., Vanmechelen, E., & Blennow, K. (2003). Cerebrospinal fluid beta-amyloid 42 is reduced before the onset of sporadic dementia: A population-based study in 85-yearolds. *Dementia and Geriatric Cognitive Disorders*, *15*(3), 169–176. doi:10.1159/000068478

Solfrizzi, V., Panza, F., Colacicco, A. M., D'Introno, A., Capurso, C., & Torres, F. (2004). Vascular risk factors, incidence of MCI, and rates of progression to dementia. *Neurology*, *63*(10), 1882–1891.

Vassar, R., Bennett, B. D., Babu-Khan, S., Kahn, S., Mendiaz, E. A., & Denis, P. (1999). Beta-secretase cleavage of Alzheimer's amyloid precursor protein by the transmembrane aspartic protease BACE. *Science*, *286*(5440), 735–741. doi:10.1126/science.286.5440.735

Verheijen, J. H., Huisman, L. G., van Lent, N., Neumann, U., Paganetti, P., & Hack, C. E. (2006). Detection of a soluble form of BACE-1 in human cerebrospinal fluid by a sensitive activity assay. *Clinical Chemistry*, *52*(6), 1168–1174. doi:10.1373/clinchem.2006.066720

Yan, R., Bienkowski, M. J., Shuck, M. E., Miao, H., Tory, M. C., & Pauley, A. M. (1999). Membraneanchored aspartyl protease with Alzheimer's disease beta-secretase activity. *Nature*, *402*(6761), 533–537. doi:10.1038/990107

Yang, L. B., Lindholm, K., Yan, R., Citron, M., Xia, W., & Yang, X. L. (2003). Elevated beta-secretase expression and enzymatic activity detected in sporadic Alzheimer disease. *Nature Medicine*, *9*(1), 3–4. doi:10.1038/nm0103-3

Zhong, Z., Ewers, M., Teipel, S., Burger, K., Wallin, A., & Blennow, K. (2007). Levels of beta-secretase (BACE1) in cerebrospinal fluid as a predictor of risk in mild cognitive impairment. *Archives of General Psychiatry*, *64*(6), 718–726. doi:10.1001/archpsyc.64.6.718

KEY TERMS AND DEFINITIONS

Alzheimer's Disease: A progressive neurodegenerative disease that is characterized by a loss of neurons and synapses in the cerebral cortex and certain subcortical regions. Which is named for German physician Alois Alzheimer, who first described it in 1906.

Amyloid β-Peptide: A peptide of 39–43 amino acids that appears to be the main constituent of amyloid plaques in the brains of Alzheimer's disease patients.

BACE1: An aspartic-acid protease important in the pathogenesis of Alzheimer's disease, and in the formation of myelin sheaths in peripheral nerve cells.

Biomarker: In general a substance used as an indicator of a biological state.

mRNA: A molecule of RNA encoding a chemical "blueprint" for a protein product.

Neurodegenerative Diseases: Degenerative nerve diseases cause worsening of many of your body's activities, including balance, movement, talking, breathing and heart function.

Chapter 16
Aβ Monomer, Oligomer and Fibril in Alzheimer's Disease

Hiroshi Mori
Department of Neuroscience, Osaka City University Medical School, Japan

ABSTRACT

*Alzheimer's disease (AD), the most prevalent disease of aged people, is a progressive neurodegenerative disorder with dementia. Amyloid-β (also known as β-protein and referred to here as Aβ) is a well-established, seminal peptide in AD that is produced from the amyloid precursor protein (APP) by consecutive digestion with the β secretase of BACE (beta-site amyloid cleaving enzyme) and gamma secretase of the presenilin complex. Abnormal cerebral accumulation of Abeta in the form of insoluble fibrils in senile plaques and cerebral amyloid angiopathy (CAA) is a neuropathological hallmark of AD. In contrast to insoluble fibrillary Aβ, a soluble oligomeric complex, ADDL, consists of low-n oligomers of Aβ, such as Aβ*56. Despite their different names, it is currently proposed that oligomeric Aβ is directly involved in synaptic toxicity and cognitive dysfunction in the early stages of AD. This chapter identifies a novel APP mutation (E693delta; referred to as the Osaka mutation) in a pedigree with probable AD, resulting in a variant Aβ lacking glutamate at position 22. Based on theoretical predictions and in vitro studies on synthetic mutant Aβ peptides, the mutated Aβ peptide showed a unique and enhanced oligomerization activity without fibrillization. This was further confirmed by PiB-PET analysis on the proband patient. Collectively, the chapter concludes that the Osaka mutation is the first human evidence for the hypothesis that oligomeric Aβ is involved in AD.*

I. INTRODUCTION

Alzheimer's disease (AD) is a well-known, progressive neurodegenerative disorder with dementia. The neuropathological features of AD include senile plaques and neurofibrillary tangles in addition to cerebral atrophy from massive neuronal loss.

DOI: 10.4018/978-1-60960-559-9.ch016

Amyloid-β (also known as β-protein and referred to here as Aβ) is a well-established, seminal peptide in AD that is produced from the amyloid precursor protein (APP) by consecutive digestion with the β-secretase of BACE and gamma-secretase of the presenilin complex. Abnormal cerebral accumulation of Aβ in the form of insoluble fibrils in senile plaques and cerebral amyloid angiopathy (CAA) is widely believed to cause AD. In contrast to insoluble Aβ fibrils, a soluble, nonfibrillary oligomeric complex is currently claimed as a new pathological Aβ species. It has been termed ADDLs (Lambert et al, 1998), low-n oligomer Aβ, dimer (Walsh et al, 2002), Abeta*56 (Lesne et al, 2006) (here, Aβ oligomer collectively together). Despite these different names, it has recently been proposed that Aβ oligomer directly causes synaptic toxicity and cognitive dysfunction in the early stages of AD (Selkoe, 2002). To discuss Aβ oligomers in depth here, the relationship among ADDLs, Aβ oligomer, single oligomers of Aβ (mainly the dimeric form), and Aβ*56 should be explained. It is not easy to compare one Aβ oligomer with other morphologically characterized nonfibrillary Aβ species such as protofibrils (Walsh, Lomakin, Benedek, Condron, & Teplow, 1997), Globulomer (Gellermann et al, 2008), AβO (Kayed et al, 2003), Paranucleus (Bitan, Kirkitadze, Lomakin, Vollers, Benedek & Teplow, 2003), Annulus (Caughey & Lansbury, 2003), amyloidspheroid (Hoshi, 2003), βamyball (Westlind-Danielsson & Arnerup, 2001), (for review in detail, see [Roychaudhuri, Yang, Hoshi & Teplow, 2009]). With these views, new concepts focusing on nonfibrillary and soluble Aβ complex based on synaptic dysfunction are emerging regarding the cause of AD. Here, I review and discuss the Aβ oligomer, particularly based on our current knowledge of patients with early onset familial AD as the sole human evidence in support of the so-called "oligomer hypothesis" and its importance to advancing the research of AD etiology.

II. A FAMILIAL CASE WITH THE EARLY ONSET ALZHEIMER'S DISEASE

A. The Osaka Mutation of Amyloid Precursor Protein

The proband was a 62-year-old woman with a history of suspected familial AD. She noticed memory disturbance at the age of 56, and she had no history or symptoms of other neurological disorders. Her Hachinski's ischemic and Mini Mental State Examination (MMSE) scores were normal. MRI and PET scans showed no cortical atrophy or abnormal metabolism, while SPECT demonstrated bilateral mild hypoperfusion in the temporal lobes. An electroencephalogram showed bilateral, intermittent, generalized slow theta activity. Thus, she was diagnosed as having mild cognitive impairment at that time. At the age of 59, she showed ideomotor apraxia, and her MMSE score was 22/30 points. According to the Diagnostic and Statistical Manual of Mental Disorders (DSM-IIIR) and the criteria of the National Institute of Neurological and Communicative Disorders and Stroke, AD and Related Disorders Association (NINCDS-ADRDA), she was diagnosed as having AD. At the age of 62, her MMSE score dropped to 5, and she exhibited cerebellar ataxia. The axial T1-weighted MRI images showed only mild parietal lobe atrophy. Genetic analysis was performed after an appropriate consultation, at which the caregiver gave informed consent to participate in this study. This study was approved by the institutional ethics committee of Osaka City University Graduate School of Medicine. Exons 16 and 17 of APP and all exons of presenilins-1 and -2 were amplified from the patient's genomic DNA by PCR. The DNA sequence of each product was analyzed using a BigDye Terminator v1.1 Cycle Sequencing Kit (Applied Biosystems, Tokyo, Japan) and an ABI PRISM 310 genetic analyzer (Applied Biosystems). Because this patient was found to have a mutation in exon 17 of the APP but not in the exons 1 or 2 of presenilin, only APP exon 17 was examined from other family members. Apolipoprotein E (ApoE) genotyping was performed by detection of the restriction site polymorphism, as described previously (Gellermann et al, 2008).

From the patient and her family members, we identified a novel mutation (hereafter referred to as the Osaka mutation) in APP exon 17. This mutation results in the deletion of codon 693 encoding glutamate (E693delta) at position 22 in the Aβ sequence (Tomiyama et al, 2008). The patient had a homozygous deletion, and her unaffected older and younger sisters showed only heterozygous deletions. The ApoE genotype appeared not to be associated with this familial case.

B. Prevalence of the Osaka Mutation

The Osaka mutation is the first deletion-type mutation to be identified in the APP. To explore if this novel mutation occurred in other members of the population, we screened 5,310 Japanese who were recruited for the Japanese Genetic Study Consortium for AD. They included patients with AD (n = 2,121), mild cognitive impairment (MCI; n = 128), dementia with Lewy bodies (n = 74), other neurological diseases (n = 446) and control subjects (n = 2,541). Clinical AD cases met the criteria of the NINCDS-ADRDA. Informed consent was obtained from all control subjects and appropriate proxies for patients. We found the Osaka mutation allele in five pedigrees in all subjects examined.

The homozygous deletion described above was rare but was found in two other pedigrees with AD (one of which exhibited mild cognitive impairment, and the other was normal); the heterozygous deletion was found in three other pedigrees. These findings strongly suggest that the Osaka mutation is a cause of AD. In addition, this mutation might represent the first recessive inheritance linked to familial AD in humans. However, any conclusion that the Osaka mutation is functionally recessive cannot be drawn from the limited information. Recently, a different recessive mutation in the APP gene was reported (Di Fede et al, 2009). However, conclusions as to whether these two mutations are recessive can only be concluded from further evidence (e.g., by model animals).

C. Characterization of the Osaka Mutation

To identify Aβ species produced from the mutant APP, we examined the molecular mass of Aβ secreted from HEK293 cells transfected with the APP construct. The resultant Aβ was found to start and end at normal positions but lack a glutamate at position 22. The secretion of the mutant Aβ1-42 and Aβ1-40 were both reduced to ~60% of wild-type Aβ levels, but the Aβ1-42/Aβ1-40 ratio was unaffected. This lowered Aβ secretion may explain why the Osaka mutation appears to be recessive, but the issue remains to be further investigated.

To examine their aggregation properties, mutant Aβ1-40deltaE and Aβ1-42deltaE peptides, which lack a glutamate at position 22, were synthesized (American Peptide Company, Sunnyvale, CA). Molecular weights and amino acid compositions of the peptides were confirmed by electrospray mass spectral analysis and amino acid analysis, respectively. The purity of the Aβ1-40deltaE and Aβ1- 42deltaE peptides, which was determined by reverse-phase HPLC, was 95.0 and 91.0%, respectively. Control wild-type Aβ1-40 and Aβ1-42 peptides were obtained from the American Peptide Company and Peptide Institute (Osaka, Japan). In a thioflavin-T (ThT) fluorescence assay, wild-type peptides showed a quick increase of fibril aggregation, whereas the mutant peptides exhibited little or no increase. On western blots, synthetic Aβpeptides were initially dissolved to 0.1 mM in the alpha-helix- promoting solvent hexafluoroisopropanol (HFIP, Sigma), and the solvent was evaporated under vacuum using a Savant Speed Vac system (GMI, Ramsey, MN). The dried peptides were resuspended to 1 mM in 0.1% NH_4OH and dispensed, in quadruplicate, into tubes containing PBS to a peptide concentration of 100 μM. The peptide solutions were incubated at 37°C for 7 days, and aliquots were taken every 24 h to monitor peptide aggregation by the ThT fluorescence assay. For western blotting, the aliquots were diluted 10-fold in SDS sample buffer and boiled for 5 min. After a further 200-fold dilution in SDS sample buffer, 4 μl (equivalent to 0.2 pmol Aβ peptide) of sample was separated by SDS-PAGE on a 12% NuPage Bis-Tris gel (Invitrogen, Tokyo, Japan) and transferred to Immobilon-P polyvinylidene difluoride (PVDF) membranes (Millipore, Tokyo, Japan). The membranes were boiled in PBS for 10 min to enhance signals and blocked overnight with 3% BSA/1% skim milk/0.1% Tween 20/150 mM NaCl/50 mM Tris-HCl, pH 7.6. Aβ peptides were probed with 6E10 or β001, followed by horseradish peroxidase (HRP)-labeled anti-mouse or anti-rabbit antibody (Bio-Rad Laboratories, Tokyo, Japan), respectively. Wild-type peptides showed a rapid decrease in the proportion of monomers, reflecting their aggregation into fibrils, but the mutant peptides only gradually decreased. However, the mutant peptides showed massive formation of SDS-stable oligomers (dimers, trimers and tetramers) immediately after solubilization.

The peptide aliquots were adsorbed onto 200-mesh Formvar-coated copper grids and negative-stained with 2% uranyl acetate. The specimens were viewed using a JEM-1200EXII electron microscope (JEOL, Tokyo, Japan), showing that wild-type Aβ1-42 peptide formed abundant fibrils during the 7-day incubation, whereas virtually no fibrillization was observed in the mutant peptide. Thus, the mutant peptides were shown to rapidly form stable oligomers but not to transform into fibrils. It has been proposed that the formation of a β-turn at positions 22 and 23 in Aβ molecules plays a crucial role in peptide aggregation (Morimoto, 2004). The Osaka mutation at position 22 may cause disruption of the secondary structure of the peptide necessary for its formation into fibrils. The lack of a polar amino acid (glutamate) should lead to increased hydrophobicity of the peptide, which may result in accelerated assembly of the peptides into oligomers.

D. Amyloid Imaging of Patients with the Osaka Mutation

The unique aggregation property of the mutant Aβ highly suggested no amyloid formation in the patient's brain. To assess this possibility, we performed PET amyloid imaging of the patients' brains with [11C]-Pittsburgh compound-B (PiB) using a PET scanner Eminence-B (Shimadzu Corp., Kyoto, Japan), which was composed of 352 detector blocks, each with a 6 x 8 array of $3.5 \times 6.25 \times 30$ mm^3 bismuth germinate oxyorthosilicate crystals, arranged as 32 crystal rings in a 208 mm axial field of view. Transmission scans were performed before PiB administration for 5 min in singles mode with a 137Cs point source to obtain attenuation correction data. Emission data were acquired over 60 min (29 frames: 6×30 s, 12×60 s, 5 × 180 s, 6 × 300 s). Images were reconstructed with segmented attenuation correction using Fourier rebinning followed by two-dimensional filtered back-projection, applying a Ramp filter cutoff at the Nyquist frequency. A three-dimensional Gaussian filter with a kernel full-width of a half maximum of 5 mm was applied to the images as a post filter.

All subjects had an intravenous bolus injection of 150-300 MBq PiB with a high specific activity (average 20-30GBq/micro mol). PiB retention data are presented as standard uptake values, as described previously (Klunk et al, 2004). Slight but significant PiB retention signals were observed in the temporal, parietal and occipital lobes and cerebellum but not in the frontal lobe, which was apparently different from most cases of AD. Thus, the absence of fibril formation of the mutant Aβ was observed *in vivo* in two homozygous patients with the Osaka mutation.

Amyloid imaging with PiB-PET is dependent on the presence of some Aβ fibrils but not on the Aβ oligomer. It is worth using for clinical data purposes because it can specifically detect the cerebral amyloid burden. These results from our patients with the Osaka mutation indirectly support the lack of Aβ fibrils, at least enough to explain the clinical course of severe illness.

III. BEYOND AMYLOID PLAQUES

The clinical concern for patients with the Osaka mutation revolves around whether they possess the variant mutation or can be classified as conventional AD. The mutation seemed to be of the recessive type by human genetic analysis, although we cannot conclude that the Osaka mutation is functionally recessive. It is widely believed that the Aβ oligomer demonstrates synaptotoxicity and is currently important at least in the early stage of the disease process, such as in mild cognitive impairment (MCI), although we cannot ultimately or exclusively specify the pathological oligomeric form yet. Despite such current knowledge, we should be aware of considerable evidence that suggests the involvement of senile plaques in the disease etiology, even if most observations are indirect or encounter the possibility that Aβ fibrils are *in vitro* admixed with non-fibrillary Aβ in a previously tested milieu. To remove ambiguity and to provide concrete evidence, the pure AD form of the Aβ oligomer without Aβ fibrils would be the best form to investigate. The pre-clinical stage that can be retrospectively referred must be further examined. The Osaka mutation is thus expected to identify the causal Aβ molecule due to the sole presence of Aβ oligomer by excluding concomitant fibrillar Aβ. One of the most critical examinations may undoubtedly be neuropathology testing of the patients with the Osaka mutation. In the mean time, model animals expressing the Osaka mutation and mimic AD should be fully examined.

There are several issues regarding the Aβ oligomer that should be addressed. Does the Aβ oligomer induce tau pathology? Does the Aβ oligomer result in cerebral atrophy by itself without Aβ fibrils? The most striking feature of the fibrillar Aβ aggregates is associated with neurotoxicity (Yankner, Dawes, Fisher, Villa-Komaroff, Oster-Granite, & Neve, 1989). Observing dystrophic neurites and spines (Spires, 2005) also revealed strong curvatures near the close plaques. Both properties are associated with the plaque hypothesis, although indirectly, and they do not exclude the possible co-occurrence of Aβ in an oligomeric form.

IV. PERSPECTIVE

There is growing evidence that reinforces the significance of Aβ oligomers. It is unclear as to the processes that control the *in vitro* and *in vivo* pathogenic formation of Aβ oligomer, though it may be simple to detect the Aβ oligomer under some conditions. It is important to understand the mechanisms of the pathogenic Aβ oligomer itself to develop diagnostic and therapeutic treatments that could target this molecule.

ACKNOWLEDGMENT

I would like to thank my many collaborators, including Drs. Takami Tomiyama, Hiroyuki Shimada, Suzuka Ataka, Hiroshi Takuma, Kennichi Ishibashi, Kiyouhisa Ohnishi, Rie Teraoka, Akiko Fukushima, Hyoue Kanemitsu, Ryozo Kuwano, Masaki Imagawa, Keiichi Yamamoto, Takami Miki, Shogo Matsuyama, Hiroyuki Iso, Tetsu Nagata, Tomoyuki Nishizaki, Yasuhiro Wada, Eito Yoshioka, Yasuyoshi Watanabe, and Drs. Yasuo Ihara, Haruhiko Akiyama, Tetsuaki Arai and Kenji Ikeda for their helpful discussion. Thanks to all of the patients, subjects and their families for their co-operation with the genetic analyses. This study was supported by the Grants-in-aid for Scientific Research on Priority Areas - Research on Pathomechanisms of Brain Disorders from MEXT of Japan, Nos. 17300114, 18023033, 20023026, and 20023026, and in part by the Alzheimer's Association (IIRG-09-132098).

REFERENCES

Bitan, G., Kirkitadze, M. D., Lomakin, A., Vollers, S. S., Benedek, G. B., & Teplow, D. B. (2003). Amyloid β-protein (Aβ) assembly: Abeta 40 and Abeta 42 oligomerize through distinct pathways. *Proceedings of the National Academy of Sciences of the United States of America*, *100*, 330–335. doi:10.1073/pnas.222681699

Caughey, B., & Lansbury, P. T. (2003). Protofibrils, pores, fibrils, and neurodegeneration: Separating the responsible protein aggregates from the innocent bystanders. *Annual Review of Neuroscience*, *26*, 267–298. doi:10.1146/annurev.neuro.26.010302.081142

Di Fede, G., Catania, M., Morbin, M., Rossi, G., Suardi, S., & Mazzoleni, G. (2009). A recessive mutation in the APP gene withdominant-negative effect on amyloidogenesis. *Science*, *323*, 1473–1477. doi:10.1126/science.1168979

Gellermann, G. P., Byrnes, H., Striebinger, A., Ullrich, K., Mueller, R., Hillen, H., & Barghorn, S. (2008). Abeta-globulomers are formed independently of the fibril pathway. *Neurobiological Disorders*, *30*, 212–220. doi:10.1016/j.nbd.2008.01.010

Hoshi, M., Sato, M., Matsumoto, S., Noguchi, A., Yasutake, K., Yoshida, N., & Sato, K. (2003). Spherical aggregates of beta-amyloid (amylospheroid) show high neurotoxicity and activate tau protein kinase I/glycogen synthase kinase-3β. *Proceedings of the National Academy of Sciences of the United States of America*, *100*, 6370–6375. doi:10.1073/pnas.1237107100

Kayed, R., Head, E., Thompson, J. L., McIntire, T. M., Milton, S. C., Cotman, C. W., & Glabe, C. G. (2003). Common structure of soluble amyloid oligomers implies common mechanism of pathogenesis. *Science*, *300*, 486–489. doi:10.1126/science.1079469

Klunk, W. E., Engler, H., Nordberg, A., Wang, Y., Blomqvist, G., & Holt, D. P. (2004). Imagingbrain amyloid in Alzheimer's disease with Pittsburgh compound-B. *Annals of Neurology*, *55*, 306–319. doi:10.1002/ana.20009

Lambert, M. P., Barlow, A. K., Chromy, B. A., Edwards, C., Freed, R., & Liosatos, M. … Klein, W. L. (1998). Diffusible, nonfibrillar ligands derived from Aβ1-42 are potent central nervous system neurotoxins. *Proceedings of the National Academy of Sciences USA, 95*, 6448–6453.

Lesne, S., Koh, M. T., Kotilinek, L., Kayed, R., Glabe, C. G., & Yang, A. (2006). A specific amyloid-β protein assembly in the brain impairs memory. *Nature*, *440*, 352–357. doi:10.1038/nature04533

Morimoto, A., Irie, K., Murakami, K., Masuda, Y., Ohigashi, H., & Nagao, M. (2004). Analysis of thesecondary structure of β-amyloid (Aβ42) fibrils by systematic prolinere placement. *The Journal of Biological Chemistry*, *279*, 52781–52788. doi:10.1074/jbc.M406262200

Roychaudhuri, R., Yang, M., Hoshi, M. M., & Teplow, D. B. (2009). Amyloid-protein assembly and Alzheimer disease. *The Journal of Biological Chemistry*, *284*, 4749–4753. doi:10.1074/jbc.R800036200

Selkoe, D. J. (2002). Alzheimer's disease is a synaptic failure. *Science*, *298*, 789–791. doi:10.1126/science.1074069

Spires, T. L., Meyer-Luehmann, M., Stern, E. A., McLean, P. J., Skoch, J., & Nguyen, P. T. (2005). Dendritic spine abnormalities in amyloid precursor protein transgenic mice demonstrated by gene transfer and intravital multiphoton microscopy. *The Journal of Neuroscience*, *25*, 7278–7287. doi:10.1523/JNEUROSCI.1879-05.2005

Tomiyama, T., Nagata, T., Shimada, H., Teraoka, R., Fukushima, A., & Kanemitsu, H. (2008). A new Amyloid β variant favoring oligomerization in Alzheimer's-type dementia. *Annals of Neurology*, *63*, 377–387. doi:10.1002/ana.21321

Walsh, D. M., Klyubin, I., Fadeeva, J. V., Cullen, W. K., Anwyl, R., & Wolfe, M. S. (2002). Naturally secreted oligomers of amyloid β protein potently inhibit hippocampal long-term potentiation in vivo. *Nature*, *416*, 535–539. doi:10.1038/416535a

Walsh, D. M., Lomakin, A., Benedek, G. B., Condron, M. M., & Teplow, D. B. (1997). Amyloid beta-protein fibrillogenesis. Detection of a protofibrillar intermediate. *The Journal of Biological Chemistry*, *272*, 22364–22372. doi:10.1074/jbc.272.35.22364

Westlind-Danielsson, A., & Arnerup, G. (2001). Spontaneous in vitro formation of supramolecular β-amyloid structures, βamyballs, by β- amyloid 1-40 peptide. *Biochemistry*, *40*, 14736–14743. doi:10.1021/bi010375c

Yankner, B. A., Dawes, L. R., Fisher, S., Villa-Komaroff, L., Oster-Granite, M. L., & Neve, R. L. (1989). Neurotoxicity of a fragment of the amyloid precursor associated with Alzheimer's disease. *Science*, *245*, 417–420. doi:10.1126/science.2474201

KEY TERMS AND DEFINITIONS

Aβ: A small protein, with the molecular size of ~4,700, derived from its precursor protein (APP). Aβ is composed of 40 to 43 amino acids. The most important and pathologically significant species is widely believed to be composed of 42 amino acids, referred to as Aβ1-42 or Aβ42. Aβ oligomer: This refers to a molecular concept for an Aβ complex or assembly that is neither monomeric nor a polymer of morphological fibrils but composed of few to several constituents of the Aβ protein. Currently, there are several names for Aβ oligomers, among which there are no clear explanations.

ADDLs: Aβ-derived diffusible ligands. Their molecular sizes are various, ranging from 17 kDa to 42 or 56 kDa. Low-n oligomer Aβ: The low-n refers to two or several Aβ molecules, but the actual number is still unclear. Aβ*56: The name for an Aβ oligomer species that is a 56-kDa soluble Aβ assembly. The Osaka mutation: An APP mutation (E693delta) lacking a glutamate at position 22 of Aβ. A variant Aβ with this mutation shows the peculiar property of enhanced oligomerization but little fibril formation.

Neuroimaging: The use of various techniques to either directly or indirectly image the structure and/or function/pharmacology of the brain. It is a relatively new discipline within medicine and neuroscience/psychology.

Neuroanatomy: The study of the anatomy of nervous tissue and neural structures of the nervous system.

Neuroscience: The scientific study of the nervous system.

Chapter 17
The Value of Quantitative EEG Measures in the Early Diagnosis of Alzheimer's Disease

Hideaki Tanaka
Department of Neurology, Dokkyo Medical University, Japan

ABSTRACT

There is growing interest in the discovery of clinically useful, robust biomarkers for Alzheimer's disease (AD) and pre-AD; the ability to accurately diagnose AD or to predict conversion from a preclinical state to AD would aid in both prevention and early intervention. This study aimed to evaluate the usefulness of a statistical assessment of cortical activity using electroencephalograms (EEGs) with normative data and the ability of such an assessment to contribute to the diagnosis of AD. 15 patients with AD and 8 patients with mild cognitive impairment (MCI) were studied. Eyes-closed resting EEGs were digitally recorded at 200 Hz from 20 electrodes placed according to the international 10/20 system on the scalp, and 20 artifact-free EEG epochs lasting 2.56 ms were selected. Each EEG epoch was down-sampled to 100 Hz and matched to the normal data sets. The selected EEGs from each subject were analyzed by standardized Low Resolution Electromagnetic Tomography (sLORETA) and statistically compared with the age-matched normal data sets at all frequencies. This procedure resulted in cortical z values for each EEG frequency with 0.39 Hz frequency resolution for each subject. Some of the AD and MCI patients presented a peak of negative z value around 20 Hz, revealing hypoactivity of the parahippocampal gyrus and the insula in the sLORETA cortical image. In addition, severe cases of AD showed decreased parietal activation. These results were in agreement with evidence from statistical neuroimaging using MRI/SPECT. Submission of normal EEG data sets to sLORETA might be useful for the detection of diagnostic and predictive markers of AD and MCI in individual patients.

INTRODUCTION

Alzheimer's disease (AD) is usually preceded by a period of cognitive decline, and this preclinical or prodromal AD state has been conceptualized as mild cognitive impairment (MCI) by Petersen et al. (Petersen et al., 1999). However, MCI remains an unsettled prognosis; some people with MCI will not develop dementia, others may "revert" to normal, and many go on to develop dementia

DOI: 10.4018/978-1-60960-559-9.ch017

(especially AD). It is clear that the discovery of clinically useful and robust biomarkers for AD and pre-AD are necessary for clinicians to accurately diagnose AD and predict the conversion of a preclinical state of AD. Such markers would be ideal means of prevention and early intervention.

Since the proposal of MCI by Petersen et al. in 1999 (Petersen et al., 1999), predictive validation of the MCI condition using spontaneous EEGs and various quantitative methods has been accumulating. The neurophysiological changes recorded by EEG activity reflect the pathological cortical dysfunction of dementing disorders and may precede any pathological changes that are detectable by neuroimaging techniques (such as MRI, SPECT, and PET). Therefore, EEG recordings might catch the subtle changes involved in MCI in a preclinical stage of dementia. However, there is still insufficient evidence for the diagnostic utility of resting EEGs in dementia, and MCI is still not a sufficient diagnostic tool to establish dementia in the initial evaluation of subjects with cognitive impairment in routine clinical practice. It is necessary to develop optimized methods for establishing the diagnostic value of EEGs in a dementia diagnosis and the predictive utility of EEGs in MCI and questionable dementia. Our study aimed to determine whether automated EEG source localization with z-transformed age-appropriate population norms could identify AD and MCI individuals with a high degree of accuracy.

METHOD

Subjects

We studied 15 patients with AD based on the diagnostic criteria of the National Institute of Neurological and Communicative Disorders and Stroke and the Alzheimer's Disease and Related Disorders Association (NINDS-ADRDA) (McKhann et al., 1984) and 8 patients with MCI based on the guidelines of Petersen et al. (Petersen et al., 1999). All patients underwent general medical, neurological, neuropsychological, and brain MRI assessments as part of the standard diagnostic work-up for dementia. All subjects were assessed for general cognitive function using the Mini-Mental State Examination (MMSE) (see Table 1).

Procedure

EEG Recording

The EEGs were recorded from the 20 electrodes (Fp1/2, Fz, F3/4, F7/8, T3/4, C3/4, Cz, P3/4, Pz, T5/6, O1/2, Oz) of the international 10/20 system using a Neurofax EEG-1518 (Nihon-Khoden,

Table 1. Subject's information

	AD	MCI
Number	15	8
Gender (male/female)	6 / 9	6 / 2
Age (years; median, range)	75, 50-89	65.5, 49-79
MMSE (score; median, range)	18, 0-24	28, 25-30
Slightly impaired (number) MMSE 21-30	4	-
Moderately impaired (number) MMSE 11-20	6	-
Severely impaired (number) MMSE 0-10	5	-

Japan). Eyes-closed resting EEGs were digitally sampled at 200 Hz and 20 artifact-free EEG epochs lasting 2.56 ms were selected.

Analysis

The global field power (GFP) (Lehmann, & Skrandies, 1980) of the 20 channels of EEG frequency data was determined by means of a Fast Fourier Transform (FFT). In addition, standardized Low Resolution Electromagnetic Tomography (sLORETA) (Pascual-Marqui, Esslen, Kochi, & Lehmann, 2002) was used to detect the three-dimensional intracerebral distribution of EEG activity.

To determine the automated EEG source localization with z-transformed age-appropriate population norms for identifying AD and MCI individuals, the following procedures were performed. Developmental equations for brain electrical activity were computed in the age range 17-80 years, based on 139 normal controls from the NYU Brain Research Labs (BRL) database. EEGs were recorded from 19 electrodes (10/20 placement system) under awake, resting, eyes-closed conditions (i.e., in the default mode). Then, signals of electrical neuronal activity were estimated at 6239 virtually implanted electrodes. This was achieved by applying sLORETA to the EEG recordings, thus computing the post-synaptic current density at 6239 voxels (5mm resolution) distributed on the cortex. These computed signals were then used to estimate the spectral densities on the cortex in the range 1.5-35 Hz with 0.39 Hz frequency resolution. Simple parametric age regression equations were computed under several scalings: absolute spectra, relative spectra, subject-wise scaling, and frequency-wise scaling. In all cases, the approximate Gaussianity of the residuals was guaranteed by using the logarithm of age, the logarithm of absolute power, and Fisher's z-transform for relative power. Each EEG epoch was down-sampled to 100 Hz to match the BRL database. The selected EEGs from each subject were analyzed by sLORETA and statistically compared at all frequencies with the age-matched BRL database. This procedure resulted in cortical z-values for each subject at each EEG frequency with 0.39 Hz frequency resolution (Figure 1).

We also quantified hippocampal volume using an MRI voxel-based specific regional analysis system developed for the study of Alzheimer's disease (VSRAD) (Hirata et al., 2005), yielding a z-score that represented the hippocampal volume.

Figure 1. Automated EEG source localization with z-transformed age-appropriate population norms

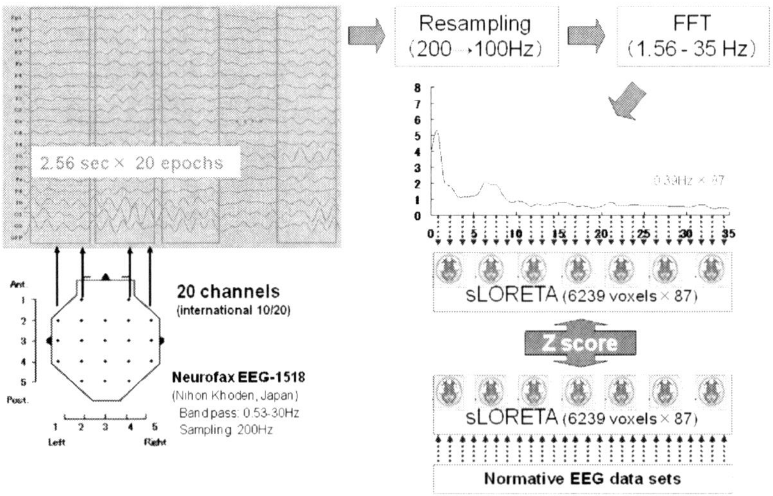

Figure 2. FFT spectrum with global field power (GFP)

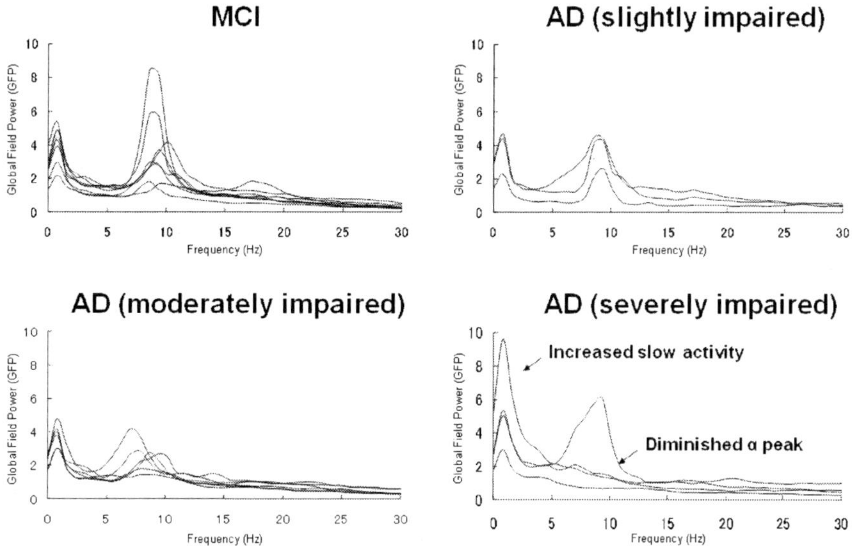

RESULTS

We classified the AD patients into 3 groups according to their MMSE scores: slightly impaired, moderately impaired, and severely impaired (see Table 1).

The FFT spectrum with GFP indicated a slowing of the alpha peak related to the severity of impairment, with most of the severely impaired AD patients exhibiting a diminished alpha peak and increased slow activity (Figure 2).

Figure 3. An example z-spectrum showing low and high frequency peaks and their EEG source localization, which corresponded to the decreased CBF region, respectively.

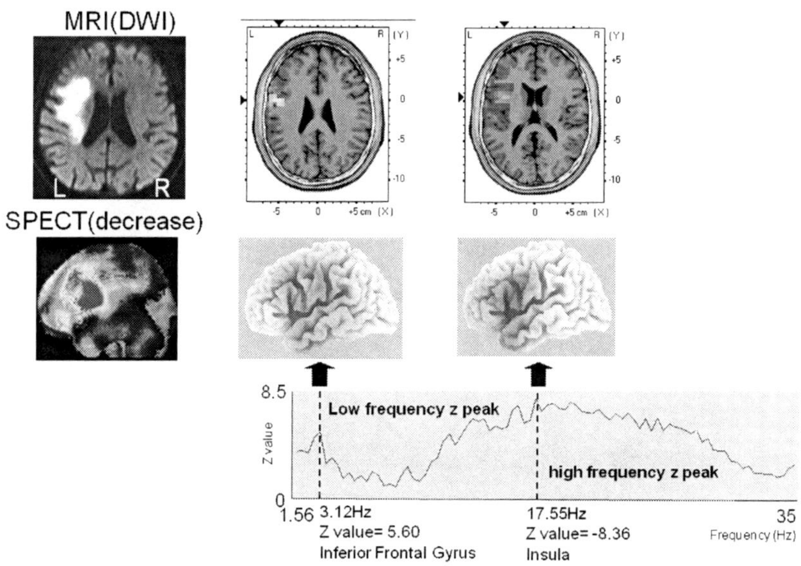

Almost all of the patients revealed double peaked z-spectra with low and high frequency bands (showing positive and negative z-values, respectively), corresponding to a decreased CBF region (Figure 3). These results led us to assess the differences from the norms in activated and deactivated lesions in both the low and high frequency bands. There was no common, significantly different pattern observed among the severely impaired cases in both low and high frequency activity. However, analysis revealed increased slow activity (functional hypoactivity) of the neocortex rather than the limbic areas (Figure 4). Three (50%) of the moderately impaired AD patients revealed increased low-frequency activity in the hippocampus, suggesting dysfunction of this region. However, two of the moderately impaired AD patients showed the opposite effect: decreased slow activity and increased fast activity compared to the normal patients in the database. These two patients were medicated with a benzodiazepine (loflazepate) and an SSRI (sertraline), drugs that generally augment beta activity (Figure 5). The slightly impaired AD patients also showed increased low-frequency activity in the hippocampus in half of the cases (Figure 6). The MCI patients did not show a pattern of low-frequency activity similar to the control, although there was a decrease in high-frequency activity in the hippocampi of five of the eight patients (Figure 7). In summary, the frequency of the low z-peak decreased and its z-value increased, although there was no corresponding tendency in the high z-peak, and the z-values from VSRAD

Figure 4. EEG source localization corresponding to low and high frequency z-peaks among severely impaired Alzheimer's disease patients

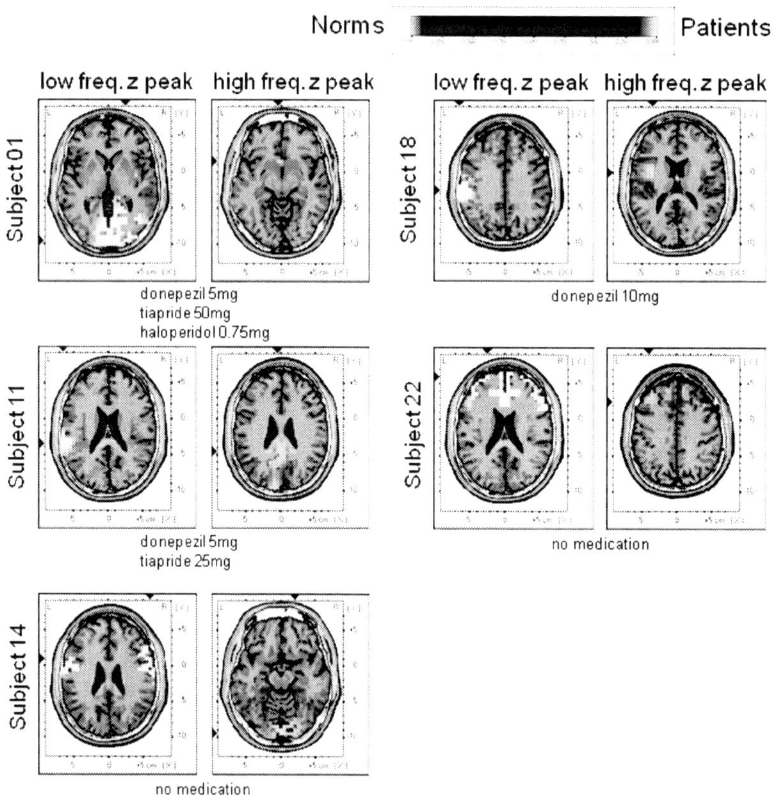

Figure 5. EEG source localization corresponding to low and high frequency z-peaks among moderately impaired Alzheimer's disease patients

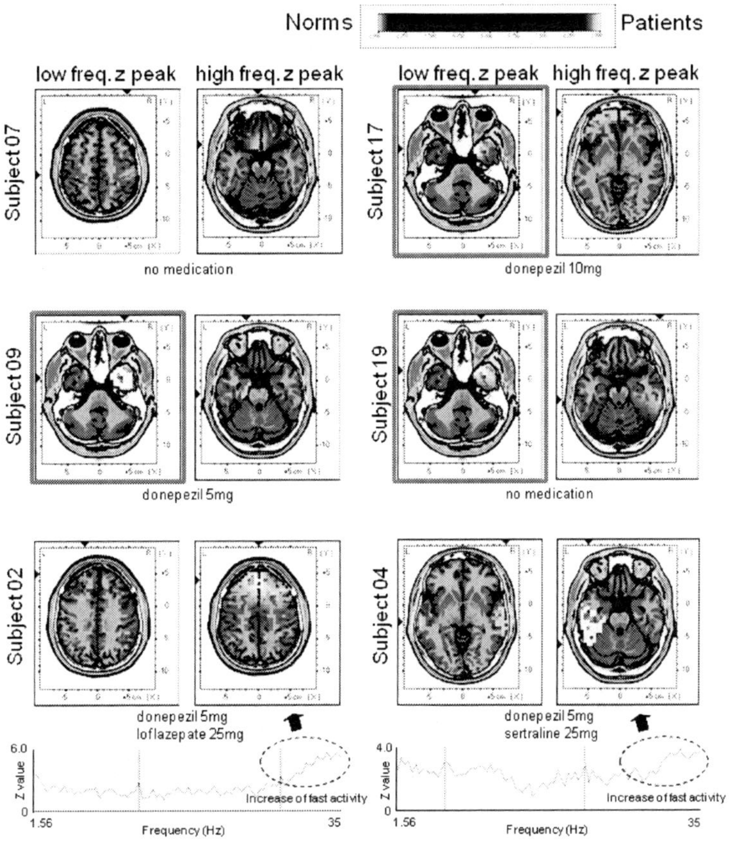

Figure 6. EEG source localization corresponding to low and high frequency z-peaks among slightly impaired Alzheimer's disease patients

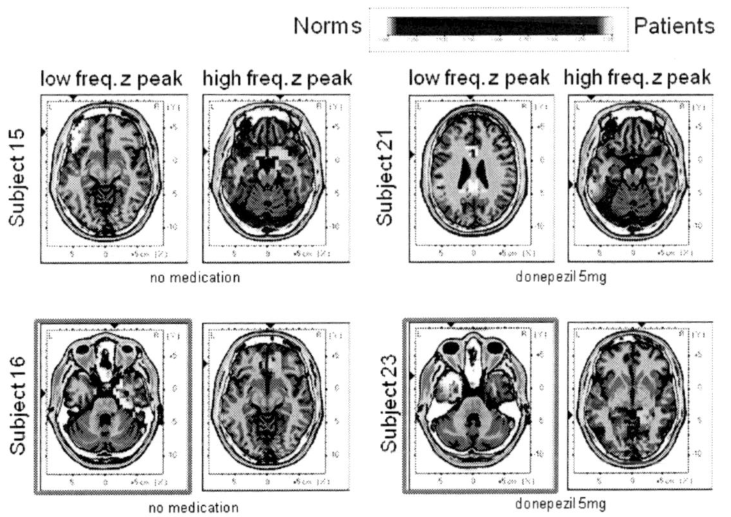

Figure 7. EEG source localization corresponding to low and high frequency z-peaks among mild cognitive impairment patients

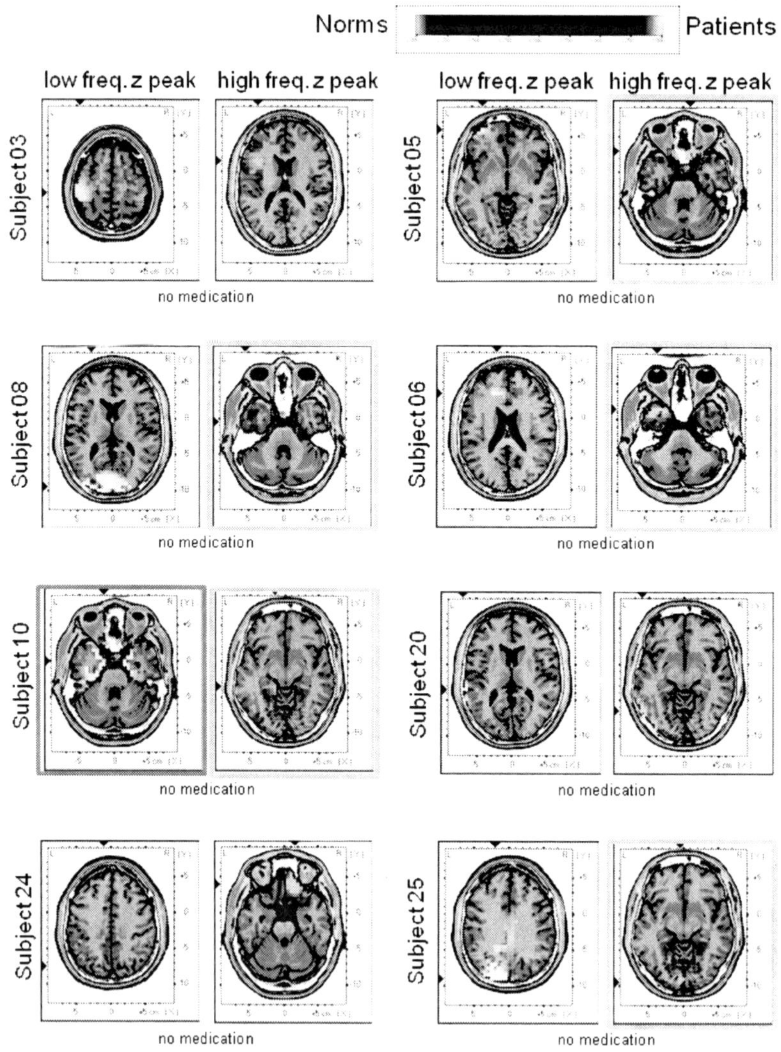

showed the same tendency as the z-values from sLORETA.

We also assessed the z-value from sLORETA focused in the parahippocampal region following VSRAD analysis, which indicated a significant negative correlation with the MMSE score in low-frequency activity ($r=-0.66$, $p<0.01$) and tended to correlate with the z-score from VSRAD ($r=0.36$, $p<0.1$).

DISCUSSION

In studies of dementia patients, theta power has been shown to be negatively correlated with perfusion, especially in the temporal–parietal and central regions (Mattia et al., 2003). In addition, a substantial number of reports in the literature have reported high inverse correlations between theta excesses, cerebral ischemia, and cerebral blood flow (Jonkman, Poortvliet, Veering, De Weerd,

& John, 1985). Observations of increased low-frequency activity in the neocortex of severely impaired AD patients support this correlation. Theta activity has also been shown to be negatively correlated with positron emission tomography (PET) glucose metabolism in the temporal–parietal region (Szelies et al., 1992) and positively correlated with hippocampal atrophy (Fernández et al., 2003). The z-value from sLORETA was focused on the parahippocampal region during low-frequency activity, which negatively correlated with the MMSE score and positively correlated with the z-score from VSRAD, supporting the idea that the increased slow activity in the parahippocampal region was caused by hippocampal atrophy. These results were in agreement with the evidence from statistical neural imaging using MRI/SPECT. The submission of normal EEG data sets to sLORETA might be useful for the identification of diagnostic and predictive markers of AD and MCI for each individual patient.

ACKNOWLEDGMENT

We thank our colleagues who recruited the patients. We also thank Dr. Pascual-Marqui from The KEY Institute for Brain-Mind Research, University Hospital of Psychiatry, Zurich, and Prof. Hirata from Department of Neurology, Dokkyo Medical University for their helpful suggestions and Mrs. Masako Saito from the second collaboration laboratory in Dokkyo Medical University for the excellent technical support.

REFERENCES

Fernández, A., Arrazola, J., Maestú, F., Amo, C., Gil-Gregorio, P., Wienbruch, C., & Ortiz, T. (2003). Correlations of hippocampal atrophy and focal low-frequency magnetic activity in Alzheimer disease: Volumetric MR imaging-magnetoencephalographic study. *AJNR. American Journal of Neuroradiology*, *24*, 481–487.

Hirata, Y., Matsuda, H., Nemoto, K., Ohnishi, T., Hirao, K., & Yamashita, F. (2005). Voxel-based morphometry to discriminate early Alzheimer's disease from controls. *Neuroscience Letters*, *382*, 269–274. doi:10.1016/j.neulet.2005.03.038

Jonkman, E. J., Poortvliet, D. C., Veering, M. M., De Weerd, A. W., & John, E. R. (1985). The use of neurometrics in the study of patients with cerebral ischaemia. *Electroencephalography and Clinical Neurophysiology*, *61*, 333–341. doi:10.1016/0013-4694(85)91023-5

Lehmann, D., & Skrandies, W. (1980). Reference-free identification of components of checkerboard-evoked multichannel potential fields. *Electroencephalography and Clinical Neurophysiology*, *48*, 609–621. doi:10.1016/0013-4694(80)90419-8

Mattia, D., Babiloni, F., Romigi, A., Cincotti, F., Bianchi, L., & Sperli, F. (2003). Quantitative EEG and dynamic susceptibility contrast MRI in Alzheimer's disease: A correlative study. *Clinical Neurophysiology*, *114*, 1210–1216. doi:10.1016/S1388-2457(03)00085-3

McKhann, G., Drachman, D., Folstein, M., Katzman, R., Price, D., & Stadlan, E. M. (1984). Clinical diagnosis of Alzheimer's disease: Report of the NINCDS-ADRDA Work Group under the auspices of Department of Health and Human Services Task Force on Alzheimer's Disease. *Neurology*, *34*, 939–944.

Pascual-Marqui, R. D., Esslen, M., Kochi, K., & Lehmann, D. (2002). Functional imaging with low-resolution brain electromagnetic tomography (LORETA): A review. *Methods and Findings in Experimental and Clinical Pharmacology*, *24*, 91–95.

Petersen, R. C., Smith, G. E., Waring, S. C., Ivnik, R. J., Tangalos, E. G., & Kokmen, E. (1999). Mild cognitive impairment: Clinical characterization and outcome. *Archives of Neurology*, *56*, 303–308. doi:10.1001/archneur.56.3.303

Szelies, B., Grond, M., Herholz, K., Kessler, J., Wullen, T., & Heiss, W. D. (1992). Quantitative EEG mapping and PET in Alzheimer's disease. *Journal of the Neurological Sciences*, *110*, 46–56. doi:10.1016/0022-510X(92)90008-9

KEY TERMS AND DEFINITIONS

Alzheimer's disease: The most common form of dementia, caused by neural death that results in an accumulation of beta amyloid peptides and tau protein.

Global Field Power: A measurement that corresponds to the spatial standard deviation and quantifies the amount of activity at each time point in the field considering the data from all recording electrodes simultaneously, resulting in a reference-independent descriptor of the potential field.

Mild Cognitive Impairment: A diagnosis given to individuals who have cognitive impairments that are beyond what is expected for their age and education but that do not interfere significantly with their daily activities.

Neuroimaging: Various techniques to either directly or indirectly image the structure or function/pharmacology of the brain. It is a relatively new discipline within medicine and neuroscience/psychology.

Standardized Low Resolution Electromagnetic Tomography (sLORETA): A method that computes 3D distributions of electric neuronal activity from surface EEGs and MEGs.

Voxel-Based Specific Regional Analysis System Developed for the Study of Alzheimer's Disease (VSRAD): A method of voxel-based morphometry (VBM) using a three-dimensional T1-weighted MRI to discriminate Alzheimer's disease (AD) from age-matched healthy controls.

Chapter 18
Apraxia

Mark Hallett
Human Motor Control Section, NINDS, National Institutes of Health, USA

ABSTRACT

Apraxia is the inability to perform skilled and/or learned movements, not explainable on the basis of more elemental abnormalities. There are several types of apraxia of which the most commonly recognized are (1) limb kinetic apraxia, the loss of hand and finger dexterity; (2) ideomotor apraxia, deficits in pantomiming tool use and gestures with temporal and spatial errors, but with knowledge of the tasks still present; (3) ideational apraxia, the failure to carry out a series of tasks using multiple objects for an intended purpose; and (4) conceptual apraxia, loss of tool knowledge, when tools and objects are used inappropriately. Apraxia can be a feature of both frontotemporal dementia and Alzheimer disease, and even a rare presenting manifestation of both. How sensitive apraxia measures would be in early detection is not well known.

I. INTRODUCTION

Apraxia is a complex disorder at the interface between cognition and movement. It is the inability to perform skilled and/or learned movements, not explainable on the basis of more elemental abnormalities (such as weakness, incoordination, language difficulty). There are several types of apraxia which complicates the recognition and clinical utility (Wheaton and Hallett, 2007). The most commonly recognized types are (1) limb kinetic apraxia (LKA), the loss of hand and finger dexterity; significantly affecting manipulative movements; (2) ideomotor apraxia (IMA), deficits in pantomiming tool use and gestures with temporal and spatial errors, but with knowledge of the tasks still present; (3) ideational apraxia, the failure to carry out a series of tasks using multiple objects for an intended purpose, a problem in the sequencing of actions; and (4) conceptual apraxia, loss of tool knowledge, when tools and objects are used inappropriately. Some experts put ideational

DOI: 10.4018/978-1-60960-559-9.ch018

and conceptual apraxia together under ideational apraxia. While LKA might be considered a motor control disorder, the other types of apraxia are commonly considered cognitive.

While most investigations of apraxia evaluate the upper limb, apraxia can affect the lower limb or oral-buccal-facial muscles.

IMA is the most commonly recognized form. The movements are spatially incorrect, and may be abnormally slow and deliberate. More often seen in tool-use pantomime (transitive movements), the abnormality may extend to gestures (intransitive movements). The deficits commonly include orientation errors (e.g., holding the limb in a posture impossible to carry out the task) and spatial and temporal errors (e.g., cutting a load of bread with jerky vertical movements instead of smooth anterior–posterior movements). Other deficits include movement errors (e.g., patients make extra and unnecessary movements or move the wrong joints). Patients may also perform "body part as object" errors (e.g., when instructed to brush their teeth, they will use a finger as if it were a toothbrush instead of pantomiming holding the toothbrush). Use of an object or tool in real life situations may be impaired as well. Characterizing the error pattern is critical in describing the abnormal performance.

Importantly, patients with IMA must know what they are told to do, and the examiner needs to be sure of this point. Patients with Wernicke aphasia, agnosia, and asymbolia must be excluded as confounds in any diagnosis. Aphasia, in particular, must be excluded as responsible, since apraxia often coexists with language impairment.

There are a number of formal scales that have been developed for apraxia. Most scales have not examined for all aspects, but some newer scales are attempting to do that. One problem is that a "complete" assessment would be very long. Hence, the newer attempts also include a brief version for screening. A recent scale, which seems complete at least for the upper limb and has been validated, is the TULIA (Test of Upper Limb Apraxia) (Vanbellingen et al, 2010). It consists of 48 items including both imitation and pantomime of non-symbolic (meaningless), intransitive (communicative) and transitive (tool related) gestures making 6 subtests.

II. CLINICAL CONDITIONS

IMA is recognized most commonly as a result of stroke and in some Parkinson-plus conditions such as corticobasal degeneration (Zadikoff & Lang, 2005; Kertesz & McMonagle, 2010; Borroni et al, 2009). These disorders have given some sense to the clinical-pathological correlation. The best evidence is for cortical lesions; whether basal ganglia lesions can cause apraxia by themselves remains controversial.

The anatomical basis for apraxia is best understood in many studies of clinical-pathological correlation (Gross & Grossman, 2008). Generally, in stroke patients, left hemisphere lesions of the parietal and premotor areas are implicated in apraxia; right hemisphere lesions are only rarely described. Early studies of IMA suggested that damage to white matter tracts was most critical; however, white matter lesions are not more common in IMA patients than controls. Subsequent studies showed that it was the pattern of white matter damage that is critical; in particular, those lesions that lead to a disconnection of the parietal and premotor areas (Borroni et al, 2008). Damage to gray matter structures, particularly the angular gyrus or the supramarginal gyrus, are common in clinical-pathological correlation (Goldenberg, 2009). Anterior lesions may produce aphasia, which makes the determination of IMA difficult or impossible. There are also some patients with IMA apparently caused by SMA damage or lateral anterior frontal lesions.

Apraxia is also a feature of many patients with dementia. Apraxia can be a feature of both frontotemporal dementia and Alzheimer disease, and even a rare presenting manifestation of both.

A recent study found that idiomotor apraxia is a common sign in Huntington disease and independent of neuropsychological decline (Hodl et al, 2008). Dementia can also be a prominent feature in corticobasal degeneration.

III. CLINICAL ISSUES

How sensitive apraxia measures would be in early detection of dementia is not well known. It certainly could well be a presenting manifestation, and one study does suggest that patients with mild cognitive impairment (MCI) who have apraxia are more likely to progress to Alzheimer disease (Crutch et al, 2007a). They investigated 23 patients with MCI and 75 healthy controls with two 3-item sequential movement tasks involving either meaningful or meaningless actions as well as a traditional gesture-to-command task. MCI patients took significantly longer than control subjects to complete the sequential movement tasks despite unimpaired performance on the traditional gesture production tasks.

On the other hand, the same group who studied the MCI patients, also looked at 37 patients with Alzheimer disease with the same 3-item sequential movement tasks in comparison with 75 healthy controls. While the Alzheimer patients were slower on the tasks, the authors found only a minimal and inconsistent influence on praxis (Crutch et al, 2007b).

A brief upper extremity apraxia scale was tested in a memory clinic (Mahieux-Laurent et al, 2009). The scale included three subtests: five symbolic gestures, five pantomimes and eight imitations of meaningless gestures. Data were collected from 419 normal subjects, 320 demented patients, and 127 patients with mild cognitive impairment. Specificity was high, and sensitivity was best for imitation of meaningless gestures, second for pantomimes and the least for symbolic gestures. The group of patients with mild cognitive impairment was half-way between demented patients and normal subjects. The authors concluded that this screening usefully contributes to clinical diagnosis.

It would also be useful to know if apraxia could differentiate among different dementias. This is also not well known or tested, although it would be suspected that apraxia would be most common in corticobasal degeneration.

IV. TREATMENT

Often it has been said that apraxia is a sign and not a symptom. However, patients with apraxia do have difficulties with many tasks of daily living. Unfortunately, there are not many well-established techniques dealing with rehabilitation of this problem. Focused rehabilitation might well be able to help, however, as demonstrated in a recent study of patients with limb kinetic apraxia in the setting of corticobasal degeneration (Kawahira et al, 2009).

REFERENCES

Borroni, B., Alberici, A., Agosti, C., Cosseddu, M., & Padovani, A. (2009). Pattern of behavioral disturbances in corticobasal degeneration syndrome and progressive supranuclear palsy. *International Psychogeriatrics*, *21*, 463–468. doi:10.1017/S1041610209008862

Borroni, B., Garibotto, V., Agosti, C., Brambati, S. M., Bellelli, G., & Gasparotti, R. (2008). White matter changes in corticobasal degeneration syndrome and correlation with limb apraxia. *Archives of Neurology*, *65*, 796–801. doi:10.1001/archneur.65.6.796

Crutch, S. J., Rossor, M. N., & Warrington, E. K. (2007a). A novel technique for the quantitative assessment of apraxic deficits: Application to individuals with mild cognitive impairment. *Journal of Neuropsychology*, *1*, 237–257. doi:10.1348/174866407X209943

Crutch, S. J., Rossor, M. N., & Warrington, E. K. (2007b). The quantitative assessment of apraxic deficits in Alzheimer's disease. *Cortex*, *43*, 976–986. doi:10.1016/S0010-9452(08)70695-6

Goldenberg, G. (2009). Apraxia and the parietal lobes. *Neuropsychologia*, *47*, 1449–1459. doi:10.1016/j.neuropsychologia.2008.07.014

Gross, R. G., & Grossman, M. (2008). Update on apraxia. *Current Neurology and Neuroscience Reports*, *8*, 490–496. doi:10.1007/s11910-008-0078-y

Hodl, A. K., Hodl, E., Otti, D. V., Herranhof, B., Ille, R., & Bonelli, R. M. (2008). Ideomotor limb apraxia in Huntington's disease: A case-control study. *Journal of Neurology*, *255*, 331–339.

Kawahira, K., Noma, T., Iiyama, J., Etoh, S., Ogata, A., & Shimodozono, M. (2009). Improvements in limb kinetic apraxia by repetition of a newly designed facilitation exercise in a patient with corticobasal degeneration. *International Journal of Rehabilitation Research. Internationale Zeitschrift fur Rehabilitationsforschung. Revue Internationale de Recherches de Readaptation*, *32*, 178–183. doi:10.1097/MRR.0b013e32831e4546

Kertesz, A., & McMonagle, P. (2010). Behavior and cognition in corticobasal degeneration and progressive supranuclear palsy. *Journal of the Neurological Sciences*, *89*(1-2), 138–143. doi:10.1016/j.jns.2009.08.036

Mahieux-Laurent, F., Fabre, C., Galbrun, E., Dubrulle, A., & Moroni, C. (2009). Validation of a brief screening scale evaluating praxic abilities for use in memory clinics. Evaluation in 419 controls, 127 mild cognitive impairment and 320 demented patients. *Revue Neurologique*, *165*, 560–567. doi:10.1016/j.neurol.2008.11.016

Vanbellingen, T., Kersten, B., Van Hemelrijk, B., Van de Winckel, A., Bertschi, M., & Muri, R. (2010). Comprehensive assessment of gesture production: A new test of upper kimb apraxia (TULIA). *European Journal of Neurology*, *17*(1), 59–66. doi:10.1111/j.1468-1331.2009.02741.x

Wheaton, L. A., & Hallett, M. (2007). Ideomotor apraxia: A review. *Journal of the Neurological Sciences*, *260*, 1–10. doi:10.1016/j.jns.2007.04.014

Zadikoff, C., & Lang, A. E. (2005). Apraxia in movement disorders. *Brain*, *128*, 1480–1497. doi:10.1093/brain/awh560

KEY TERMS AND DEFINITIONS

Apraxia: The inability to perform skilled and/or learned movements, not explainable on the basis of more elemental abnormalities.

Conceptual Apraxia: Loss of tool knowledge, when tools and objects are used inappropriately.

Corticobasal Degeneration: A degenerative neurological condition characterized by asymmetrical parkinsonism, dystonia, myoclonus, cortical sensory loss and apraxia; pathologically, there is excess accumulation in the brain of a protein called tau.

Ideational Apraxia: The failure to carry out a series of tasks using multiple objects for an intended purpose, a problem in the sequencing of actions.

Ideomotor Apraxia (IMA): Deficits in pantomiming tool use and gestures with temporal and spatial errors, but with knowledge of the tasks still present.

Limb Kinetic Apraxia (LKA): The loss of hand and finger dexterity significantly affecting manipulative movements.

Chapter 19
Pharmacokinetic Challenges against Brain Diseases with PET

Hiroshi Watabe
Department of Molecular Imaging in Medicine Osaka University Graduate School of Medicine 2-2 Yamadaoka Suita, Japan

Keisuke Matsubara
Akita Research Institute of Brain and Blood Vessels, Japan

Yoko Ikoma
Department of Clinical Neuroscience, Karolinska Institute, Sweden

ABSTRACT

Positron emission tomography (PET) is an imaging technology used to visualize distribution of particular ligands inside living organisms. The ligand is labeled by a positron-emitting isotope, such as ^{11}C, ^{15}O, ^{13}N and ^{18}F, and injected into subjects. By detecting γ-rays emitted from the ligand, in vivo biodistribution and kinetics of the ligand can be depicted with high sensitivity. By altering the target ligand for PET, one can see different distributions and time courses of the target. PET provides several biological and functional images inside the body, rather than simply an anatomical image. Therefore, PET can potentially detect biological changes that occur long before anatomical changes begin. PET has been widely used for neuroreceptor and neurotransmitter studies by tracing radioligands, which have selective affinity for a particular site. For example, the dopamine and serotonin receptors are highly related to brain disorders. By analyzing the pharmacokinetics of these ligands using PET, it is possible to noninvasively detect abnormalities in the brain. However, signals from PET contain many different types of information, and it is important to interpret the signals appropriately and choose the proper technique to analyze PET data. This chapter discusses several analytical methods for PET data.

INTRODUCTION

Positron emission tomography (PET) is an advanced imaging techniques used to visualize the interior of living bodies. PET scanning is initiated by the injection of a specific ligand labeled by a radioisotope, such as ^{11}C, ^{13}N, ^{15}O and ^{18}F, that emits positrons (we call this ligand a 'radioligand'). Each positron annihilates an electron, and two γ rays of 511 keV energy are simultaneously emitted in opposite directions. The two emitted photons are

DOI: 10.4018/978-1-60960-559-9.ch019

detected by γ-ray detectors in coincidence. The line connecting the two detectors is called the line-of-response (LOR), which encompasses the source of the photons. By combining multiple LORs with a mathematical image reconstruction algorithm, a tomographic image of the three-dimensional distribution of the radioligand can be generated. A contemporary PET system uses a scintillation crystal, such as bismuth germinate (BGO), lutetium oxyorthosilicate (LSO), or gadolinium orthosilicate (GSO), as the γ-ray detector, and the scanner is ring shaped with more than 10,000 small pieces of scintillation crystals cylindrically aligned (see Figure 1). The half life (time for the specific activity of the radioisotope to decrease by half) of the positron-emitted radioisotope used in PET is usually short (2 min for ^{15}O, 10 min for ^{13}N, 20 min for ^{11}C, and 110 min for ^{18}F). Thus, it is necessary for each site to have a cyclotron (Figure 2) to generate the radioligand. One advantage of PET is the ability to employ radioligands that are molecular analogs of ligands naturally present inside the human body.

By visualizing the three dimensional distribution and time course of the radioligand by PET, we can noninvasively obtain information of the injected radioligand. Note that depending on the radioligand, PET scanning can sometimes last for a few hours, and a patient must lie in a fixed position during the scan. It is difficult to ask children and patients with dementia not to move during the scan, and motion correction techniques must be considered when using PET (Woo et al., 2004). The image obtained by PET represents certain functions related to the injected radioligand. For instance, images of ^{15}O -water are related to blood flow, and images of ^{11}C –raclopride, which is an antagonist for the D2 dopamine neuroreceptor, represent the map of the D2 dopamine neuroreceptor inside the body. Therefore, by altering the radioligand, we are able to measure different functions related to the ligand (Table 1). Although the spatial resolution of the PET scan-

Figure 1. Photograph of the inside of a PET scanner. It consists of a ring-shaped gantry with many scintillation crystals.

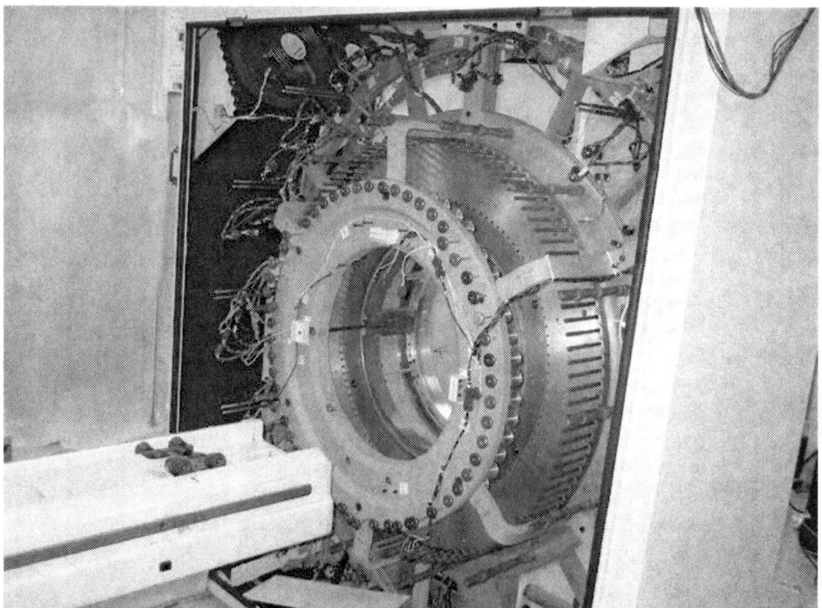

Figure 2. Photograph of the inside of a cyclotron. The cyclotron generates a proton or deuteron beam, which collides with the appropriate target (for example, water with enriched ^{18}O to generate ^{18}F).

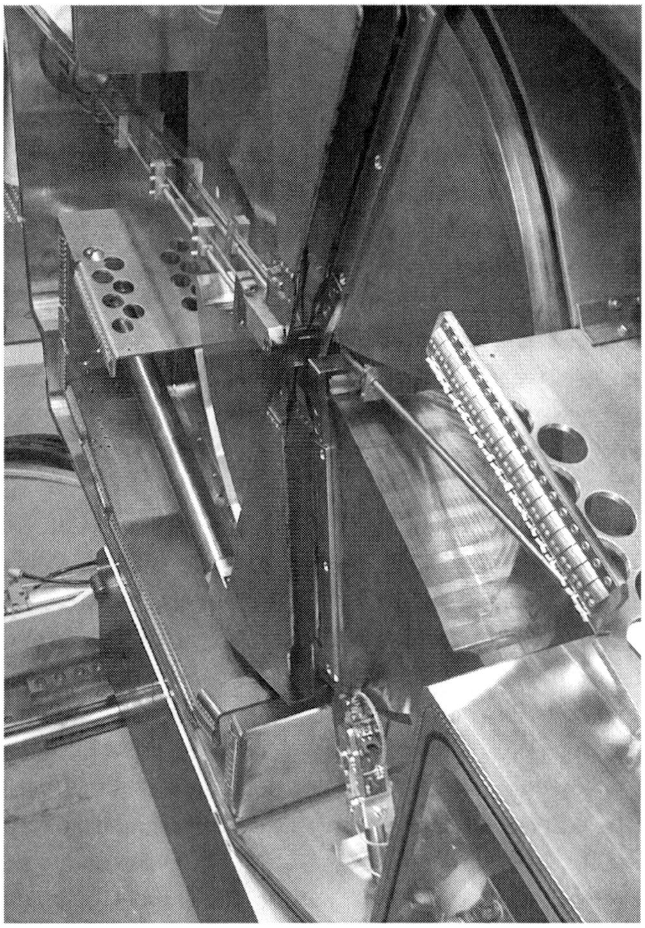

Table 1. Examples of radioligands for PET. Each radioligand behaves differently inside the body, and PET can visualize the radioligand and, consequently, the function related to the radioligand.

target	radioligand
Blood flow	$H_2{}^{15}O$
Blood volume	$C^{15}O$
Oxygen	$^{15}O_2$
Glucose	^{18}F-FDG
Dopamine D1 receptor	^{11}C-SCH23390
Dopamine D2 receptor	^{11}C-raclopride
Serotonin 1A receptor	^{11}C-WAY100635
Serotonin 2A receptor	^{11}C-MDL100,907
Benzodiazepine receptor	^{11}C-Flumazenil
Serotonin transporter	^{11}C-MPIQ

ner is not high compared with other imaging modalities (e.g., X-ray CT and MRI), it has a very high sensitivity to detect the specific ligand in a quantitative manner. Consequently, PET has the potential to sensitively detect certain diseases by identifying functional changes that occur prior to anatomical changes. Therefore, many PET radioligands have been developed and applied to detect and evaluate several neurological disorders, such as Alzheimer's disease, Parkinson's disease, schizophrenia, and stroke.

To properly interpret a PET image with a certain radioligand, it is important to have knowledge of not only the pharmacokinetics of the radioligand but also the principles of PET. Detection of γ rays is truly a statistical event, and uncertainty in the PET data is unavoidable. Moreover, signals from the PET image represent a combination of information, such as binding to specific neuroreceptors, free ligand, binding to proteins, and metabolization to other compounds. PET cannot distinguish between γ rays from the injected radioligand and those from its metabolites. Thus, determining the useful information is sometimes a methodological challenge in PET imaging. When distinguishing between non-metabolites and metabolites, one often uses the mathematical model called the 'compartment model' (Watabe, Ikoma, Kimura, Naganawa, & Shidahara, 2006), which describes how a drug and its metabolites travel in the body. It is assumed that the injected radioligand travels between "compartments" in tissue and plasma as an input function, and PET data is assumed to be the composition of multiple compartments. The relationship between compartments is expressed by rate constants that are regarded as the kinetic parameters of the targeted ligand. Quantification of kinetic parameters in the compartment model is a common approach used to analyze PET data. In general, nonlinear regression analysis is required to solve the equations derived from the compartment model, and difficulties are often faced when obtaining kinetic parameters with stability. Thus, some assumptions, simplifications, and ingenuities may be required to obtain kinetic parameters. Indeed, many investigators have developed techniques to analyze PET data to obtain useful information for detecting neurological disorders.

In this chapter, several techniques and applications of PET for pharmacokinetic analysis will be discussed.

STANDARD UPTAKE VALUE (SUV)

One of the simplest techniques to analyze PET data is to compute the standard uptake value (SUV), which is obtained by normalizing PET data by the injected dose and body mass. The SUV of a PET image with radioligands to depict amyloid deposition, such as ^{11}C–PIB (Klunk et al., 2004) and ^{11}C–BF-227 (Kudo et al., 2007), successfully differentiated between healthy controls and patients with Alzheimer's disease.

CBF AND CMRO2 USING ^{15}O2 AND $H_2{}^{15}O$ SUBJECTS

One of the earliest applications for the compartment model is the model for $H^{15}O_2$ and $^{15}O_2$ (Subramanyam, Alpert, Hoop, Brownell, & Taveras, 1978; Frackowiak, Lenzi, Jones, & Heather, 1980; Mintun, Raichle, Martin, & Herscovitch, 1984). Cerebral blood flow (CBF) and the cerebral metabolite rate of oxygen ($CMRO_2$) are sensitive indices to detect brain damage, and PET can quantitate CBF and $CMRO_2$ using $H_2{}^{15}O$ (we often use gaseous $C^{15}O_2$ instead of $H_2{}^{15}O$ due to the rapid exchange of $H_2{}^{15}O$ by carbonate dehydratase in the lung) and $^{15}O_2$. Fig. 3 shows the compartment model that represents the circulation of oxygen and water inside the body. Based on this model, a mathematical formulation is derived. $^{15}O_2$, $^{15}CO_2$ and $C^{15}O$ (carbon monoxide to depict blood volume) are separately inhaled by a patient, and PET data are acquired. There are two approaches for administration of radioactive gases, one is continuous inhalation, and the other is bolus inhalation. The beauty of continuous inhalation is the mathematical simplicity. By continuous supply of ^{15}O gases, a steady state of radioactivity inside the body is achieved. Under this steady state, the mathematical formulation for the compartment model becomes simple because no differential equations are required. Conversely, the bolus inhalation approach requires more complex mathematics, but it shortens the study time and, therefore, the radiation exposure to a patient.

Figure 3. Compartment model for oxygen and water to analyze the behavior of $H_2{}^{15}O$ and $^{15}O_2$

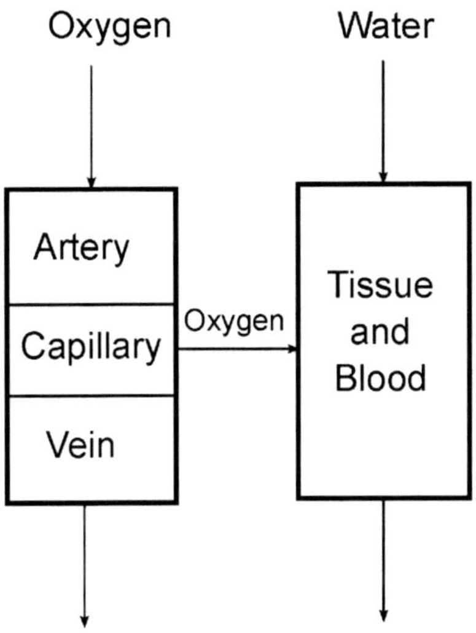

DUAL INJECTION STUDY FOR CBF AND $CMRO_2$

As described above, conventional PET study for CBF and $CMRO_2$ requires separate inhalations of radioactive gases of $^{15}O_2$ and $^{15}CO_2$. Kudomi et al. (Kudomi et al., 2005) developed a protocol of dual tracer injections in which inhalations of $^{15}O_2$ and $^{15}CO_2$ are carried out in short intervals. By this protocol, the time duration for PET examination can be shortened. As shown in Figure 4, the radioactivity of $^{15}O_2$ still exists at the time of $^{15}CO_2$ inhalation, and mathematical formulas that take into account the residual radioactivity that is utilized to calculate CBF and $CMRO_2$.

^{18}F-FDOPA MODEL

Parkinson's disease (PD) is caused by nigral degeneration and striatal dopamine deficiency and characterized by motor disorders, such as resting tremor, bradykinesia and rigidity dementia. A patient with PD often develops dementia. It is difficult to detect PD by routine brain CT or MRI scan (Johansen, White, Sando, & Aasly, 2010). ^{18}F-FDOPA is an analog of the endogenous precursor of dopamine, and PET with ^{18}F-FDOPA can detect PD in early stages (Sioka, Fotopoulos, & Kyritsis, 2010). As shown in Figure 5, ^{18}F-FDOPA has

Figure 4. Example of the time activity curve in brain measured by PET for dual injections of $^{15}O_2$ and $^{15}CO_2$. $^{15}O_2$ was injected at time 0, and $^{15}CO_2$ was injected 5 min later.

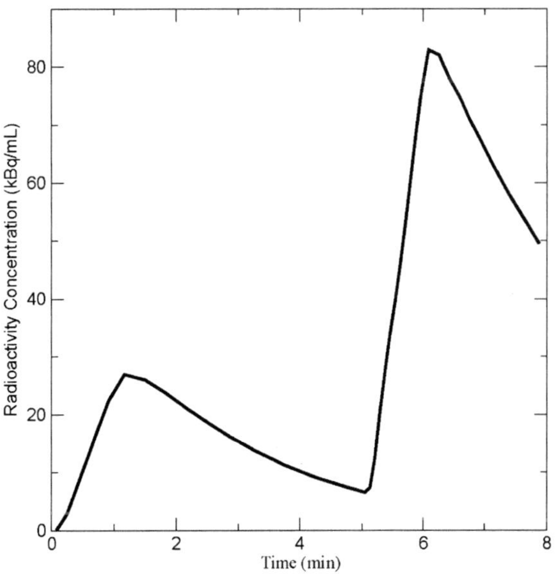

Figure 5. Metabolic paths for FDOPA in dopaminergic neurons. FDOPA is decarboxylated to fluorodopamine (FDA) by the enzyme dopa decarboxylase (DDC). FDA is partially trapped in synaptic vesicles through the vesicle monoamine transporter (VMAT). FDA is also metabolized to FDOPAC, FMT and FHVA by monoamine oxidase (MAO) and catechol-O-methyltransferase (COMT). FDOPA is also O-methylated by COMT to form OMFD.

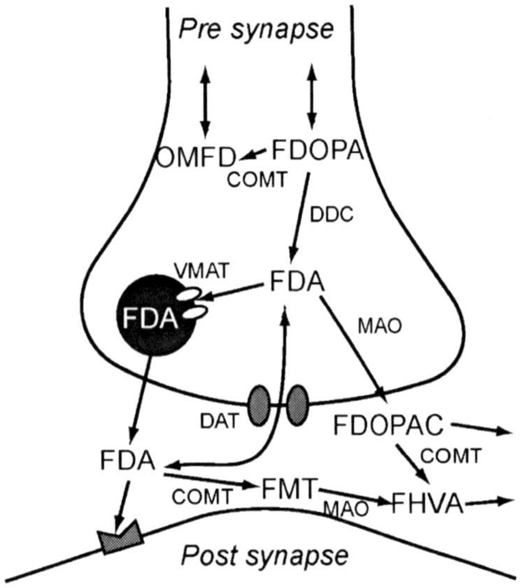

complex pathways in the neuron. Therefore, the compartment model, which describes all pathways for ^{18}F-FDOPA, contains multiple compartments and many rate constants (Figure 6) (Matsubara, Watabe, Hayashi, Minato, & Iida, 2010). Unfortunately, it is too complicated to estimate all rate constants in the compartment model by PET, and many investigators have developed simpler techniques to diagnose PD. The most popular approach for analyzing ^{18}F -FDOPA uses Gjedde-Patlak graphical analysis (Gjedde, 1981; Patlak, Blasberg, & Fenstermacher, 1983). In this method, PET data is analyzed via simple regression line models, and the slope of the line represents the amount of dopamine synthesis. Kumakura et al. developed multiple regression techniques to estimate the loss of the decarboxylated metabolites and showed that estimation of the loss was more sensitive at detecting PD compared with using the synthesis of dopamine (Kumakura, Gjedde, Danielsen, Christensen, & Cumming, 2006).

REFERENCE TISSUE MODEL

One drawback of the compartment analysis model is the requirement of an arterial input function, which represents the time course of radioactivity concentration in the plasma after injection of the radioligand. To measure the input function, frequent arterial blood sampling and (on some occasions) analysis of metabolites are required, which is a burden for patients and examiners.

Figure 6. Detail of the FDOPA compartment model describing all of the metabolic pathways of ^{18}F–FDOPA

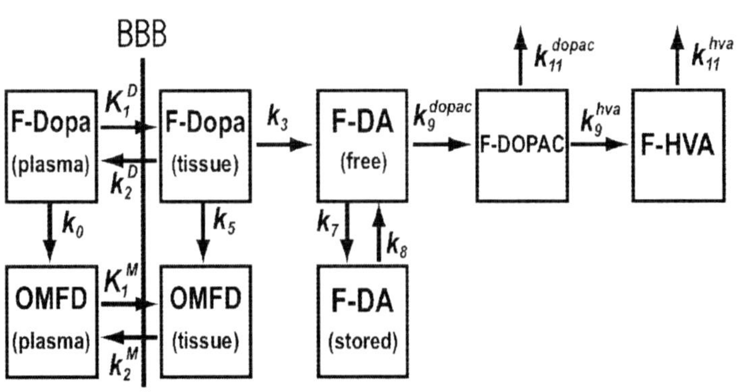

Figure 7. Reference tissue model. Two regions are considered: the target and reference regions. In this model, the reference region has only one compartment for free ligand, and the target region has two compartments of binding (Cb) and free (Cf) ligands.

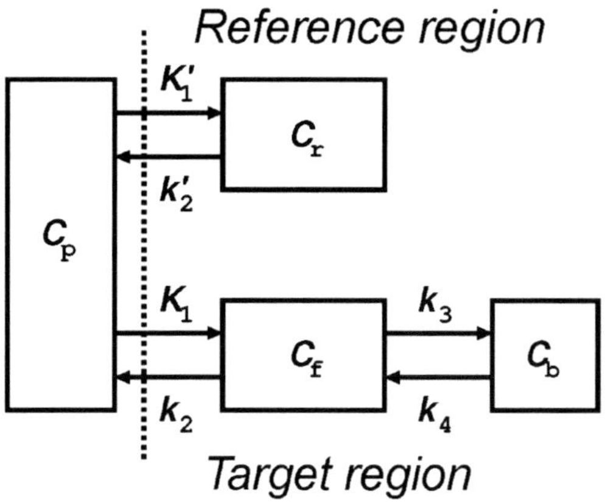

However, with the reference tissue method (Lammertsma & Hume, 1996), one can avoid arterial blood sampling by means of employing a reference region as an alternative to the arterial input function in PET imaging. In the reference region method, two regions, the target region and the reference region, are considered (Figure 7). Both regions share the same arterial input function (C_p in Figure 7) and C_p is mathematically eliminated if data from the two regions are combined. There are many radioligands that can be adapted to the reference tissue model. ^{11}C-raclopride is the suitable radioligand for the reference tissue model. The region of the basal ganglia has high concentrations of D2 dopamine receptor, and the cerebellar region has negligible amounts of D2 dopamine receptor. In the target region, there are two compartments, one for binding and one for free ligand. In the reference region, there is only one compartment for the free ligand (Figure 7). Note, however, that it is not necessary that the reference region have only one compartment (Endres, Bencherif, Hilton, Madar, & Frost, 2003).

APPROACH FOR NEURORECEPTOR COMPETITION STUDY

Although the PET scanner can only detect the location and intensity of injected radioligand, it is possible to detect changes of endogenous compounds indirectly by PET. Figure 8 shows a schematic diagram for competition between the radioligand and the endogenous ligand, and the compartment model explains this competition (Endres et al., 1997). The radioligand binding to the specific receptor site is replaced by the endogenous ligand, which eventually causes a decline of the signal in the PET image. Therefore, by comparing PET images of two conditions for different occupancy of the radioligand, it is possible to investigate synaptic interaction between the radioligand and the endogenous ligand. Many studies have been conducted using this principle to understand neurotransmitter behavior and drug action (Talbot & Laruelle, 2002).

Similar to PET with ^{15}O studies, there are two approaches for injecting radioligand in competition studies: continuous infusion and bolus injection.

In the continuous infusion technique, after achieving the equilibrium condition, the binding

Figure 8. Schematic diagram for competition between radioligand and endogenous ligand (left). Two conditions, less endogenous ligand (above) and more endogenous ligand (bottom), are considered. The compartment model used to explain this competition is shown (right).

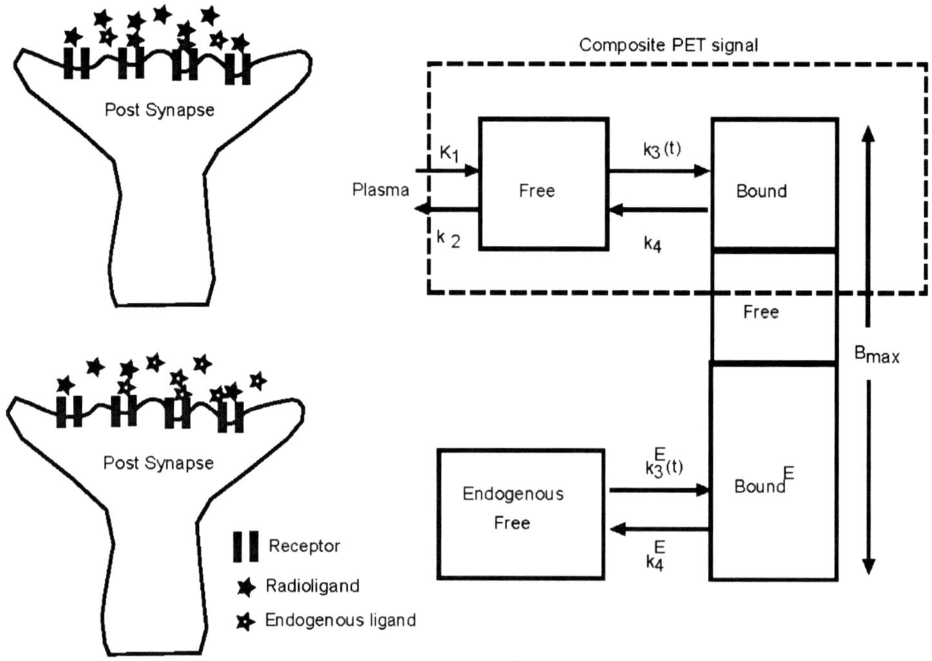

potential (BP_{ND}) of the radioligand (i.e., the ability to bind to a specific region) can be easily calculated by using PET counts in the target region (the region in which the radioligand specifically binds) and in the reference region (the region with no specific binding) (Watabe et al., 2000). In the bolus injection, it is necessary to analyze time courses of PET data to fully understand pharmacokinetics of the radioligand. However, the bolus injection technique has greater sensitivity, allowing it to detect changes in BP_{ND} under different conditions (Endres & Carson, 1998). Conventionally, to obtain BP_{ND} under different conditions, we must perform PET scans on different days. Ikoma et al. developed a technique that enables multiple injections with a single PET scan (Ikoma et al., 2009, 2010). By this technique, the whole study can be shortened dramatically (Figure 9).

CONCLUSION

PET is a very attractive tool for early detection of brain disorders. To strengthen the power of PET, it is important to understand the pharmacokinetics of the radioligand, and one must choose the appropriate technique to analyze the PET data.

REFERENCES

Endres, C., Bencherif, B., Hilton, J., Madar, I., & Frost, J. (2003). Quantification of brain mu-opioid receptors with 11C carfentanil: Reference-tissue methods. *Nuclear Medicine and Biology*, *30*(2), 177–186. doi:10.1016/S0969-8051(02)00411-0

Figure 9. Parametric images of BP_{ND} (top) and time activity curves of basal ganglia (specific binding site) and cerebellum (reference region site) measured by PET (bottom). Three doses of ^{11}C-raclopride were injected in 50-min intervals. By altering the specific activity of ^{11}C-raclopride for each injection, occupancy of the D2 dopamine receptor by ^{11}C-raclopride was changed, and the technique successfully estimated BP_{ND} for each injection of ^{11}C-raclopride.

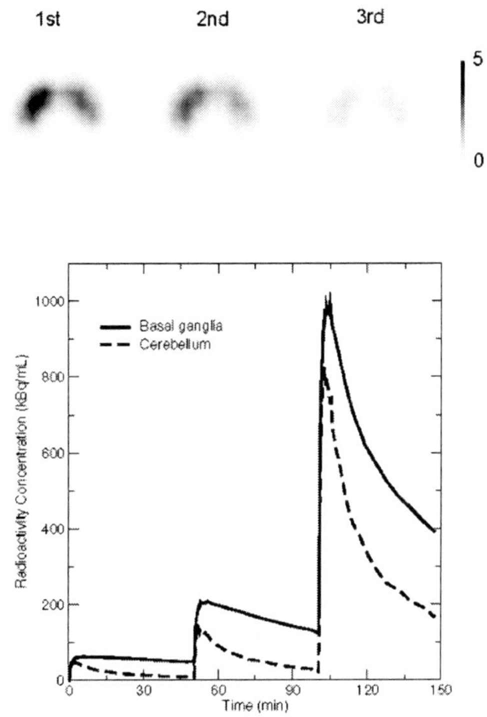

Endres, C., & Carson, R. (1998). Assessment of dynamic neurotransmitter changes with bolus or infusion delivery of neuro-receptor ligands. *Journal of Cerebral Blood Flow and Metabolism*, *18*(11), 1196–1210. doi:10.1097/00004647-199811000-00006

Endres, C., Kolachana, B., Saunders, R., Su, T., Weinberger, D., & Breier, A. (1997). Kinetic modeling of 11C raclopride: Combined PET-microdialysis studies. *Journal of Cerebral Blood Flow and Metabolism*, *17*(9), 932–942. doi:10.1097/00004647-199709000-00002

Frackowiak, R. S., Lenzi, G. L., Jones, T., & Heather, J. D. (1980). Quantitative measurement of regional cerebral blood flow and oxygen metabolism in man using 15o and positron emission tomography: Theory, procedure, and normal values. *Journal of Computer Assisted Tomography*, *4*(6), 727–736. doi:10.1097/00004728-198012000-00001

Gjedde, A. (1981). High-and low-affinity transport of D-glucose from blood to brain. *Journal of Neurochemistry*, *36*(4), 1463–1471. doi:10.1111/j.1471-4159.1981.tb00587.x

Ikoma, Y., Watabe, H., Hayashi, T., Miyake, Y., Teramoto, N., & Minato, K. (2009). Quantitative evaluation of changes in binding porential with a simplified reference tissue model and multiple injections of 11c raclopride. *NeuroImage, 47*(4), 1639–1648. doi:10.1016/j.neuroimage.2009.05.099

Ikoma, Y., Watabe, H., Hayashi, T., Miyake, Y., Teramoto, N., & Minato, K. (2010). Measurement of density and affinity for dopamine d(2) receptors by a single positron emission tomography scan with multiple injections of (11)c raclopride. *Journal of Cerebral Blood Flow and Metabolism, 30*, 663–667. doi:10.1038/jcbfm.2009.239

Johansen, K. K., White, L. R., Sando, S. B., & Aasly, J. O. (2010). Biomarkers: Parkinson disease with dementia and dementia with lewy bodies. *Parkinsonism & Related Disorders, 16*(5), 307–315. doi:10.1016/j.parkreldis.2010.02.015

Klunk, W., Engler, H., Nordberg, A., Wang, Y., Blomqvist, G., & Holt, D. (2004). Imaging brain amyloid in Alzheimer's disease with Pittsburgh compound-b. *Annals of Neurology, 55*(3), 306–319. doi:10.1002/ana.20009

Kudo, Y., Okamura, N., Furumoto, S., Tashiro, M., Furukawa, K., & Maruyama, M. (2007). 2-(2-(2-dimethylaminothiazol-5-yl)ethenyl)-6-(2-(fluoro)ethoxy)benzoxazole: A novel pet agent for in vivo detection of dense amyloid plaques in Alzheimer's disease patients. *Journal of Nuclear Medicine, 48*(4), 553–561. doi:10.2967/jnumed.106.037556

Kudomi, N., Hayashi, T., Teramoto, N., Watabe, H., Kawachi, N., & Ohta, Y. (2005). Rapid quantitative measurement of CMRO(2) and CBF by dual administration of (15)O-labeled oxygen and water during a single PET scan-a validation study and error analysis in anesthetized monkeys. *Journal of Cerebral Blood Flow and Metabolism, 25*, 1209–1224. doi:10.1038/sj.jcbfm.9600118

Kumakura, Y., Gjedde, A., Danielsen, E., Christensen, S., & Cumming, P. (2006). Dopamine storage capacity in caudate and putamen of patients with early Parkinson's disease: Correlation with asymmetry of motor symptoms. *Journal of Cerebral Blood Flow and Metabolism, 26*(3), 358–370. doi:10.1038/sj.jcbfm.9600202

Lammertsma, A., & Hume, S. (1996). Simplified reference tissue model for pet receptor studies. *NeuroImage, 4*(3 Pt 1), 153–158. doi:10.1006/nimg.1996.0066

Matsubara, K., Watabe, H., Hayashi, T., Minato, K., & Iida, H. (2010). Evaluation of bias of the influx constant estimated by patlak analysis for (18F) FDOPA PET: Influence of metabolites for (18F) FDOPA (Japanese). *Transactions of the Japanese Society for Medical and Biological Engineering, 48*(1), 66–74.

Mintun, M., Raichle, M., Martin, W., & Herscovitch, P. (1984). Brain oxygen utilization measured with O-15 radiotracers and positron emission tomography. *Journal of Nuclear Medicine, 25*(2), 177–187.

Patlak, C., Blasberg, R., & Fenstermacher, J. (1983). Graphical evaluation of blood-to-brain transfer constants from multiple-time uptake data. *Journal of Cerebral Blood Flow and Metabolism, 3*(1), 1–7.

Sioka, C., Fotopoulos, A., & Kyritsis, A. P. (2010). Recent advances in PET imaging for evaluation of Parkinson's disease. *European Journal of Nuclear Medicine and Molecular Imaging.*

Subramanyam, R., Alpert, N. M., Hoop, B., Brownell, G. L., & Taveras, J. M. (1978). A model for regional cerebral oxygen distribution during continuous inhalation of 15O2, C15O, and C15O2. *Journal of Nuclear Medicine, 19*(1), 48–53.

Talbot, P. S., & Laruelle, M. (2002). The role of in vivo molecular imaging with PET and SPECT in the elucidation of psychiatric drug action and new drug development. *European Neuropsychopharmacology, 12*(6), 503–511. doi:10.1016/S0924-977X(02)00099-8

Watabe, H., Endres, C., Breier, A., Schmall, B., Eckelman, W., & Carson, R. (2000). Measurement of dopamine release with continuous infusion of (11C)raclopride: Optimization and signal-to-noise considerations. *Journal of Nuclear Medicine, 41*(3), 522–530.

Watabe, H., Ikoma, Y., Kimura, Y., Naganawa, M., & Shidahara, M. (2006). PET kinetic analysis–compartmental model. *Annals of Nuclear Medicine, 20*(9), 583–589. doi:10.1007/BF02984655

Woo, S., Watabe, H., Choi, Y., Kim, K., Park, C., & Bloomfield, P. (2004). Sinogram-based motion correction of PET images using optical motion tracking system and list-mode data acquisition. *IEEE Transactions on Nuclear Science, 51*(3), 782–788. doi:10.1109/TNS.2004.829786

KEY TERMS AND DEFINITIONS

Binding Potential: Kinetic parameter representing the strength of binding for a ligand. The binding potential is a function of the concentration of neuroreceptor available and is also related to the dissociation rate of the ligand from the neuroreceptor.

Cerebral Blood Flow (CBF): In PET, this is measured by $H_2{}^{15}O$. CBF is utilized to diagnose brain diseases such as stroke and dementia.

Cerebral Metabolic Rate of Oxygen ($CMRO_2$): In PET, this is measured by $^{15}O_2$ and $H_2{}^{15}O$. Oxygen consumption is a basic metabolic process of the brain, and $CMRO_2$ is an important index used to investigate brain damage.

Cyclotron: A particle accelerator. It is used to generate positron-emitting radioisotopes. A charged particle is accelerated by a magnetic field and high frequency voltage and finally collides with a target to produce nuclear reactions.

Dopamine: A catecholamine neurotransmitter. There are many diseases related to dopamine, such as Parkinson's disease, schizophrenia, and autism.

Endogenous Ligand: Chemical compound that originates from within an organism.

Kinetic Parameter: A parameter that represents some kinetic feature of the pharmaceutical. The rate constant between compartments for the compartment model is one kind of kinetic parameter.

Neuroreceptor: A neural signal from one neuron passes to another neuron across a synapse. The synapse is a small gap between neurons. From one neuron (presynaptic neuron), a particular chemical (neurotransmitter) is emitted, and the other side of the neuron at the synapse (postsynaptic neuron) receives the neurotransmitter through a neuroreceptor, which is a chemically gated ion channel in the neuron membrane.

PET: Positron emission tomography allows the inside of a living body to be imaged by detecting γ rays from radioligands that emit positrons.

Positron: An electron with a positive charge. The positron collides with an electron, and by this collision, the positron and the electron annihilate each other to produce two γ rays of 511 keV, which are emitted in opposite directions.

Chapter 20
Motion Perception in Healthy Humans and Cognitive Disorders

Takao Yamasaki
Department of Clinical Neurophysiology, Neurological Institute, Graduate School of Medical Sciences, Kyushu University, Japan

Shozo Tobimatsu
Department of Clinical Neurophysiology, Neurological Institute, Graduate School of Medical Sciences, Kyushu University, Japan

ABSTRACT

To elucidate how the dorsal visual pathway is functionally altered in mild cognitive impairment (MCI) and Alzheimer's disease (AD) patients, first, the neural basis of motion perception in healthy young adults was examined by using visual event-related potentials (ERPs) and functional magnetic resonance imaging (fMRI) with coherent motion stimuli such as radial optic flow (OF) and horizontal motion (HO). Nonspecific, motion-related N170 from V5/MT and OF-specific P200 with an inferior parietal lobule (IPL) origin were obtained in ERPs. fMRI revealed the close relationship between IPL activity and OF stimuli. Next, coherent motion perception was assessed by the psychophysical thresholds for patients with AD and MCI, as well as ERPs for MCI patients. MCI patients manifested a selective elevation of the OF threshold, while AD patients exhibited higher psychophysical thresholds for both OF and HO. In ERPs, the P200 latency for OF (but not the N170 latency for OF and HO) was significantly prolonged in MCI patients. These findings indicate that patients with AD and MCI have impaired coherent motion processing due to higher levels of the dorsal pathway. In particular, OF processing related to the IPL is selectively impaired in patients with MCI. Therefore, a combined approach with psychophysics and ERPs using coherent motion (particularly OF) can be useful to discriminate MCI and AD patients from older but healthy adults.

DOI: 10.4018/978-1-60960-559-9.ch020

Figure 1. Parallel visual pathways in humans. d-d pathway, dorso-dorsal pathway; v-d pathway, ventro-dorsal pathway; LGN, lateral geniculate nucleus; V1, 2, 3, 4 and 6 are the primary, secondary, tertiary, quaternary and senary visual cortices, respectively; V5/MT, quinary visual cortex/middle temporal area; MST, medial superior temporal area; IPL, inferior parietal lobule, SPL, superior parietal lobule; and IT, inferior temporal cortex.

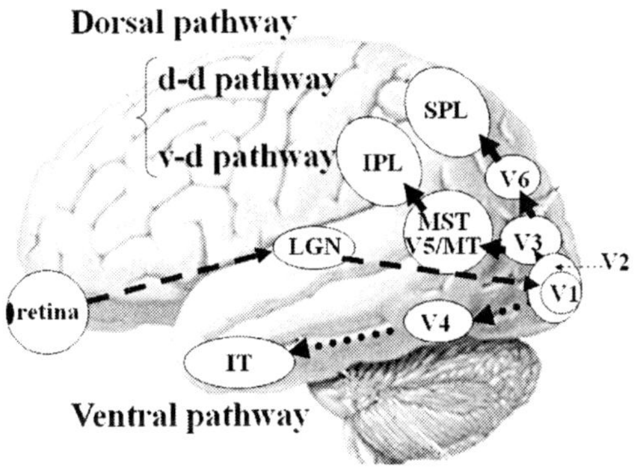

INTRODUCTION

The Parallel Visual Pathways in Humans

Two major parallel visual pathways exist in humans, namely the parvocellular (P) and magnocellular (M) pathways (Livingstone, & Hubel, 1988; Tobimatsu, & Celesia, 2006). Both systems begin in the retina and project to the primary visual cortex (V1) via the lateral geniculate nucleus. From V1, the P-pathway projects to the ventral stream, which includes V4 and the inferior temporal cortex. This system is responsible for processing form and color because it can detect stimuli with high spatial frequency and color (Livingstone & Hubel, 1988; Tobimatsu, & Celesia, 2006). Conversely, after V1, the M-pathway projects to the dorsal stream, which includes V3a, V5/MT, MST, V6 and the posterior parietal lobule. This system plays an important role in detecting motion as it responds to high temporal stimuli (Livingstone, & Hubel, 1988; Tobimatsu, & Celesia, 2006). Recently, the dorsal stream was shown to be divided into two functional streams in primates: the dorso-dorsal (d-d) and ventro-dorsal (v-d) streams (Rizzolatti, & Matelli, 2003). The former consists of V6 and the superior parietal lobule (SPL), whereas the latter is formed by V5/MT and the inferior parietal lobule (IPL).

Figure 2. Local and global motion processing. (a) Local motion processing in V1. V1 neurons have a small receptive field and can detect rightward singular motion. (b) Global motion processing in the higher visual areas, including V5/MT and the parietal lobules. Neurons in the higher visual areas have a large receptive field and can detect rightward group motion. Therefore, we can perceive rightward coherent motion.

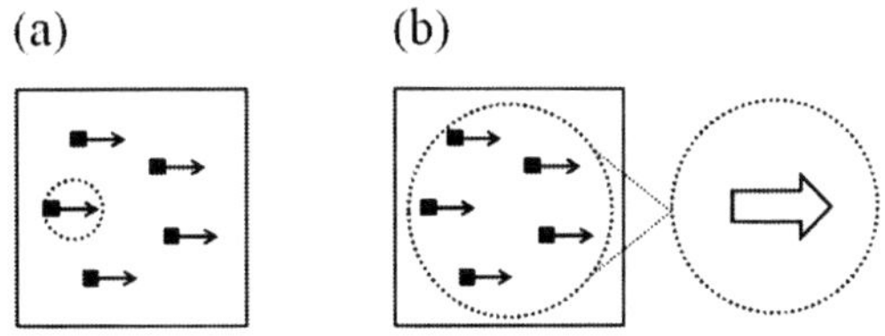

Motion Perception in Humans

Motion information is mainly processed by the dorsal stream (Livingstone, & Hubel, 1988; Tobimatsu, & Celesia, 2006). It is well-known that the higher level dorsal stream, including V5/MT, integrates local motion signals from V1 into global motion (Snowden, Treue, Erickson, & Andersen, 1991) (Figure 2). Therefore, coherent motion stimuli have been widely used to investigate global motion processing in psychophysical, electrophysiological and neuroimaging studies (Newsome, & Paré, 1988; Niedeggen, & Wist, 1999; Morrone et al., 2000). There are several types of global motion, including radial optic flow (OF) and horizontal motion (HO; Figure 3). In particular, radial OF, the visual motion seen during observer self-movement, is important for

Figure 3. Visual motion stimuli in this study. (a) HO stimulus that moves leftward or rightward. (b) OF stimulus that moves radially and outward.

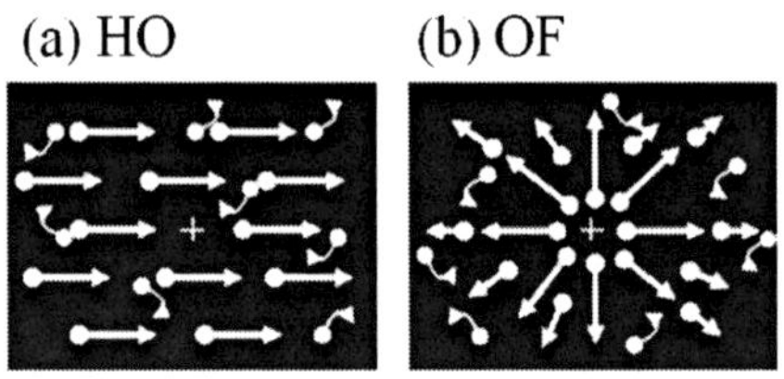

daily life because it provides cues about the direction and 3D structure of the visual environment (Warren, & Hannon, 1988). However, it remains uncertain how OF and HO are processed within the two distinct dorsal streams in humans.

Visuospatial Impairment in Cognitive Disorders

Alzheimer's disease (AD) is a neurodegenerative disease that is the most frequent type of dementia (Ferri et al., 2005). Many patients with AD have visuospatial impairment early in the course of the disease (Henderson, Mack, & Williams, 1989), and this impairment is associated with possible dysfunction of the dorsal pathway (Kiyosawa et al., 1989). Mild cognitive impairment (MCI) has been considered as an intermediate cognitive state between healthy aging and dementia (Bennett, Schneider, Bienias, Evans, & Wilson, 2005) and frequently converts to AD (conversion rate, 10–15% per year) (Petersen, Smith, Waring, Ivnik, Tangalos, & Kokmen, 1999). MCI also causes visuospatial impairment (Mapstone, Teresa, Steffenella, & Duffy, 2003). However, it remains unknown how the dorsal pathway is functionally altered in AD and MCI.

Therefore, to elucidate this issue, we first examined the neural basis of motion perception in humans (in particular, how OF and HO are differently processed within the two distinct dorsal streams in healthy young adults), by using visual event-related potentials (ERPs) and functional magnetic resonance imaging (fMRI) with coherent OF and HO stimuli (Yamasaki, Goto, & Tobimatsu, 2006; Yamasaki, Fujita, Kamio, & Tobimatsu, 2009). Then, coherent motion perception was assessed by determining the psychophysical thresholds for MCI and AD (Yamasaki et al., 2006), as well as the ERPs for MCI.

METHODS

Motion Perception in Healthy Young Adults

ERP and fMRI in response to coherent motion (HO and OF) stimuli were recorded in healthy young adults. Visual stimuli consisted of 400 white square dots randomly presented on a black background. The white dots moved at a velocity of 5.0°/s. HO contained dots that moved leftward or rightward, and OF contained dots that moved radially in an outward pattern (Figure 3). The coherent level was 90% in both stimuli. A high-density 128-channel ERP was recorded using the Geodesic electroencephalogram system, NetAmps 200 (EGI, Eugene, Oregon).

fMRI was recorded using a 1.5 T Magnetom SYMPHONY (Siemens, Erlangen, Germany) whole body MRI system. Image processing and statistical analyses were performed using SPM2 (from the Wellcome Department of Cognitive Neurology, London, UK).

Motion Perception in Healthy Old Adults and Cognitive Disorders

First, the motion coherence thresholds for HO and OF motions were determined in healthy old adults and in patients with MCI and AD using a left/right two-alternative forced-choice discrimination technique (Harvey, 1986). Coherent motion patterns were intermixed with random motion, and the percentage of coherently and randomly moving dots varied between trials for

Figure 4. ERP responses in healthy young adults. Two major components (N170 and P200) are obtained. The N170 component is evoked by both stimuli, but the P200 is only elicited by OF.

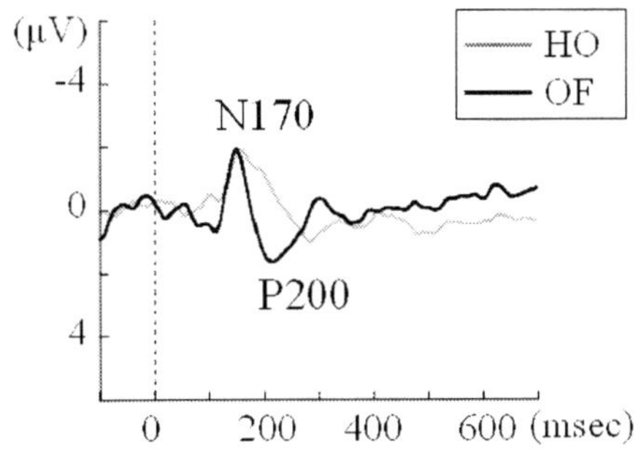

the determination of motion coherent thresholds. In the HO condition, subjects indicated whether the coherent motion was to the left or right. In the OF condition, subjects indicated whether the focus of expansion or contraction was on the left or right. Perceptual thresholds were defined as the percentages of coherent motion in stimuli ([coherently moving dots]/[coherently moving dots + random dots]) × 100), yielding 82.0% correct responses and reflecting a Weibull fit to psychophysical responses (Harvey, 1986).

Next, a high-density 128-channel ERP for coherent OF and HO stimuli was recorded in healthy old adults and in patients with MCI using the Geodesic electroencephalogram system, NetAmps 200 (EGI, Eugene, Oregon).

RESULTS AND DISCUSSION

Motion Perception in Healthy Young Adults

With ERPs, two major components (N170, P200) were obtained (Figure 4). The N170 had a V5/MT origin and was evoked by both stimuli. In contrast, the P200 had an IPL (BA 40) origin and was only elicited by OF. These findings suggest that the N170 component is a nonspecific, motion-related component originating from V5/MT, while the P200 is an OF-specific component generated by the IPL.

With regard to fMRI, activations of the v-d stream, including IPL (BA 39/40), were found in the OF minus HO condition (Figure 5a). On the contrary, the HO minus OF condition showed the activation of the d-d stream, including SPL (BA 7; Figure 5b). These results demonstrate that the dorsal pathway can be separated into two distinct functional streams in healthy young adults. SPL (the d-d stream) is more related to HO motion processing, and IPL (the v-d stream) is important for OF motion processing.

Motion Perception in Healthy Old Adults and Those with Cognitive Disorders

The HO motion threshold was significantly higher in AD but not in MCI patients compared with

Figure 5. fMRI responses in healthy young adults. (a) Activations of the v-d stream, including IPL (BA 39/40), are found in the OF minus HO condition. (b) The HO minus OF condition shows the activation of the d-d stream, including SPL (BA 7).

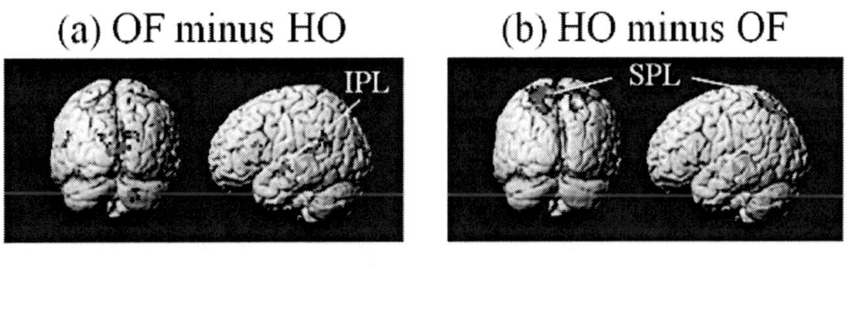

healthy old adults. In contrast, the significant elevation of the OF motion threshold was observed in both AD and MCI patients compared with healthy old adults. These findings imply that motion processing is more severely impaired in AD than in MCI patients, and impaired OF motion perception may occur early in the course from MCI to AD.

Similar to healthy young adults, two major components (N170 and P200) were obtained with ERPs. There was no significant difference in N170 latency for both OF and HO stimuli between healthy old adults and MCI patients. Conversely, significant prolongation of P200 latency for OF was observed in MCI patients. These results indicate that MCI patients have selective impairment of OF perception that is related to the v-d pathway (IPL).

CONCLUSION

AD and MCI patients have impaired coherent motion processing due to the higher level of the dorsal pathway. In particular, OF processing related to the v-d pathway (IPL) is selectively impaired in MCI patients. Therefore, a combined approach with psychophysics and ERPs using coherent motion (particularly OF) can be useful in discriminating MCI and AD patients from healthy older adults early in the disease course.

ACKNOWLEDGMENT

This study was supported in part by Grants-in-Aid for Scientists, No. 18890131 and No. 20591026, from the Ministry of Education, Culture, Sports, Science and Technology in Japan. We would like to thank Drs. Jun-ichi Kira, Takayuki Taniwaki, Yasumasa Ohyagi, Yoshinobu Goto, Takashi Yoshiura, Katsuya Ogata, Shinji Munetsuna, Ikue Ijichi and Yuka Miyanaga for their research assistance.

REFERENCES

Bennett, D. A., Schneider, J. A., Bienias, J. L., Evans, D. A., & Wilson, R. S. (2005). Mild cognitive impairment is related to Alzheimer disease pathology and cerebral infarctions. *Neurology*, *64*, 834–841.

Ferri, C. P., Prince, M., Brayne, C., Brodaty, H., Fratiglioni, L., & Ganguli, M. (2005). Global prevalence of dementia: A Delphi consensus study. *Lancet*, *366*, 2112–2117. doi:10.1016/S0140-6736(05)67889-0

Harvey, L. O. (1986). Efficient estimation of sensory thresholds. *Behavior Research Methods, Instruments, & Computers*, *18*, 623–632. doi:10.3758/BF03201438

Henderson, V. W., Mack, W., & Williams, B. W. (1989). Spatial disorientation in Alzheimer's disease. *Archives of Neurology*, *46*, 391–394.

Kiyosawa, M., Bosley, T. M., Chawluk, J., Jamieson, D., Schatz, N. J., & Savino, P. J. (1989). Alzheimer's disease with prominent visual symptoms clinical and metabolic evaluation. *Ophthalmology*, *96*, 1077–1086.

Livingstone, M., & Hubel, D. (1988). Segregation of form, color, movement, and depth: Anatomy, physiology, and perception. *Science*, *240*, 740–749. doi:10.1126/science.3283936

Mapstone, M., Teresa, M., Steffenella, M., & Duffy, C. J. (2003). A visuospatial variant of mild cognitive impairment. Getting lost between aging and AD. *Neurology*, *60*, 802–808.

Morrone, M. C., Tosetti, M., Montanaro, D., Fiorentini, A., Cioni, G., & Burr, D. C. (2000). A cortical area that responds specifically to optic flow, revealed by fMRI. *Nature Neuroscience*, *12*, 1322–1328. doi:10.1038/81860

Newsome, W. T., & Paré, E. B. (1988). A selective impairment of motion perception following lesions of the middle temporal area (MT). *The Journal of Neuroscience*, *8*, 2201–2211.

Niedeggen, M., & Wist, E. R. (1999). Characteristics of visual evoked potentials generated by motion coherence onset. *Brain Research. Cognitive Brain Research*, *8*, 95–105. doi:10.1016/S0926-6410(99)00009-9

Petersen, R. C., Smith, G. E., Waring, S. C., Ivnik, R. J., Tangalos, E. G., & Kokmen, E. (1999). Mild cognitive impairment: clinical characterization and outcome. *Archives of Neurology*, *56*, 303–308. doi:10.1001/archneur.56.3.303

Rizzolatti, G., & Matelli, M. (2003). Two different streams form the dorsal visual system: anatomy and functions. *Experimental Brain Research*, *153*, 146–157. doi:10.1007/s00221-003-1588-0

Snowden, R. J., Treue, S., Erickson, R. G., & Andersen, R. A. (1991). The response of area MT and V1 neurons to transparent motion. *The Journal of Neuroscience*, *11*, 2768–2785.

Tobimatsu, S., & Celesia, G. G. (2006). Studies of human visual pathophysiology with visual evoked potentials. *Clinical Neurophysiology*, *117*, 1414–1433. doi:10.1016/j.clinph.2006.01.004

Warren, W. H., & Hannon, D. J. (1988). Direction of self-motion is perceived from optic flow. *Nature*, *336*, 162–163. doi:10.1038/336162a0

Yamasaki, T., Fujita, T., Kamio, Y., & Tobimatsu, S. (2009). Visual motion processing in autism spectrum disorder. *Clinical EEG (Electroencephalography)*, *51*, 463–469.

Yamasaki, T., Goto, Y., & Tobimatsu, S. (2006). Evoked potentials related to motion perception and face recognition. *Clinical EEG (Electroencephalography)*, *48*, 413–418.

KEY TERMS AND DEFINITIONS

Alzheimer's Disease (AD): A progressive neurodegenerative disorder with characteristic clinical (memory loss, disorientation for time and place and visuospatial impairment) and pathological (cerebral atrophy, amyloid β and neurofibrillary tangles) features.

Coherent Motion: Global motion signal that is apparent from the integration of locally moving elements.

Dorsal Visual Pathway: Is known as the "where" pathway. This pathway stretches from the primary visual cortex (V1) in the occipital lobe forward into the parietal lobe. It is interconnected with the parallel ventral pathway (the "what" pathway), which runs downward from V1 into the temporal lobe. The dorsal pathway is characterized by high temporal resolution, high contrast sensitivity, color insensitivity, and low spatial resolution. Thus, this pathway is important for perception of motion, global structure and stereopsis and is related to control of action "on-line".

Event-Related Potentials (ERPs): A procedure that measures electrical activity of the brain related to higher processes. ERPs have excellent time resolution (milliseconds).

Functional Magnetic Resonance Imaging (fMRI): Measures the hemodynamic response (change in blood flow) related to neural activity in the brain. fMRI provides excellent spatial resolution (millimeters).

Inferior Parietal Lobule (IPL): This region lies below the horizontal portion of the intraparietal sulcus and behind the lower part of the postcentral sulcus. The IPL is further divided into the supramarginal and angular gyri.

Mild Cognitive Impairment (MCI): A diagnosis given to individuals who have cognitive impairments beyond those expected for their age and education that do not interfere significantly with their daily activities. MCI is considered to be the boundary or transitional stage between normal aging and dementia.

Optic Flow (OF): The pattern of apparent motion of objects, surfaces, and edges in a visual scene caused by the relative motion between an observer and the scene. There are several types of OF, such as radial (expansion and contraction), circular and spiral motion.

Chapter 21
Neuronal Transcytosis of WGA Conjugated Protein: A New Approach to Amyloid-β In Vivo

Yoshiki Takeuchi
Department of Anatomy and Neurobiology, Faculty of Medicine, Kagawa University, Japan

Yoshiki Matsumoto
Department of Anatomy and Neurobiology, Faculty of Medicine, Kagawa University, Japan

Takanori Miki
Department of Anatomy and Neurobiology, Faculty of Medicine, Kagawa University, Japan

Katsuhiko Warita
Department of Anatomy and Neurobiology, Faculty of Medicine, Kagawa University, Japan

Zhi-Yu Wang
Department of Anatomy and Neurobiology, Faculty of Medicine, Kagawa University, Japan

Tomiko Yakura
Department of Anatomy and Neurobiology, Faculty of Medicine, Kagawa University, Japan

Jun-Qian Liu
Department of Anatomy and Neurobiology, Faculty of Medicine, Kagawa University, Japan

ABSTRACT

Neuronal transcytosis was observed at the stage when no neurotransmitter was released after the injection of wheat germ agglutinin-conjugated horseradish peroxidase (WGA-HRP; WGA = 22 kDa, HRP = 40 kDa) into the vagus nerve. The co-injection of Rab3A-siRNA with WGA-HRP into the vagus nerve was performed to further examine this phenomenon. This co-injection resulted in the transcytosis of WGA-HRP, both of the passing type, by which it crossed the synapses, and of the secretion type followed by endocytosis of postsynaptic membranes. These findings raised the possibility in vivo that WGA plays an important role in the transcytosis of protein. Therefore, WGA may be a valuable tool for therapeutic drug targeting via transcytosis. The ability of WGA-conjugated Amyloid β (WGA-Aβ) to decrease amyloid deposits in Alzheimer's disease was investigated. The conjugation of WGA to amyloid-β (1-40) (Aβ; 5 kDa) was confirmed. WGA-Aβ was then shown to move to terminals by axonal flow in vivo as well as WGA-HRP. WGA-Aβ was also observed in the nodose ganglion cells and terminals after injections of fluorescent Aβ (FAβ) into the vagus nerve and fluorescent WGA (FWGA) into the common carotid artery. These studies suggested that WGA-Aβ could be localized to solitary neurons via transcytosis.

DOI: 10.4018/978-1-60960-559-9.ch021

INTRODUCTION

A biological analysis of functional implications at the cellular and molecular levels is useful for understanding normal and pathological brain conditions. In the nervous system, axonal transport and synaptic transmission are exclusively essential for brain function. Many studies commonly used wheat germ agglutinin (WGA) -conjugated horseradish peroxidase (HRP) as a neuronal tracer. Recently, WGA-HRP has been indicated to undergo non-vesicular synaptic transport at the stage when no neurotransmitter was released (Takeuchi, 2009) in contrast to vesicular synaptic transport (von Bartheld, 2004). These findings seem to be based on the specificity of protein conjugation to WGA (Kaji, 2006). Therefore, the present study was performed to investigate whether WGA conjugates amyloid-β (Aβ) and whether its conjugation undergoes axonal flow or transcytosis *in vivo*, as a unique method for the treatment of Alzheimer's disease.

MATERIALS AND METHODS

Male Wistar rats weighing 180-236 g were anesthetized with intraperitoneal injection of chloral hydrate (490 mg/kg) for all surgical procedures. The experimental procedures were conducted in accordance with the National Institutes of Health (NIH) Guide for the Care and Use of Laboratory Animals. The Kagawa University Animal Care and Use Committee approved the procedures, and all efforts were made to minimize the number of animals used and their suffering.

1) Experiments of WGA-HRP

A 4% solution of WGA-HRP (0.4-2.0 μl) or a working solution of 1 nM Rab3A-siRNA containing 4% WGA-HRP was injected into the vagus nerve on one side using a 10-μl Hamilton microsyringe (Reno, Nevada, U.S.A.). After a survival period of 12-72 h, the animals were sacrificed by perfusion with 0.1 M phosphate buffer (pH 7.4) followed by a fixative of 1% paraformaldehyde and 1.25% glutaraldehyde in 0.1 M phosphate buffer. The blocks containing the nucleus of the solitary tract (NST) and dorsal motor nucleus (DMV) of the vagus nerve were processed for visualization of HRP-reaction products (RP) according to the heavy metal-intensified DAB methods. The blocks were then postfixed in buffered 1% osmium tetroxide for 2 h, block-stained in saturated uranyl acetate for 1 h, dehydrated in a graded acetone or an alcohol series and embedded in an epoxy resin mixture. The NST region was identified by the examination of toluidine blue-stained or unstained 1-μm-thick sections. Ultrathin sections of the region were cut and observed without further lead staining using a JEM 200CX electron microscope.

2) Experiments of WGA-Aβ

A solution of fluorescent (F) WGA (1.5-2.0 μl) (Alexa 594-conjugated WGA; Invitrogen, USA), FAβ (1.5-2.0 μl) (Alexa 488-conjugated Aβ; Invitrogen, USA) or FWGA containing FAβ was injected into the vagus nerve on one side using a Hamilton microsyringe fitted with a 33-gauge needle in a volume of 5 μL. Further experiments involved the injection of FAβ into the vagus nerve and FWGA into the common carotid artery. For tissue cryosection analysis, the brain stem and nodose ganglions of the animals were processed with 0.1 M phosphate buffer perfusion and a 4% PFA fixative solution, dehydrated in a solution of graded sucrose in 0.1 M phosphate buffer and embedded in an O.C.T. compound. The sliced NST region and nodose ganglions were placed onto slide glasses and processed for nuclear counter staining with 50 ng/ml Hoechst 33258 (Sigma-Aldrich) for 10 min. All slides were mounted in fluorescence mounting medium (DAKO); the localization of molecules was then detected by an epi-illumination fluorescence microscope (DP-72, Olympus) or a confocal laser scanning microscope (Radiance

*Figure 1. Electron micrograph of anterograde transport of WGA-HRP at the synapse (At: axon terminal, Dend: Dendrite). The HRP-RP (asterisk mark, *) frequently forms a large mass containing a membranous substance. A large irregular shaped mass of the HRP-RP passes through synapses (passing type). Permission to reprint this figure was obtained from ref. (Takeuchi, 2009). Calibration bar = 0.5 μm*

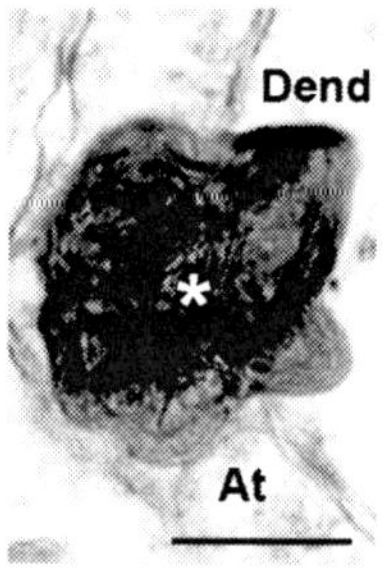

*Figure 2. Electron micrograph of HRP-RP (asterisk mark, *) in the terminals (At: axon terminal) and secondary neurons (Dend: Dendrite) after co-injection of Rab3A-siRNA with WGA-HRP. Secretion followed by endocytosis of the dendrite is better seen in the terminal (secretion type). Permission to print this figure was obtained from ref. (Takeuchi, 2009). Calibration bar = 0.2 μm.*

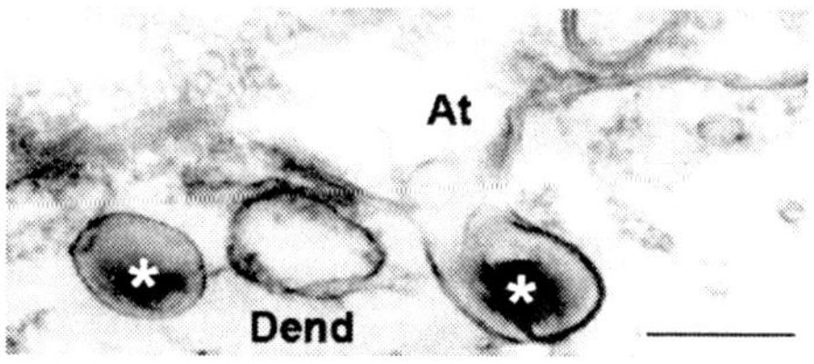

2100 rainbow system, Zeiss) and photographed. All images were analyzed using NIS-elements software (Nikon).

RESULTS

In the terminals of the NST, electron-dense HRP-RP showed various types of lysosomal-like structures and was characterized by the presence of membranous substance crossing synapses (Figure 1). Neuronal transcytosis of WGA-HRP was induced at the stage when no neurotransmitter was released. Based on neurotransmitter release suppression by siRNA interference methods, Rab3A-siRNA was co-injected with WGA-HRP into the vagus nerve. Furthermore this experiments were performed neuronal transcytosis of WGA-HRP including secretion followed by endocytosis of postsynaptic neurons (Figure 2).

The co-injection of FAβ with FWGA into the vagus nerve resulted in double-labeling of these substances in ganglion cells and terminals. FWGA was strongly associated with the plasma membrane. Interestingly, two FWGA granules were frequently co-localized with one FAβ granule (Figure 3). On the other hand, injections of FAβ into the vagus nerve and FWGA into the common carotid artery on same side showed the uptake of FWGA from blood vessel. Vessel-injected FWGA and axon-injected FAβ were demonstlated similar co-localization in the ganglion cytoplasm (data not shown). In addition, vessel-injected FWGA co-localized with axon-injected FAβ in the NST cytoplasm (data not shown). Furthermore, as was seen with co-injection into the vagus nerve, FAβ was conjugated to two FWGA-granules in the NST region (Figure 4). These results suggested the neuronal transcytosis of WGA-Aβ from terminals to solitary neurons.

DISCUSSION

WGA-conjugated proteins, particularly HRP, that could pass through synapses (diacrine like transport) showed the following characteristics: (1) formation of a mass of the HRP-RP, (2) no diffusion into the synaptic cleft, and (3) correspondence to the stage when no neurotransmitter was released. Further studies involving the co-injection of WGA-HRP with Rab3A-siRNA indicated the following additional characteristics: (4) the exis-

Figure 3. The cellular localization of FWGA (A: red) and FAβ (B: green). In the merged images, yellow indicates the overlapping expression of FAβ with FWGA in the ganglion cytoplasm (arrows). After injection into the vagus nerve, a pair of FWGA-granules conjugated with one FAβ-granule (arrows). In another experiment, he vessel-injected FWGA demonstrated a similar conjugation with FAβ (data not shown). Calibration bar = 10 μm.

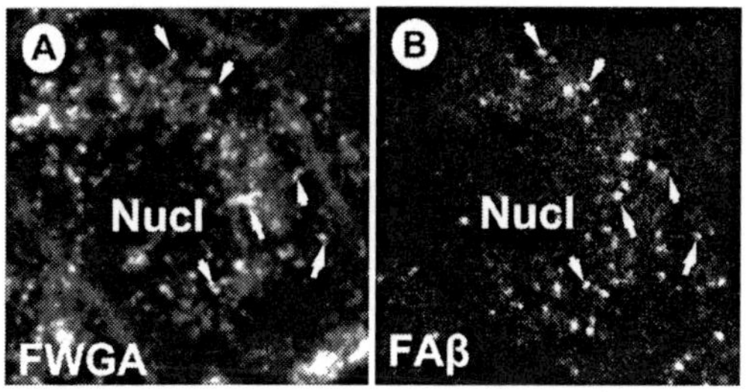

tence of a secretion type (apocrine like transport) and (5) gene-targeted animals were unnecessary. In the fluorescent studies, WGA was also shown to conjugate Aβ in the nerve cell body and move to the terminals, suggesting its movement occurred via transcytosis to secondary neurons *in vivo.*

Immunoblot analysis demonstrated that lectin (WGA)-HRP binds to specific carbohydrate moieties attached to glycoproteins and glycolipids expressed on surface plasma membranes (Schmidt, 1985). WGA has been used as an effective tracer in neuronal systems for a number of lectins because of the common expression of WGA receptors on the surface plasma membranes of most neurons (Yoshihara, 2002). Furthermore, proteoglycans and glycosaminoglycans have been proposed to facilitate amyloid fibril formation and/or stabilize the plaque aggregates (Fraser, 2001). These findings might give insight into the detailed molecular binding sites between WGA and Aβ.

The present study raised the possibility that *in vivo,* WGA plays an important role in the decrease of amyloid deposits in Alzheimer's disease, which is induced by WGA conjugation with Aβ followed by transport to the axon terminals. Electron mi-

Figure 4. The morphological conformation of FWGA (A: red) and FAβ (B: green) was detected and co-localized (C: merged color) in the NST region. The vessel-injected FWGA also co-localized with FAβ in a similar conjugation (data not shown). Calibration bar = 5 μm.

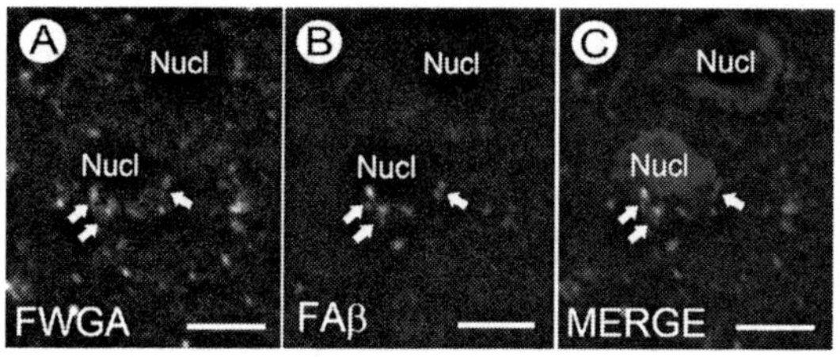

croscopic observations of neuronal transcytosis of WGA-Aβ are currently in progress.

ACKNOWLEDGMENT

The author's gratefully acknowledge the skillful technical assistance of Mr. Wakashi Nagata and Mrs. Mizue Fukutomi. This investigation was supported by a grant for Science Research from the Japanese Ministry of Education (No. 18591292 for YT, No. 21791036 for YM) and the Kagawa University Characteristic Prior Research Fund 2009.

REFERENCES

Fraser, P. E., Darabie, A. A., & McLaurin, J. (2001). Amyloid-β interactions with chondroitin sulfate-derived monosaccharides and disaccharides: Implications for drug development. *The Journal of Biological Chemistry, 276,* 6412–6419. doi:10.1074/jbc.M008128200

Kaji, H., & Isobe, T. (2006). Large-scale analysis of glycoproteins by LC-MS method. *Trends in Glycoscience and Glycotechnology, 18,* 313–332.

Schmidt, M. L., & Trojanowski, J. Q. (1985). Immunoblot analysis of horseradish peroxidase conjugates of wheat germ agglutinin before and after retrograde transport in the rat peripheral nervous system. *The Journal of Neuroscience*, *5*, 2779–2785.

Takeuchi, Y., Matsumoto, Y., Miki, T., Yokoyama, T., Warita, K., & Wang, Z. Y. (2009). Anterograde synaptic transport of neuronal tracer enzyme (WGA-HRP): Further studies with Rab3A-siRNA in the rat. *Biomedical Research*, *20*, 149–154. doi:10.4103/0970-938X.54832

von Bartheld, C. S. (2004). Axonal transport and neuronal transcytosis of trophic factors, tracers, and pathogens. *Journal of Neurobiology*, *58*, 295–314. doi:10.1002/neu.10315

Yoshihara, Y. (2002). Visualizing selective neural pathways with WGA transgene: Combination of neuroanatomy with gene technology. *Neuroscience Research*, *44*, 133–140. doi:10.1016/S0168-0102(02)00130-X

KEY TERMS AND DEFINITIONS

Axonal Transport: The essential brain functions for the movement of macromolecules from viruses, fluorescence substances, amino acids and neuronal tracers. The movement can occur retro- or anterogradely along the axons.

Neuronal Transcytosis: The process by which macromolecules from viruses, fluorescence substances, amino acids and neuronal tracers are transported across the pre- or post-synaptic membrane of an axon terminal.

Nodose Ganglion: Inferior ganglion consisting of sensory cell bodies of the vagus nerve. The sensory fibers reach nucleus of the solitary tract (NST) via the nodose ganglion. The nodose ganglion cells contain amyloid polypeptides (called IAPP, or amylin), and these molecules may regulate cross-polymerization, creating the fibrils of Amyloid-beta of Alzheimer's disease.

Post-Synaptic Membrane: A neuronal network consisting of synapses. A synapse has a small cleft that fits with a neighboring neuron. The pre-synaptic end contains neurotransmitters, and the post-synaptic end contains receptors on the surface of its neuronal membrane.

Rab3A: A Ras-related protein. Brain-specific Ras-related proteins can activate Akt and promote cell survival signal transduction, and the major protein family of rab3A can regulate membrane transport as well as associate with synaptic vesicles that are transported in the neuron.

Small Interfering RNA (siRNA): A gene silencing system that has rapidly become a standard tool for regulating the expression of specific genes *in vivo*. Although siRNA or RNAi therapy has not been commonly applied for clinical use, recent advances in these fields will overcome technical problems for the in vivo delivery of these molecules.

Wheat Germ Agglutinin (WGA): The most well known lectin. WGA can selectively bind N-acetyl-D-glucosamine (GlcNAc)- and O-GlcNAc-modified proteins. O-GlcNAc modification and related proteins can affect synaptic vesicle release and post-synaptic signal transduction. These modifications of WGA (GlcNAc) are linked to important neurodegenerative disorders such as Alzheimer's disease.

Chapter 22
Functional Optical Hemodynamic Imaging of the Olfactory Cortex in Patients with Parkinson's Disease

Masayuki Karaki
Department of Otorhinolaryngology, Japan & Health Sciences School of Nursing, Faculty of Medicine, Kagawa University, Japan

Eiji Kobayashi
Department of Otorhinolaryngology, Japan & Health Sciences School of Nursing, Faculty of Medicine, Kagawa University, Japan

Ryuichi Kobayashi
Department of Otorhinolaryngology, Japan & Health Sciences School of Nursing, Faculty of Medicine, Kagawa University, Japan

Kosuke Akiyama
Department of Otorhinolaryngology, Japan & Health Sciences School of Nursing, Faculty of Medicine, Kagawa University, Japan

Tetsuo Toge
Health Sciences School of Nursing, Faculty of Medicine, Kagawa University, Japan

Nozomu Mori
Department of Otorhinolaryngology, Japan & Health Sciences School of Nursing, Faculty of Medicine, Kagawa University, Japan

ABSTRACT

Olfactory dysfunction is a frequent non-motor symptom in Parkinson's disease (PD). This symptom is considered to be an early manifestation of the disease. The aim of this study was to establish the cortical basis of olfactory function in patients with PD. This study was conducted on ten healthy, normosmic subjects and seven patients with PD (one with subjective olfactory dysfunction and nine without subjective olfactory dysfunction). We employed a 22-channel near-infrared spectroscopy (NIRS) device with eight light-incident fibers and seven light-detector fibers, each with an inter-optode distance of 2.5 centimeters on the frontal head. Isovaleric acid was used as the odor stimulant. We measured the change in total hemoglobin concentrations (totalHb) from pre-baseline values and compared the results obtained for healthy normosmic subjects and patients with PD. In all healthy normosmic subjects and three patients with PD, isovaleric acid caused remarkable changes in (totalHb), especially in the lower areas of the frontal cortex. However, in four patients with PD, isovaleric acid caused no changes. This

DOI: 10.4018/978-1-60960-559-9.ch022

result indicates that subjective symptoms are different from objective test results in patients with PD. These activated areas may be related to the orbitofrontal cortex corresponding to the olfactory cortices. This study suggests that normosmic subjects with PD already have damage to their olfactory function.

INTRODUCTION

Olfactory dysfunction is a frequent non-motor symptom in Parkinson's disease (PD) that is considered to be an early manifestation of the disease. Olfactory dysfunction in PD has been previously reported in some studies (Ross et al, 2008; Kranick & Duda, 2008; Doty, 2007). In a general clinical setting, many methods used in the evaluation of olfactory function are subjective tests (Kondo et al, 1998; Doty et al, 1984). On the other hand, functional magnetic resonance imaging (fMRI) (Sobel et al, 1998; Hummel et al, 2003) and positron emission tomography (PET) (Doty et al, 1984) are objective methods that can be used to evaluate olfactory function. Objective olfactory testing is very rare. Recently, near-infrared spectroscopy (NIRS) has been used to study the functional activation in various areas of the brain (Kusaka et al, 2004; Hoshi & Tamura, 1993). NIRS is a noninvasive method for detecting changes in oxygenated hemoglobin [oxyHb], deoxygenated hemoglobin [deoxyHb] and total hemoglobin [totalHb]. NIRS is useful as a clinical testing device because of its convenience and compact size. In a previous study, we used multi-channel NIRS (MNIRS) to perform functional brain imaging of olfactory activity (Savic, 2004). The aim of this study was to establish the cortical basis of olfactory function in patients with PD.

Figure 1. Comparisons between the maximum changes in [totalHb] of normosmic subjects and patients with PD

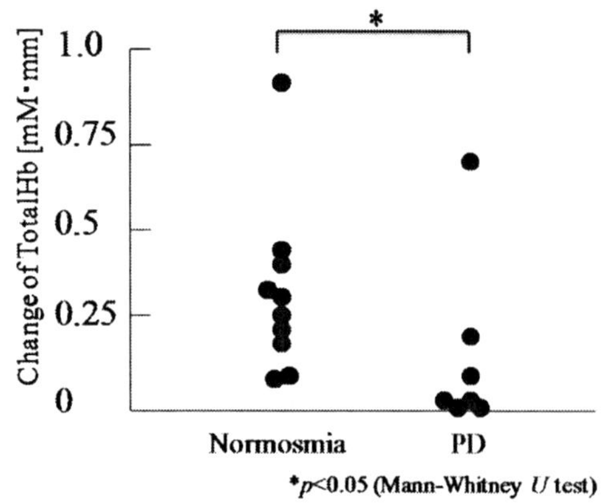

MATERIALS AND METHODS

Multi-Channel Near-Infrared Spectroscopy

The 22-channel near-infrared spectroscopy device (Hitachi Medico Co., Japan) that we employed has seven light-incident fibers and eight light-detector fibers, each with an inter-optode distance of 2.5 centimeters. The light sources were two 0.5 mW continuous laser diodes with wavelengths of 780 and 830 nm. Figure 1 shows the 22 measurement positions in which the 15 fibers were placed in a 5 centimeter by 10 centimeter field over the frontal cortex. These channels could measure changes in concentrations of oxyHb, deoxyHb and totalHb from the pre-baseline values.

Subjects

This study was conducted on ten normosmic subjects (four males and six females: mean age, 28.9 years; range, 22-39 years) and seven PD patients (five males and two females: mean age, 66.8 years; range, 58-77 years). Among the PD patients, one had subjective olfactory dysfunction. All subjects understood the aim of this study and gave informed consent for participation, and the study's protocol was approved by the local ethics committee. T&T olfactometry was done in all subjects. The results showed that all of the normosmic subjects and three patients with PD had normal olfactory function. However, four patients with PD had olfactory dysfunction (grade 2 to grade 4). T&T olfactometry tests categorize the grade from one to five. Normal olfactory function is grade 1. T&T olfactometry is widely used for clinical olfactory testing in Japan (Kondo et al, 1984).

Experimental Procedure

Functional imaging tests were performed on subjects who were awake and sitting in a comfortable chair. During the experiments, subjects closed their eyes and had their ears covered. Isovaleric acid was used as an odor stimulant. Isovaleric acid, which smells like sweat, is used for T&T olfactometry. The intensity of the odorant in T&T olfactometry is generally divided into eight grades, weakest (Level -2) to strongest (Level 5). In this study, isovaleric acid was used at the strongest intensity [Level 5]. A cotton pack containing the isovaleric acid was placed before a participant's nose for five seconds for olfactory stimulation. All subjects breathed through their nose during measurements. No subjects had nasal obstruction.

Methods for Evaluation

We measured changes in [totalHb] from pre-baseline values. The maximum changes in [totalHb] of healthy normosmic subjects and subjects with PD were compared. Statistical analysis was carried out using Mann-Whitney U tests.

RESULTS

Table 2 shows the results of T&T olfactometry and the change in [totalHb] in normosmic subjects. None of the normosmic subjects demonstrated olfactory dysfunction. All changes in [totalHb] were

Table 1. Subject information

Normosmic subjects				
Subjects	**Sex**	**Age**	**Subjective olfactory dysfunction**	**T&T olfactogram**
Sub1	Female	25	No	Grade 1
Sub2	Male	24	No	Grade 1
Sub3	Male	24	No	Grade 1
Sub4	Male	39	No	Grade 1
Sub5	Male	28	No	Grade 1
Sub6	Female	22	No	Grade 1
Sub7	Male	31	No	Grade 1
Sub8	Male	38	No	Grade 1
Sub9	Female	25	No	Grade 1
Sub10	Female	22	No	Grade 1
Patients with PD				
Subjects	**Sex**	**Age**	**Subjective olfactory dysfunction**	**T&T olfactogram**
Sub1	Female	58	no	Grade 1
Sub2	Male	77	no	Grade 2
Sub3	Male	61	no	Grade 1
Sub4	Male	59	no	Grade 1
Sub5	Female	75	no	Grade 4
Sub6	Female	67	yes	Grade 4
Sub7	Male	71	no	Grade 3

Table 2. Results of normosmic subjects

Subjects	Subjective olfactory dysfunction	T&T olfactogram	Max Change of [TotalHb] (mM·mm)
Sub1	No	Grade 1	0.40
Sub2	No	Grade 1	0.34
Sub3	No	Grade 1	0.43
Sub4	No	Grade 1	0.31
Sub5	No	Grade 1	0.18
Sub6	No	Grade 1	0.28
Sub7	No	Grade 1	0.13
Sub8	No	Grade 1	0.11
Sub9	No	Grade 1	0.89
Sub10	No	Grade 1	0.23

Table 3. The results of patients with PD

Subjects	Subjective olfactory dysfunction	T&T olfactogram	Max Change of [TotalHb] (mM·mm)
Sub1	no	Grade 1	0.70
Sub2	no	Grade 2	0.03
Sub3	no	Grade 1	0.02
Sub4	no	Grade 1	0.11
Sub5	no	Grade 4	0.04
Sub6	yes	Grade 4	0.05
Sub7	no	Grade 3	0.21

over 0.1 mM·mm. These results show changes in the hemodynamics of the frontal cortex after isovaleric acid stimulation. The increased changes were seen in the lower area of the frontal cortex.

Table 3 shows the results of T&T olfactometry and the change in [totalHb] in patients with PD. Only one subject had subjective olfactory dysfunction. However, in four subjects the maximum change in [totalHb] was under 0.1 mM·mm.

Figure 1 shows the maximum changes in [totalHb] in normosmic subjects compared with those of patients with PD during isovaleric acid stimulation in the frontal cortex. A significant difference was seen between the two groups.

DISCUSSION

This study was undertaken to establish to the cortical basis of olfactory function in patients with PD. In normosmic subjects, isovaleric acid caused hemodynamic changes in the lower regions of the frontal cortex. The same changes were seen in the same area in three patients with PD. These active areas may be related to the orbitofrontal cortex corresponding to the olfactory cortices. Several studies using PET and fMRI have shown that the orbitofrontal cortex is the main olfactory cortex (Diordjevic et al, 2005; Koizuka et al, 1994). On the other hand, isovaleric acid caused no changes in four of the PD patients. Because only one of these four patients presented olfactory symptoms, these results suggest that normosmic subjects with PD already have functional damage to the olfactory cortices.

MNIRS is a convenient and non-invasive method for functional brain imaging of olfactory activity that does not require a large amount of space. We will therefore continue to use MNIRS to explore further changes in olfactory function in patients with PD.

ACKNOWLEDGMENT

This research is supported by Kagawa University Characteristic Prior Research fund 2010.

REFERENCES

Diordjevic, J., Zatorre, R. J., Petrides, M., Boyle, J. A., & Jones-Gotman, M. (2005). Functional neuroimaging of odor imagery. *NeuroImage*, *24*, 791–801. doi:10.1016/j.neuroimage.2004.09.035

Doty, R. L. (2007). Olfaction in Parkinson's disease. *Parkinsonism & Related Disorders*, *13*(3), S225–S228. doi:10.1016/S1353-8020(08)70006-3

Doty, R. L., Shaman, P., Kimmelman, C. P., & Dann, M. S. (1984). University of Pennsylvania smell identification test: A rapid quantitative olfactory function test for the clinic. *The Laryngoscope*, *94*, 176–178. doi:10.1288/00005537-198402000-00004

Hoshi, Y., & Tamura, M. (1993). Dynamic multi-channel near-infrared optical imaging of human brain activity. *Journal of Applied Physiology*, *75*, 1842–1846.

Hummel, T., Damm, M., Vent, J., Schmidt, M., Theissen, P., Larsson, M., & Klussmann, J. P. (2003). Depth of olfactory sulcus and olfactory function. *Brain Research*, *975*, 85–89. doi:10.1016/S0006-8993(03)02589-7

Kobayashi, E., Kusaka, T., Karaki, M., Kobayashi, R., Ito, S., & Mori, N. (2007). Functional optical hemodynamic imaging of the olfactory cortex. *The Laryngoscope*, *117*, 541–546. doi:10.1097/MLG.0b013e31802ffe2a

Koizuka, I., Yano, H., Nagahara, M., Mochizuki, R., Seo, R., & Shimada, K. (1994). Functional imaging of the human olfactory cortex by magnetic resonance imaging. *Journal of Oto-Rhino-Laryngology*, *56*, 273–275.

Kondo, H., Matsuda, T., Hashiba, M., & Baba, S. (1998). A study of the relationship between the T&T olfactometer and the University of Pennsylvania Smell Identification Test in a Japanese population. *American Journal of Rhinology*, *12*, 353–358. doi:10.2500/105065898780182390

Kranick, S. M., & Duda, J. E. (2008). Olfactory dysfunction in Parkinson's disease. *Neuro-Signals*, *16*(1), 35–40. doi:10.1159/000109757

Kusaka, T., Kawada, K., Okubo, K., Nagano, K., Namba, M., & Okada, H. (2004). Noninvasive optical imaging in the visual cortex in young infants. *Human Brain Mapping*, *22*, 122–132. doi:10.1002/hbm.20020

Ross, G. W., Petrovitch, H., Abbott, R. D., Tanner, C. M., Popper, J., & Masaki, K. (2008). Association of olfactory dysfunction with risk for future Parkinson's disease. *Annals of Neurology*, *63*(2), 167–173. doi:10.1002/ana.21291

Savic, B. (2004). Imaging of olfaction and gestation. *Nutrition Reviews*, *62*, 224–241.

Sobel, N., Prabhakaran, V., Desmond, J. E., Glover, G. H., Goode, R. L., & Sullivan, E. V. (1998). Sniffing and smelling: Separate subsystems in the human olfactory cortex. *Nature*, *392*, 282–286. doi:10.1038/32654

KEY TERMS AND DEFINITIONS

Hemoglobin: The iron-containing oxygen-transport metalloprotein in the red blood cells of vertebrates and the tissues of some invertebrates.

Isovaleric Acid: A natural fatty acid found in a wide variety of plants and essential oils. Isovaleric acid has a strong pungent cheesy or sweaty smell, but its volatile esters have pleasing scents and are used widely in perfumery.

Near-Infrared Spectroscopy: A spectroscopic method that uses the near infrared region of the electromagnetic spectrum (from about 800 nm to 2500 nm). Typical applications include pharmaceuticals, medical diagnostics (including blood sugar and oximetry), food and agrochemical quality control, and combustion research.

Olfactory Dysfunction: A lack of functioning olfaction, in other words, an inability to perceive odors.

Orbitofrontal Cortex: A region of the prefrontal cortex in the frontal lobes of the brain that is involved in the cognitive processing of decision-making.

Parkinson's Disease: A degenerative disorder of the central nervous system that often impairs the sufferer's motor skills, speech, and other functions.

T&T Olfactometry: An olfactory testing method that is widely used in Japan.

Chapter 23
Basic Study on the Effect of Scent on Arousal Level Using Multi-Channel Near-Infrared Spectroscopy (MNIRS)

Shun'ichi Doi
Faculty of Engineering, Kagawa University, Japan

Takahiro Wada
Faculty of Engineering, Kagawa University, Japan

Eiji Kobayashi
Faculty of Engineering, Kagawa University, Japan

Masayuki Karaki
Faculty of Engineering, Kagawa University, Japan

Nozomu Mori
Faculty of Engineering, Kagawa University, Japan

ABSTRACT

Long term monotonous driving has been often found to decrease the driver's arousal level and effect his/hers property of perception, cognition and judgment. It is preferable to apply arousal assist for the driver instead of huge stimulus such as warning sound and vibration to the driver while driving. On the other hand, the effect of the scent is also reported as an environmental stimulus for driver.

In this study, the seven kinds of scent were used as olfactory stimulation and the influence of scent on the driver's psychosomatic state was examined using a fixed-based driving simulator by measuring biological measurements including electrocardiogram and finger plethysmograph. As for brain activity of olfactory cortex, the multi-channel near-infrared spectroscopy (MNIRS) has been shown to enable the evaluation of changes in hemodynamic. The MNIRS was also used to monitor the activity of the frontal cortex as mirrored by hemodynamic responses subjected to olfactory stimulation.

DOI: 10.4018/978-1-60960-559-9.ch023

As a result, it is verified that not only characteristics of the scent but also the driver's preference and subjective judgment of scent changes affect on the each driving performance. The brain activity change by olfactory stimulation and the brain blood flow change by other stimulation were also investigated. The effects of the functional brain imaging of olfactory activity were measured and the comfortable scent for the individual subject was verified to be effective for maintaining the arousal level.

INTRODUCTION

Monotonous and drowsy driving is a major cause of accidents in situations involving long-term highway driving. To assist the driver and prevent an accident, the use of arousal assistance for the driver is preferable to a huge stimulus such as a warning sound or vibration. There are various reports concerning the effects of arousal upon a driver and its role in maintaining his or her awareness of traffic environments. (Hirata, 2001).

In this study, we examined the effect of scent on the driver's psychosomatic state by using a driving simulator and measuring biological indicators by methods such a electrocardiogram, electrooculogram and finger plethysmograph. With respect to brain activity in the olfactory cortex, the multi-channel near-infrared spectroscopy (MNIRS) system can be used to evaluate changes in hemodynamics(Kobayashi et al, 2007). The MNIRS system was used to monitor the activity of the frontal cortex as mirrored by the hemodynamic responses in response to olfactory stimulation. In addition, changes in brain activity in response to olfactory stimulation and changes in blood flow in the brain in response to other stimuli were investigated.

Table 1. Experimental overview

	Experiment 1: driving simulator	Experiment 2: seated position
Task	Simulated drive (Straight road)	Sitting with eye-mask
Test duration	20 minutes	10 minutes 45 seconds
Measurement items	Subjective judgment・Electrocardiogram	
	Finger plethysmograph・Lateral displacement on DS	Electroencephalogram Blood flow
Subjects	11(Sub A~K) Average age 23.0 10 males:1 female	5 (Sub. A~E) Average age 22.4 4 males:1 female
Supplying Timing	For a duration of 15 seconds after the vehicle in the DS oversteps the lateral line	Cyclic (supplied for 15 seconds and shutoff for 45 seconds)
Scent	Four scents were selected through subjective judgment	

EXPERIMENTAL PROCEDURE

1. Experiment 1 on Driving Simulator

In this study, two kinds of experiments were executed, as described in Table 1. In experiment 1, the subject drove along a straight road for 20 minutes at 60 km/h using a driving simulator (DS) (DS-2000, Mitsubishi Precision co. Ltd) (Figure 1). Under this condition, almost all subjects tended to become somnolent. We attempted to maintain

Figure 1. Driving simulator

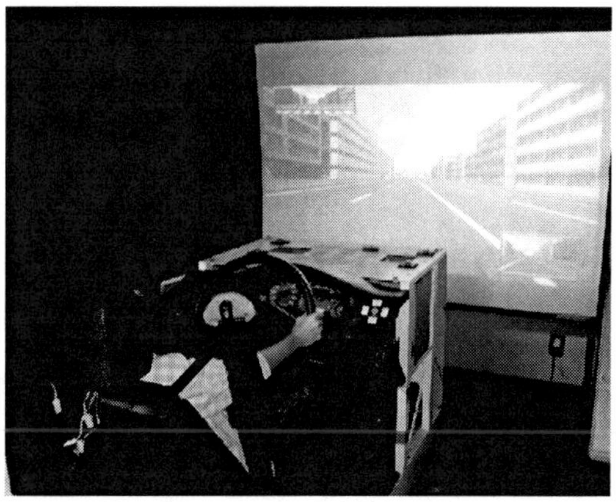

wakefulness by supplying scents to the subject. Four kinds of scents were used in the experiments, which were selected individually using a preliminary questionnaire. The generator of the scents was 'Aromax silent' (Air-aroma Inc). To remove lingering scents, the subject used a nasal cannula. When the subject became sleepy, as indicated by the vehicle behavior on the DS and watching the overstep of the sideline, the experimenter supplied a scent for 15 seconds.

2. Experiment 2 on Seating Condition

Blood flow was measured to estimate the effect of the scent on the driver's psychosomatic state. The measuring device was a multi-channel near-infrared spectroscopy (NIRS) system (Hitachi Medical Corporation) with 22-channel electrodes. Both the generation of scent and variety of scents were the same as in Exp. 1. The supply time was 15 seconds, and the shutoff time was 45 seconds (Figure 2).

3. Variety of Scents

In this experiment, a variety of scents were used. These scents were peppermint, lavender, lemon, sandalwood, vanilla, rose, and jasmine. The filtering of the scents was based on earlier studies.

4. Subjects

The subjects included 11 adults (10 males and 1 female) ranging in age from 20 to 25 (average age = 22.6). The study was conducted during the same period of the day to account for circadian rhythms.

5. Measuring Items

In addition to subjective judgment, lateral displacement of the vehicle in the DS, electrocardiogram, finger plethysmograph, electroencephalogram and blood flow were measured.

Figure 2. Supply timing (Experiment 2)

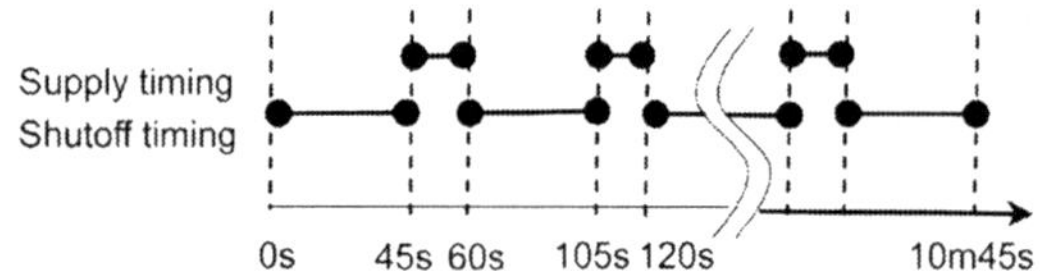

Electrocardiograms were measured using PowerLab (AD Instruments, Inc.) The heartbeat interval (RRI) was determined over a 180-second period as a moving average for every 18-second segment, and the RRI time-series for each subject was compared with those for the other subjects. In addition, LF/HF was calculated using a wavelet transform. A large LF/HF value indicates stress. Finger plethysmograph (CCI, Inc.) was used to measure blood flow changes at the forefinger. The recorded signals were analyzed by chaos analysis, which calculates the Maximum Lyapunov exponent. Considered a measurement for stress, a larger Maximum Lyapunov exponent value indicates increased levels of stress in the subject. Electroencephalograms were measured using FM-515A (FUTEC, Inc.). The α, β and θ waves were measured and compared as a ratio to the total wave amount, which was taken as a moving average for every 18 segment over a 180-second period sliding period.

TASTE FOR SCENT

1. Subjective Judgment

Subjective evaluations were performed by having the subjects sniff seven scents and fill out a seven-stage questionnaire that categorized his or her response to each scent as Comfortable/Uncomfortable and Excitement/Remission. There was variation in the taste of each subject for each scent. The average of the subjective judgment for each of the 11 subjects is shown in Figure 3, with the X-Y plane as Comfortable–Excitement. (Min et al, 2005; Min et al, 2003).

Figure 3. Average of subjective judgments

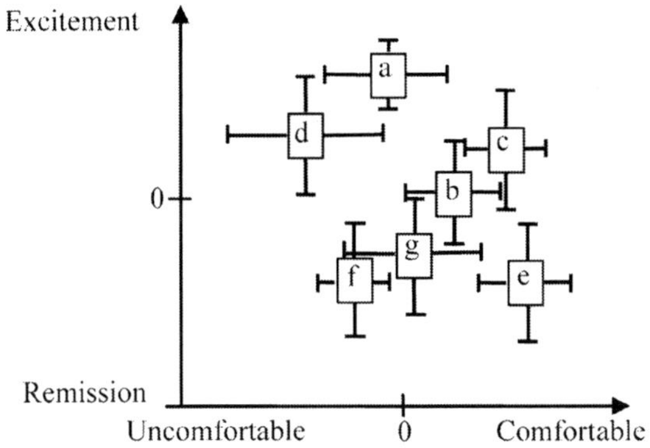

2. Select of Scents

Table 2 shows the scents that were supplied to the individual subjects in this study. Each subject was exposed to four different scents, based upon their responses in the questionnaire. Each scent elicits one of four states in the subject: comfort and excitement (the Comfortable-Excitement condition), comfort and remission (the Comfortable-Remission condition), discomfort and excitement (the Uncomfortable-Excitement condition), or discomfort and remission (the Uncomfortable-Remission condition).

Table 2. Scent attribution selected by subjects

	Comfortable		Uncomfortable	
	Excitement	Remission	Excitement	Remission
A	Lemon	Vanilla	Peppermint	Jasmine
B	Peppermint	Jasmine	Sandalwood	Vanilla
C	Peppermint	Vanilla	Sandalwood	Jasmine
D	Lemon	Rose	Peppermint	Lavender
E	Lemon	Vanilla	Peppermint	Rose
F	Vanilla	Jasmine	Sandalwood	Lavender
G	Peppermint	Lemon	Sandalwood	Rose
H	Sandalwood	Vanilla	Peppermint	Rose
I	Sandalwood	Lavender	Lemon	Jasmine
J	Jasmine	Vanilla	Lemon	Rose
K	Lavender	Sandalwood	Lemon	Rose

EXPERIMENTAL RESULTS ON THE DRIVING SIMULATOR

1. Comparison of the Excitement and Remission Conditions

1) Exposure to the "Comfortable-Excitement" and "Comfortable-Remission" scents:

Using subject G as an example (Figure 4), the RRI time-series revealed that arousal was maintained under the "Comfortable-Excitement" condition, but that there was an increased level of sleepiness, indicated by a lengthening in the RRI, under the "Comfortable-Remission" condition. Nine of the eleven subjects were able to maintain their arousal level when exposed to "Excitement" scents.

Next, the state of stress was estimated using a time-series of Maximum Lyapunov exponent data (Figure 5 (a)) and a time-series of LF/HF data (Figure 5 (b)). There was no significant difference in stress level between the "Excitement" and "Remission" conditions. These tendencies were shown in eight of the eleven subjects.

When the "Comfortable-Excitement" condition was compared with the "Comfortable-Remission" condition, there was little difference in

Figure 4. RR-Interval (Subject G) for "Comfortable-Excitement" and "Comfortable-Remission" conditions

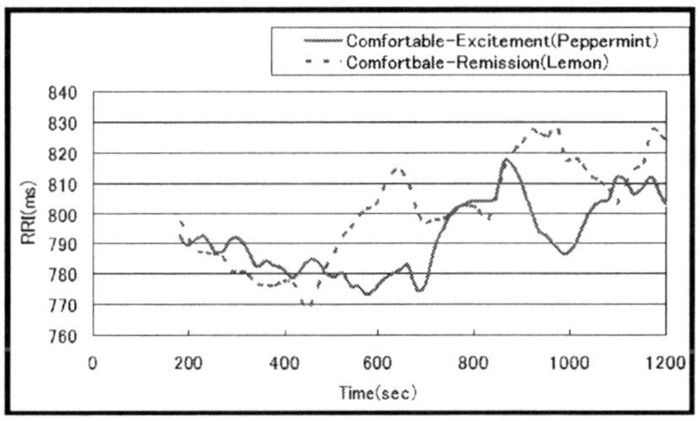

Figure 5. (a) Maximum Lyapunov exponent in Subject G for "Comfortable-Excitement" and "Comfortable-Remission" conditions. (b) The LF/HF ratio for Subject G for "Comfortable-Excitement" and "Comfortable-Remission" conditions

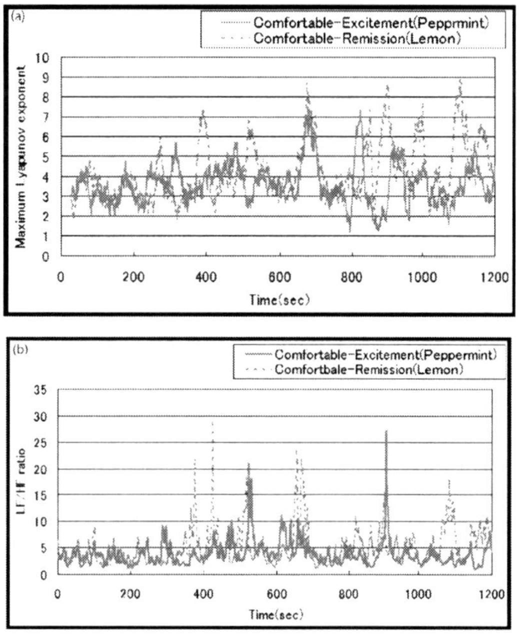

the stress levels of the subjects, which is consistent with description of these scents as "comfortable" for the subjects. If the subjects were provided scents also categorized as "excitement" scents, they maintained wakefulness.

2) Exposuretothe"Uncomfortable-Excitement" and "Uncomfortable-Remission" scents:

Using subject H as an example (Figure 6), the RRI time-series revealed that arousal was maintained under both the "Uncomfortable-Excitement" and "Uncomfortable-Remission" conditions. Thus, "uncomfortable" scents appear to help maintain wakefulness. This tendency was shown for six out of the eleven subjects. In contrast, three subjects experienced this effect of maintained wakefulness only under the "Uncomfortable-Excitement" condition.

Figure 6. RR-Interval (Subject H) for "Uncomfortable-Excitement" and "Uncomfortable-Remission"

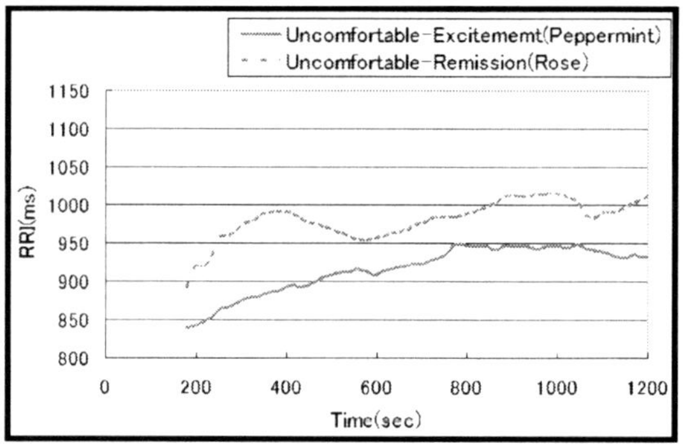

Next, the state of stress was estimated using a time-series of Maximum lyapunov exponent data (Figure 7). There was no significant difference in the stress level between the "Excitement" and "Remission" conditions. Similar results were seen with the LF/HF data. When the "Uncomfortable-Excitement" condition was compared with the "Uncomfortable-Remission" condition, there was little difference in the stress levels of the subjects. If the subjects were provided scents also categorized as "excitement" scents, they maintained wakefulness.

Figure 7. Maximum Lyapunov exponent (Subject H) for "Uncomfortable-Excitement" and "Uncomfortable-Remission"

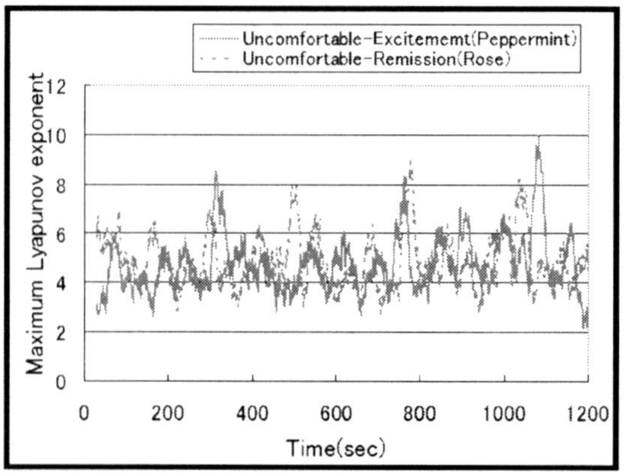

Figure 8. RR-Interval (Subject G) for "Comfortable-Excitement" and "Uncomfortable-Excitement"

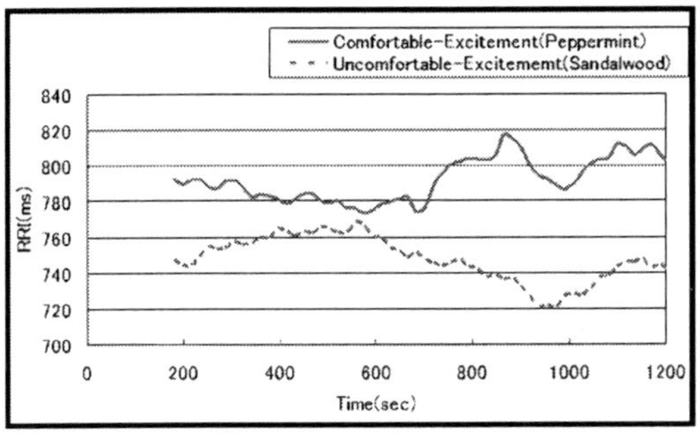

Figure 9. Maximum Lyapunov exponent (Subject G) for "Comfortable-Excitement" and "Uncomfortable-Excitement"

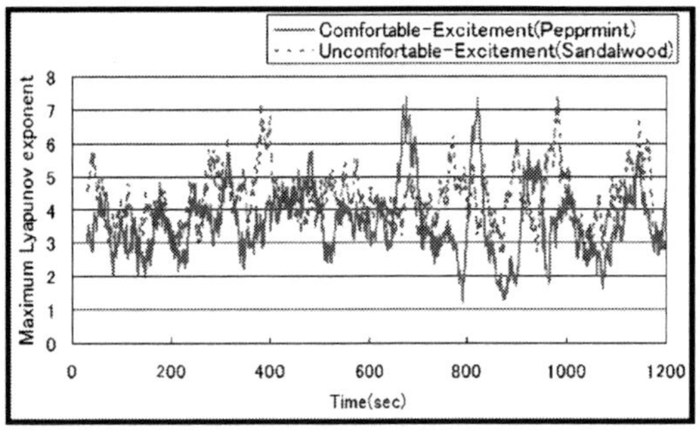

2. Comparison of the Comfortable and Uncomfortable Conditions

1) Exposure to the "Comfortable-Excitement" and "Uncomfortable-Excitement" scents:

Using subject G as an example (Figure 8), the RRI time-series revealed that arousal was maintained under both the "Comfortable-Excitement" and "Uncomfortable-Excitement" conditions. Seven out of the eleven subjects were able to maintain their arousal level when exposed to both of these scent conditions.

Next, the state of stress was estimated using a time-series data of Maximum Lyapunov exponent data (Figure 9). The uncomfortable condition caused much stress in the subjects. Similar results were seen with the LF/HF data. This tendency was shown for six out of eleven subjects.

When the "Comfortable-Excitement" condition was compared with the "Uncomfortable-Excitement" condition, there was little difference in the wakefulness levels of the subjects. If the subjects were provided scents also categorized as "uncomfortable" scents, they experienced high stress levels.

2) Exposure to the "Comfortable-Remission" and "Uncomfortable-Remission" scents:

Using subject G as an example (Figure 10), the RRI time-series revealed that there was an increased level of sleepiness, indicated by a lengthening in the RRI, under the "Comfortable-Remission" condition, but that wakefulness was maintained under the "Uncomfortable-Remission" condition. The latter observation is consistent with the description of the scents as "uncomfortable" for the subjects. These tendencies were also shown in five out of eleven subjects. Next, the state of stress was estimated using a time-series of Maximum Lyapunov exponent (Figure 11). The uncomfortable condition caused much stress in the subjects. Similar results were seen with the LF/HF data. This tendency was shown for seven out of eleven subjects. In addition, although these

Figure 10. RR-Interval (Subject G) for "Comfortable-Remission" and "Uncomfortable-Remission"

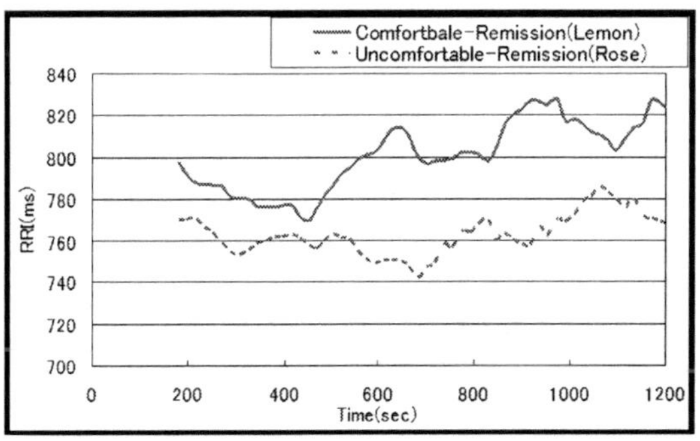

Figure 11. Maximum Lyapunov exponent (Subject G) for "Comfortable-Remission" and "Uncomfortable-Remission"

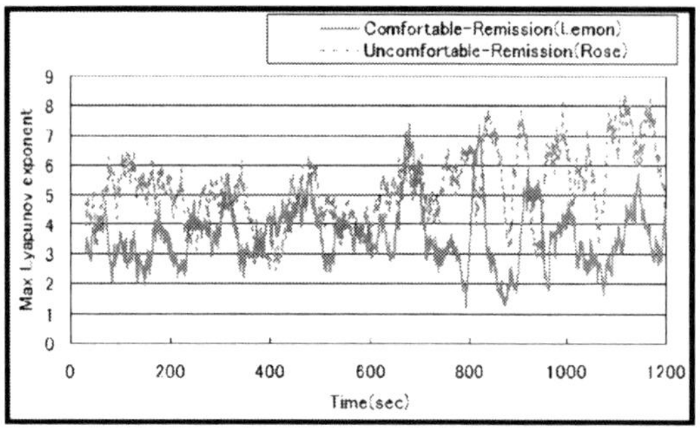

scents caused much stress for the subjects, the scents also helped the subjects

In summary, the subjects felt little stress when supplied with comfortable scents but much stress when supplied with uncomfortable scents. With respect to the effects on arousal, the subjects could maintain wakefulness when supplied with excitement scents, but there were mixed results when supplied with remission scents. Some subjects were still able to maintain wakefulness when supplied with the remission scents because they hated their smell, but that condition also resulted in much stress for the subjects. Based on these results, exposure to comfortable and excitement scents to subjects while driving is the optimal condition.

EXPERIMENTAL RESULTS ON SEATING CONDITIONS

An example of the time-series data from the electroencephalogram is shown in Figure 12. A drop in the α wave below 50% accompanied by an increase in the θ wave indicated that the subject was falling asleep, given as times Ta and Tb. All subjects, regardless of their individual scent preferences, fell asleep fastest under the Comfortable-Remission condition. All remission scents resulted in an earlier onset of sleepiness.

Figure 12. (a) Electroencephalogram (Subject A) for "Comfortable-Excitement". (b) Electroencephalogram (Subject A) for "Comfortable-Remission"

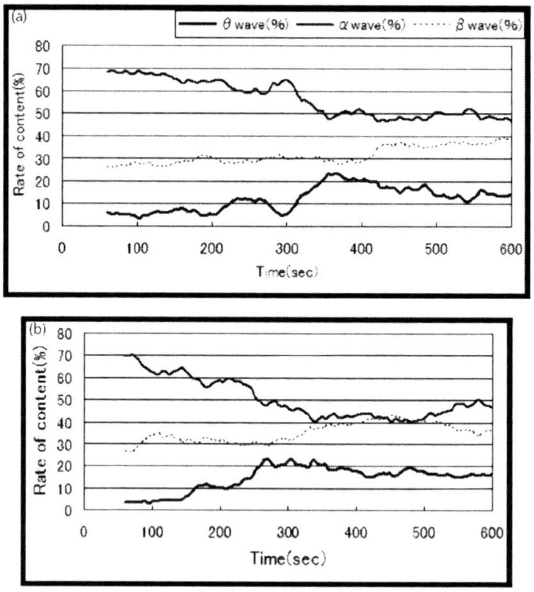

SENTS ADOPTABLE FOR EACH SUBJECT

According to the above results, the preferable condition involves supplying comfortable and excitement scents to maintain wakefulness during driving. The effect of the scent is, however, altered by individual preference. Therefore, when determining which scents should be adopted, the selection was limited to "Comfortable-Excitement" and "Uncomfortable-Excitement" because, as shown above, the remission scents resulted in sleepiness. Here, the subjects were divided into three classes based on their subjective judgment with respect to their answers to the questionnaire. The first class, which included subject H, was "Subject prefers scents that give a remission effect" (Figure 13 (A)). The second class, which included subject E, was "Subject prefers scents that give an excitement effect" (Figure 13 (B)). The third class, which included subject G, was "Subjects fit into neither category" (Figure 13 (C)).

Figure 13. Subject classification 1

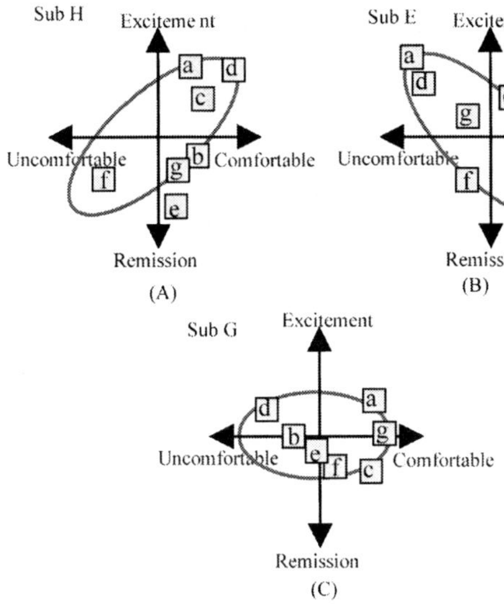

1.Preference for "Excitement" scents

Three subjects belong to this class. They tended to fall asleep under the comfortable conditions (Figure 14). The time-series of Maximum Lyapunov exponent data revealed that the subjects did not experience any stress regardless if the scent was comfortable or uncomfortable (Figure 15) because the scents were all considered to be "excitement" scents by the subjects. Therefore, when these subjects were supplied "Uncomfortable-Excitement" scents, they maintained wakefulness and had a comfortable feeling.

Figure 15. Maximum Lyapunov exponent (Subject H) for "Comfortable-Excitement" and "Uncomfortable-Excitement"

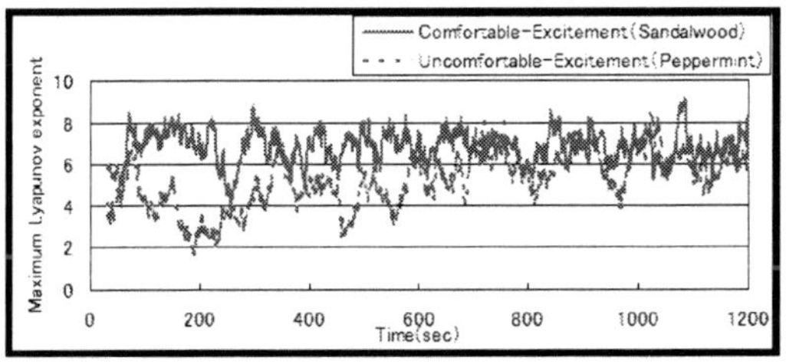

Figure 14. RRI (Subject H) for "Comfortable-Excitement" and "Uncomfortable-Excitement"

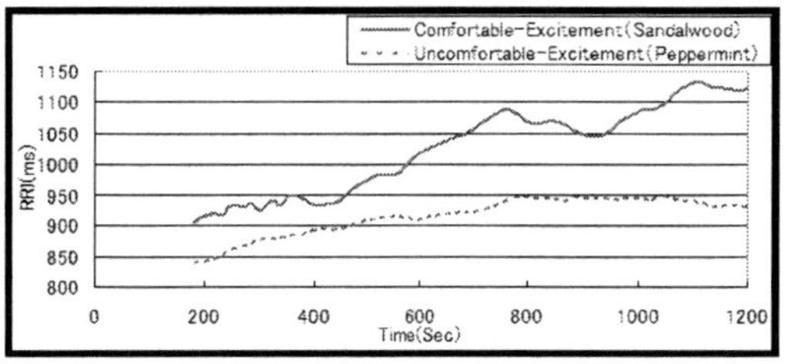

2.Preference for "Remission" Scents/No Preference for Either "Remission" or "Excitement" Scents

Those subjects who preferred scents that gave a remission effect were further classified into two categories. In the questionnaire, the subjects were exposed to scents that elicited a level of excitement that was either higher or lower under the Comfortable-Excitement condition than under the Uncomfortable-Excitement condition. Based on their responses, the subjects had a strong preference (a) or a weak preference (b) for remission scents (Figure 16).

Using subject F as an example, the RRI time-series data and Maximum Lyapunov exponent are shown in Figures 17 and 18, respectively. Subjects belonging to class (A) tended to fall asleep under the uncomfortable condition. Because they have strong preference for remission scents, they should not be given scents that create the "Uncomfortable-Excitement" condition. In addition, they felt a high level of stress under the "Uncomfortable"

Figure 16. Subject classification 2

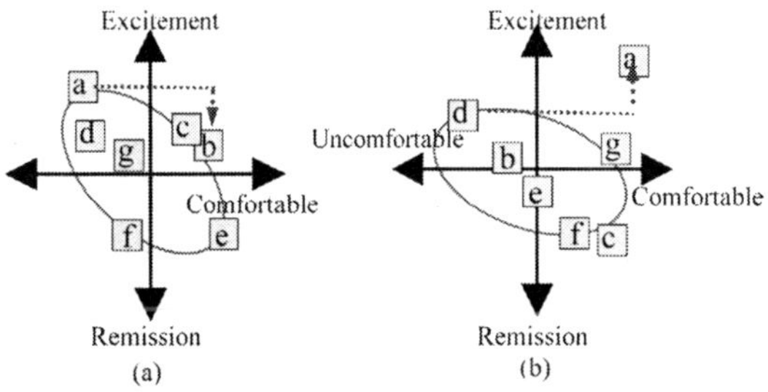

Figure 17. RRI (Subject F) for "Comfortable-Excitement" and "Uncomfortable-Excitement"

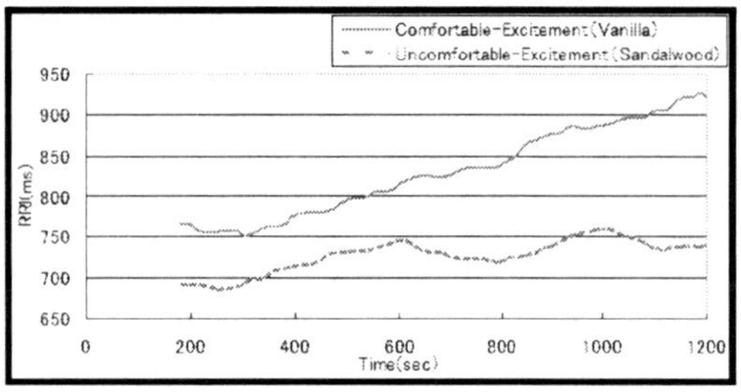

Figure 18. Maximum Lyapunov exponent (Subject F) for "Comfortable-Excitement" and "Uncomfortable-Excitement"

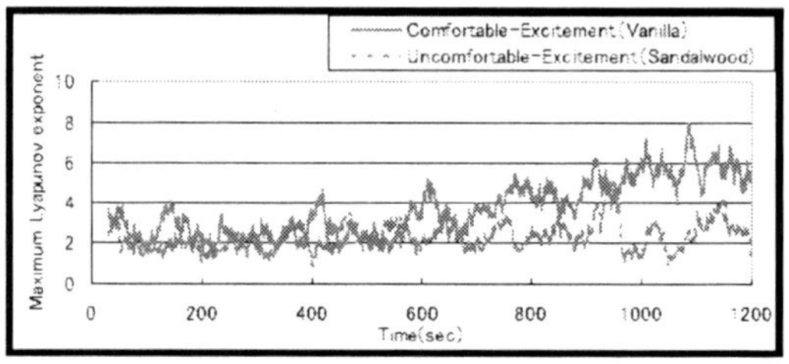

condition. Thus, this group should be supplied Comfortable-Excitement scents while driving.

Using subject C as an example, a topographic image pattern of every five seconds, demonstrating the hemodynamic changes in the frontal head, is shown in Figure 19. The subject was supplied a scent between 0 and 15 seconds. Under the control condition (no scent), there was no change. Under the Comfortable-Excitement condition, a hemodynamic change occurred for a long period of time. Under the Uncomfortable-Excitement condition, however, this change had only a brief duration.

Using subject B as an example, the change in blood flow in the right cephalic (a) and left cephalic veins (b) is shown in Figure 20. The subject was supplied a scent between times Ta and Tb for 15 seconds. These data were similar to those shown in Figure 19. Based on these results, supplying a comfortable scent to the driver is good for maintaining wakefulness. Because subject C belongs to group A ("Subject prefers scents that give a remission effect"), he or she should not be given scents that create the "Uncomfortable-Excitement" condition. Based upon the measurement of blood flow, none of the subjects preferred excitement scents. These subjects experienced a long reaction time under both the "Comfortable-Excitement" and "Uncomfortable –Excitement" conditions.

Figure 19. Blood flow changes in the frontal head (Subject C)

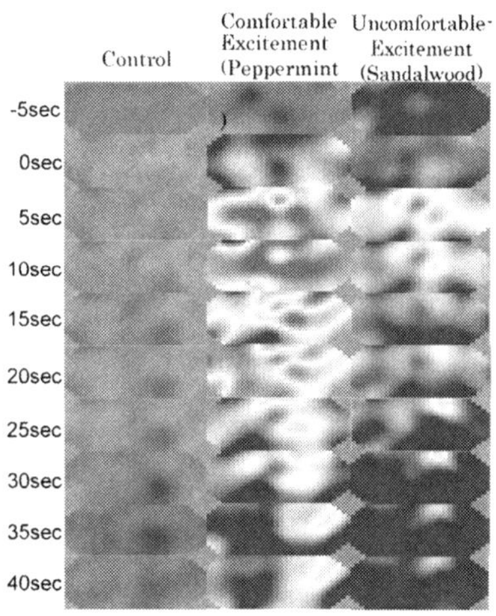

7. CONCLUSION

In this study, we examined the effect of scent on the driver's psychosomatic state using a driving simulator and taking biological measurements.

After being exposed to a variety of scents, the subjects were divided into three groups:

A. Subjects prefer scents that give a remission effect;
B. Subjects prefer scents that give an excitement effect;
C. Subjects fit into neither category

The subjects in group A were further classified into two categories: (a) subjects more likely to

Figure 20. Time history of blood flow change (Subject B)

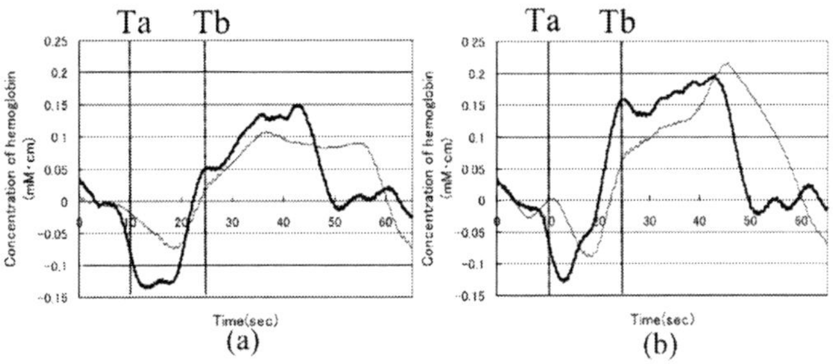

prefer remission scents or (b) subjects with only a weak preference for remission scents. The subjects in subgroup experienced stress under the "Uncomfortable" condition and tended to fall asleep under the "Remission" condition. In addition, they should not be provided scents that create the "Uncomfortable-Excitement" condition because they felt uncomfortable. Based on these results, subjects belonging to group A should be given Comfortable-Excitement scents while driving.

On the other hand, the subjects in groups C and B tended to maintain wakefulness under the excitement condition but experienced stress under the uncomfortable condition. Based on these results, these subjects should be given Comfortable-Excitement scents while driving. The subjects in group B tended to fall asleep under the "Comfortable-Excitement" condition because they preferred excitement scents. They also experienced stress only under the "Uncomfortable-Remission" condition. Based on these results, these subjects should be given mildly uncomfortable and excitement scents while driving.

In conclusion, not only the characteristics of the scent, but also the driver's preference and subjective judgment of that scent, affected the performance of each driver. The effects of the functional brain imaging of olfactory activity were also measured, which verified that the comfortable scent selected by the individual subject would be effective for maintaining the arousal level while driving.

ACKNOWLEDGMENT

This research was supported by the Kagawa University Characteristic Prior Research Fund 2009. This work was also supported in part by the Kagawa University Presidential Grant for Complex Medical Engineering activities. The authors are indebted to the students of their laboratories for their generous help and experimental support, particularly Messrs. Shin'ya Hiroike and Kousuke Kamesawa.

REFERENCES

Hirata, Y. (2001). A study of the effective way to release scent to maintain alertness. *JSAE Review*, *22*, 331–336. doi:10.1016/S0389-4304(01)00105-9

Kobayashi, E. (2007). Functional optical hemodynamic imaging of the olfactory cortex. *The Laryngoscope*, *117*, 1–6. doi:10.1097/MLG.0b013e31802ffe2a

Min, B.-C. (2003). Analysis of mutual information content for EEG responses to odor stimulation for subjects classified by occupation. *Chemical Senses*, *28*(9), 741–749. doi:10.1093/chemse/bjg066

Min, K.-Y., Chung, S.-C., & Min, B.-C. (2005). Physiological evaluation on emotional change induced by imagination. *Applied Psychophysiology and Biofeedback*, *30*(2). doi:10.1007/s10484-005-4310-0

KEY TERMS AND DEFINITIONS

Arousal Assist: Air aroma which is used in air-conditioning for aiming to assist the driver and prevent an accident in monotonous and drowsy driving in the case of long term highway driving.

Electrocardiogram (ECG): Tansthoracic interpretation of the electrical activity of the heart over time captured and externally recorded by skin electrodes. It is a noninvasive recording produced by an electrocardiographic.

Electrooculogram (EOG): An electrophisiological test of function of the outer retina and retinal pigment epithelium in which the change in the electrical potential between the cornea and the ocular.

Maximum Lyapunov Exponent: In mathematics the Lyapunov exponent of a dynamical system is a quantity that characterizes the rate of separation of infinitesimally close trajectories. Quantitatively, two trajectories in phase space with initial separation is defined by λ (Lyapunov exponent). The rate of separation can be different for different orientations of initial separation vector. Thus, there is a whole spectrum of Lyapunov exponents—the number of them is equal to the number of dimensions of the phase space. It is common to just refer to the largest one, i.e. to the Maximal Lyapunov exponent (MLE), because it determines the predictability of a dynamical system. A positive MLE is usually taken as an indication that the system is chaotic.

MNIRS (Multi-Channel Near-Infrared Spectroscopy): Spectroscopy to monitor the activity of the frontal cortex as mirrored by hemodynamic. MNIRS enables evaluation of changes in hemodynamics related to brain activity by olfactory stimulation.

Olfactory Cortex: A group of cortical areas of the cerebrum that receive sensory input from the olfactory bulb via the olfactory tract, includes the piriform cortex and parts of the olfactory tubercle, amygdale.

Plethysmograph: A measuring changes in volume within an organ finger or lobe usually resulting from fluctuations in the amount of blood.

Chapter 24
A Speech Prosody-Based Approach to Early Detection of Cognitive Impairment in Elderly Subjects:
A Preliminary Study

Shohei Kato
Graduate School of Engineering, Department of Computer Science and Engineering, Nagoya Institute of Technology, Japan

Sachio Hanya
Graduate School of Engineering, Department of Computer Science and Engineering, Nagoya Institute of Technology, Japan

Akiko Kobayashi
Ifcom Co., Ltd., Japan

Toshiaki Kojima
Ifcom Co., Ltd., Japan

Hidenori Itoh
Graduate School of Engineering, Department of Computer Science and Engineering, Nagoya Institute of Technology, Japan

Akira Homma
Tokyo Dementia Care Research and Training Center, Japan

ABSTRACT

This chapter presents a novel approach for early detection of cognitive impairment in the elderly. The approach incorporates the use of speech sound analysis and multivariate statistical techniques. The focus is on the prosodic features of speech. One hundred and fifteen Japanese subjects (32 males and 83 females between the ages of 38 and 99 years) participated in this study. The authors collected speech sounds from segments of dialogue during an HDS-R examination. The segments correspond to speech sounds from answers to questions about time orientation and number counting. One hundred and thirty prosodic features were extracted from each of the speech sounds. These prosodic features consisted of spectral and pitch features (53), formant features (56), intensity features (19), and speech rate and response time (2). These features were refined by principal component analysis and/or feature selection. In addition, the authors calculated speech prosody-based cognitive impairment rating (SPCIR) by multiple linear regression analysis. The results indicate that a moderately significant correlation exists

DOI: 10.4018/978-1-60960-559-9.ch024

between the HDS-R score and the synthesis of several selected prosodic features. Consequently, the adjusted coefficient of determination ($\bar{R}^2 = 0.50$) suggests that prosody-based speech sound analysis could potentially be used to detect cognitive impairment in elderly subjects.

INTRODUCTION

Japan has a rapidly aging society and in 2005 had 2.05 million elderly patients with dementia. The number of patients with dementia is expected to increase to more than 3 million over the next 10 years (Awata, 2009). Thus, the Ministry of Health, Labour and Welfare (MHLW) has begun projects to improve dementia treatment and quality of life. These projects are focused on the development of early detection methods for dementia that are both sensitive and specific.

To screen for dementia and cognitive impairment, a questionnaire test such as the Mini-Mental State Examination (MMSE) (Folstein, Folstein, & McHugh, 1975), Revised Hasegawa's Dementia Scale (HDS-R) (Katoh et al., 1991), Clinical Dementia Rating (CDR) (Morris, 1993), or Memory Impairment Screen (MIS) (Buschke et al., 1999) is commonly used, in addition to a neurophysiological test (e.g., using MRI, FDG-PET, and CSF biomarkers). Questionnaire tests have some disadvantages and their use is limited in the clinic. The MMSE, HDS-R, and CDR are more time-consuming that a general practitioner's consultation. In general, the questionnaire cannot completely dismiss the influence of education, social class, and gender difference on the results. In addition, there is a possibility that practitioner subjectivity may affect the scoring. Thus, we believe that the development of a simple, non-invasive examination that is objective and combined with a physiological test could enable the early detection of dementia in a broad population.

In a pilot study, we focused on speech sounds during the subject's answers to the questionnaire. Taler et al. reported language (Taler & Phillips, 2007), grammatical, and emotional prosodic impairment (Taler, Baum, Chertkow, & Saumier, 2008), as well as mild cognitive impairment (MCI), in elderly patients with Alzheimer's disease (AD). Hoyte et al. (Hoyte, Brownell, & Wingfield, 2009) reported that the components of speech prosody are useful for detecting the syntactic structure of speech. These reports suggest the possibility of using speech prosodic feature analysis to screen for dementia. This paper presents a novel approach to the early detection of cognitive impairment in the elderly that uses speech sound analysis in combination with a multivariate statistical technique. In this paper, we focused on the prosodic features of speech sound. We expect that the computation and information technology of this approach will enable general practitioners to easily screen for dementia. In our preliminary study, we examined the relationship between the HDS-R score and speech prosodic features. In addition, we addressed the effectiveness of speech prosody in discriminating between elderly individuals with normal cognitive abilities (NL) and patients with cognitive impairment (CI).

METHOD

Design

We recorded the speech sound of elderly patients while they provided answers for an HDS-R questionnaire test. We focused on questions about time orientation and numbering. In addition, we collected speech sounds while the patients were talking about the topics of hometown, childhood, and school.

Table 1. Category breakdown of the speech data (N=115)

Age	30's	40's	50's	60's	70's	80's	90's	Total
Male	3 (1)	0 (0)	15 (5)	32 (11)	21 (7)	12(5)	7 (3)	90 (32)
Female	0 (0)	20 (7)	45 (15)	24 (8)	28 (10)	87 (33)	25 (10)	229 (83)
Subtotal	3 (1)	20 (7)	60 (20)	56 (19)	49 (17)	99 (38)	32 (13)	319 (115)

Value in bracket means the number of subjects.

Participants

One hundred and fifteen Japanese subjects (32 males and 83 females between the ages of 38 and 99) participated in this study. With some exceptions, we collected three samples of speech sound from each of the participants. The number of total sound data points was 319, as shown in Table 1. The sound data contained 205 samples of speech by elderly patients whose HDS-R score was 30-24 (NL) and 114 samples from patients with cognitive impairment whose HDS-R score was 23-11 (CI).

MEASUREMENT

Prosodic Feature Extraction

Speech has three components: prosody, tone, and phoneme. Past research indicates that the prosodic component has important non-verbal information such as emotional expressions (Cowie et al., 2001; Scherer, Johnstone, & Klasmeyer, 2003; Cho, Kato, & Itoh, 2009). In accordance with our hypothesis, cognitive impairment was observed in the elderly (Taler & Phillips, 2007; Taler et al., 2008). In this study, we considered 130 different acoustic correlates related to both segmental and suprasegmental information from speech signals. We used a computational data mining strategy based on a statistical-analytical approach. We extracted as many features as possible and disregarded irrelevant features using a feature selection technique. These features were phrase-level statistics corresponding to fundamental frequency (F0), harmonic components (Fl) and their time-series behavior (53 features), formant and its time-series behavior (56 features), power envelope and its time-series behavior (19 features), speech rate, and response time (2 features). Prosodic analysis was performed in 23-ms frames and passed through a Hamming window (1024 points). Voice waveforms (sampled at 44.1 kHz with 16 bits) were extracted using a short-time Fourier transform (STFT) every 11 ms.

Spectral and Pitch Features

The set of 53 spectral features is comprised of statistical properties and time-series behaviors of fundamental frequency (F0) and the harmonic component (F_l).

1-7. Amplitude of F0 contour during t sec after the beginning of the phrase (t = 0.05, 0.10-0.35). The F0 contour is recorded in the interquartile range.
8. Spectral centroid.
9. Power ratio of F0 component to whole harmonic component.
10-48. Power ratio of the sum of harmonic components from F0 to F_l to whole harmonic component (l = 2, 3-40).
49. Power ratio between odd and even harmonic components.
50-53. Standard deviation, mean, maximum, and minimum value of the F0 contour.

Formant Features

Formant features consist of 56 values of frequency and bandwidth for the first 4 formants of distinguishing or meaningful frequency components within human speech.

54.-57. Standard deviation of the first, second, third, and fourth formant frequencies.
58.-61. Mean value of the first, second, third, and fourth formant frequencies.
62.-65. Maximum value of the first, second, third, and fourth formant frequencies.
66.-69. Minimum value of the first, second, third, and fourth formant frequencies.
70.-73. Median value of the first, second, third, and fourth formant frequencies.
74.-77. Difference between the maximum and minimum value of the first, second, third, and fourth formant frequencies.
78.-81. Gradient of the linear regression line of the first, second, third, and fourth formant frequencies.
82.-85. Standard deviation of the first, second, third, and fourth formant bandwidths.
86.-89. Mean value of the first, second, third, and fourth formant bandwidths.
90.-93. Maximum value of the first, second, third, and fourth formant bandwidths.
94.-97. Minimum value of the first, second, third, and fourth formant bandwidths.
98.-101. Median value of the first, second, third, and fourth formant bandwidths.
102.-105. Difference between the maximum and minimum values of the first, second, third, and fourth formant bandwidths.
106.-109. Gradient of the linear regression line of the first, second, third, and fourth formant bandwidths.

Intensity (Energy) Features

We extracted 19 energy features with the statistical properties of the power envelope.

110. Gradient of the linear regression line of the power envelope.
111.-117. Median value of the first derivative of the power envelope during the t seconds after the beginning of the phrase (t = 0.05, 0.10-0.35).
118.-124. Ratio of the power at t seconds after the beginning of the phrase to the maximum power (t = 0.05, 0.10-0.35).
125.-128. Standard deviation, mean, maximum, and minimum value of the short-time power.

Speech Rate and Response Time

In addition, we measured two features concerning speech rate and response time to answers in the questionnaire.

129. Average duration for a single mora.
130. Time taken to respond to the questionnaire.

Automatic Feature Selection

In our strategy for feature extraction, all of the prosodic features described above may not be equally useful and important for discrimination between NL and CI. This creates the need for systematic feature selection. In this study, we used the forward stepwise (FSW) method (Draper & Smith, 1998), which is the most popular form of feature selection in statistics and consists of a combination of the forward selection and backward elimination methods. FSW is an algorithm that adds the best feature (or deletes the worst feature) during each round. We chose a model selection method based on the Akaike's information criterion (AIC) (Akaike, 1974), which is a measure of the goodness of fit of an estimated statistical model. Using this criterion in the FSW, we were able to develop an estimation accuracy model with high accuracy and avoid over-fitting to training data. The AIC is defined as:

$$\mathrm{AIC} = -2\ln L + 2k, \quad (1)$$

Table 2. Category breakdown of the speech data (N=115)

	$SPCIR_{FE}$	$SPCIR_{FSW\text{-}AIC}$	$SPICR_{PCA\text{-}FSW\text{-}AIC}$
# of regressors	130	19	55
R	0.78	0.67	0.77
$\bar{R}^2$	0.37	0.41	0.50
S.E.	4.57	4.43	4.08

where k is the number of parameters in the estimated model, and L is the maximized value of the likelihood function for the estimated model. Under the assumption that the model errors are normally and independently distributed, this becomes (up to an additive constant, which depends only on n and not on the model):

$$\text{AIC}=n\cdot\ln(\text{RSS}/n)+2k, \quad (2)$$

where n is the number of data points (sample size), and RSS is the residual sum of squares from the estimated model. In this study, the RSS was obtained by calculating the sum of the square error of the difference between the estimated and observed HDS-R scores. FSW selects the best subset of all features to minimize the AIC score.

When determining the model parameters using the maximum likelihood estimation, it is possible to increase the likelihood by adding additional parameters; however, this also may result in over-fitting of the data. This represents a tradeoff between precision and complexity in the model. In addition to Schwarz's BIC (Schwarz, 1978), the AIC resolves this problem by introducing a penalty term [corresponding to the second term in Equation (2)] for the number of parameters in the model. This penalty discourages over fitting, but it should be avoided so that the feature may be effectively eliminated. In this paper, we introduce a pre-processing method that synthesizes prosodic features by principal component analysis (PCA) prior to feature selection. This method is a combination of principal component regression (Massy, 1965) and automatic feature selection.

In the following section, the correlation between HDS-R score and synthesis of selected prosodic features is described by experimental results of multiple regression analysis through three manners of feature selection: forward stepwise method with AIC (FSW-AIC), PCA pre-processed forward stepwise method with AIC (PCAFSW-AIC), and forced entry method without feature selection (FE).

RESULTS AND DISCUSSION

This section describes the correlation between HDS-R and speech prosody in elderly patients using 319 speech voice samples (N=115), each with 130 prosodic features. We calculated the speech prosody-based cognitive impairment rating (SPCIR) by multiple linear regression using prosodic features (as regressors) selected by the feature selection method mentioned above. $SPCIR_{FE}$, $SPCIR_{FSW\text{-}AIC}$, and $SPCIR_{PCA\text{-}FSW\text{-}AIC}$ were calculated from the feature set chosen by FE, FSW-AIC, and PCA-FSW-AIC, respectively. Table 2 shows the results of the analysis, and the scatter plots of HDS-R and the SPCIRs are shown in Figures 1-4. Table 3 shows the dominant regressors obtained from each of the feature selection methods.

$SPCIR_{FE}$ apparently has a larger correlation with HDS-R (R = 0.78); however, the adjusted coefficient of determination declined ($\bar{R}^2$ =0.37). This method detected few dominant regressors, suggesting over-fitting of the samples and multicollinearity due to a large number of regressors.

$SPCIR_{FSW\text{-}AIC}$ avoids the disadvantages of over-fitting and increases the number of dominant regressors; however, it does not give a satisfactory HDS-R (R = 0.67) correlation and an adjusted coefficient of determination ($\bar{R}^2$ = 0.41).

Figure 1. Dataflow of four methods of automatic feature selection

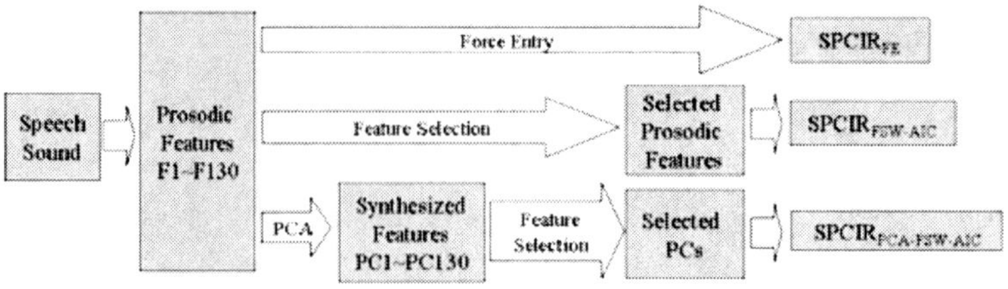

Figure 2. Scatter plot of HDS-R and $SPCIR_{FE}$ ($\bar{R}^2 = 0.37$)

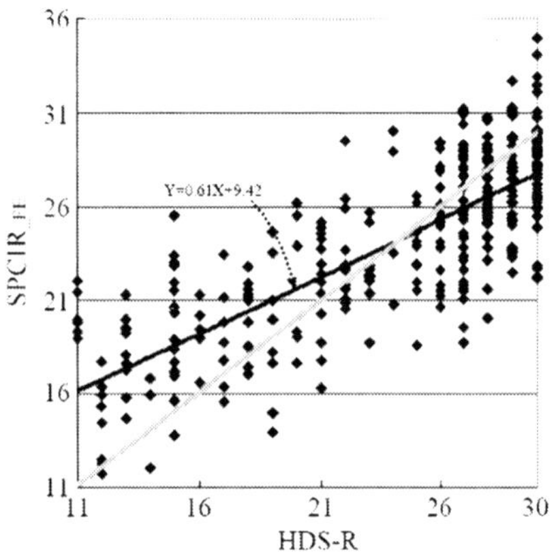

Figure 3. Scatter plot of HDS-R and $SPCIR_{FSW-AIC}$ ($\bar{R}^2 = 0.41$)

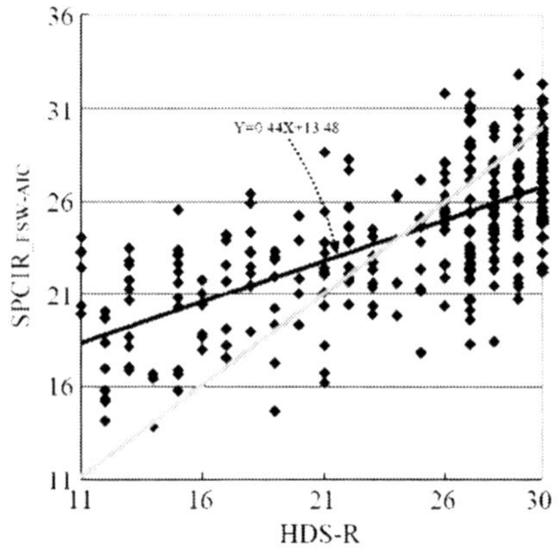

Figure 4. Scatter plot of HDS-R and $SPCIR_{PCA-FE}$ ($\bar{R}^2 = 0.38$)

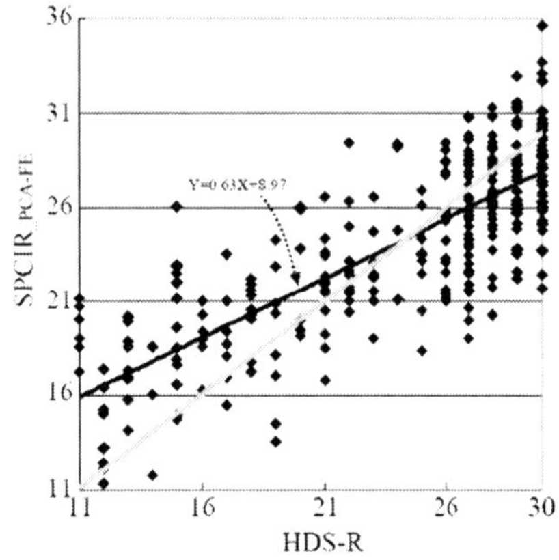

$SPCIR_{FSW-AIC}$ uses only 19 total regressors due to the penalty term of AIC, which was based on model complexity. There might be effective features for estimation of HDS-R in the 111 regressors that were not chosen by FSW-AIC.

$SPCIR_{PCA-FSW-AIC}$, with the PCA pre-processed forward stepwise method in combination with AIC, solved the above-mentioned problems. In this method, principal components of 130 features were used as regressor candidates during feature selection, and 55 PCs were used as regressors in multiple regression. As shown in Table 3, the principal components with higher variance (i.e., PC2, PC7, PC4) were dominant regressors; however, the low-variance principal components, such as PC77, PC115 and PC103, were also important for estimation of HDS-R. Finally, we obtained the scatter plot shown in Figure 4, which suggests a positive linear relationship between HDS-R and SPCIR. The results indicate a moderately significant correlation (R = 0.77) between the HDS-R score and the appropriate synthesis of several

Figure 5. Scatter plot of HDS-R and SPCIR$_{PCA\text{-}FSW\text{-}AIC}$ ($\bar{R}^2$ = 0.50)

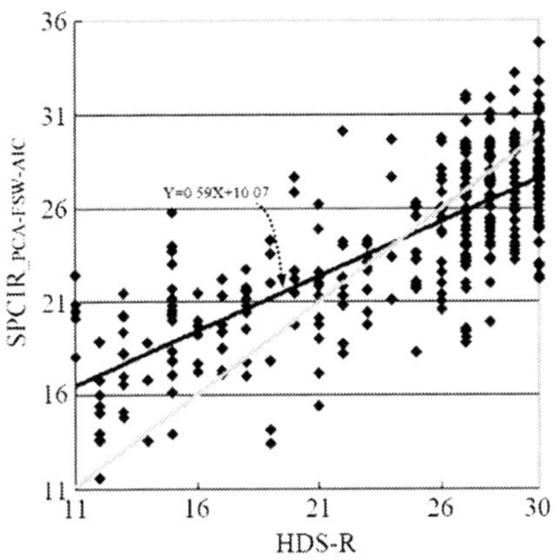

selected prosodic features. Consequently, the adjusted coefficient of determination ($\bar{R}^2$ = 0.50) suggests that prosody-based speech sound analysis could potentially be used to detect cognitive impairment in elderly patients.

Table 3. Dominant regressors used to estimate HDS-R

Method	Dominant Regressors	
SPICR$_{FE}$		130 regressors in total
	*** F129	
	** F110	
	* F57, F33, F78	
SPI-CR$_{FSW\text{-}AIC}$		19 regressors in total
	*** F129, F128	
	** F118, F130, F57, F8, F1010, F59	
	* F110, F72, F69, F73	
SPI-CR$_{PCA\text{-}FSW\text{-}FE}$		55 regressors in total
	*** PC2, PC7, PC12, PC4, PC26, PC52, PC54	
	** PC34, PC3, PC30, PC9, PC77, PC15, PC61, PC115	
	* PC22, PC40. PC13, PC31, PC103, PC14, PC1, PC46, PC129, PC100	

***: with significance level of 0.001
**: with significance level of 0.01
*: with significance level of 0.05

CONCLUSION AND FUTURE WORK

Our study presented a novel approach to detect cognitive impairment in elderly patients. This approach uses prosody-based speech sound analysis and a multivariate statistical technique. Before clinical data examination, we collected 319 speech voice samples from 115 Japanese participants and extracted 130 prosodic features from each of the samples. We then analyzed the correlation between the HDSR score and synthesis of selected prosodic features by multiple linear regression in combination with sophisticated feature selection. We uncovered a moderately significant correlation. Thus, this speech prosody-based approach may be used to detect cognitive impairment in elderly patients.

In future studies, more expansive multimodality data collection will be performed using non-invasive neurophysiological measurements such as near-infrared spectroscopy (NIRS). Clinical trials will also be evaluated, and the technique proposed here will be used as a screening tool for dementia.

ACKNOWLEDGMENT

This work was supported, in part, by SENTAN and the Japan Science and Technology Agency (JST).

REFERENCES

Akaike, H. (1974). A new look at the statistical model identification. *IEEE Transactions on Automatic Control*, *19*(6), 716–723. doi:10.1109/TAC.1974.1100705

Awata, S. (2009). Role of the dementia medical center in the community. *Japanese Journal of Geriatrics*, *46*, 203–206. doi:10.3143/geriatrics.46.203

Buschke, H., Kuslansky, G., Katz, M., Stewart, W. F., Sliwinski, M. J., & Eckholdt, H. M. (1999). Screening for dementia with the Memory Impairment Screen. *Neurology*, *52*(2), 231–238.

Cho, J., Kato, S., & Itoh, H. (2009). *Comparison of sensibilities of Japanese and Koreans in recognizing emotions from speech by using Bayesian Networks*. In IEEE International Conference on Systems, Man, and Cybernetics, (pp. 2945-2950).

Cowie, R., Douglas-Cowie, E., Tsapatsoulis, N., Votsis, G., Kollias, S., & Fellenz, W. (2001). Emotion recognition in human-computer interaction. *IEEE Signal Processing Magazine*, *18*(1), 32–80. doi:10.1109/79.911197

Draper, N., & Smith, H. (1998). *Applied regression analysis* (3rd ed.). John Wiley & Sons.

Folstein, M. F., Folstein, S. E., & McHugh, P. R. (1975). Mini-mental state: A practical method for grading the cognitive state of patients for the clinician. *Journal of Psychiatric Research*, *12*(3), 189–198. doi:10.1016/0022-3956(75)90026-6

Hoyte, K., Brownell, H., & Wingfield, A. (2009). Components of speech prosody and their use in detection of syntactic structure by older adults. *Experimental Aging Research*, *35*(1), 129–151. doi:10.1080/03610730802565091

Katoh, S., Simogaki, H., Onodera, A., Ueda, H., Oikawa, K., & Ikeda, K. (1991). Development of the revised version of Hasegawa's Dementia Scale (HDS-R). *Japanese Journal of Geriatric Psychiatry*, *2*(11), 1339–1347.

Massy, W. F. (1965). Principal components regression in exploratory statistical research. *Journal of the American Statistical Association*, *60*(309), 234–256. doi:10.2307/2283149

Morris, J. C. (1993). The Clinical Dementia Rating (CDR): Current version and scoring rules. *Neurology*, *43*(11), 2412–2414.

Scherer, K. R., Johnstone, T., & Klasmeyer, G. (2003). Vocal expression of emotion. In Davidson, R. J., Goldsmith, H., & Scherer, K. R. (Eds.), *Handbook of the affective sciences* (pp. 433–456). Oxford University Press.

Schwarz, G. E. (1978). Estimating the dimension of a model. *Annals of Statistics*, *6*(2), 461–464. doi:10.1214/aos/1176344136

Taler, V., Baum, S. R., Chertkow, H., & Saumier, D. (2008). Comprehension of grammatical and emotional prosody is impaired in Alzheimer's disease. *Neuropsychology*, *22*(2), 188–195. doi:10.1037/0894-4105.22.2.188

Taler, V., & Phillips, N. (2007). Language performance in Alzheimer's disease and mild cognitive impairment: A comparative review. *Journal of Clinical and Experimental Neuropsychology*, *30*(5), 501–556. doi:10.1080/13803390701550128

KEY TERMSAND DEFINITIONS

Adjusted Coefficient of Determination: Used in the context of statistical models whose main purpose is the prediction of future outcomes on the basis of other related information. It provides a measure of model accuracy.

Feature selection: The technique of selecting a subset of relevant features for building robust learning models.

Formants: The spectral peaks of the sound spectrum of the voice. Formant is also used to mean an acoustic resonance and, in speech science and phonetics, is the resonance of the human vocal tract.

Fundamental Frequency: The lowest frequency in a harmonic series. The fundamental frequency of a periodic signal is the inverse of the period length. This determines sound pitch.

Principal Component Analysis (PCA): A mathematical procedure that transforms a number of possibly correlated variables into a smaller number of uncorrelated variables called principal components.

Speech Prosody: One of the major components of human voice, in addition to tone and phoneme. It is a universal characteristic of human speech and elicits important non-verbal information, such as emotion, mind, and mental condition of talker.

Speech Prosody-Based Cognitive Impairment Rating (SPCIR): A novel computational scale used to screen cognitive impairment in elderly patients. It is calculated using multiple linear regression combined with prosodic features extracted from human speech.

Chapter 25
Non-Linear Analysis of Plethysmograms and the Effect of Communication on Dementia in Elderly Individuals

Mayumi Oyama-Higa
Osaka Univiersity, Japan

Tiejun Miao
Osaka Univiersity, Japan

Yoko Hirohashi
Osaka Univiersity, Japan

Yuko Matsumoto-Mizuno
Osaka Univiersity, Japan

ABSTRACT

The authors of this chapter measured plethysmography and calculated the Largest Lyapunov Expornent (LLE) using non-linear analysis. They found that the value of LLE was significantly related to the severity of dementia and the communication skill in the ADL index for 144 elderly individuals. The authors developed a mathematical model to analyze the results by studying the information extracted from the plethysmogram data. Furthermore, data were collected when the central nerve was blocked by general anesthesia to evaluate the mathematical model. The pulse wave data indicated that the authors included information from the nucleus of the brain origin. In other words, they obtained conclusive evidence of dementia using the LLE and communication skills. The authors measured pulse waves while elderly individuals had a conversation. They calculated the activation of the sympathetic nerve and the parasympathetic (LF/HF, HF) response simultaneously. LLE that was activated by communication had a low HF, and the HF was high in individuals who were not activated. In other words, an effect of communication was observed in conscious elderly individuals. Communication scientifically indicated the mental activity of elderly individuals.

DOI: 10.4018/978-1-60960-559-9.ch025

Figure 1. Method of recording finger wave pulses

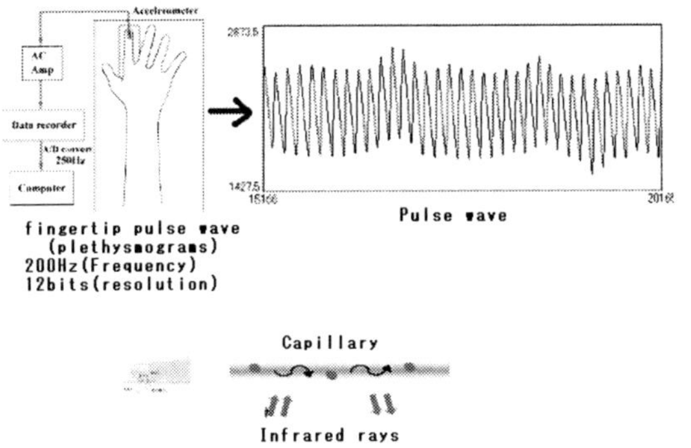

Figure 2. Schematic representation of the model

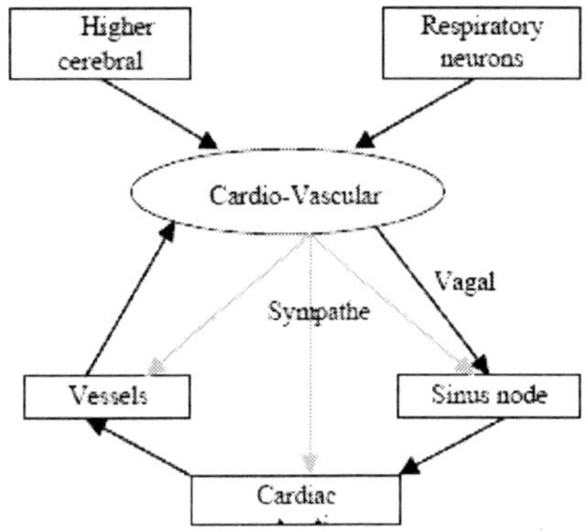

INTRODUCTION

Biogenic information, such as heartbeat, blood pressure, and blood flow, is coded in complex systems. The dynamic rhythm of the biogenic information is neither constant, such as that of a metronome, nor random. Most of the natural world has chaos in the dynamic rhythm.

The blood flow in capillaries of the finger was examined by infrared rays. Figure 1 shows the method of measurement of finger plethysmography using a sampling rate of 200 Hz and a 12-bit resolution.

In a given time series ($\underline{x}(i)$, with i=1…N), the phase space is reconstructed using a method of delays. Assuming that we create a d-dimensional phase space using a τ constant delay lag, the vectors in the space are formed by d-tuples from the time series and are given by

$$\mathbf{x}(i)=(x(i),\ldots,x(i-(d-1)\tau))=\{x_k(i)\} \quad (1)$$

where $x_k(i)=x(i-(k-1)\tau)$, with k=1,..., d. To correctly reconstruct the phase space, the parameters of delay lag τand embedding dimension d should be carefully chosen. For the reconstructed phase space, one of the important complexity measures is the LLE. The LLE characterizes how a set of infinite orthonormal small distances evolves according to its dynamics. For a chaotic system, there is at least one positive Lyapunov exponent ($\lambda_1>$ 0 is the largest exponent). The defining property of chaos is dependent on the initial conditions. Given an initial infinitely small distance $\Delta x(0)$, its evolution obeys

$$\Delta x(t) = \Delta x(0)e^{\lambda_1 t} \quad (2)$$

For an M-dimensional dynamical system, there are M Lyapunov exponents. We estimated only λ_1 using the algorithm of Sano and Sawada (1985; paraneters: d-dimensional phase space d= 4. τ: time delay 50 ms).

MATHEMATICAL MODEL

To understand changes in chaos in the finger plethysmograms, a mathematical model was proposed. Figure 2 shows a schematic description of the model used in this paper. The model consists of a feedback loop and physiological factors (Miao et al 2006). The pressure receptors sense and transmit neural afferent signals to the cardio-vascular center. Neural efferent signals are created and then sent to effectors. Influences come from respiratory centers and from higher cerebral regions.

Pulsation of the blood in the ear was represented as a response function to pulsation in the

Figure 3. LLE in the plethysmograms was explained in relation to the decreased chaoticity. A high Lyapunov exponent was theoretically predicted due to excitations of the central nervous system.

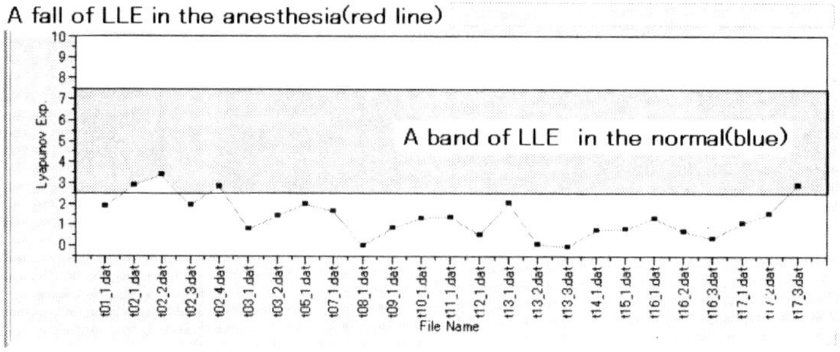

radial artery, and a proportional relationship between finger plethysmogram and artery blood pressure was approximated. Thus, for the sake of simplifying unimportant details, our model concentrated on the dynamics of blood pressure in finger plethysmograms without a loss of generalization.

VERIFICATION FROM ANESTHETIZING EXPERIMENT

We used anesthetized subjects to verify the hypothetical mathematical model. The patient who participated in the experiment was a 71-year-old male. He was put into deep anesthesia during cancer surgery.

The surgery took place at Rakuwakai Otowa Hospital, Kyoto on December 12, 2008. The participant provided informed consent.

The subject slept comfortably in a hospital bed in a relaxed manner. His hands were gently placed on the side of his body and were in a relaxed, semi-open position with the palms turned downward. A photoelectric plethysmography sensor was placed on the distal phalanx of second finger. Finger plethysmograms were recorded continuously for all processes before, during and after the surgery by an instrument (BACS2000; CCI). Signals were digitized at a 200-Hz sampling rate with resolution of 12 bits and transferred via an A/D converter to a PC for data processing.

The time course of anesthesia is shown in Figure 3. Pulse waves were continuously measured from 9:10 to 14:25. The patient was initially anesthetized by injection and then anesthetized by suction. Figure 8 shows the LLE during the operation. Noise caused by the radio-knife was omitted, and 23 pulse waves were calculated. The LLE was occupied by blocking information in the center system during anesthesia. A small value (from 0 to 1) was obtained for the able-bodied person's exponent and was changed from 3 to 5 using the same parameter. When the patient woke up, the t21 and t23 were interesting. In addition, an uptrend was observed due to the voice of the patient.

Chaotic dynamics in finger plethysmograms were observed in relation to the anesthesia process. The LLE of the plethysmograms was significant and may be used to characterize mental/physical status. Lower values of Lyapunov exponents were observed, indicating a blocked or depressed effect of anesthesia on the central neural system. We found that a smaller value could be used to estimate the laparotomy and the 50% O2 change, depicting an effect of mental comedown. The LLE increased once the patient regained consciousness. To understand how the chaos arises and to explain the changes in the LLE of the finger plethysmograms,

Figure 4. Evaluation of the LLE and (A) communication skills and (B) severity of dementia in elderly patients

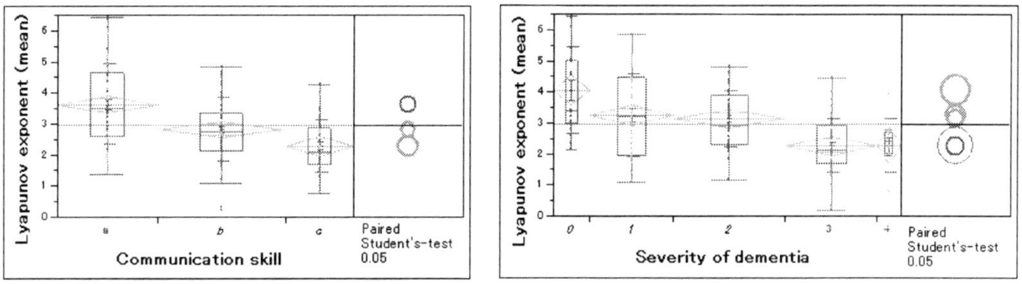

a mathematical model of the baroreflex feedback and autonomous interactions was proposed. According to the model, a decrease in the LLE of the plethysmograms occurred in relation to the decreased chaos, and depression or blockade of the central nervous system was predicted in higher cerebral regions. A high Lyapunov exponent was theoretically predicted to be caused by excitations of the central nervous system.

STUDIES OF ELDERLY SUBJECTS WITH DIFFERENT COMMUNICATION SKILLS

Subjects: Data were obtained from 179 subjects (40 male, 139 female) at three nursing homes in Shiga prefecture, Japan.

Indices: Data were evaluated based on the ADL index of communication skills (three-graded evaluation), which is composed of seven items and estimated by a care manager. We examined the relationship between the data and the LLE calculated from fingertip pulse waves.

Results: Five grades indicating the severity of dementia were evaluated by a physician. Data were evaluated using the ADL index. We examined the relationship between the data and the LLE calculated from fingertip pulse waves.

Fifteen subjects with high cognition were selected and measurements were taken again after 9 months (August 2004) (Figure 5). Compared to the first measurements taken in November 2003, the LLE values increased in some subjects and decreased in others. These results suggest that changes in the LLE always occur. However, more information is necessary to understand the causes of very low values.

Figure 5. LLE measurements after 9 months (15 subjects). Subject e7 died prior to the second measurement.

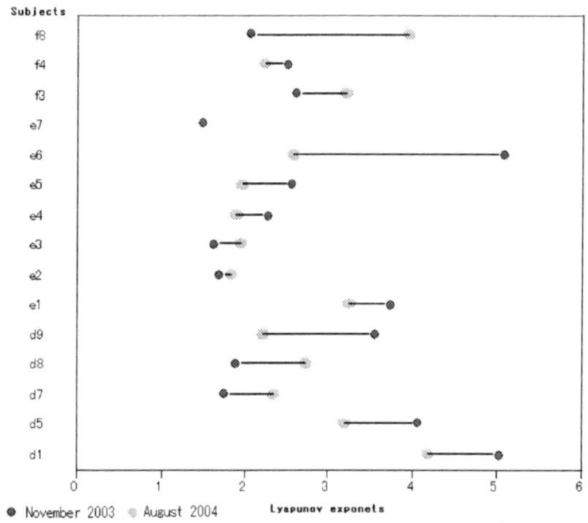

In constellation graphs, the right side indicates a small LLE and the left side indicates the LLE (Figures 6 and 7). Because of the large quantity of data, five representative cases for each rank in the index (i.e. dementia, 0–4; communication skills, a–c) are shown.

Figure 6. Correlation between the severity of dementia (0–4) and the LLE. One line denotes one subject.

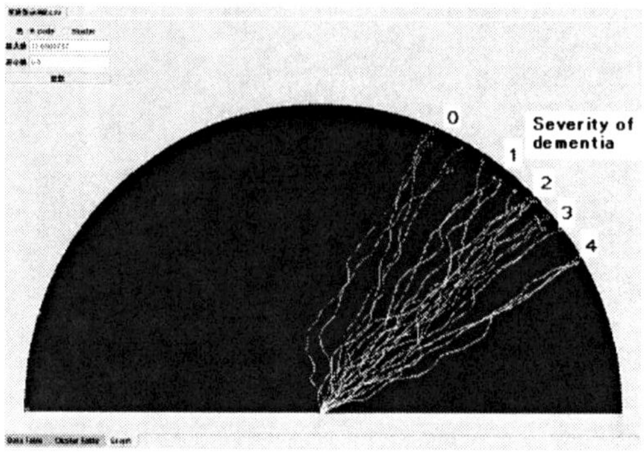

Figure 7. Correlation between communication skills (a–c) and the LLE

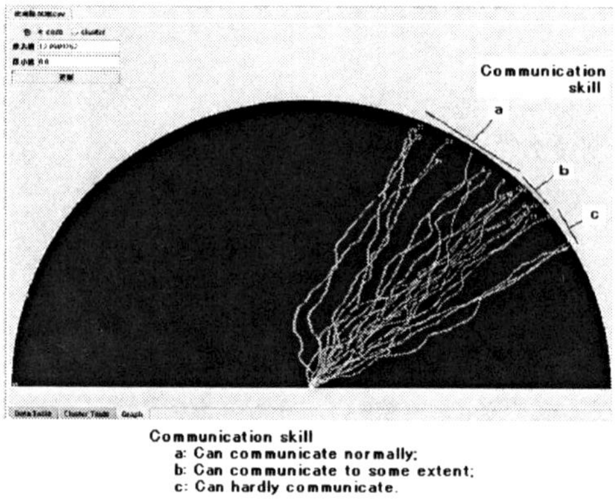

MEASUREMENT OF THE EFFECT OF COMMUNICATION-DEPENDENT REHABILITATION

After determining the correlation between communication and the degree of dementia, we predicted that communications skills would increase the LLE of patients with dementia. We then tested whether the LLE of a patient with dementia was altered.

A patient with a high degree of dementia was chosen. An experienced care manager, who was familiar with elderly individuals, communicated with the patient.

The pulse wave device was initially placed on the finger. Communication began after two minutes and was measured for 7-10 minutes.

The sympathetic and the parasympathetic response were measured from the pulse wave simultaneously. Reactions were slow due to sleepiness when the parasympathetic value was high.

The sex, age, level of care needed, disease, and communications and states of the measurement are shown for 22 patients. Seven of the 22 people reacted to the care manager's voice. Seven people had a high parasympathetic response and seemed to be in a sleep state. An effective pulse wave was not obtained in the remaining eight subjects.

Modulation of the LLE, the sympathetic nerve, and the parasympathetic response in patients who saw the communication is shown in the graph. A and B are representative of these patients. C and D are examples of patients with a high parasym-

Figure 8. Correlation between the LLE and HF/LR of four patients

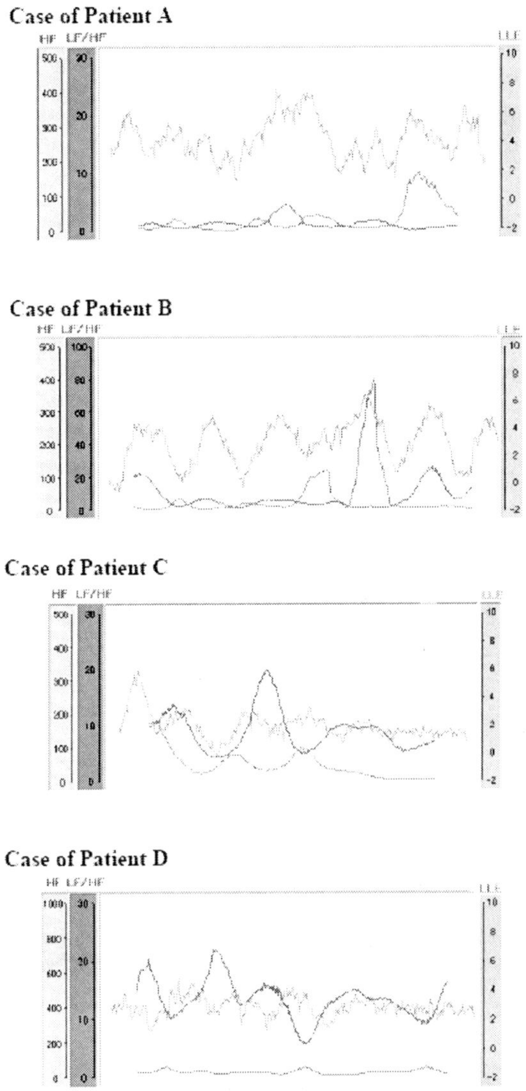

pathetic response. The communication effect is not remarkable because patients were sleepy.

HF indicates a parasympathetic value. LF/HF indicates a sympathetic value.

CONCLUSION

Patients with dementia tend to have a low LLE value. The LLE decreased when the dementia became more severe according to communications skill based on the ADL index. A decrease in communication skills is related to dementia. Communication is an important element that modulates the LLE. The present study measured the pulse wave of 22 patients with dementias. The experimental method examined how the LLE was modulated as the care manager spoke with the patient. Measurements could not be made in eight patients due to vibration of the finger. However, large alterations in the LLE were observed in seven patients. In these patients, the parasympathetic responses and substantial changes were not seen in the LLE. These responses are indicative of a sleep state. Communication affects the LLE.

It is thought that communication is useful for the recovery of patients with dementia or the prevention of dementia.

ACKNOWLEDGMENT

We would like to thank Dr. Maho Imoto, Rakuwakai Otowa Hospital, who provided useful and helpful assistance during the experiments.

REFERENCES

Imanishi, A., & Oyama-Higa, M. (2006). *The relation between observers' psychophysiological conditions and human errors during monitoring task*. 2006 IEEE Conference on Systems, Man, and Cybernetics, Taipei, Taiwan, (pp. 2035–2039).

Miao, T., Shimoyama, O., & Oyama-Higa, M. (2006). *Modelling plethysmogram dynamics based on baroreflex under higher cerebral influences*. 2006 IEEE Conference on Systems, Man, and Cybernetics, Taipei, Taiwan, (pp. 2868–2873).

Oyama-Higa, M., & Miao, T. (2006). *Discovery and application of new index for cognitive psychology*. 2006 IEEE Conference on Systems, Man, and Cybernetics, Taipei, Taiwan, (pp. 2040–2044).

Oyama-Higa, M., Miao, T., & Mizuno-Matsumoto, Y. (2006). *Analysis of dementia in aged subjects through chaos analysis of fingertip pulse waves*. 2006 IEEE Conference on Systems, Man, & Cybernetics, Taipei, Taiwan, 2863–2867.

Sano, M., & Sawada, Y. (1985). Measurement of the Lyapunov spectrum from a chaotic time series. *Physical Review Letters*, *55*, 1082. doi:10.1103/PhysRevLett.55.1082

Takens, F. (1985). *Dynamical systems and bifurcations* (Braaksma, B. L. J., Broer, H. W., & Takens, F., eds). (LNM 1125). Heidelberg, Germany: Springer.

Tsuda, I., Tahara, T., & Iwanaga, I. (1992). Chaotic pulsation in capillary vessels and its dependence on mental and physical conditions. *International Journal of Bifurcation and Chaos in Applied Sciences and Engineering*, *2*, 313–324. doi:10.1142/S0218127492000318

KEY TERMS AND DEFINITIONS

ADL Index: Activity of Daily Living Index.

Anesthesia: Yhe state of nerve paralysis.

HRV: Heart rate variability.

Largest Lyapunov Exponent: A coefficient that describes the rate at which nearby trajectories in phase space converge or diverge.

Non-Linear Analysis: Analysis using non-linear methods.

Plethysmograms: A wave pulse at the finger tip.

Chapter 26
Diffusion Tensor Imaging for Dementia

Kei Yamada
Department of Radiology, Graduate School of Medical Science, Kyoto Prefectural University of Medicine, Japan

Kentaro Akazawa
Department of Radiology, Graduate School of Medical Science, Kyoto Prefectural University of Medicine, Japan

Tsunehiko Nishimura
Department of Radiology, Graduate School of Medical Science, Kyoto Prefectural University of Medicine, Japan

ABSTRACT

Magnetic resonance MR tractography based on diffusion tensor imaging (DTI) was first introduced to the medical imaging community a decade ago. Since then, it has been successfully applied to a number of neurological conditions. It has been most commonly applied to the pre-operative planning of brain tumors. The other areas with active research additionally include stroke, multiple sclerosis and dementia, providing valuable information that would not be available through other imaging techniques. Tractography was first introduced with the deterministic streamline technique and has evolved to use more sophisticated probabilistic approaches. In this chapter, the authors will describe the clinical application of this tractographic technique to patients with dementia.

I. INTRODUCTION

Diffusion-tensor imaging (DTI)-based tractography is one of the most remarkable advances in the field of neuroimaging in the past decade. This method offers *in vivo* localization of neuronal fiber tracts, which was not previously possible. As a clinical tool, this technique primarily targets intracranial space-occupying lesions, i.e., brain tumors and vascular malformations (Mori, 1999; Witwer, 2002; Wiegell, 2000; Nimsky, 2006; Yamada, 2003; Yamada, 2004). Further, DTI has been shown to be robust by many reports.

DOI: 10.4018/978-1-60960-559-9.ch026

II. BASICS OF DTI AND TRACTOGRAPHY

Water-diffusion anisotropy (directionality) in the white matter of the brain is defined on the basis of axonal alignment (Wiegell, 2000). Water preferentially diffuses in a direction parallel to the axon's longitudinal axis but is relatively restricted in the perpendicular axis. This phenomenon can be represented mathematically by the so called diffusion ellipsoid, or tensor (Figure 1).

The tensor has three eigenvalues. The long one pointing along the axonal direction is λ1, and the two small axes have lengths λ2 and λ3 (Figure 2). The diffusivity along the principal axis λ1 is also called longitudinal, axial, or parallel diffusivity.

The tensors of cerebral white matter can be reconstructed to track three-dimensional macroscopic fiber orientation in the brain. The translation of the longest axis of the tensor (v1) into neural trajectories can be achieved by various algorithms (Figure 3 and Figure 4).

Figure 1. Diffusion ellipsoids (tensors). When there is no directionality, the fractional anisotropy (FA) is zero (spherical). A typical tensor of a white matter bundle will have the shape of a cigar. When there are crossing fibers, the ellipsoid becomes flattened, resulting in "pancake" tensors (lower left).

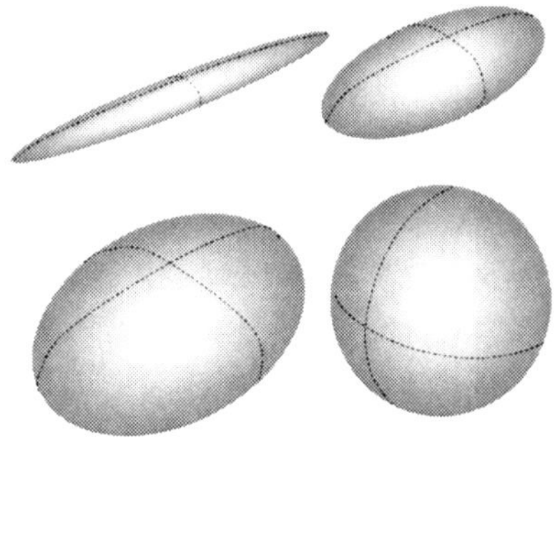

Figure 2. Diffusion constants of a given ellipsoid are shown in this figure. λ1 represents diffusivity in the longest axis of this tensor. The v1 represents the vector orientation of λ1.

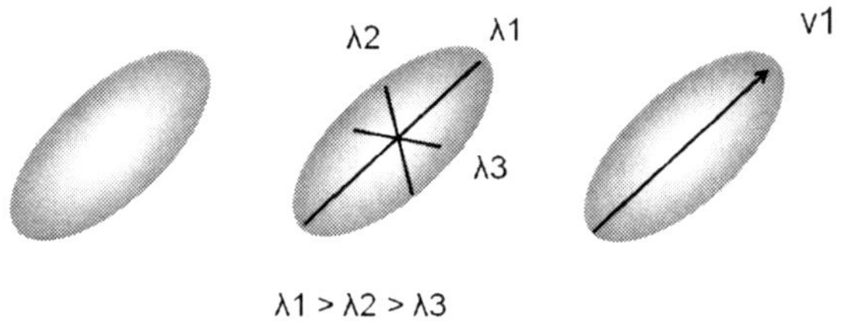

Figure 3. Tracking starts at a pixel (or ROI). The FACT program tracks the ellipsoids as long as the adjacent vectors are strongly aligned.

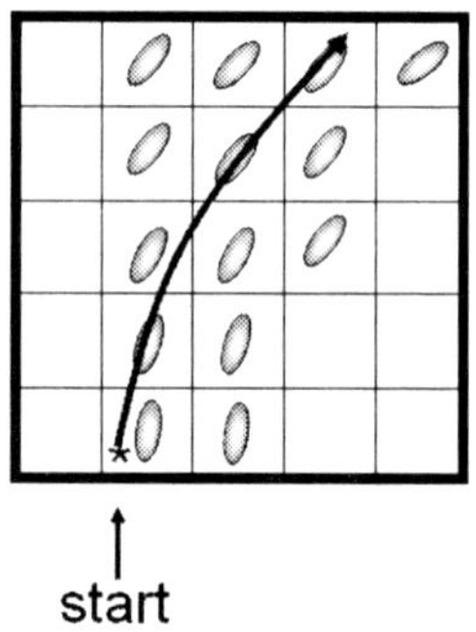

Figure 4. When vector orientation becomes random, as judged quantitatively by the inner products of these vectors, tracking is terminated. The program also terminates when the diffusion ellipsoids approach a spherical shape.

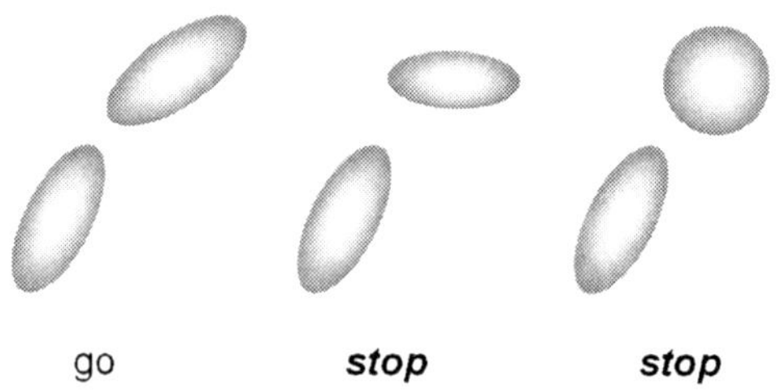

III. LIMITATIONS OF TRACTOGRAPHY

Perhaps the most important limitation of tractography is that it has not yet been fully validated.

Attempts to validate this technique have been made in the past (Qazi, 2009; Lin, 2001; Ciccarelli, 2003; Parker, 2002; Okada, 2006), and most of these efforts have been based on comparisons of tractographic images and known neuroanatomy. A study that evaluated deterministic tractography in patients who underwent intra-operative electrophysiological tests indicated that tractography appears to underestimate fiber tracts (Kinoshita, 2005). Thus, this tool has to be used with caution, knowing that we are observing only a fraction of reality.

IV. CLINICAL APPLICATION

Tractography has been used not only for assessing neuroanatomy (Yamamoto, 2005; Yamada, 2007), but also extensively for diseases such as brain tumors (Figure 5) (Nimsky, 2006; Kinoshita, 2005; Yamada, 2003), stroke (Nagakane, 2008; Yamada, 2003; Yamada, 2004; Konishi, 2005; Yamada, 2006; Murakami, 2008; Hosomi, 2008) and neurodegenerative diseases (Yoshida, 2004; Yoshikawa, 2004; Shiga, 2005). Application to dementia is also one of the most rapidly growing fields. The targets of these investigations include Alzheimer's disease (AD) (Hanyu, 1998; Takahashi, 2002; Taoka, 2006; Yasmin, 2008; Bozzali, 2002), frontotemporal lobar degeneration (FTLD) (Matsuo, 2008; Yoshiura, 2006), and dementia with Lewy bodies (DLB) (Bozzali, 2005). These studies typically measured the mean diffusivity (MD = 1/3 of the trace of the tensor) and FA of various regions using manual ROI placement; in more recent studies, they often use tract-based analysis.

In patients with AD and FTLD, various areas of the brain have been shown to be involved, including the posterior cingulate, arcuate fasciculus, inferior occipitofrontal fascicles and uncinate fascicles (UF). Among these areas, UF is most commonly investigated (Figure 5) (Taoka, 2006; Yasmin, 2008; Matsuo, 2008). The UF is the largest connection between the temporal and frontal lobes, and its traumatic disruption is known to result in severe memory impairment. In patients with AD and FTLD, the degree of damage to the relevant fiber tracts, as estimated by DTI, is known to correlate with the severity of the disease process (Taoka, 2006; Matsuo, 2008).

The MD and FA measurement alone, however, does not provide specific information in discriminating the different pathological substrates (e.g., demyelination vs. axonal loss vs. neuronal dysfunction) (Bozzali, 2007). For example, AD and DLB are characterized by different pathophysiological processes, at least in their pure forms. More specifically, AD is characterized by neuronal loss, whereas DLB is characterized by neuronal dysfunction. Bozzali et al. studied patients with AD (Bozzali, 2002) and DLB (Bozzali, 2005) in

Figure 5. This 66-year-old woman had a right frontal brain tumor and was referred to our facility for treatment. MRI study showed a ring-enhanced mass in the right frontal lobe that involved part of the precentral gyrus. She underwent pre-operative fiber tracking of sensory and motor tracts, and the tumor was completely resected with the aid of intra-operative neuronavigation and electrical subcortical stimulation. The pyramidal (cortico-spinal) tract is colored in purple and the sensory tract in green. The tumor posteriorly compresses both the pyramidal and sensory tract.

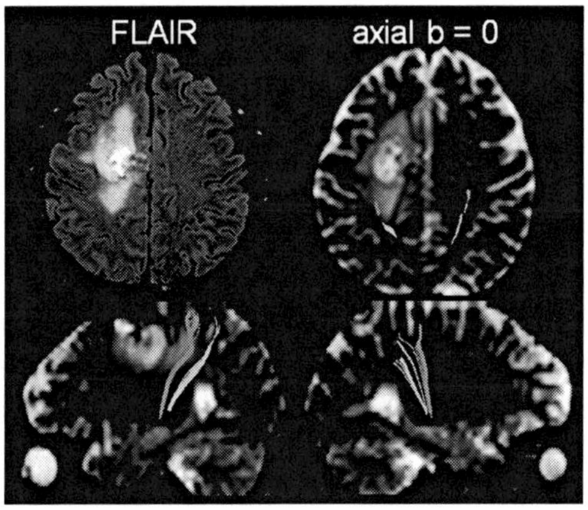

different investigations, and found very similar patterns of MD and FA changes in regions such as the corpus callosum and pericallosal areas. Thus, any definitive interpretation of these MD/FA changes in terms of different pathological substrates seems difficult. Conversely, lesion distribution was much more disease-specific (Bozzali, 2007) and thus may be clinically useful in discriminating the two conditions.

A previous AD investigation was done using not only the FA and MD but also radial diffusivity, based on the assumption that radial diffusivity would reflect myelin integrity (Choi, 2005). Indeed, that study successfully demonstrated increased radial diffusivity at the frontal lobes, which the authors concluded was due to demyelination. This assumption, however, is purely speculative, as there is no pathological proof. Future studies are needed to confirm this correlation.

Differentiation between the AD and vascular dementia (VaD) can be a clinical burden. Clinical diagnosis of VaD is made by established criteria, but it is not specific or sensitive. Tractography has been used in attempts to overcome this problem, and the results indicate that it may be a promising tool (Zarei, 2009). The study found a significant reduction of the FA at the forceps minor in VaD patients, suggesting that the damage to the transcallosal prefrontal connection could be an important marker for VaD.

Figure 6. Tractography of the left uncinate fasciculus of a normal volunteer is shown in this figure. The tract is demonstrated as a bright yellow bundle. (A: anterior side; Post: posterior side; and S: superior side). The vector elements of the color maps are designated by red (x element, left to right), green (y element, anteroposterior), and blue (z element, superoinferior) colors. The intensities of the color map are scaled in proportion to the FA.

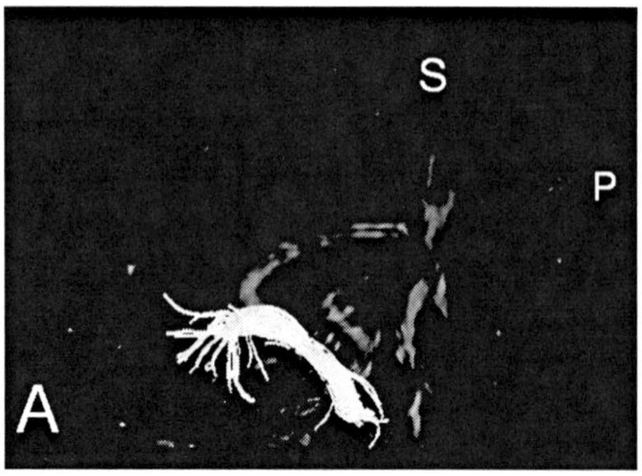

V. CONCLUSION

Diffusion tensor imaging and tractography has been shown to be a promising tool in assessing the white matter of brains in patients with dementia, and its clinical application is expanding. However, the pathological substrates underlying the changes that we observed with this technique still await validation (Yamada, 2009).

REFERENCES

Bozzali, M., & Cherubini, A. (2007). Diffusion tensor MRI to investigate dementias: A brief review. *Magnetic Resonance Imaging*, *25*, 969–977. doi:10.1016/j.mri.2007.03.017

Bozzali, M., Falini, A., Cercignani, M., Baglio, F., Farina, E., & Alberoni, M. (2005). Brain tissue damage in dementia with Lewy bodies: An in vivo diffusion tensor MRI study. *Brain*, *128*, 1595–1604. doi:10.1093/brain/awh493

Bozzali, M., Falini, A., Franceschi, M., Cercignani, M., Franceschi, M., & Schiatti, E. (2002). White matter damage in Alzheimer's disease assessed in vivo using diffusion tensor magnetic resonance imaging. *Journal of Neurology, Neurosurgery, and Psychiatry*, *72*, 742–746. doi:10.1136/jnnp.72.6.742

Choi, S. J., Lim, K. O., Monteiro, I., & Reisberg, B. (2005). Diffusion tensor imaging of frontal white matter microstructure in early Alzheimer's disease: A preliminary study. *Journal of Geriatric Psychiatry and Neurology*, *18*, 12–19. doi:10.1177/0891988704271763

Ciccarelli, O., Toosy, A. T., Parker, G. J., Wheeler-Kingshott, C. A., Barker, G. J., Miller, D. H., & Thompson, A. J. (2003). Diffusion tractography based group mapping of major white-matter pathways in the human brain. *NeuroImage*, *19*, 1545–1555. doi:10.1016/S1053-8119(03)00190-3

Hanyu, H., Sakurai, H., Iwamoto, T., Takasaki, M., Shindo, H., & Abe, K. (1998). Diffusion-weighted MR imaging of the hippocampus and temporal white matter in Alzheimer's disease. *Journal of the Neurological Sciences*, *156*, 195–200. doi:10.1016/S0022-510X(98)00043-4

Hosomi, A., Nagakane, Y., Yamada, K., Kuriyama, N., Mizuno, T., Nishimura, T., & Nakagawa, M. (2009). Assessment of arcuate fasciculus with diffusion-tensor tractography may predict the prognosis of aphasia in patients with left middle cerebral artery infarcts. *Neuroradiology*, *51*, 549–555. doi:10.1007/s00234-009-0534-7

Kinoshita, M., Yamada, K., Hashimoto, N., Kato, A., Izumoto, S., & Baba, T. (2005). Fiber-tracking does not accurately estimate size of fiber bundle in pathological condition: Initial neurosurgical experience using neuronavigation and subcortical white matter stimulation. *NeuroImage*, *25*, 424–429. doi:10.1016/j.neuroimage.2004.07.076

Konishi, J., Yamada, K., Kizu, O., Ito, H., Sugimura, K., & Yoshikawa, K. (2005). MR tractography for the evaluation of functional recovery from lenticulostriate infarcts. *Neurology*, *64*, 108–113.

Lin, C. P., Tseng, W. Y., Cheng, H. C., & Chen, J. H. (2001). Validation of diffusion tensor magnetic resonance axonal fiber imaging with registered manganese-enhanced optic tracts. *NeuroImage*, *14*, 1035–1047. doi:10.1006/nimg.2001.0882

Matsuo, K., Mizuno, T., Yamada, K., Akazawa, K., Kasai, T., & Kondo, M. (2008). Cerebral white matter damage in frontotemporal dementia assessed by diffusion tensor tractography. *Neuroradiology*, *50*, 605–611. doi:10.1007/s00234-008-0379-5

Mori, S., Crain, B. J., Chacko, V. P., & van Zijl, P. C. (1999). Three-dimensional tracking of axonal projections in the brain by magnetic resonance imaging. *Annals of Neurology*, *45*, 265–269. doi:10.1002/1531-8249(199902)45:2<265::AID-ANA21>3.0.CO;2-3

Murakami, A., Morimoto, M., Yamada, K., Kizu, O., Nishimura, A., Nishimura, T., & Sugimoto, T. (2008). Fiber-tracking techniques can predict the degree of neurologic impairment for periventricular leukomalacia. *Pediatrics*, *122*, 500–506. doi:10.1542/peds.2007-2816

Nagakane, Y., Yamada, K., Ohara, T., Yoshikawa, K., Kuriyama, N., & Takayasu, N. (2008). Acute lenticulostriate infarction presenting with skip lesions may reflect the selective vulnerability of gray and white matter. *Stroke*, *39*, 494–496. doi:10.1161/STROKEAHA.107.484337

Nimsky, C., Ganslandt, O., Merhof, D., Sorensen, A. G., & Fahlbusch, R. (2006). Intraoperative visualization of the pyramidal tract by diffusion-tensor-imaging-based fiber tracking. *NeuroImage*, *30*, 1219–1229. doi:10.1016/j.neuroimage.2005.11.001

Okada, T., Mikuni, N., Miki, Y., Kikuta, K., Urayama, S., & Hanakawa, T. (2006). Corticospinal tract localization: integration of diffusion-tensor tractography at 3-T MR imaging with intraoperative white matter stimulation mapping-preliminary results. *Radiology*, *240*, 849–857. doi:10.1148/radiol.2403050916

Parker, G. J., Stephan, K. E., Barker, G. J., Rowe, J. B., MacManus, D. G., & Wheeler-Kingshott, C. A. (2002). Initial demonstration of in vivo tracing of axonal projections in the macaque brain and comparison with the human brain using diffusion tensor imaging and fast marching tractography. *NeuroImage*, *15*, 797–809. doi:10.1006/nimg.2001.0994

Qazi, A. A., Radmanesh, A., O'Donnell, L., Kindlmann, G., Peled, S., & Whalen, S. (2009). Resolving crossings in the corticospinal tract by two-tensor streamline tractography: Method and clinical assessment using fMRI. *NeuroImage*, *47*(2), T98–T106. doi:10.1016/j.neuroimage.2008.06.034

Shiga, K., Yamada, K., Yoshikawa, K., Mizuno, T., Nishimura, T., & Nakagawa, M. (2005). Local tissue anisotropy decreases in cerebellopetal fibers and pyramidal tract in multiple system atrophy. *Journal of Neurology*, *252*, 589–596. doi:10.1007/s00415-005-0708-0

Takahashi, S., Yonezawa, H., Takahashi, J., Kudo, M., Inoue, T., & Tohgi, H. (2002). Selective reduction of diffusion anisotropy in white matter of Alzheimer disease brains measured by 3.0 Tesla magnetic resonance imaging. *Neuroscience Letters*, *332*, 45–48. doi:10.1016/S0304-3940(02)00914-X

Taoka, T., Iwasaki, S., Sakamoto, M., Nakagawa, H., Fukusumi, A., & Myochin, K. (2006). Diffusion anisotropy and diffusivity of white matter tracts within the temporal stem in Alzheimer disease: Evaluation of the tract of interest by diffusion tensor tractography. *AJNR. American Journal of Neuroradiology*, *27*, 1040–1045.

Wiegell, M. R., Larsson, H. B., & Wedeen, V. J. (2000). Fiber crossing in human brain depicted with diffusion tensor MR imaging. *Radiology*, *217*, 897–903.

Witwer, B. P., Moftakhar, R., Hasan, K. M., Deshmukh, P., Haughton, V., & Field, A. (2002). Diffusion-tensor imaging of white matter tracts in patients with cerebral neoplasm. *Journal of Neurosurgery*, *97*, 568–575. doi:10.3171/jns.2002.97.3.0568

Yamada, K. (2009). Diffusion tensor tractography should be used with caution. *Proceedings of the National Academy of Sciences of the United States of America*, *106*, E14. doi:10.1073/pnas.0812352106

Yamada, K., Ito, H., Nakamura, H., Akada, W., Kubota, T., & Goto, M. (2004). Stroke patients' evolving symptoms assessed by tractography. *Journal of Magnetic Resonance Imaging*, *20*, 923–929. doi:10.1002/jmri.20215

Yamada, K., Kizu, O., Ito, H., & Nishimura, T. (2004). Tractography for an arteriovenous malformation. *Neurology*, *62*, 669.

Yamada, K., Kizu, O., Kubota, T., Ito, H., Matsushima, S., Oouchi, H., & Nishimura, T. (2007). The pyramidal tract has a predictable course through centrum semiovale: A diffusion-tensor based tractography study. *Journal of Magnetic Resonance Imaging*, *26*, 519–524. doi:10.1002/jmri.21006

Yamada, K., Kizu, O., Mori, S., Ito, H., Nakamura, H., & Yuen, S. (2003). Clinically feasible diffusion-tensor imaging for fiber tracking. *Radiology*, *227*, 295–301. doi:10.1148/radiol.2271020313

Yamada, K., Mori, S., Nakamura, H., Ito, H., Kizu, O., & Shiga, K. (2003). Fiber-tracking method reveals sensorimotor pathway involvement in stroke patients. *Stroke*, *34*, E159–E162. doi:10.1161/01.STR.0000085827.54986.89

Yamada, K., Nagakane, Y., Yoshikawa, K., Kizu, O., Ito, H., & Kubota, T. (2007). Somatotopic organization of thalamocortical projection fibers as assessed by MR tractography-initial observations. *Radiology*, *242*, 840–845. doi:10.1148/radiol.2423060297

Yamada, K., Shiga, K., Kizu, O., Ito, H., Akiyama, K., Nakagawa, M., & Nishimura, T. (2006). Oculomotor nerve palsy evaluated by diffusion-tensor tractography. *Neuroradiology, 48*, 434–437. doi:10.1007/s00234-006-0070-7

Yamamoto, T., Yamada, K., Nishimura, T., & Kinoshita, S. (2005). Tractography to depict three layers of visual field trajectories to the calcarine gyri. *American Journal of Ophthalmology, 140*, 781–785. doi:10.1016/j.ajo.2005.05.018

Yasmin, H., Nakata, Y., Aoki, S., Abe, O., Sato, N., & Nemoto, K. (2008). Diffusion abnormalities of the uncinate fasciculus in Alzheimer's disease: Diffusion tensor tract-specific analysis using a new method to measure the core of the tract. *Neuroradiology, 50*, 293–299. doi:10.1007/s00234-007-0353-7

Yoshida, T., Shiga, K., Yoshikawa, K., Yamada, K., & Nakagawa, M. (2004). White matter loss in the splenium of the corpus callosum in a case of posterior cortical atrophy: A diffusion tensor imaging study. *European Neurology, 52*, 77–81. doi:10.1159/000079750

Yoshikawa, K., Nakata, Y., Yamada, K., & Nakagawa, M. (2004). Early pathological changes in the Parkinsonian brain demonstrated by diffusion tensor MRI. *Journal of Neurology, Neurosurgery, and Psychiatry, 75*, 481–484. doi:10.1136/jnnp.2003.021873

Yoshiura, T., Mihara, F., & Koga, H. (2006). Mapping of subcortical white matter abnormality in Alzheimer's disease using diffusion-weighted magnetic resonance imaging. *Academic Radiology, 13*, 1460–1464. doi:10.1016/j.acra.2006.09.042

Zarei, M., Damoiseaux, J. S., Morgese, C., Beckmann, C. F., Smith, S. M., & Matthews, P. M. (2009). Regional white matter integrity differentiates between vascular dementia and Alzheimer disease. *Stroke, 40*, 773–779. doi:10.1161/STROKEAHA.108.530832

KEYWORDS AND DEFINITIONS

Alzheimer: Senile dementia of most common type.

Diffusion Tensor Imaging: Water molecular diffusivity expressed using mathematical model, known as tensor.

MRI: Magnetic resonance imaging.

Neuroanatomy: Anatomy of the nervous tissue.

Neuroimaging: Imaging of the nervous system.

Tractography: A method that enables visualization of nerve fiber tract.

Chapter 27
The Important Role of Lipids in Cognitive Impairment

Jia Yu
Neuroscience Research Institute & Department of Neurobiology; Key Laboratory for Neuroscience Ministry of Education; Key Laboratory for Neuroscience Ministry of Public Health, Health Science Center, Peking University, China & Beijing Geriatric Hospital, China

Zheng Chen
Beijing Geriatric Hospital, China

Jiangyang Lu
Department of Pathology, First Affiliated Hospital of General Hospital of PLA, China

Tingting Liu
Neuroscience Research Institute & Department of Neurobiology; Key Laboratory for Neuroscience Ministry of Education; Key Laboratory for Neuroscience Ministry of Public Health, Health Science Center, Peking University, China

Liang Zhou
Neuroscience Research Institute & Department of Neurobiology; Key Laboratory for Neuroscience Ministry of Education; Key Laboratory for Neuroscience Ministry of Public Health, Health Science Center, Peking University, China

Xinying Liu
Neuroscience Research Institute & Department of Neurobiology; Key Laboratory for Neuroscience Ministry of Education; Key Laboratory for Neuroscience Ministry of Public Health, Health Science Center, Peking University, China

Miao Sun
Neuroscience Research Institute & Department of Neurobiology; Key Laboratory for Neuroscience Ministry of Education; Key Laboratory for Neuroscience Ministry of Public Health, Health Science Center, Peking University, China

Weizhong Xiao
Department of Neurology, Third Hospital of Peking University, China

Dongsheng Fan
Department of Neurology, Third Hospital of Peking University, China

Dehua Chui
Neuroscience Research Institute & Department of Neurobiology; Key Laboratory for Neuroscience Ministry of Education; Key Laboratory for Neuroscience Ministry of Public Health, Health Science Center, Peking University, China & Department of Neurology, Third Hospital of Peking University, China

DOI: 10.4018/978-1-60960-559-9.ch027

ABSTRACT

The current knowledge base on circulating serum and plasma risk factors of the cognitive decline of degenerative Alzheimer's Disease is linked to cholesterol homeostasis and lipoprotein disturbances (i.e., total cholesterol, 24S-hydroxy-cholesterol, lipoprotein(a), or apolipoprotein E. Lipoprotein lipase (LPL) is also expressed in the brain, with the highest levels found in the pyramidal cells of the hippocampus, suggesting a possible role for LPL in the regulation of cognitive function. Little is currently known, however, about the specific role of LPL in the brain. The authors of this chapter have generated an LPL-deficient mouse model that was rescued from neonatal lethality by somatic gene transfer. The levels of the presynaptic marker synaptophysin were reduced in the hippocampus while the levels of the post-synaptic marker PSD-95 remained unchanged in the LPL-deficient mice. The decreased frequency of mEPSC in LPL-deficient neurons indicated that the number of presynaptic vesicles was decreased, which was consistent with the decreases observed in the numbers of total vesicles and docking vesicles. These findings indicate that LPL plays an important role in learning and memory function, possibly by influencing presynaptic function.

I. INTRODUCTION

While a number of genetic and environmental factors have been demonstrated to be linked with the development of Alzheimer's Disease (AD), the single greatest risk factor is aging. Several lines of evidence suggest a role for age-related increases in neuropathology in the development of AD and that the age-related accrual of AD pathology promotes the progression of AD. Most studies linking pathology with the onset of AD have focused solely on the role of AD-related pathology.

The principle indication that lipids may play an important role in amyloid precursor protein (APP) processing and β-amyloid peptide (Aβ) production was provided by a common feature shared by the proteins involved in APP processing, which is that they are all integral membrane proteins. Moreover, Aβ cleavage by γ-secretase occurs in the middle of the membrane, suggesting that the lipid environment influences Aβ production and hence AD pathogenesis. The current knowledge base on circulating serum and plasma risk factors of cognitive decline of degenerative AD is linked to cholesterol homeostasis and lipoprotein disturbances (i.e., total cholesterol (TC), 24S-hydroxy-cholesterol, lipoprotein(a) (Lp(a)), or apolipoprotein E (APOE)). Lipoprotein lipase (LPL) is predominantly expressed in adipose and muscle, where it plays a crucial role in the metabolism of triglyceride-rich plasma lipoproteins. LPL is also expressed in the brain, with its highest levels found in the pyramidal cells of the hippocampus, suggesting a possible role for LPL in the regulation of cognitive function. Little is currently known, however, about the specific role of LPL in the brain. We sought to investigate the role of LPL in the brain, specifically with respect to learning and memory. Behavioral studies have not been performed in adult *LPL* gene targeted mice because of neonatal lethality. Viable adult LPL-deficient mice were generated by rescue through the somatic gene transfer of a beneficial mutant form of LPL. In the present study, we report a significant impairment in learning and memory in LPL-deficient animals and demonstrate alterations in presynaptic morphology. Our findings demonstrate that LPL plays a role in cognitive function in the central nervous system (CNS).

II. MATERIALS AND METHODS

Detailed methods can be found in the online Supplemental Methods. LPL-deficient mice in a C57BL/6J background were rescued by intramuscular administration of an adenoviral vector encoding a human LPL mutant, LPL^{S447X}. Learning and memory were examined by both water maze and step-down passive avoidance tests. Quantification was carried out by image analysis. The ultrastructure of synapses in the hippocampus was examined by transmission electron microscopy. The results were expressed as mean ± SEM. The statistical significance for differences between the two groups was evaluated with an unpaired Student's *t* test, and *p* values <0.05 were regarded as significant.

III. RESULTS

The hippocampus-dependent learning and memory of LPL-deficient mice were studied by performance in the water maze and step-down passive avoidance tests. During the training sessions (days 1 and 2) for the water maze test, LPL-deficient mice spent a significantly longer amount of time than WT mice to find the terminal escape platform. There were no differences in the number of entries into the non-exit arms on day 1 of training between the two genotypes. The number of no-exit arm entries by the LPL-deficient mice significantly increased on day 2 of training. From days 3 to 7, both the latency to escape the platform and the frequency of entries into the no-exit arms by the LPL-deficient mice were significantly increased compared with those by the WT mice. There was a significant correlation between the latency to escape the platform and the number of errors. No changes in swim speed were observed during the training period. Taken together, these observations suggest that the increase in latency to platform is most likely due to the impairment of navigational strategy in the LPL-deficient mice. We further used a step-down inhibitory avoidance task to study the role of LPL in learning and memory. A significant decrease in the latency to step-down was observed in the LPL-deficient mice during the training trial. Similarly, a shortened retention time was observed in the LPL-deficient mice.

Transmission electron microscopy (TEM) revealed a significant decrease in the number of presynaptic vesicles in the hippocampi, along with a severe depletion of synaptic vesicles in the presynaptic terminals, of LPL-deficient mice (Figure 1). The numbers of total vesicles (TV) per terminal and docked vesicles (DV, defined as the vesicles within 50 nm of the plasma membrane in an active zone) were significantly reduced when compared with controls. The number of vesicles per terminal (DV/μm) and docked vesicles per square micrometer of synapse area (TV/μm^2) were all reduced accordingly ($p<0.001$). The levels of the presynaptic marker synaptophysin were also reduced in the hippocampus while the levels of the post-synaptic marker PSD-95 remained unchanged in the LPL-deficient mice. By an electrophysiological examination, LPL-deficient neurons had a decreased frequency of mEPSC, indicating that presynaptic vesicle numbers were decreased. This observation was consistent with the decrease in total vesicle and docking vesicle numbers seen by TEM. Although there is no difference between the single-evoked EPSCs produced by the WT and LPL-deficient neurons, impaired paired-pulse facilitation and the smaller size of the RRP suggests that not enough vesicles could be supplied by the LPL-deficient neurons to support a continuous stimulus.

IV. DISCUSSION

The aim of the current study was to investigate the role of LPL in the CNS in vivo. We used viable adult LPL-deficient mice and demonstrated that these mice display impaired hippocampus-dependent learning and memory, indicating that

*Figure 1. Ultrastrucural changes of synapses from WT and LPL-deficient neonatal mice detected by transmission electron microscopy. Synaptic vesicles within the presynaptic part are highlighted by arrows; the edges of the active zone/ postsynaptic density complexes are marked by arrowheads. (A), (B) and (C) are representative photos showing the total and docked synaptic vesicles in the hippocampal terminals of WT mice; while (D), (E) and (F) are those of LPL deficient ones. The table below shows the morphological analysis of synapses in CA3 regions of hippocampi from WT and LPL-deficient mice. Abreviations are L, active zone length (μm); DV, Number of docked vesicles per active zone; DV/μm, number of docked vesicles per micrometer of active zone length; TV, total vesicle number per terminal; TV/μm², total vesicle number per micrometer square of synapse area. Numbers are mean ±SEM. 30 synapses from each mouse were analyzed in WT group, n=4); 50 synapses from each mouse were analyzed in LPL deficiency group, n=4). ***p<0.001. (Liu and Chui, 2008; Xian et al, 2009)*

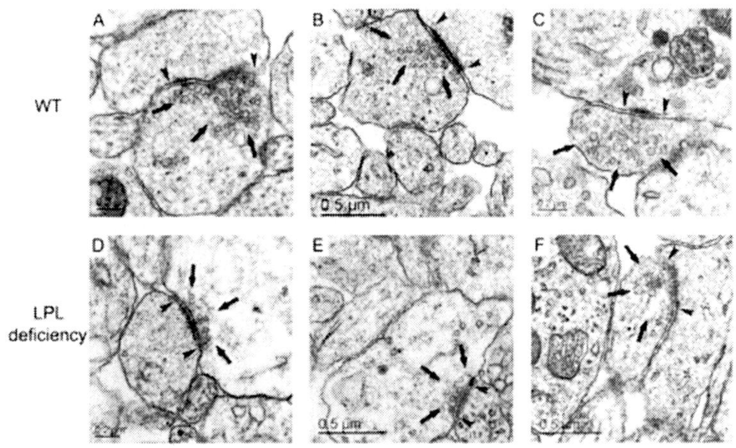

	L (μm)	DV	DV/μm	TV	TV/μm²
WT	0.34±0.02	4.45±0.28	13.36±0.82	29.24±3.45	71.08±8.50
LPL deficiency	0.37±0.02	2.55±0.23***	7.49±0.66***	15.59±1.22***	27.89±3.08***

LPL plays an important role in cognitive function. We then wanted to determine if there was a structural basis for this dysfunction. There was no obvious difference in neuronal counts or neuronal apoptosis. Ultrastructural analysis, however, revealed a severe depletion of synaptic vesicles at the presynaptic terminals of hippocampal neurons in LPL-deficient mice. Consistent with this observation, decreased levels of the presynaptic marker synaptophysin were detected. The reduction of synaptophysin and synaptic vesicles in the hippocampus in LPL-deficient mice could be involved in the impairment of learning and memory function.

With respect to the declining cognitive functions in AD patients, recent discoveries have shifted research to a wider focus on synaptic vesicle cycle lipids and lipid-based regulatory mechanisms from a focus centered only on a protein-based mechanism. Some kinds of lipids have been shown to interact with lipid-binding proteins and consequently affect the synaptic vesicle cycle. In the process of vesicle exocytosis, phosphatidylinositol-4,5-bisphosphate-DAG-mediated signaling and lipid-protein interactions have been shown to be involved in the regulation of several synaptic vesicle cycle stages, such as vesicle priming and fusion. In addition, cholesterol is enriched in secretory and synaptic vesicles as well as the exocytic domains of neurosecretory cell plasma membranes. Cholesterol binds to synaptophysin and modulates its interaction with synaptobrevin, one of the essential vesicular SNARE proteins, which facilitates vesicle trafficking.

V. CONCLUSION

These findings indicate that LPL plays an important role in learning and memory function, possibly by influencing presynaptic function.

ACKNOWLEDGMENT

This project was supported by the National Natural Science Foundation of China (No. 30670414 and No. 30973145) and the National Hightech Research and Development program of China (973- project No. 2006CB500705).

REFERENCES

Liu, T., & Chui, D. H. (2008). Role of lipids and lipid-associated proteins in Alzheimer s disease. *Nervous Diseases and Mental Health*, *8*(5), 329–334.

Xian, X., Liu, T., Yu, J., Wang, Y., Miao, Y., & Zhang, J. (2009). Presynaptic defects underlying impaired learning and memory function in lipoprotein lipase deficient mice. *The Journal of Neuroscience*, *29*(14), 4681–4685. doi:10.1523/JNEUROSCI.0297-09.2009

KEY TERMS AND DEFINITIONS

Alzheimer's Disease (AD): The most common form of dementia. This incurable, degenerative, and terminal disease was first described by the German psychiatrist and neuropathologist Alois Alzheimer in 1906 and was named after him.

Amyloid Precursor Protein (APP): An integral membrane protein expressed in many tissues and concentrated in the synapses of neurons. Its primary function is not known though it has been implicated as a regulator of synapse formation and neural plasticity. APP is best known and most commonly studied as the precursor molecule that, after proteolysis, generates amyloid beta (Aβ), a 39- to 42-amino acid peptide. The amyloid fibrillar form of Aβ is the primary component of amyloid plaques found in the brains of Alzheimer's disease patients.

Hippocampus: A curved elevation of gray matter extending the entire length of the floor of the temporal horn of the lateral ventricle. The hippocampus, subiculum, and Dentate Gyrus constitute the hippocampal formation. Sometimes authors include the Entorhinal Cortex in the hippocampal formation.

Learning: A relatively permanent change in behavior that is the result of past experience or practice. The concept includes the acquisition of knowledge.

Lipoprotein Lipase (LPL): An enzyme of the hydrolase class that catalyzes the reaction of triacylglycerol and water to yield diacylglycerol and a fatty acid anion. The enzyme hydrolyzes triacylglycerols in chylomicrons, very-low-density lipoproteins, low-density lipoproteins, and diacylglycerols. LPL is found on capillary endothelial surfaces, especially in mammary, muscle, and adipose tissue. Genetic deficiency of this enzyme causes familial hyperlipoproteinemia Type I.

Memory: A complex mental function having four distinct phases: (1) memorizing or learning, (2) retention, (3) recall, and (4) recognition. Generally, the clinical subdivisions include immediate, recent, and remote memory.

Synapse: A structure in the nervous system that permits a neuron to pass an electrical or chemical signal to another cell. Synapses are essential to neuronal function: neurons are specialized cells that pass signals to individual target cells, a function that is carried out through its synapses. At a synapse, the plasma membrane of the signal-passing neuron (the *presynaptic* neuron) comes into close apposition with the membrane of the target (*postsynaptic*) cell. Both the presynaptic and postsynaptic sites contain extensive arrays of molecular machinery that link the two membranes together and carry out the signaling process. In many synapses, the presynaptic part is located on an axon, but some presynaptic sites are located on a dendrite or soma.

Chapter 28
Noninvasive Detection of Misfolded Proteins in the Brain Using [^{11}C]BF-227 PET

Nobuyuki Okamura
Department of Pharmacology, Tohoku University, Japan

Shozo Furumoto
Department of Pharmacology & Cyclotron and Radioisotope Center, Tohoku University, Japan

Manabu Tashiro
Cyclotron and Radioisotope Center, Tohoku University, Japan

Katsutoshi Furukawa
Institute of Development, Aging and Cancer, Tohoku University, Japan

Hiroyuki Arai
Institute of Development, Aging and Cancer, Tohoku University, Japan

Yukitsuka Kudo
Innovation of New Biomedical Engineering Center, Tohoku University, Japan

Kazuhiko Yanai
Department of Pharmacology, Tohoku University, Japan

ABSTRACT

Alzheimer's disease (AD) and many other neurodegenerative disorders belong to the family of protein misfolding diseases. These diseases are characterized by the deposition of insoluble protein aggregates containing an enriched β-sheet structure. To evaluate PET amyloid-imaging tracer [^{11}C]BF-227 as an agent for in vivo detection of various kinds of misfolded protein, a [^{11}C]BF-227 PET study was performed in patients with various protein misfolding diseases, including AD, frontotemporal dementia (FTD), dementia with Lewy bodies (DLB), sporadic Creutzfeldt-Jakob disease (sCJD) and Gerstmann-Sträussler-Scheinker disease (GSS). BF-227 binds to β-amyloid fibrils with high affinity. Most of the AD patients showed prominent retention of [^{11}C]BF-227 in the neocortex. In addition, neocortical retention of BF-227 was observed in the subjects with mild cognitive impairment who converted to AD during

DOI: 10.4018/978-1-60960-559-9.ch028

follow-up. DLB patients had elevated [^{11}C]BF-227 uptake in the neocortex. However, FTD and sCJD patients showed no cortical retention of [^{11}C]BF-227. Patients with multiple system atrophy had elevated BF-227 binding in the putamen. Finally, GSS patients had elevated BF-227 uptake in the cerebellum and other brain regions. This chapter confirms that BF-227 can selectively bind to α-synuclein and prion protein deposits using postmortem brain samples. Based on these findings, [^{11}C]BF-227 is not necessarily specific for β-amyloid in AD patients. However, this tracer could be used to detect various types of protein aggregates in the brain.

INTRODUCTION

Alzheimer's disease (AD) is the most common cause of dementia in the elderly. AD currently affects 4 million people in the United States and 15 million people globally. This disease begins insidiously with mild memory problems and progresses to the development of functional impairment in multiple cognitive domains within a few years. It is important to develop diagnostic methods that have adequate sensitivity and specificity to distinguish those who are likely to develop AD from those memory-impaired individuals who will not. The pathological hallmarks of AD are the deposition of senile plaques (SPs) and neurofibrillary tangles (NFTs) (Vickers et al., 2000). SPs and NFTs are mainly composed of β-amyloid (Aβ) protein and hyperphosphorylated tau protein, respectively. Aβ is a 4 kDa 39–43 amino acid metalloprotein product derived from the proteolytic cleavage of the amyloid precursor protein (APP) by β- and γ-secretases. The abnormal accumulation of SPs has been implicated as a central event in the etiology and the pathogenesis of AD and precedes the cognitive deterioration observed in AD (Okamura et al., 2008). Tau proteins accumulate in the neuronal cytoplasm and form NFTs with age. The initial lesions leading to NFTs occur in the transentorhinal cortex, followed by involvement of the entorhinal cortex and hippocampus, progressing to the neocortex. In vivo detection of SPs and NFTs in the brain enables the detection of AD patients in the pre-symptomatic stage. Noninvasive measurement of the amount of Aβ and tau deposits in the living brain is desirable for preventive interventions and assessment of therapeutic effects.

The density of SPs in brain tissue can be measured by molecular imaging techniques using positron emission tomography (PET) and a specific radiotracer. As Aβ deposits in the AD brain generally include the β-sheet fibrillar structure, many β-sheet binding agents have been developed as Aβ binding radiotracers for PET imaging. Currently, the most successful amyloid-binding agent is N-methyl-[^{11}C]2-(4'-methylaminophenyl)-6-hydroxybenzothiazol (PIB), which has been shown to possess a high affinity for Aβ fibrils. PIB-PET studies in human subjects have shown a robust difference between the retention pattern in AD patients and healthy controls, with AD cases showing significantly higher retention of PIB in the neocortical areas of the brain affected by Aβ deposition (Klunk et al., 2004). PIB retention in the neocortical areas is correlated with the Aβ plaque load (Ikonomovic et al., 2008). Benzoxazole derivatives are also promising alternatives for amyloid-imaging probes (Okamura et al., 2004; Furumoto et al., 2007). A PET study using ^{11}C-labeled 2-(2-[2-dimethylaminothiazol-5-yl]ethenyl)-6-(2-[fluoro]ethoxy) benzoxazole (BF-227) demonstrated retention of this tracer in the cerebral cortices of AD patients but not in those of normal subjects. AD patients were clearly distinguishable from normal individuals using neocortical uptake of [^{11}C]BF-227 (Kudo et al., 2007). Neocortical retention of BF-227 was observed in the subjects with mild cognitive impairment (MCI). BF-227 PET showed higher specificity and sensitivity than FDG-PET and voxel-based morphometric analysis of MRI for differentiating between AD patients and normal controls, and between MCI converters and non-converters (Waragai et al., 2009; Furukawa et al., 2010). A voxel-by-voxel analysis demonstrated a higher retention of [^{11}C]BF-227, mainly in the posterior association cortex of AD patients and MCI converters. This distribution pattern corresponds well with the distribution of neuritic plaque deposits in postmortem AD brains. These findings suggest that [^{11}C]BF-227 is a promising PET probe for in vivo detection of dense amyloid deposits in AD patients.

AD and many other neurodegenerative disorders, including frontotemporal dementia (FTD), progressive supranuclear palsy, corticobasal degeneration, Parkinson's disease (PD), dementia with Lewy bodies (DLB), multiple system atrophy, and prion disease, belong to the family of protein misfolding diseases characterized by protein self-aggregation and deposition (Table 1). The tissue deposits observed in the brain in these diseases usually contain an enriched β-sheet structure, suggesting a potential target for non-invasive imaging using β-sheet binding agents. Thus, molecular PET imaging has the potential to be extended to this wide spectrum of protein misfolding diseases (Okamura et al., 2005; Okamura et al., 2009). The purpose of this study was to evaluate the clinical utility of [^{11}C]BF-227 PET for the noninvasive detection of misfolded proteins in the brain.

EXPERIMENT

Subjects

[^{11}C]BF-227 PET study was performed in 12 elderly normal controls, 14 patients with Alzheimer's disease (AD) and 12 subjects with mild cognitive impairment (MCI). The [^{11}C]BF-227 PET study was additionally performed in patients with frontotemporal dementia (FTD), dementia with Lewy bodies (DLB), multiple system atrophy (MSA), sporadic *Creutzfeldt-Jakob disease* (sCJD) and *Gerstmann-Sträussler-Scheinker* disease (GSS). The MCI subjects were divided into two groups: MCI converters (n=6) and MCI non-converters (n=7). The MCI converters were defined as patients who eventually developed AD within a mean follow-up of 27.0±7.9 months (range 14–30 months). The MCI non-converters were defined as having a transient memory loss or remaining cognitively stable through at least a two-year follow-up (27.7±2.2 months; range 25–30 months).

Table 1. Protein misfolding diseases and their fibrillar deposits

Protein	Fibrillar deposits	Diseases
Amyloid-β	Senile plaque Cerebrovascular amyloid	Alzheimer's disease Down syndrome Cerebral amyloid angiopathy
Tau	Neurofibrillary tangle Pick body Tufted astrocytes Astrocytic plaque	Alzheimer's disease Frontotemporal lobar degeneration Progressive supranuclear palsy Corticobasal degeneration
α-synuclein	Lewy body Glial cytoplasmic Inclusions	Parkinson's disease Dementia with Lewy bodies Multiple system atrophy
Prion	Prion plaque	Creutzfeldt-Jakob disease Gerstmann-Sträussler-Scheinker disease

Method

[^{11}C]BF-227 was synthesized from its precursor by N-methylation in dimethyl sulfoxide using [^{11}C]methyl triflate, as previously described (Kudo et al., 2007). The [^{11}C]BF-227 PET study was performed using a SET-2400W PET scanner (Shimadzu, Kyoto, Japan). After intravenous injection of 211–366 MBq [^{11}C]BF-227, dynamic PET images were obtained for 60 min (23 sequential scans; 5 scans × 30 s, 5 scans × 60 s, 5 scans × 150 s, and 8 scans × 300 s) with closed eyes. The standardized uptake value (SUV) was calculated by normalizing tissue concentrations by injected dose and body weight. Regions of interest (ROIs) were placed on co-registered axial MR images. The ROI information was then copied onto the PET images, and regional SUV values were sampled. The ratio of regional SUV to cerebellar SUV (SUVR) between 40 and 60 min post administration was calculated as an index of [^{11}C]BF-227 retention. For the analysis of prion disease data, we calculated regional to pons SUV ratio (SUVRp). For the analysis of MSA patient data, the distribution volume of [^{11}C]BF-227 was calculated by Logan's graphical analysis using arterial blood sample data. The protocol of this study was approved by the Committee on Clinical Investigation at Tohoku University School of Medicine and by the Advisory Committee on Radioactive Substances at Tohoku University. Written informed consent was obtained from all patients and control subjects after a complete description of the study. The clinical study was performed in accordance with the Declaration of Helsinki.

RESULTS

A PET study using [^{11}C]BF-227 demonstrated the retention of this tracer in the cerebral cortices of AD patients and MCI converters to AD but not in normal subjects or MCI non-converters (Figure 1). The average neocortical SUVR in BF-227 PET was significantly higher in the AD patients and MCI converters than in the normal subjects and MCI non-converters (Figure 2). We further examined BF-227 PET scans in patients with FTD, PD and DLB. Although imaging in FTD and PD patients showed normal distribution of BF-227 in the brain, DLB patients had moderate neocortical retention of BF-227 (Figure 1). Intriguingly, imaging from MSA patients showed BF-227 retention in the putamen, cerebral cortex and subcortical white matter. Microscopic examination indicates that BF-227 selectively binds to intracellular α-synuclein deposits, called glial cytoplasmic inclusions (GCIs), in MSA brain sections (Figure 3). Finally, significantly higher retention of BF-227 was detected in the cerebellum of GSS patients compared with that of normal controls and AD patients (Figure 4). In contrast, sCJD patients showed no obvious BF-227 retention in the cerebellum. Selective binding of BF-227 to prion protein plaques was confirmed using brain samples from autopsy-confirmed GSS cases (Figure 4).

DISCUSSION

Our study demonstrated that [^{11}C]BF-227 PET is useful for the in vivo detection of Aβ and prion protein plaques in the human brain. BF-227 PET achieved high diagnostic accuracy in discriminating between MCI converters and non-converters. This result strongly suggests that [^{11}C]BF-227 PET would be useful to predict conversion from MCI to AD. Regarding the binding of PET imaging agents to prion proteins, a previous PET study demonstrated a moderate level of FDDNP retention and no remarkable PIB retention in the brain of familial CJD patients (Boxer et al., 2007). Another PET study also demonstrated that PIB was not specifically retained in two sCJD patients (Villemagne et al., 2009). In comparison with these previous studies, BF-227 successfully

Figure 1. [^{11}C]BF-227 PET images in an elderly normal control, a patient with Alzheimer's disease (AD), a MCI non-converter, a MCI converter, a patient with frontotemporal dementia (FTD) and a patient with dementia with Lewy bodies (DLB).

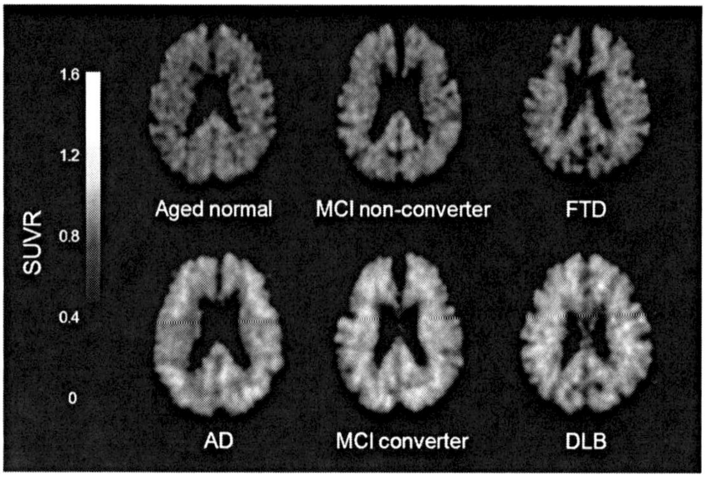

*Figure 2. Average neocortical SUVR values in elderly normal controls (AN), MCI non-converters (MCI-NC), MCI converters (MCI-C), and patients with Alzheimer's disease (AD). *p<0.05, ANOVA followed by a Bonferroni multiple comparisons test.*

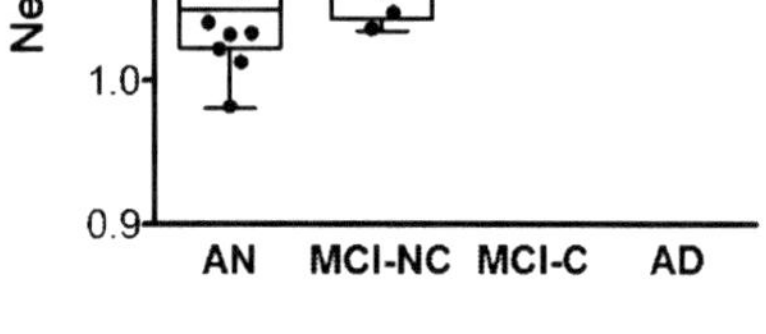

visualized prion protein plaques in the brains of GSS patients. Histopathological studies indicate a higher density of prion protein plaques in GSS patients than in familial CJD patients (Okamura et al., 2010). Therefore, the differences between our findings and those of previous studies would mainly depend upon the amount of prion protein fibrils in the brain. The difference might also be attributable to higher binding affinity of BF-227 to prion protein plaques compared to the other PET probes. Further analysis is necessary to compare the variable binding affinity of different PET probes for prion protein fibrils.

PET and microscopic studies also demonstrated that BF-227 has a potential ability to bind to and detect α-synuclein protein deposits in the brain. Previous PIB-PET studies have shown neocortical tracer accumulation in the brains of DLB patients. However, an in vitro binding study indicated that PIB failed to stain Lewy bodies in DLB brain sections. Considering the smaller size and lower density of Lewy bodies within the brains of DLB subjects relative to amyloid plaques, the contribution of Lewy bodies to the PET signals would be negligible. A recent study demonstrated that [^{18}F]BF-227 binds α-synuclein fibrils (Kd = 9.63 nM) with high affinity (Fodero-Tavoletti et al., 2009). Moreover, BF-227 labeled Lewy bodies and GCIs in fluorescence and immunohistochemical analyses of human brain sections, suggesting that BF-227 has higher binding affinity to α-synuclein deposits than PIB. Elevated BF-227 uptake was

Figure 3. (A): [^{11}C]BF-227 PET images in a normal control subject (Control) and a patient with multiple system atrophy (MSA). (B and C): Microscopic images of BF-227 staining (B) and α-synuclein immunostaining (C) of the cerebellar white matter of a MSA case. Bar = 100 μm.

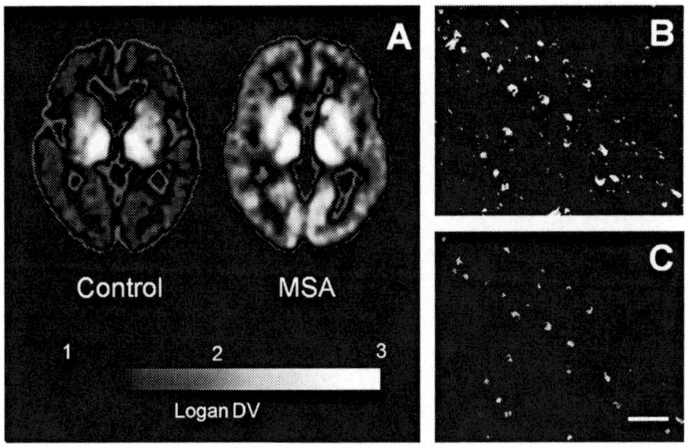

Figure 4. (A): The regional to pons SUV ratio (SUVRp) values in the cerebella of 10 normal controls, 17 patients with Alzheimer's disease (AD), 2 patients with sporadic Creutzfeldt-Jakob disease (sCJD), and 3 patients with Gerstmann-Sträussler-Scheinker disease (GSS). (B and C): Microscopic images of BF-227 staining (B) and PrP immunostaining (C) of the cerebellar cortex of a GSS case. Bar = 25 μm.

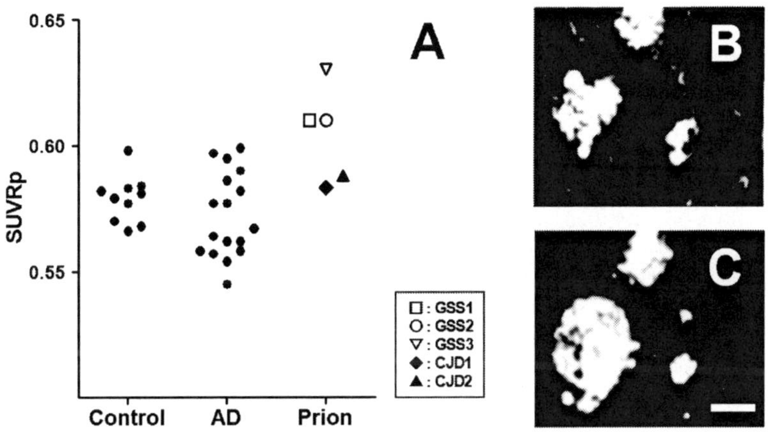

observed in the brains of MSA patients, which contain more α-synuclein deposits than those of DLB patients (Kikuchi et al., 2010). Further clinical studies of patients with α-synucleinopathy will clarify the potential of BF-227 for noninvasive detection of α-synuclein deposits in the human brain. From these findings, we conclude that BF-227 PET provides a potential method to facilitate both early diagnosis and noninvasive monitoring of protein misfolding diseases.

ACKNOWLEDGMENT

Part of this study was supported by the Health and Labor Sciences Research Grants for Translational Research from the Ministry of Health and the

Grant-in-Aid for Scientific Research on Priority Areas, Integrative Brain Research, from the Ministry of Education, Culture, Sports, Science, and Technology of Japan (20019006). We appreciate the technical assistance of Dr. R. Iwata, Dr. S. Watanuki, M. Miyake and Dr. Y. Ishikawa in the clinical PET studies, and Dr. K. Sugi and Dr. S. He in the imaging analysis. We also thank Dr. M. Higuchi for supporting the staining of human brain sections.

REFERENCES

Boxer, A. L., Rabinovici, G. D., Kepe, V., Goldman, J., Furst, A. J., & Huang, S. C. (2007). Amyloid imaging in distinguishing atypical prion disease from Alzheimer disease. *Neurology*, *69*, 283–290. doi:10.1212/01.wnl.0000265815.38958.b6

Fodero-Tavoletti, M. T., Mulligan, R. S., Okamura, N., Furumoto, S., Rowe, C. C., & Kudo, Y. (2009). In vitro characterisation of BF227 binding to alpha-synuclein/Lewy bodies. *European Journal of Pharmacology*, *617*, 54–58. doi:10.1016/j.ejphar.2009.06.042

Furukawa K., Okamura, N., Tashiro, M., Waragai, M., Furumoto, S., Iwata, R., … Arai, H. (2010). Amyloid PET in mild cognitive impairment and Alzheimer's disease with BF-227: Comparison to FDG-PET. *Journal of Neurology*.

Furumoto, S., Okamura, N., Iwata, R., Yanai, K., Arai, H., & Kudo, Y. (2007). Recent advances in the development of amyloid imaging agents. *Current Topics in Medicinal Chemistry*, *7*, 1773–1789. doi:10.2174/156802607782507402

Ikonomovic, M. D., Klunk, W. E., Abrahamson, E. E., Mathis, C. A., Price, J. C., & Tsopelas, N. D. (2008). Post-mortem correlates of in vivo PIB-PET amyloid imaging in a typical case of Alzheimer's disease. *Brain*, *131*, 1630–1645. doi:10.1093/brain/awn016

Kikuchi, A., Takeda, A., Okamura, N., Tashiro, M., Hasegawa, T., Furumoto, S., … Itoyama, Y. (2010). In vivo visualization of α-synuclein deposition by [^{11}C]-BF-227 PET in multiple system atrophy. *Brain*.

Klunk, W. E., Engler, H., Nordberg, A., Wang, Y., Blomqvist, G., & Holt, D. P. (2004). Imaging brain amyloid in Alzheimer's disease with Pittsburgh Compound-B. *Annals of Neurology*, *55*, 306–319. doi:10.1002/ana.20009

Kudo, Y., Okamura, N., Furumoto, S., Tashiro, M., Furukawa, K., & Maruyama, M. (2007). 2-(2-[2-Dimethylaminothiazol-5-yl]ethenyl)-6-(2-[fluoro]ethoxy)benzoxazole: A novel PET agent for in vivo detection of dense amyloid plaques in Alzheimer's disease patients. *Journal of Nuclear Medicine*, *48*, 553–561. doi:10.2967/jnumed.106.037556

Okamura, N., Fodero-Tavoletti, M. T., Kudo, Y., Rowe, C. C., Furumoto, S., & Arai, H. (2009). Advances in molecular imaging for the diagnosis of dementia. *Expert Opinion on Medical Diagnostics*, *3*, 705–716. doi:10.1517/17530050903133790

Okamura, N., Furumoto, S., Arai, H., Iwata, R., Yanai, K., & Kudo, Y. (2008). Imaging amyloid pathology in the living brain. *Current Medical Imaging Reviews*, *4*, 56–62. doi:10.2174/157340508783502840

Okamura, N., Shiga, Y., Furumoto, S., Tashiro, M., Tsuboi, Y., Furukawa, K., … Doh-Ura, K. (2010). In vivo detection of prion amyloid plaques using [^{11}C]BF-227 PET. *European Journal of Nuclear Medicine and Molecular Imaging*.

Okamura, N., Suemoto, T., Furumoto, S., Suzuki, M., Shimadzu, H., & Akatsu, H. (2005). Quinoline and benzimidazole derivatives: Candidate probes for in vivo imaging of tau pathology in Alzheimer's disease. *The Journal of Neuroscience*, *25*, 10857–10862. doi:10.1523/JNEUROSCI.1738-05.2005

Okamura, N., Suemoto, T., Shimadzu, H., Suzuki, M., Shiomitsu, T., & Akatsu, H. (2004). Styrylbenzoxazole derivatives for in vivo imaging of amyloid plaques in the brain. *The Journal of Neuroscience*, *24*, 2535–2541. doi:10.1523/JNEUROSCI.4456-03.2004

Vickers, J. C., Dickson, T. C., Adlard, P. A., Saunders, H. L., King, C. E., & McCormack, G. (2000). The cause of neuronal degeneration in Alzheimer's disease. *Progress in Neurobiology*, *60*, 139–165. doi:10.1016/S0301-0082(99)00023-4

Villemagne, V. L., McLean, C. A., Reardon, K., Boyd, A., Lewis, V., & Klug, G. (2009). ^{11}C-PiB PET studies in typical sporadic Creutzfeldt-Jakob disease. *Journal of Neurology, Neurosurgery, and Psychiatry*, *80*, 998–1001. doi:10.1136/jnnp.2008.171496

Waragai, M., Okamura, N., Furukawa, K., Tashiro, M., Furumoto, S., & Funaki, Y. (2009). Comparison study of amyloid PET and voxel-based morphometry analysis in mild cognitive impairment and Alzheimer's disease. *Journal of the Neurological Sciences*, *285*, 100–108. doi:10.1016/j.jns.2009.06.005

KEY TERMS AND DEFINITIONS

Alzheimer's Disease: The most common form of dementia.

Mild Cognitive Impairment (MCI): A diagnosis given to individuals who have cognitive impairments beyond that expected for their age and education but that do not interfere significantly with their daily activities.

Neurofibrillary Tangles: Pathological protein aggregates found within neurons in cases of Alzheimer's disease.

Positron Emission Tomography (PET): A nuclear medicine imaging technique that produces a three-dimensional image or picture of functional processes in the body.

Prion: An infectious agent that is primarily composed of protein.

Protein Misfolding Diseases: Clinically and pathologically diverse disorders in which specific proteins accumulate in cells or tissues of the body.

Senile Plaques: Extracellular deposits of amyloid in the gray matter of the brain.

Tau: A neuronal microtubule-associated protein found predominantly on axons.

α-Synuclein: The primary structural component of Lewy body fibrils.

β-Amyloid: A 39-43 amino acid peptide that appears to be the main constituent of senile plaques in the brains of Alzheimer's disease patients.

Chapter 29

Quantitative Analysis of Amyloid β Deposition in Patients with Alzheimer's Disease Using Positron Emission Tomography

Manabu Tashiro
Cyclotron Nuclear Medicine, Tohoku University, Japan

Nobuyuki Okamura
Department of Pharmacology, Tohoku University Graduate School of Medicine, Japan

Shoichi Watanuki
Cyclotron Nuclear Medicine, Tohoku University, Japan

Shozo Furumoto
Radiopharmaceutical Chemistry, Cyclotron and Radioisotope Center, Tohoku University, Japan & Department of Pharmacology, Tohoku University Graduate School of Medicine, Japan

Katsutoshi Furukawa
Department of Geriatrics and Gerontology, Institute of Development, Aging and Cancer, Tohoku University, Japan

Yoshihito Funaki
Radiopharmaceutical Chemistry, Cyclotron and Radioisotope Center, Tohoku University, Japan

Ren Iwata
Radiopharmaceutical Chemistry, Cyclotron and Radioisotope Center, Tohoku University, Japan

Yukitsuka Kudo
Innovation of New Biomedical Engineering Center, Tohoku University Hospital, Japan

Hiroyuki Arai
Department of Geriatrics and Gerontology, Institute of Development, Aging and Cancer, Tohoku University, Japan

Hiroshi Watabe
Department of Molecular Imaging in Medicine, Osaka University Graduate School of Medicine, Japan

Kazuhiko Yanai
Cyclotron Nuclear Medicine, Tohoku University, Japan & Radiopharmaceutical Chemistry, Cyclotron and Radioisotope Center, Tohoku University, Japan

DOI: 10.4018/978-1-60960-559-9.ch029

ABSTRACT

Positron emission tomography (PET) is a sensitive technique for functional and molecular imaging. In Japan, the incidence of cognitive disorders is increasing at an accelerated pace, partly due to the increasing size of the elderly population. Basic and clinical studies on dementia have become very important. In vivo detection of amyloid beta (Aβ) deposits could be useful for early diagnosis of Alzheimer's disease (AD). "Aβ imaging" by PET has been recognized as one of the most important methods for the early diagnosis of AD. Clinical PET studies have been conducted using several probes, such as [^{18}F]FDDNP, [^{11}C]SB-13 and [^{11}C]Pittsburgh compound-B ([^{11}C]PIB). [^{11}C]PIB is the most commonly used probe.

In this chapter, a novel imaging probe, 2-[2-(2-dimethylaminothiazol-5-yl)-ethenyl]-6- [2-(fluoro)ethoxy] benzoxazole ([^{11}C]BF-227), is reported. To the authors' knowledge, [^{11}C]BF-227 is the first Aβ imaging probe to be used in Japan. The purpose of this chapter is to examine methods for quantitative analysis of Aβ deposition in the human brain using PET and [^{11}C]BF-227. Six AD patients and six healthy control subjects were used in the present study. Dynamic PET images were obtained over 60 min. Blood samples were obtained from the radial arteries.

The results were analyzed using Logan graphical analysis and full kinetic analysis. A significantly higher distribution volume ratio (DVR) value was observed in AD patients in cortical regions, e.g., the cingulate, frontal, temporal, parietal and occipital regions, than in control subjects. Satisfactory correlation of these values to the semiquantitative standardized uptake values (SUV) was obtained.

These findings suggest that [^{11}C]BF-227 is a promising PET probe for clinical evaluation of early Aβ deposition in AD patients.

INTRODUCTION

Positron Emission Tomography

Positron emission tomography (PET) is a technique used for functional and molecular imaging based on nuclear medicine technology. Nuclear medicine techniques date back to the early 20th century. Nuclear medicine was originally developed as a "tracer technique" by the Nobel laureate, Dr. George de Hevesy. In our study, the term "tracer" means an extremely small amount of radioisotope that is administered to the subject to permit imaging certain biological phenomena in the living body. A tracer is sometimes also called a "probe". Probes detect the presence of a certain biological substances in small amounts (often at the "nano-" to "pico-" molar scale) (Tashiro, 2010). The tracer technique was later established as a nuclear medicine technique in the late 20th century, mainly due to advancements in radiolabeling techniques and signal detection devices such as PET.

Using PET, a wide range of biological information can be obtained from the living human brain, such as the cerebral metabolic rate of glucose (CMRglc), regional cerebral blood flow (rCBF) and pharmacokinetic information regarding receptor-transmitter interactions such as those in the dopaminergic and histaminergic neuronal systems (Yanai & Tashiro, 2007; Tashiro, 2010). CMRglc is often measured using a radioactive analogue of glucose, [^{18}F]fluorodeoxyglucose ([^{18}F]FDG). In brain regions that have increased glucose consumption, an increased demand for glucose and oxygen causes dilation of cerebral capillaries, which can be measured as an increase in the regional cerebral blood flow (rCBF)(Tashiro, 2008). The rCBF is measured using radiolabeled water ([^{15}O]H_2O), though other radiation-free techniques, such as functional magnetic resonance imaging (fMRI) and near-infrared light spectroscopy (NIRS), are also available. Currently, PET is useful for visualization and quantification of various molecular phenomena, such as neurotransmission, DNA synthesis, and production of physiological and pathological proteins, in living organisms. To our knowledge, PET is one of the most sensitive imaging techniques. (Figure 1)

In Japan, the incidence of cognitive disorders is increasing at an accelerated pace, partly due to the increasing size of the elderly population. Basic and clinical studies on dementia have become increasingly important. In functional neuroimaging of early Alzheimer's disease (AD), it is commonly known that a decrease in the CMR_{glc} often starts in the posterior cingulate gyrus and propagates to the temporo-parietal and other regions, as visualized by [^{18}F]FDG PET (Minoshima, 1994; Furukawa, 2009; Ishii, 2009). In this stage of dementia, many nerve cells are damaged and the density of healthy neurons is reduced in the gray matter, resulting in low [^{18}F]FDG uptake. However, the regional metabolic reduction is not easily detected and is widespread during early disease stages, e.g., mild cognitive impairment (MCI)(Furukawa, 2009; Ishii, 2009). Neuronal damage is associated with high deposition of amyloid β (Aβ) protein in the brain, and massive neuronal loss is often preceded by high Aβ deposition. An early diagnosis of mild AD can be established if a tracer that specifically binds to Aβ proteins is used.

Amyloid β Imaging with PET

"Aβ imaging" using PET and an Aβ-specific probe has been recognized as one of the most important methods for the diagnosis of early AD. This is, in part, due to the excellent sensitivity of the PET

Figure 1. Information available from the human brain. Information regarding glucose and oxygen metabolism obtained using [^{18}F]FDG PET and [^{15}O]O_2 PET. Currently, regional cerebral blood flow is measured using various methods, such as [^{15}O]H_2O PET, functional MRI (fMRI) and near infrared light spectroscopy (NIRS). Interaction of neurotransmitters and receptors is measured using PET and various radiotracers labeled with ^{18}F and ^{11}C nuclides.

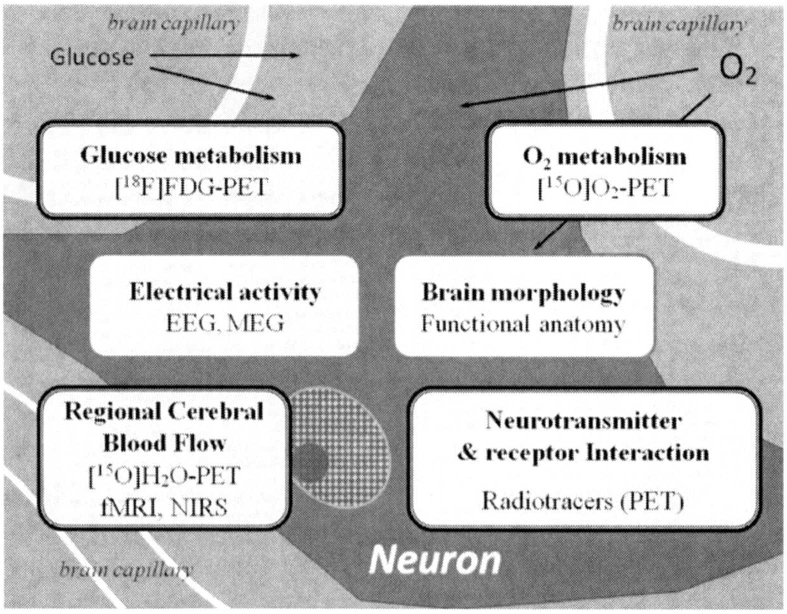

technique (Nordberg, 2004). It is important that Aβ deposition detection occur as soon as possible to allow initiation of medication before the symptoms of dementia worsen. It is believed that deposition and aggregation of Aβ begins before patients manifest clinical symptoms. Numerous candidate compounds have been tested for Aβ imaging, and several compounds were selected for clinical studies (Furumoto, 2007). Clinical PET studies have been conducted using several probes, such as [^{18}F]FDDNP (Shoghi-Jadid, 2002), [^{11}C]SB-13 (Verhoeff, 2004), and [^{11}C]Pittsburgh compound-B ([^{11}C]PIB)(Klunk, 2004), in addition to others (Figure 2). Among these compounds, [^{11}C]PIB is the most commonly used (Klunk, 2004; Mintun, 2005; Price, 2005). Many studies have clearly demonstrated that [^{11}C]PIB binds to Aβ fibrils, enabling noninvasive assessment of Aβ deposition in the brain of AD patients (Klunk, 2004).

Considering the importance of Aβ imaging, our group developed a novel PET tracer, 2-(2-[2-demethylaminothiazol-5-yl] ethenyl)-6-(2-[Fluoro]ethoxy)benzoxazole (BF-227), which is the first compound used for human studies in Japan (Kudo, 2007). Our clinical study demonstrated that this compound is able to detect Aβ deposition primarily in the posterior association area of AD patients. Accumulation in the frontal area is not prominent (Kudo, 2007). Interestingly, in contrast to [^{11}C]PIB, [^{11}C]BF-227 preferentially detects senile plaques containing dense amyloid fibrils. This provides unique and specific information regarding Aβ pathology in AD patients (Kudo, 2007). In addition, we compared the ability of [^{11}C]BF-227 PET, structural MRI, and FDG PET to diagnose and track the severity of AD. [^{11}C]BF-227 PET was more sensitive than MRI in the diagnosis of AD and the detection of converters from MCI to AD (Waragai, 2009). These studies indicate that [^{11}C]BF-227 PET is a useful method for the early diagnosis of AD and prediction of converters from MCI to AD (Furukawa, 2009; Waragai, 2009).

Though these PET studies succeeded in establishing [^{11}C]BF-227 as a useful tracer, they used standardized uptake values (SUV) as a tool for clinical evaluation. This is a semi-quantitative measure that corrects for the injected dose and body size of the subject. Precise quantitative examination may provide a better rationale for the use of this method as a clinical tool, similar to studies of [^{11}C]PIB (Mintun, 2005; Price, 2005). However, we have not conducted the precise examination of [^{11}C]BF-227 pharmacokinetics in the human brain using data from arterial samples. In this paper,

Figure 2. Chemical structures of amyloid imaging agents, FDDNP, SB-13, PIB, and BF-227

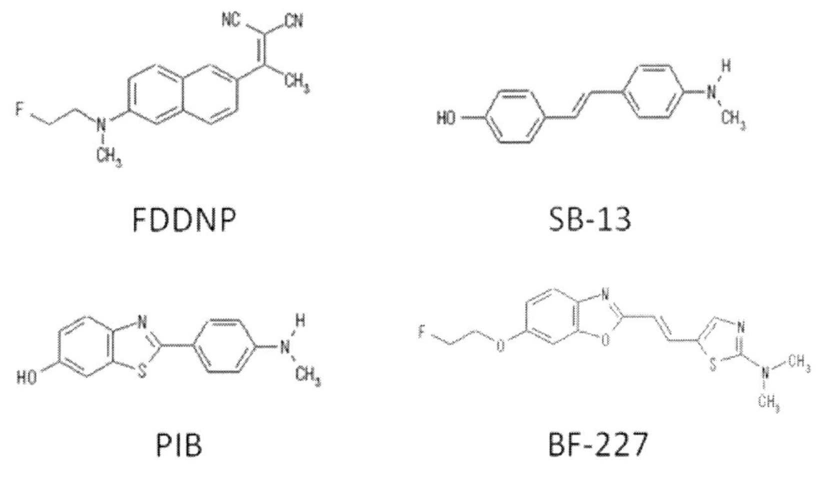

quantification methods for Aβ imaging with PET are briefly overviewed and the preliminary results of the [^{11}C]BF-227 PET study are discussed.

MATERIALS AND METHODS

Subjects

In the present study, 6 AD patients (mean age: 73 years) and 6 healthy volunteers (mean age: 61 years) were recruited. PET scans were initiated simultaneously with [^{11}C]BF-227 injection and data from 23 time frames (30 sec×5, 60 sec×5, 150 sec×5, 300 sec×8) were obtained. Serial arterial blood sampling was also performed (10 sec×12, 20 sec×3, 60 sec×2, 150 sec×2, 300 sec×2, 600 sec×4). The metabolite fraction in the blood was also examined at 5, 15, 30 and 60 min post-injection, and the fraction data were used for correction of input functions. PET data were co-registered to the individual MRI T1 images to define regions of interest (ROIs) in the cortex and subcortical deep nuclei (Figure 3a,b).

This study was approved by the ethics committee of Tohoku University Graduate School of Medicine, and informed consent was obtained from each subject.

Method

The distribution volume (DV) and binding potential (BP) values of [^{11}C]BF-227 were estimated using a full kinetic compartmental model based on the 1-tisssue (1TM) and 2-tissue models (2TM) (Figure 3d). Graphical analysis methods were also applied using 2 types of Logan graphical analysis; one used the time-activity curve (TAC) of arterial plasma data as an input function for analysis (LGA)(Logan, 1990) and the other used

Figure 3. Regions of interest (ROIs) defined in the cerebral cortex and subcortical deep nuclei of a healthy volunteer subject taken by MRI (a) and the co-registered PET (b). The results of linearization using Logan graphical analysis (c) and time activity curves in plasma and brain tissue for compartmental model analysis (d) are demonstrated.

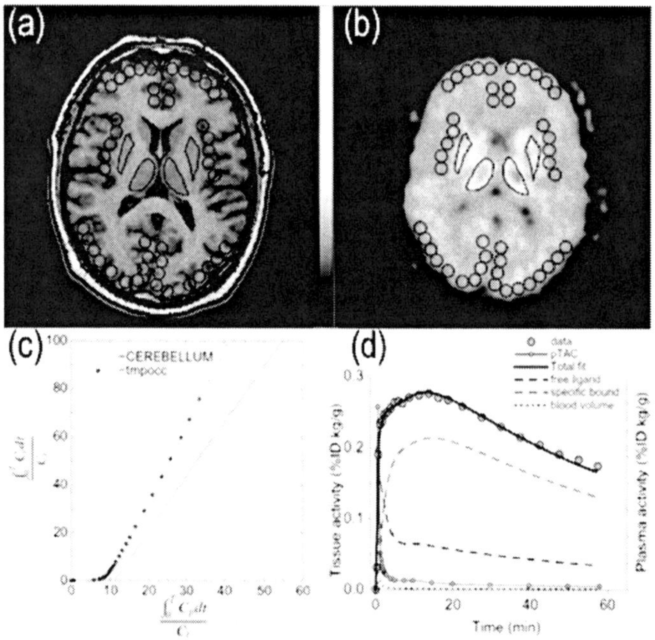

the TAC of reference brain tissue (cerebellum) (LGAR) (Logan, 1996) (Figure 3c). PMOD software (version 3.0; PMOD Technologies, Zurich, Switzerland) was used for calculation. The results of the compartmental model analysis and graphical analysis were compared to the SUV and the SUV ratios of the cerebellar SUV (cerebellar SUVR). Correlations derived from these different methods were examined.

RESULTS

The plasma TAC was not different between AD patients and control subjects. However, a difference was observed in the tissue TAC between AD patients and control subjects. [11C]BF-227 accumulation was significantly higher in the cerebral cortex than in the cerebellum of AD patients, whereas there was no difference in control subjects (Figure 4).

Our analysis determined that the 2TM described the pharmacokinetics of [11C]BF-227 better than 1TM (Figure 5). The DV and BP values of [11C]BF-227 were significantly higher in AD patients than in control subjects, and the most prominent difference was observed in the temporo-occipital and lateral temporal regions. The DV values from the 2TM and LGA (r^2 >0.95 in all regions) methods were similar. In addition, the results of LGA and LGAR were also similar, and the LGA values were similar to the SUV and cerebellar SUVR (r^2 >0.94 in all regions).

DISCUSSION

Currently, Aβ imaging using PET has been recognized as one of the most effective methods for diagnosing early AD and for predicting potential converters from MCI to AD (Nordberg, 2004; Klunk, 2006). Several promising probes, such as

Figure 4. Time activity curves (TAC) of the cerebral cortex and cerebellum of healthy controls (Control) and Alzheimer's disease patients (AD patient). Open circles indicate TAC in the cerebellum and closed squares indicate TAC in the cerebral cortical tissues, e.g., the temporo-occipital cortex (temp-occ) and lateral temporal cortex (ltm). [11C]BF-227 accumulation was significantly higher in the cerebral cortex than in the cerebellum of AD patients, whereas there was no difference in control subjects.

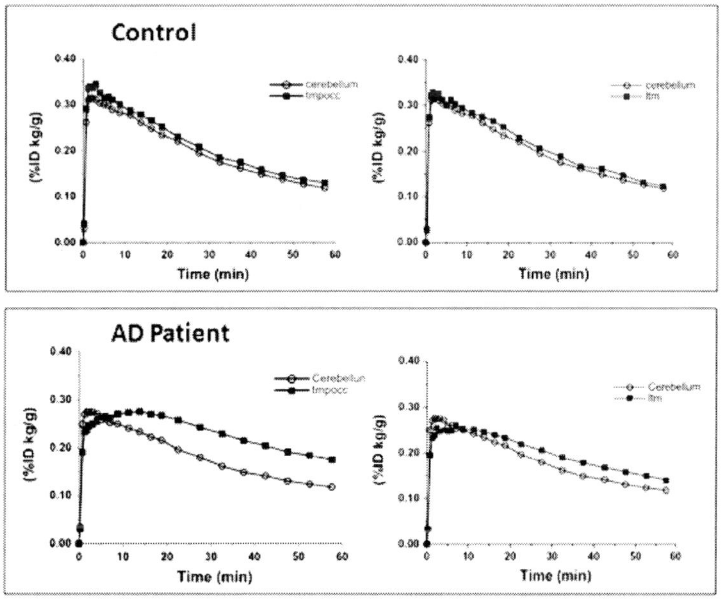

Figure 5. Analysis of the time-activity curve in the temporoparietal cortex of an Alzheimer's disease patient based on the 1-tissue (LEFT) and 2-tissue compartmental models (RIGHT). The 2-tissue model gave more accurate results.

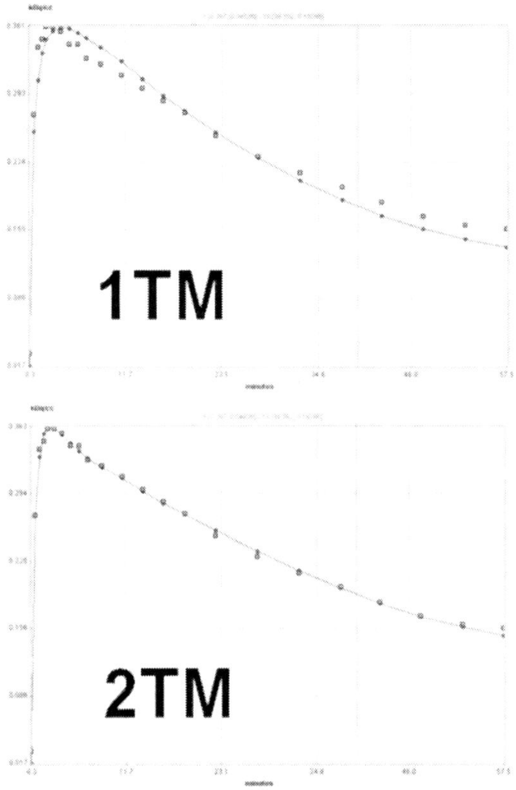

[^{18}F]FDDNP (Shoghi-Jadid, 2002), [^{11}C]SB-13 (Verhoeff, 2004) and [^{11}C]PIB (Klunk, 2004), have been tested in clinical studies, and [^{11}C]PIB is regarded as the most successful Aβ imaging probe. Though an initial study was performed without arterial blood sampling and mainly used SUV for clinical evaluation (Klunk, 2004), the results of a quantitative study were reported in detail (Price, 2005).

Initial studies using [^{11}C]BF-227 have been conducted in a similar manner. Kudo and colleagues reported that this compound was able to detect Aβ deposition primarily in the posterior association area of AD patients, suggesting that [^{11}C]BF-227 may be able to preferentially detect senile plaques containing dense amyloid fibrils. This is in contrast to [^{11}C]PIB, which provides unique and specific information regarding Aβ pathology in AD patients (Kudo, 2007). In addition, we performed a comparative study between [^{11}C]BF-227 PET and structural MRI for the diagnosis and tracking of AD pathology. The results demonstrated that PET with [^{11}C]BF-227 was more sensitive than MRI for detection of voxel-based morphometry (VBM) (Waragai, 2009). Another study demonstrated that [^{11}C]BF-227 was more sensitive than FDG PET for diagnosis of AD and detection of converters from MCI to AD (Furukawa, 2009). Thus, these studies suggest that Aβ PET imaging is more sensitive than detection of hippocampal atrophy and reduced metabolism of glucose.

The pharmacokinetics of [^{11}C]PIB have been thoroughly examined using various quantification methods, such as full kinetic analysis and graphical analysis (Mintun, 2005; Price, 2005). In full kinetic analysis, the commonly used compartmental models are the 3-compartment model (2-tissue compartmental model: 2TM), in which one blood compartment and 2 tissue compartments with specific and non-specific binding are assumed (Figure 6), and the 2-compartmental model (1-tissue compartmental model: 1TM), in which one tissue compartment represents both specific and non-specific binding (Mintun, 2005; Price, 2005). When the tracer rapidly penetrates the blood-brain barrier (BBB) in the tissue compartment, the 1-tissue compartmental model is more appropriate for describing its kinetics. In the analysis of [^{11}C]PIB, 2TM is more appropriate for describing the kinetics of tracer binding to Aβ in the human brain (Mintun, 2005; Price, 2005). Price and colleagues reported that Logan graphical analysis (LGA) was more useful and robust than 2TM analysis. However, in the cerebellum, in which the reference regions are assumed to be free of mature Aβ plaques, 2TM analysis was more appropriate (Price, 2005). Though many [^{11}C]PIB studies employ DVR values for clinical

Figure 6. Basic compartmental models describing the distribution and binding of radiotracers: 2-tissue model (TOP) and 1-tissue model (BOTTOM). Abbreviations: C_p, plasma concentration; C_{f+ns}, concentration of free and nonspecifically bound tracers in the brain tissue; C_b, concentration of specifically bound tracers in the brain tissue.

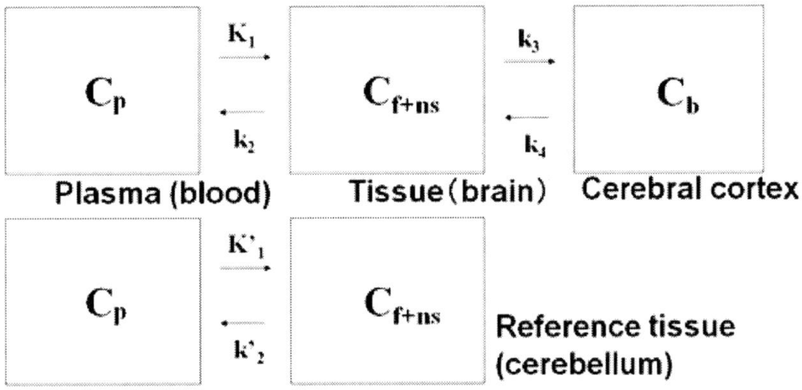

evaluation, the use of BP was also proposed in the paper by Mintun and colleagues (Mintun, 2005).

Similar to [^{11}C]BF-227, compartmental analysis indicated that 2TM analysis was a better fit than 1TM when analyzing data from [^{11}C]PIB (Price, 2005). Linearization by the LGA method was also successful when analyzing the [^{11}C]PIB data. A significant correlation between the DV values calculated by 2TM and LGA analysis (and LGAR, as well) suggests that Logan methods are fully applicable to the quantification of [^{11}C]BF-227. A significant correlation of the results of Logan methods to the SUV (and SUVR) suggests that clinical evaluation of Aβ deposition using [^{11}C]BF-227 PET is possible using LGA (and LGAR), SUV, and SUVR. These results reconfirm the reliability of the results from our recent studies (Kudo, 2007; Furukawa, 2009; Waragai, 2009).

In summary, we demonstrated that [^{11}C]BF-227 is a promising tracer for Aβ imaging, diagnosing AD patients and detecting potential converters from MCI to AD. In addition to the study on AD diagnosis, recent clinical applications of [^{11}C]BF-227 PET have successful. For instance, PET imaging was used to visualize pathological prion proteins in prion diseases (Okamura, 2009) and to image α-synuclein deposition in multiple system atrophy (Kikuchi, 2010).

Future studies should be performed to obtain more accurate data. However, correction for the partial volume effect should be considered. This partial volume correction (PVC) is important because of local atrophy in AD patients and the relatively high accumulation of [^{11}C]BF-227 in the white matter, as observed using [^{11}C]PIB PET (Meltzer, 1999; Price, 2005). A practical correction method has been proposed for the analysis of [^{11}C]PIB data, and it was demonstrated that the difference of the results with and without PVC correction was negligible in [^{11}C]PIB PET (Meltzer, 1999; Price, 2005). In future studies, development of a simplified protocol will be important. Omission of serial blood sampling is practical and would be helpful for clinical use. In a [^{11}C]PIB PET study, Lopresti and colleagues demonstrated that the TAC taken from the ROIs of bilateral carotid arteries defined in MRI co-registered PET images could be successfully used as an input function to obtain reliable results with acceptable errors (Lopresti, 2005).

ACKNOWLEDGMENT

This study was partly supported by grant-in-aids from the Ministry of Health, Welfare and Labor for Amyloid imaging and a grant for education and research for molecular imaging (JST). The authors thank to all the staff of the Cyclotron and Radioisotope Center, Tohoku University for the operation of the cyclotron and administering of patient care.

REFERENCES

Furukawa, K., Okamura, N., Tashiro, M., Waragai, M., Furumoto, S., & Iwata, R. (2009). Amyloid PET in mild cognitive impairment and Alzheimer's disease with BF-227: Comparison to FDG-PET. *Journal of Neurology*, *257*, 721–727. doi:10.1007/s00415-009-5396-8

Furumoto, S., Okamura, N., Iwata, R., Yanai, K., Arai, H., & Kudo, Y. (2007). Recent advances in the development of amyloid imaging agents. *Current Topics in Medicinal Chemistry*, *7*, 1773–1789. doi:10.2174/156802607782507402

Ishii, H., Ishikawa, H., Meguro, K., Tashiro, M., & Yamaguchi, S. (2009). Decreased cortical glucose metabolism in converters from CDR 0.5 to Alzheimer's disease in a community: The Osaki-Tajiri Project. *International Psychogeriatrics*, *21*, 148–156. doi:10.1017/S1041610208008132

Kikuchi, A., Takeda, A., Okamura, N., Tashiro, M., Hasegawa, T., & Furumoto, S. (2010). In vivo visualization of α-synuclein deposition by carbon-11-labeled 2-(2-[2-dimethylaminothiazol-5-yl]ethenyl)-6-(2-[fluoro]ethoxy)benzoxazole positron emission tomography in multiple system atrophy. *Brain*, *133*, 1772–1778. doi:10.1093/brain/awq091

Klunk, W. E., Engler, H., Nordberg, A., Wang, Y., Blomqvist, G., & Holt, D. P. (2004). Imaging brain amyloid in Alzheimer's disease with Pittsburgh Compound-B. *Annals of Neurology*, *55*, 306–319. doi:10.1002/ana.20009

Klunk, W. E., Mathis, C. A., Price, J. C., Lopresti, B. J., & DeKosky, S. T. (2006). Two-year follow-up of amyloid deposition in patients with Alzheimer's disease. *Brain*, *129*, 2805–2807. doi:10.1093/brain/awl281

Kudo, Y., Okamura, N., Furumoto, S., Tashiro, M., Furukawa, K., & Maruyama, M. (2007). 2-(2-[2-Dimethylaminothiazol-5-yl]ethenyl)-6-(2-[fluoro]ethoxy)benzoxazole: A novel PET agent for in vivo detection of dense amyloid plaques in Alzheimer's disease patients. *Journal of Nuclear Medicine*, *48*, 553–561. doi:10.2967/jnumed.106.037556

Logan, J., Fowler, J. S., Volkow, N. D., Wang, G. J., Ding, Y. S., & Alexoff, D. L. (1996). Distribution volume ratios without blood sampling from graphical analysis of PET data. *Journal of Cerebral Blood Flow and Metabolism*, *16*, 834–840. doi:10.1097/00004647-199609000-00008

Logan, J., Fowler, J. S., Volkow, N. D., Wolf, A. P., Dewey, S. L., & Schlyer, D. J. (1990). Graphical analysis of reversible radioligand binding from time-activity measurements applied to [N-11C-methyl]-(-)-cocaine PET studies in human subjects. *Journal of Cerebral Blood Flow and Metabolism*, *10*, 740–747.

Lopresti, B. J., Klunk, W. E., Mathis, C. A., Hoge, J. A., Ziolko, S. K., & Lu, X. (2005). Simplified quantification of Pittsburgh Compound B amyloid imaging PET studies: A comparative analysis. *Journal of Nuclear Medicine*, *46*, 1959–1972.

Meltzer, C. C., Kinahan, P. E., Greer, P. J., Nichols, T. E., Comtat, C., & Cantwell, M. N. (1999). Comparative evaluation of MR-based partial-volume correction schemes for PET. *Journal of Nuclear Medicine*, *40*, 2053–2065.

Minoshima, S., Foster, N. L., & Kuhl, D. E. (1994). Posterior cingulate cortex in Alzheimer's disease. *Lancet*, *344*, 895. doi:10.1016/S0140-6736(94)92871-1

Mintun, M. A. (2005). Utilizing advanced imaging and surrogate markers across the spectrum of Alzheimer's disease. *CNS Spectrums*, *10*, 13–16.

Nordberg, A. (2004). PET imaging of amyloid in Alzheimer's disease. *The Lancet Neurology*, *3*, 519–527. doi:10.1016/S1474-4422(04)00853-1

Okamura, N., Shiga, Y., Furumoto, S., Tashiro, M., Tsuboi, Y., & Furukawa, K. (2009). In vivo detection of prion amyloid plaques using [(11) C]BF-227 PET. *European Journal of Nuclear Medicine and Molecular Imaging*, *37*, 934–941. doi:10.1007/s00259-009-1314-7

Price, J. C., Klunk, W. E., Lopresti, B. J., Lu, X., Hoge, J. A., & Ziolko, S. K. (2005). Kinetic modeling of amyloid binding in humans using PET imaging and Pittsburgh Compound-B. *Journal of Cerebral Blood Flow and Metabolism*, *25*, 1528–1547. doi:10.1038/sj.jcbfm.9600146

Shoghi-Jadid, K., Small, G. W., Agdeppa, E. D., Kepe, V., Ercoli, L. M., & Siddarth, P. (2002). Localization of neurofibrillary tangles and beta-amyloid plaques in the brains of living patients with Alzheimer disease. *The American Journal of Geriatric Psychiatry*, *10*, 24–35.

Tashiro, M., Itoh, M., Fujimoto, T., Masud, M. M., Watanuki, S., & Yanai, K. (2008). Application of positron emission tomography to neuroimaging in sports sciences. *Methods (San Diego, Calif.)*, *45*, 300–306. doi:10.1016/j.ymeth.2008.05.001

Tashiro, M., Miyake, M., Masud, M. M., Ogura, M., Watanuki, S., & Yanai, K. (2010). Nano-bio-imaging with radiopharmaceuticals and its application to health sciences. *Annals of nanoBME*, *3*, 73-87.

Verhoeff, N. P., Wilson, A. A., Takeshita, S., Trop, L., Hussey, D., & Singh, K. (2004). In-vivo imaging of Alzheimer disease beta-amyloid with [11C] SB-13 PET. *The American Journal of Geriatric Psychiatry*, *12*, 584–595.

Waragai, M., Okamura, N., Furukawa, K., Tashiro, M., Furumoto, S., & Funaki, Y. (2009). Comparison study of amyloid PET and voxel-based morphometry analysis in mild cognitive impairment and Alzheimer's disease. *Journal of the Neurological Sciences*, *285*, 100–108. doi:10.1016/j.jns.2009.06.005

Yanai, K., & Tashiro, M. (2007). The physiological and pathophysiological roles of neuronal histamine: An insight from human positron emission tomography studies. *Pharmacology & Therapeutics*, *113*, 1–15. doi:10.1016/j.pharmthera.2006.06.008

KEY TERMS AND DEFINITIONS

[^{11}C]BF-227: The first radiolabeled compound used for PET Aβ imaging in Japan.

[^{11}C]Pittsburgh Compound-B ([^{11}C]PIB): The most common radiolabeled compound used for PET imaging of Amyloid β.

Amyloid β Imaging (Aβ Imaging): A method for the early diagnosis of mild AD using a probe that specifically binds to Aβ proteins in vivo.

Full Kinetic Analysis: A type of mathematical technique used to estimate pharmacokinetic properties of radiolabeled tracers in biological organisms. This is an accurate method; however, the analytic procedure is sometimes complex and time-consuming. This is partly because this method uses non-linear analysis based on the minimum square method. Therefore, an appropriate compartmental model should be selected in advance.

Logan Graphical Analysis: A type of mathematical technique used to estimate pharmacokinetic properties of radiolabeled tracers in biological organisms. This method is convenient because a proper compartmental model is not required. Results are plotted as the distribution volume value.

Neuroimaging: Use of various techniques to either directly or indirectly image the structure and function/pharmacology of the brain. It is a relatively new discipline within the medicine and neuroscience/psychology communities.

Neuroscience: The scientific study of the nervous system.

Positron Emission Tomography (PET): A functional and molecular neuroimaging technique based on nuclear medicine technology that measures various types of biological information, such as regional cerebral metabolic rate for glucose, cerebral blood flow and pharmacology.

Chapter 30
Neuroimaging in Alzheimer's Disease

Hidenao Fukuyama
Human Brain Research Center, Kyoto University Graduate School of Medicine, Japan

ABSTRACT

The diagnosis of Alzheimer's disease (AD) is often based on clinical and pathological data. Positron emission tomography (PET) using the tracer 18F-FDG revealed findings specific to AD-mainly the posterior part of the brain and the association cortices of the parietal and occipital lobes were affected by a reduction in glucose metabolism. Recent advances in the development of tracers for amyloid protein, which is the key protein in the pathogenesis of AD, enables the pattern of deposition of amyloid protein in the brain to be visualized. Various tracers have been introduced to visualize other aspects of AD pathology. Recent clinical interests on dementia have focused on the early detection of AD and variation of Parkinson's disease, namely dementia with Lewy body disease (DLB), because the earlier the diagnosis, the better the prognosis. The differential diagnosis of mild AD or mild cognitive impairment (MCI) as well as DLB has been studied using PET and MRI as part of the NIH's Alzheimer disease Neuroimaging initiative (ADNI). At present, many countries are participating in the ADNI, which is yielding promising results. This chapter's study will improve the development of new drugs for the treatment of dementia patients by enabling the evaluation of the effect and efficacy of those drugs.

I. INTRODUCTION

Various aspects of Alzheimer's disease (AD) have been investigated from a variety of research fields, including genetics, biochemistry, behavior and imaging. Neuroimages of AD patients have been obtained by positron emission tomography (PET) using different tracers and magnetic resonance imaging (MRI). Recently, the AD neuroimaging initiative (ADNI) has been started in U.S.A.,

DOI: 10.4018/978-1-60960-559-9.ch030

and the J-ADNI started two years ago in Japan. These imaging modalities are regarded as not only diagnostic biomarkers, but also as a tool to investigate the pathophysiology of the disease, such as inflammation and amyloid protein accumulation.

II. PET AND SPECT IMAGING

Fluorine-18 Labeled Deoxyglucose (FDG)-PET

In the early 1980's, FDG-PET was applied to neuro-degenerative disorders to clarify the energy metabolism of the brain. AD showed a typical reduction in glucose metabolism by FDG-PET as well as in cerebral blood flow (CBF) and oxygen metabolism in the posterior association cortices (Fukuyama, Ogawa, Yamauchi, Yamaguchi, Kimura, Yonekura & Konishi, 1994). Statistical analysis demonstrated the reduction of metabolism and CBF in the posterior cingulated cortex and precuneus (Minoshima, Frey, Koeppe, Foster & Kuhl, 1995). This finding is also specific to the early phase of AD, which involved mild cognitive impairment (MCI) of the amnestic type. These observations have been confirmed by single photon emission CT (SPECT) and FDG-PET, and they were clearly shown using statistical image manipulations, such as 3D-SSP (Figure 1) or SPM.

Based on this background work, AD can be diagnosed easily using PET or SPECT combined with clinical and psychological data. Because the functional state of the brain is damaged in several specific regions, this particular pattern of damage supports the correct diagnosis. These types of image analyses have been used in clinical trials for the early diagnosis on AD in studies performed all over the world.

III. NEW TRACERS FOR AD DIAGNOSIS

C11-Labeled PK11195 Imaging for Microglial Activation

McGeer et al. proposed that a mild inflammatory process was involved in the pathology of AD (Lee, Sparatore, Del Soldato, McGeer & McGeer, 2009). Their hypothesis was based upon the observation that the incidence of AD is relatively

Figure 1. CBF reduction in statistical images. The parietal and temporal lobes as well as the posterior cigulate cortex and precunes showed reduced CBF. These images were taken from statistical parametric mapping (Friston, Frith, Liddle&Frackowiak, 1991) and 3D-SSP (Minoshima, Frey, Koeppe, Foster&Kuhl, 1995). The use of these findings on SPECT CBF or FDG-PET makes the diagnosis of AD and MCI easy. The arrow indicates the posterior cigulate cortex and precuneus.

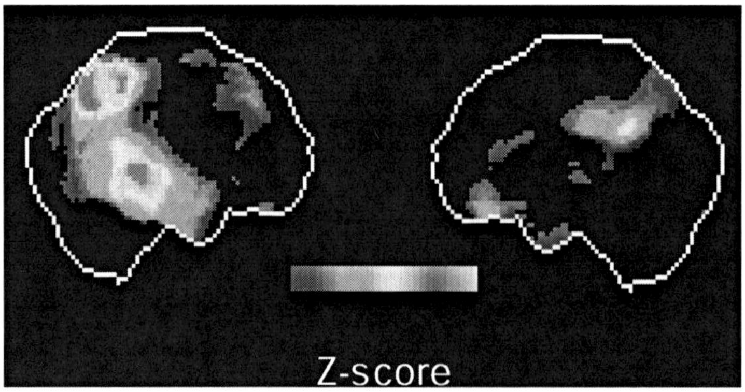

Figure 2. PK11195 image of AD patient

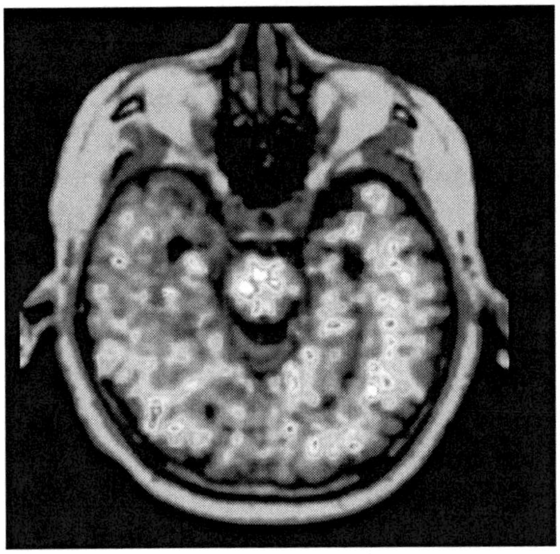

small in patients with rheumatoid arthritis who are administered aspirin compared with its frequency in the normal population and the pathology caused by activated microglial reactions in the affected brain. Based on that proposal, R. Banati attempted to visualize the activated microglia by PK11195 in AD patients (Figure 2) (Cagnin, Brooks, Kennedy, Gunn, Myers, Turkheimer, Jones & Banati, 2001).

The left temporal lobe is affected by the accumulation of tracer, showing left temporal lobe damage (Courtesy of Dr. Richard Banati, Hammersmith Hospital, London, UK).

Although the cause and pathophysiological implications of this mild inflammatory process remain unresolved, amyloid deposition and Alzheimer fibrillary tangle formation might be related to this pathology.

The role of inflammation with regard to pathogenesis of AD remains unclear. Activated microglia have been shown in the degenerative lesions, which are affected by slowly progressive tissue necrosis. In some cases, degenerative lesions can be cleared up by an unknown physiological process to maintain the tissue in its normal state. Whether this observation represents a pathological process that aggravates the plaque and tangle formation or simply a reactive process in degenerative tissues remains to be determined.

Amyloid Imaging

The amyloid hypothesis of AD is now the most prevalent hypothesis for explaining the pathogenesis of AD. Therefore, imaging tracers for amyloid are important to evaluate the efficacy of treatment in vivo. Many tracers have been tried, and Pittsburg compound B (PIB) is widely used at present (Klunk, Engler, Nordberg, Wang, Blomqvist, Holt, et al., 2004) because PIB is highly sensitive and has a reduced level of non-specificity.

A problem associated with amyloid imaging is that the amyloid deposition itself is not necessarily specific to AD pathology, with some individuals in the normal population having amyloid deposition without AD. An early diagnosis for AD may be possible using amyloid imaging, but the above-mentioned potential for false positive results prevents its usefulness for an accurate diagnosis of AD. A more specific tracer or combination of tracers, such as PK11195 and FDG, may improve the accuracy of diagnosing AD in the early stage of cognitive decline, such as during the development of MCI.

IV. LEWY BODY DISEASE AND PARKINSON'S DISEASE

A. Lewy Body Disease

Professor K. Kosaka hypothesized that the deposition of Lewy bodies in the cerebral cortex caused dementia (Kosaka, 1990), similar to that seen in AD with some modified symptoms such as frequent visual hallucinations and unstable symptoms within the course of one day. The deposition of alpha-synclein begins in the brain stem and migrates up through the midbrain, resulting in Parkinson's disease, and finally settles in the cerebral cortices, resulting in cognitive decline.

There are still controversies with regard to Lewy body disease as a separate disease entity. Some have claimed this condition is the combination of AD and Parkinson's disease. Dr. Orimo specifically found generalized Lewy body deposition in the autonomic nervous system by pathological research and showed cardiac noradrenergic damage by I-123 labeled MIBG (Orimo, Amino, Itoh, Takahashi, Kojo, et al., 2005). Parkinson's disease itself has a tendency to exhibit damage in the autonomic nervous system and have a poor accumulation of MIBG during its later stages (Fukuyama, 2009). Furthermore, amyloid deposition was proven to accumulate in the brain of Lewy body disease. Thus, these features make the separation of Lewy body disease from Parkinson's disease or Alzheimer's disease problematic (Gomperts, Rentz, Moran, Becker, Locascio, Klunk, et al., 2008).

B. Parkinson's Disease

The improvement of Parkinson's disease patients has been remarkable these days, due to treatment by several different drugs, including not only levodopa, but also dopamine agonists, a COMT inhibitor and MAO-B inhibitors. As a result, patients survive over ten years after diagnosis, with motor complications.

Mild cognitive decline has been noticed among these patients. We observed the cognitive decline in the early phase of Parkinson's disease (Sawamoto, Honda, Hanakawa, Fukuyama & Shibasaki, 2002). Patients who have had the disease for over 10 years, however, have shown symptoms similar to AD or Lewy body disease, with the poor accumulation of MIBG. This observation indicates that there are generalized damages to the autonomic nervous system, as well as midbrain dopaminergic and cortical cell damage.

V. ALZHEIMER DISEASE NEUROIMAGING INITIATIVE

The accurate diagnosis of AD is essential for the evaluation of its treatment. Previously, the diagnosis of AD was confirmed by pathological findings, such as the presence of tangles and plaques. Biochemical studies on amyloid protein, the main protein involved in the pathogenesis of AD, and its precursors revealed the possibility of developing drugs for AD treatment that would eliminate amyloid from the brain or inhibit amyloid synthesis in the brain. NIH leads the diagnostic standard for such pharmaceutical developments by searching for biomarkers of AD in vivo. Although this initiative is still on-going, several reports that show promising results for the diagnosis and treatment of AD have already been published.

ACKNOWLEDGMENT

A part of this study was supported by a Grant-in-Aid for Scientific Research (B), the Japan and AA Science Platform Program of the Japan Society for the Promotion Science.

REFERENCES

Cagnin, A., Brooks, D. J., Kennedy, A. M., Gunn, R. N., Myers, R., & Turkheimer, F. E. (2001). In-vivo measurement of activated microglia in dementia. *Lancet*, *358*, 461–467. doi:10.1016/S0140-6736(01)05625-2

Friston, K. J., Frith, C. D., Liddle, P. F., & Frackowiak, R. S. (1991). Comparing functional (PET) images: The assessment of significant change. *Journal of Cerebral Blood Flow and Metabolism*, *11*, 690–699.

Fukuyama, H. (2009). Is (123)I-MIBG cardiac scintigraphy a surrogate marker for Parkinson's disease? *European Journal of Nuclear Medicine and Molecular Imaging.*

Fukuyama, H., Ogawa, M., Yamauchi, H., Yamaguchi, S., Kimura, J., Yonekura, Y., & Konishi, J. (1994). Altered cerebral energy metabolism in Alzheimer's disease: A PET study. *Journal of Nuclear Medicine*, *35*, 1–6.

Gomperts, S. N., Rentz, D. M., Moran, E., Becker, J. A., Locascio, J. J., & Klunk, W. E. (2008). Imaging amyloid deposition in Lewy body diseases. *Neurology*, *71*, 903–910. doi:10.1212/01.wnl.0000326146.60732.d6

Klunk, W. E., Engler, H., Nordberg, A., Wang, Y., Blomqvist, G., & Holt, D. P. (2004). Imaging brain amyloid in Alzheimer's disease with Pittsburgh Compound-B. *Annals of Neurology*, *55*, 306–319. doi:10.1002/ana.20009

Kosaka, K. (1990). Diffuse Lewy body disease in Japan. *Journal of Neurology*, *237*, 197–204. doi:10.1007/BF00314594

Lee, M., Sparatore, A., Del Soldato, P., McGeer, E., & McGeer, P. L. (2009). Hydrogen sulfide-releasing NSAIDs attenuate neuroinflammation induced by microglial and astrocytic activation. *Glia*, *58*, 103–113. doi:10.1002/glia.20905

Minoshima, S., Frey, K. A., Koeppe, R. A., Foster, N. L., & Kuhl, D. E. (1995). A diagnostic approach in Alzheimer's disease using three-dimensional stereotactic surface projections of fluorine-18-FDG PET. *Journal of Nuclear Medicine*, *36*, 1238–1248.

Orimo, S., Amino, T., Itoh, Y., Takahashi, A., Kojo, T., & Uchihara, T. (2005). Cardiac sympathetic denervation precedes neuronal loss in the sympathetic ganglia in Lewy body disease. *Acta Neuropathologica*, *109*, 583–588. doi:10.1007/s00401-005-0995-7

Sawamoto, N., Honda, M., Hanakawa, T., Fukuyama, H., & Shibasaki, H. (n.d.). Cognitive slowing in Parkinson's disease: A behavioral evaluation independent of motor slowing. *The Journal of Neuroscience*, *22*, 5198–5203.

KEY TERMS AND DEFINITIONS

Magnetic Resonance Imaging (MRI): An imaging device that detects the magnetic spin yielding the free induction decay in the strong static magnetic field activated by a radiofrequency pulse. Various kinds of sequences are available to visualize changes in the brain tissue, such as within a damaged brain: T1-, T2- or FLAIR-weighted images; water diffusion (diffusion-weighted image) and fast image acquisition (echo planner imaging technique).

Neuroimaging: The use of various techniques to either directly or indirectly image a structure in the brain.

Neuroscience: The scientific study of the nervous system.

Positron Emission Tomography (PET): An imaging device that uses positron emitter imaging, such as F-18- or C11-labeled compounds. It is the most sensitive tool to detect minute amount of substances in the brain.

Chapter 31
In Vivo Optical Imaging of Brain and its Application in Alzheimer's Disease

Jinho Kim
Department of Bio and Brain Engineering, KAIST, Korea

Yong Jeong
Department of Bio and Brain Engineering, KAIST, Korea & Department of Neurology, Samsung Medical Center, Korea

ABSTRACT

Brain imaging has become an essential tool for research, clinical trials and neurological practice. Advances in imaging techniques have enabled scientists to observe the brain in vivo. Investigation of the brain provides several levels of analysis from molecular and cellular to systems and cognition. In vivo imaging techniques such as MRI, PET and optical imaging have become highly advanced and are capable of providing anatomical and physiological information. Microscopic and other intravital optical techniques have been developed during the past decades and have enabled in vivo studies of genetic, molecular and cellular events in the brain through cranial windows. This chapter introduces the applications of intravital microscopy of intrinsic signals and voltage sensing and two-photon microscopy of neuronal and vascular function.

Recently, various in vivo optical brain imaging techniques have been developed. Here, the authors introduce some of these systems and their application to in vivo brain imaging in a mouse model of Alzheimer's disease (AD). Two-photon laser scanning microscopy (TPLSM) is specialized for fluorescence imaging in deep tissue with sub-micron resolution and has scanning capabilities, intrinsic optical signal imaging detects the relative changes in oxy- and deoxy-hemoglobin concentration following sensory stimulation and voltage-sensitive dye imaging can directly image the changes of the membrane potential after neural stimulation.

DOI: 10.4018/978-1-60960-559-9.ch031

I. TWO-PHOTON LASER SCANNING MICROSCOPY

The concept of two-photon (or multi-photon) excitation of fluorescence was first introduced by Nobel laureate Maria Göppert-Mayer in 1963 (Peticolas, Goldsborough, & Rieckhoff, 1963). The first laser scanning microscope that used this concept was reported in 1990 (Denk, Strickler & Webb, 1990). Since then, TPLSM has been used for *in vivo* tissue imaging, particularly in brain imaging. This device utilizes the two-photon effect; a fluorescent probe is excited not by a single photon of visible light, but by nearly simultaneous two photons of lower-energy (infrared). Fluorescently labeled specimens are illuminated by a Ti:sapphire femto-second pulsed laser of near infrared light, and emit the specified emission wavelength light.

Because TPLSM uses a long-wavelength light source (over 700 nm to 1,000 nm) and because light with longer wavelengths can penetrate deeper into samples, deep tissue imaging (theoretically up to 1 mm) becomes possible. Furthermore, simultaneous photon absorption significantly reduces photo-bleach and/or photo-damage in peripheral planes that are not in focus. These features of TPLSM allow *in vivo* fluorescence imaging with high temporal and spatial resolution.

1) Cranial Window and Structural Imaging

For *in vivo* brain imaging by the above-mentioned TPLSM, a cranial window is required because the skull is not sufficiently transparent. The open-skull and thinned-skull cranial window methods are primarily used with various minor modifications. For an open-skull window, 2 × 2 mm or 3 × 3 mm craniotomy on the region of interest is performed, and the cortex is covered with 1-1.5% agarose and a glass cover slip. The margin is secured by cyanoacrylate glue, and dental cement is applied around the cover slip to provide a well for a water-immersion lens. In a thinned-skull cranial window, the region of interest is gently thinned with a high-speed hand-drill, typically to a thickness at which cerebral blood flow can be clearly visualized when water is applied. Once the skull is thinned, dental cement is applied to make a well for water immersion of the lens.

The vascular structure is imaged through the cranial window. To better visualize the vessel, a fluorescent probe tagged with dextran is injected into the tail vein. Dextran tagging prevents the dye from crossing the vessel wall. As seen in Figure 1(a), fluorescein isothiocyanate (FITC)-dextran (2 MDa) was injected, and the cerebral vasculature images were obtained through the cranial window.

Amyloid plaques are one of hallmarks of the AD brain, and they can be imaged and quantified through cranial windows with appropriate probes. Thioflavin S and methoxy-X04 are common probes used for amyloid plaque detection. Figure 1(b) shows thioflavin S imaging and methoxy-X04 imaging for amyloid plaque and cerebrovascular amyloid angiopathy in a mouse model of AD. Methoxy-X04 is more advantageous than thioflavin S because it crosses the blood brain barrier; therefore, it can be systemically administered (Nagayama, Zeng, Xiong, Fletcher, Masurkar et al., 2007).

2) Functional Imaging

In addition to structural imaging, it is possible to observe some functional characteristics of the brain using TPLSM. For example, Figure 1(c) shows the calculation of red blood cell (RBC) velocity in cerebral micro-vessels in a mouse brain. Because RBCs do not incorporate dextran-conjugated dyes, they produce a blank signal inside the fluorescent lumen of the blood vessel. During repeated scanning of a line along the vessel, RBCs leave streaks that can be analyzed as distance traveled over time to yield velocity. RBC velocity can be calculated in other vessels, but faster scanning speeds are required for larger vessels, particularly for arteries (Kim & Jeong, 2009).

Figure 1. (a) Cerebral blood vessel morphology as detected by TPLSM. Maximum projection image (left) and z-axis transparent projection (right), scale bar = 50 µm. (b) Amyloid plaques and perivascular amyloid deposition (arrow) detection using thioflavin S (left). FITC-dextran was injected via the tail vein to visualize cerebral vessels. Prominent cerebral amyloid angiopathy and dense amyloid plaques were detected with methoxy-X04 (right). (c) Time-lapse line scanning of RBCs in cerebral capillaries. Each column represents a capillary, and black streaks represent RBCs. The bottom of each column shows the RBC velocity (left). Velocities were mapped into a capillary network (right) that displays direction as well as velocity. (d) Calcium staining with Oregon-green BAPTA 1-AM and detection of spontaneous neuronal calcium spikes.

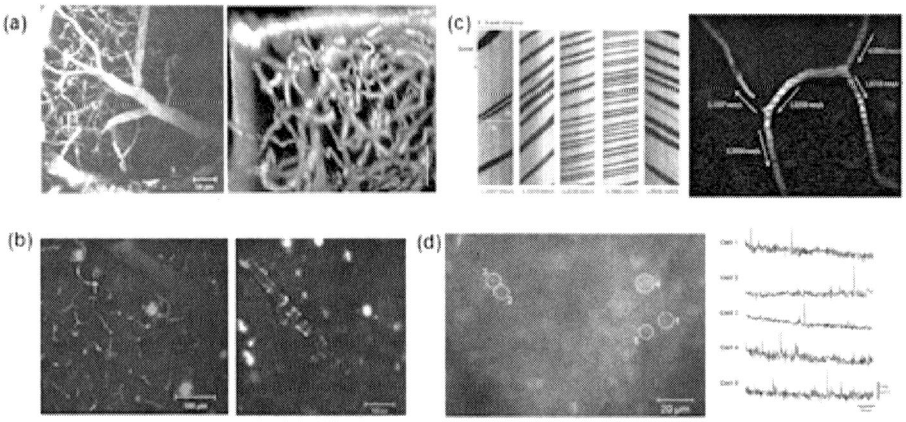

Neuronal activities can also be observed with TPLSM by injecting a calcium-specific dye into the cortex. For single-cell imaging, dyes are injected directly into the cell using a patch pipette (Stosiek, Garaschuk, Holthoff, & Konnerth, 2003), and to visualize a cluster of cells, dyes are injected into the parenchyma by a multi-cell bolus loading method (Klunk, Bacskai, Mathis, Kajdasz, & McLellan, et al., 2002). In Figure 1(d), a calcium-specific dye, Oregon green BAPTA 1-AM, was injected into the cortex using multi-cell bolus loading, and spontaneous calcium signals were recorded. Calcium signal detection using TPLSM has advantages over other modalities for detection of neuronal firing because it provides resolution at the single-cell level (within an approximately 0.5 mm by 0.5 mm field of view). Therefore, it provides a sufficient amount of temporal and spatial information about calcium signaling in a group of neurons.

3) TPLSM Imaging of AD Brains

As mentioned above, amyloid plaques and cerebral amyloid angiopathy (CAA) can be imaged using TPLSM with targeting fluorescent probes such as thioflavin S and methoxy-X04. Therefore, it is possible to perform longitudinal studies in mice to detect changes in the amyloid burden over time. This augments the significance of studies of amyloid burden detection and simultaneously reduces the sample sizes. AD brain imaging using TPLSM in mice is commonly performed. One study found that plaque formation is a more rapid process than expected and that plaque formation leads to abnormal structural changes in dendrites (Meyer-Luehmann, Spires-Jones, Prada, Garcia-Alloza, & de Calignon, et al., 2008). Furthermore, researchers have found that neurons in the proximity of the plaques and astrocytes are hyperactive in AD mouse brains (Busche, Eichhoff, Adelsberger, Abramowski, & Wiederhold, et al., 2008; Kuchibhotla, Lattarulo, Hyman, & Bacskai, 2009).

II. INTRINSIC OPTICAL SIGNAL IMAGING

Intrinsic optical signal (IOS) imaging utilizes various endogenous molecules in the body, primarily oxy- (HbO) and deoxy-hemoglobin (HbR). Briefly, IOS imaging detects changes in the reflectance level of specific wavelengths of light. Every intrinsic molecule has a specific light absorption spectrum, and, according to that spectrum, each molecule absorbs specific intensity of light of a specific wavelength. Light with a wavelength of 570 nm is absorbed by both oxy- and deoxy-hemoglobin, and light with a wavelength of 610 nm is absorbed only by HbR (Sheth, Nemoto, Guiou, Walker, & Pouratian, et al., 2003). Therefore, a decrease in the reflection of light of 570 nm indicates increased absorption by both oxy- and deoxy-hemoglobin, which, in turn, indicates an increase in the total hemoglobin (HbT) concentration. Likewise, a decrease in the reflectance of 610-nm light indicates an increase in HbR concentration and vice versa. Figure 2 shows a 570-nm IOS map of a hindpaw drawn on the reference image of mouse cortex. Images were taken for 40 seconds at 10 Hz with a charge-coupled device (CCD) camera, and 20 msec, 2mA electric stimulation pulses were given to the hindpaw at 2.5 Hz, starting at 10 sec time point for 2 s. Relative changes in reflectance were calculated using the following equation:

$$\Delta R/R\ (\%) = (R_t - R_{avg}) / R_{avg}\ X100\ (\%) \qquad (1)$$

R_{avg} is the average background reflectance level, and R_t is the reflectance level in a specific time frame. Response values are defined by the area under the graph of the time series (ΔR/R) for every pixel, and the maximum response value is recorded. By setting the threshold to the maximum response value, we were able to draw IOS imaging response maps, as shown in Fig. 2. A time series graph of each map is also presented. This provides information on vascular function, as changes in the HbT concentration imply changes in the cerebral blood volume (CBV), and CBV changes are driven by vessel dilation. Therefore, by comparing patterns of HbT fluctuation from IOS imaging and neuronal activity between AD mice and control mice, it may be possible to detect

Figure 2. IOS response map (HbT; 570 nm) with thresholds of 30%, 50% and 70% (blue, yellow and red, respectively) of the maximum response value (see text). The graph on the right side is the relative reflectance change in response to the stimulation (black column). Scale bar = 500 µm.

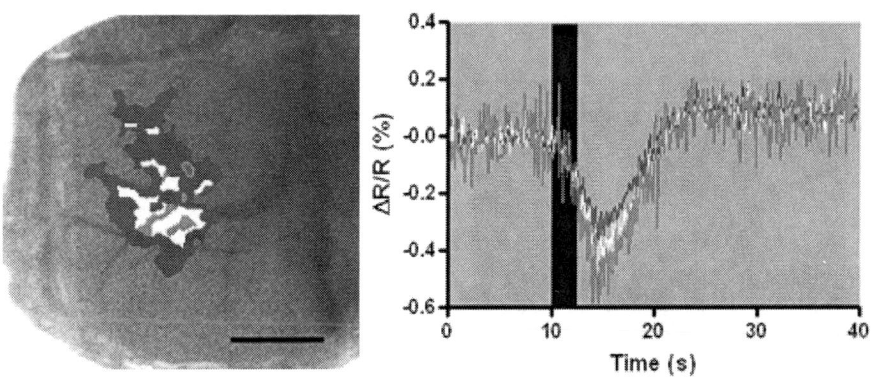

functional neurovascular defects in AD mice (Iadecola, 2004).

III. VOLTAGE-SENSITIVE DYE IMAGING

A voltage-sensitive dye (VSD) is a fluorescent dye used to detect changes in the membrane potential. VSDs bind to cell membranes and change their conformation depending on the membrane potential, with a resultant shift in fluorescence spectra (Lippert, Takagaki, Xu, Huang, & Wu, 2007). This technique enables the detection of membrane potential change with high temporal resolution. Figure 3 shows an example of VSD imaging. Imaging was performed at 100 Hz for 5 seconds with a CCD camera, and hindpaw stimulation was applied with a single 10-msec electric pulse of 20 mA. The fluorescence change was calculated by Equation (1), except for the notation (F instead of R), and the maximum response value was evaluated by calculating the peak value in each pixel of the image.

VSD images have an advantage over conventional electrophysiology because they provide spatial information about neuronal activity from a macroscopic perspective rather than evaluating single cell activity or a non-selective field potential.

FUTURE DIRECTIONS

For decades, research on neuronal and cerebral vascular function was conducted using *in vitro* cultured cells or brain slices in *ex vivo* systems. However, many of the *in vitro* studies produced indiscernible results that could not be reproduced in *in vivo* systems. This may be because the *ex vivo* system is not in a normal physiological condition. Therefore, the need for *in vivo* studies has increased; however, this has been hampered by various technical limitations. Electrophysiology is an *in vivo* technique that provides limited spatial information. However, this drawback can be overcome by the use of optical imaging techniques. Nevertheless, the *in vivo* optical imaging techniques discussed in the current chapter also have limitations, such as invasiveness and possible inflammation during surgical preparation. Overcoming these problems will make the *in vivo* experiments more representative physiologic conditions, which will eventually lead to the development of indispensable methods for translational research.

Figure 3. VSD imaging was performed for the IOS response area at 570 nm (red box on the bottom left image [scale bar = 100 μm]). The graph shows the fluorescence change after stimulation was performed at the 2-second time point (the first second was discarded to eliminate equipment noise).

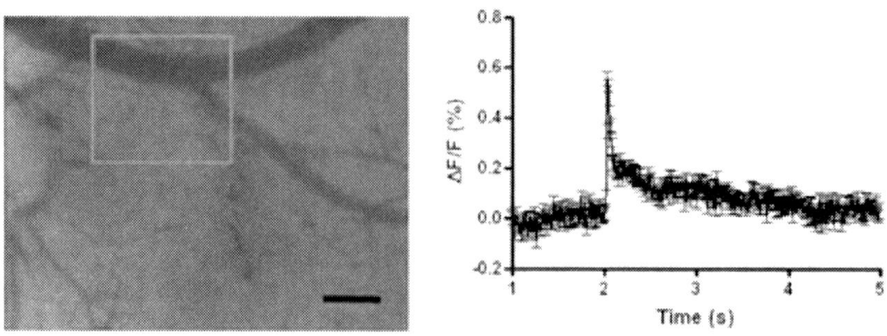

REFERENCES

Busche, M. A., Eichhoff, G., Adelsberger, H., Abramowski, D., Wiederhold, K. H., & Haass, C. (1686-1689). … Garaschuk, O. (2008). Clusters of hyperactive neurons near amyloid plaques in a mouse model of Alzheimer's disease. *Science*, 321.

Denk, W., Strickler, J. H., & Webb, W. W. (1990). Two-photon laser scanning fluorescence microscopy. *Science*, *248*, 73–76. doi:10.1126/science.2321027

Iadecola, C. (2004). Neurovascular regulation in the normal brain and in Alzheimer's disease. *Nature Reviews. Neuroscience*, *5*, 347–360. doi:10.1038/nrn1387

Kim, J., & Jeong, Y. (2009). *Measurement of vascular function in mice brain using two-photon laser scanning microscopy*. Presented at the 4th Asian Pacific Symposium on BioPhotonics 2009.

Klunk, W. E., Bacskai, B. J., Mathis, C. A., Kajdasz, S. T., McLellan, M. E., & Frosch, M. P. (2002). Imaging Abeta plaques in living transgenic mice with multiphoton microscopy and methoxy-X04, a systemically administered Congo red derivative. *Journal of Neuropathology and Experimental Neurology*, *61*, 797–805.

Kuchibhotla, K. V., Lattarulo, C. R., Hyman, B. T., & Bacskai, B. J. (2009). Synchronous hyperactivity and intercellular calcium waves in astrocytes in Alzheimer mice. *Science*, *323*, 1211–1215. doi:10.1126/science.1169096

Lippert, M. T., Takagaki, K., Xu, W., Huang, X., & Wu, J. Y. (2007). Methods for voltage-sensitive dye imaging of rat cortical activity with high signal-to-noise ratio. *Journal of Neurophysiology*, *98*, 502–512. doi:10.1152/jn.01169.2006

Meyer-Luehmann, M., Spires-Jones, T. L., Prada, C., Garcia-Alloza, M., de Calignon, A., & Rozkalne, A. (2008). Rapid appearance and local toxicity of amyloid-beta plaques in a mouse model of Alzheimer's disease. *Nature*, *451*, 720–724. doi:10.1038/nature06616

Nagayama, S., Zeng, S., Xiong, W., Fletcher, M. L., Masurkar, A. V., & Davis, D. J. (2007). In vivo simultaneous tracing and Ca(2+) imaging of local neuronal circuits. *Neuron*, *53*, 789–803. doi:10.1016/j.neuron.2007.02.018

Peticolas, W. L., Goldsborough, J. P., & Rieckhoff, K. E. (1963). Double photon excitation in organic crystals. *Physical Review Letters*, *10*, 43–45. doi:10.1103/PhysRevLett.10.43

Sheth, S., Nemoto, M., Guiou, M., Walker, M., Pouratian, N., & Toga, A. W. (2003). Evaluation of coupling between optical intrinsic signals and neuronal activity in rat somatosensory cortex. *NeuroImage*, *19*, 884–894. doi:10.1016/S1053-8119(03)00086-7

Stosiek, C., Garaschuk, O., Holthoff, K., & Konnerth, A. (2003). In vivo two-photon calcium imaging of neuronal networks. *Proceedings of the National Academy of Sciences of the United States of America*, *100*, 7319–7324. doi:10.1073/pnas.1232232100

KEY TERMS AND DEFINITIONS

Alzheimer's Disease: The most common form of dementia. The pathological hallmarks are amyloid plaques and neurofibrillary tangles.

Cerebral Amyloid Angiopathy: A form of angiopathy in which amyloid deposits form in the walls of the blood vessels within the central nervous system.

Cerebral Blood Vessels: Blood vessels in the brain.

Dementia: Refers to the loss of cognitive function due to changes in the brain by degenerative or other diseases, leading to interference with normal activities.

***In Vivo* Imaging:** Imaging techniques conducted in live animals.

Intravital Microscopy: A technique used to observe biological systems *in vivo*.

Intrinsic Optical Signal: A signal arising from changes in the absorption (or reflection) of light by intrinsic properties of tissues.

Two-Photon Microscopy: Microscopy that uses the two-photon phenomenon. This is defined as simultaneous excitation by two or more photons, usually in near-infra red wavelength by a femtosecond laser. This enables deep-tissue fluorescence imaging.

Section 3

Chapter 32 The Relationship between Knee Extension Strength and Activities of Daily Living in Patients with Dementia

Makoto Suzuki
Faculty of Medical Technology, Niigata University of Health and Welfare, Japan

Hikari Kirimoto
Faculty of Medical Technology, Niigata University of Health and Welfare, Japan

Atsushi Inamura
Department of Health Support, Setagaya Municipal Kitazawa En, Japan

Yoshitsugu Omori
Department of Rehabilitation Medicine, St. Marianna University, Yokohama City Seibu Hospital, Japan

Sumio Yamada
School of Health Sciences, Nagoya University, Japan

ABSTRACT

The purpose of this study was to examine the test-retest reliability of hand-held dynamometer measurements in patients with dementia and determine if predictions about a patient's ability to perform daily activities can be made from knee extension strength measurements. This study was composed of two rounds of data collection. Sixty patients with dementia were enrolled in the first round to assess the reliability of hand-held dynamometer measurements, and 54 patients with dementia were enrolled in the second round for predicting their ability to perform daily activities. Knee extensor strength was measured twice, separated by a three minute interval, with hand-held dynamometer. The authors also assessed daily activities related to the patient's lower extremities, including dressing the lower body, using the toile, transferring to the bed/toilet/shower, and walking. Lower extremity activities of the Functional Independence Measure were assessed by the nursing home caregiver that had the most regular contact with each subject. When the Functional Independence Measure score of each lower extremity function was ≥6 points, the subject

DOI: 10.4018/978-1-60960-559-9.ch032

was considered to be independent. The intraclass correlation coefficient was 0.97. Bland-Altman plots showed the 95% difference value to be within 2 SDs of the mean. The curves of negative and positive predictive values revealed the following threshold levels: 0.8 Nm/kg was the best predictor for dressing the lower body and using the toilet; 1.2 Nm/kg was the best predictor for transferring to the bed/toilet/shower; and 0.6 Nm/kg was the best predictor for gait performance. Strength measurements taken with a hand-held dynamometer were reliable in patients with dementia, and normalized knee extensor strength was found to be a predictor of the ability to perform activities of daily living.

INTRODUCTION

Lower limb weakness can prevent a person from performing activities of daily living, such as walking, sit-to-stand transfer, climbing steps, and dressing the lower-body (Bohannon, 1995; Cheng et al., 1998; Lamoureux et al., 2002; Moreland et al., 2004; Wolfson et al., 1995; Corrigan and Bohannon, 2001; Azegami et al., 2007; Puthoff and Nielsen, 2007). As people age, they undergo an overall decline in muscle mass (Lexell et al., 1988; Sato et al., 1984; Janssen et al., 2000). This generalized loss of skeletal muscle is considered to be a major factor in the impairment of muscle strength in older adults (Janssen et al., 2002). Muscle weakness that is associated with aging is obvious in locations where the population is dramatically aging, such as Japan, the United States and Europe (Okamoto, 1992; Ory et al., 2003; Franceschi et al., 2007). Lower extremity dysfunction related to every-day life activities is also common among older adults (Boyle et al., 2007; Bennett et al., 1996; Waite et al., 2005). In particular, lower extremity dysfunction is common in elderly people with dementia (Goldman et al., 1999; Wilson et al., 2000) and increases in frequency and severity as the disease progresses (Goldman et al., 1999; Wilson et al., 2000; Scarmeas et al., 2004). For people with dementia, as well as their caregivers, lower extremity functional decline may be the most problematic aspect of the condition, as loss of function in the lower extremities is associated with cognitive decline (Bennett et al., 1998; Scarmeas et al., 2005) and death (Wilson et al., 2003; Bennett et al., 1998). Dysfunction in a patient's lower limbs also increases the need for care and increases the risk of institutionalization. Such care accounts for the majority of disease-related costs for patients with dementia (Kinosian et al., 2000; Taylor et al., 2000).

Various methods can be used to assess muscle strength, including manual muscle testing, isokinetic and isometric dynamometry, and 1- and 2-repetition maximum testing. Because the use of fixed dynamometers is time-consuming, these instruments are not suitable for routine application in clinical practice. Furthermore, in patients with dementia, impaired balance, a diminished ability to concentrate, and an apprehension toward unfamiliar devices may impede these measurements (Brill et al., 1995). For ease of measurement, a hand-held dynamometer (HHD) may be used to quantify maximal strength and may offer several advantages over free weights, including ease of transport, time efficiency and lower costs. Isometric strength assessment of patients with dementia by means of a HHD is becoming increasingly popular due to its technical simplicity, low cost, and objectivity relative to other methods of strength testing (Brill et al., 1995). Intraclass correlation coefficients used to characterize the reliability of strength testing by HHD have been shown to range between 0.84 and 0.99, which is considered sufficient (Schaubert and Bohannon, 2005; Suomi et al., 1993). However, there is limited evidence about the reliability of strength assessment by HHD in patients with dementia (Thomas and Hageman, 2003). Furthermore, little is known about the relationship between knee extension strength and lower extremity function, and the threshold level of strength for accurately predicting lower extremity dysfunction in patients with dementia is unknown. Thus, predicting the level of muscle strength that enables patients with dementia to carry out lower extremity functions independently remains difficult. If investigators could predict the lower extremity functions of patients with dementia from measurements of knee muscle strength, better training regimens for regaining lower extremity functions could be designed for an aging society. Therefore, this study was designed to examine the test-retest reliability of HHD measurements of knee extension strength in patients with dementia (Suzuki et al., 2009) and to use these measurements as an index of lower extremity muscle strength that could be used to predict lower extremity function (unpublished data).

RELIABILITY OF KNEE EXTENSION STRENGTH MEASUREMENTS OBTAINED IN PATIENTS WITH DEMENTIA

METHODS

Subjects

Subject eligibility criteria included the presence of dementia, nursing home residency, absence of delirium or palsy, and the desire to participate in the study. Dementia was diagnosed according to the clinical criteria of the National Institute of Neurological and Communicative Disorders and the Stroke-Alzheimer Disease and Related Disorders Association (NINCDS-ADRDA) (Makhann et al., 1984). Individuals were excluded from the study if they could not push against the dynamometer with their leg with physical guidance. This study was performed according to the Declaration of Helsinki. All subjects and their families were informed about the aims of the study and the testing procedure prior to participation. Written informed consent was obtained from each subject and/or the subject's family. In this study, 60 people with dementia (14 men, 46 women) were recruited from a nursing home. The characteristics of the subjects are presented in Table 1.

Knee Extension Strength

Knee extension strength was assessed with a HHD (μTas MT-1, ANIMA, Japan). The dynamometer pad is 55×55 mm, and its front side is curved to fit the shape of the areas to be measured on the extremities. The measurement range of this dynamometer is 0.1 to 999.9 N, with a recording interval of 0.1 N.

For knee extensor assessments, subjects were seated in an elevated hard chair with knees flexed 90°, feet dangling over the floor, and arms on their thighs. Before the start of the strength testing, the therapist took the subject's leg and guided it in the appropriate direction several times in accordance with the testing protocol to familiarize the subject with the feel of pushing against the dynamometer. The dynamometer was then placed perpendicular to the leg just above the malleoli. Subjects were told to push against the dynamometer by attempting to

Table 1. Characteristics of patients satisfying eligibility criteria for study of reliability of knee extension strength measurements

Age (years)	86.6 ± 6.2
Sex (N)	
Female	46
Male	14
Body weight (kg)	45.6 ± 8.4
Lower leg length (m)	0.38 ± 0.03
Mini-Mental State Examination	11 (6 − 15)
Dementia Behavior Disturbance Scale	21 (16 − 35)

Values are mean ± SD or median (interquartile range).

straighten their knees. They were asked to increase force gradually to a maximum voluntary effort. They were then instructed to maintain maximum effort for five additional seconds. Throughout the session, each subject was given consistent verbal encouragement and praise as reinforcement. The examiner measured the strength of each subject twice, with the tests separated by a three-minute interval. During all tests, the dynamometer was stabilized by the examiner with both hands. Bilateral limbs were assessed for extension, and the starting limb was randomized.

Statistical Analysis

Statistical analyses to assess reliability were performed for the first and second measurement within the same day. Two different mathematical approaches were used for intra-subject analysis. The intraclass correlation coefficient (ICC) was used for variance estimation. ICC values in the range of 0.80–1.00 indicate that the test has "excellent repeatability," and ICC values in the range of 0.60–0.80 suggest "good repeatability." Values below 0.60 indicate "poor repeatability" (Bartko, 1966). Bland-Altman plots of the mean and standard deviation (SD) of differences between trials were used to determine the coefficient of repeatability (Bland and Altman, 1986). The plot of differences against the mean allowed for the investigation of any possible relationship between the measurement error and the true value. If the mean difference is zero and 95% of the values lie within 2 SDs of the mean difference, the data can indicate that the test has repeatability.

All statistical procedures were carried out with SPSS software (version 12.0) with a significance level set at $P < 0.05$.

RESULTS

The knee extensor muscle strengths of the 60 subjects in this study ranged from 1.4 to 90.0 Nm (average, 30.9 Nm; SD, 20.1 Nm). The normalized knee extensor strengths for the 60 subjects in this study ranged from 0.04 to 1.76 Nm/kg (average, 0.67 Nm/kg; SD, 0.40 Nm/kg). The first and second measurements of isometric knee extensor strength are presented in Figure 1 and Table 2. The ICC for knee extensor strength between the two successive strength assessments was 0.97, indicating excellent reproducibility. A Bland-Altman plot graphically displays the difference against the mean of the two measurements (Figure 2). The mean difference of all subjects between the two measurements was –0.8 Nm (Figure 2). Ninety-five percent of difference values (57/60) were within 2 SDs of the mean. However, the distribution of test-retest differences increased slightly with isometric knee extensor strength.

Figure 1. Isometric knee extensor strength with line of equality

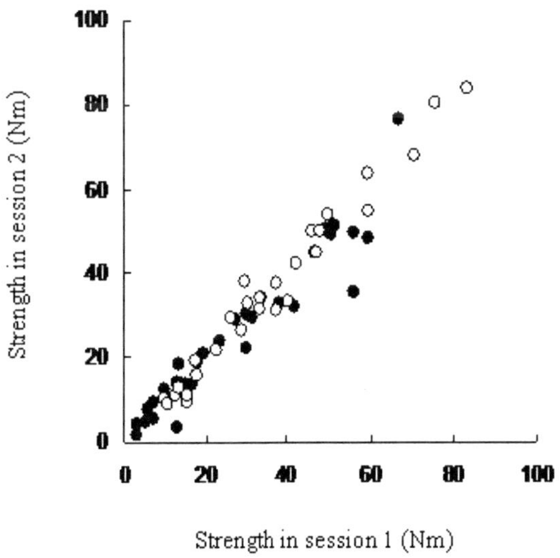

Table 2. Knee extensor muscle strength of the study subjects

Subjects	Non-normalized Knee Extensor Muscle Strength (Nm)		Normalized Knee Extensor Muscle Strength (Nm/kg)		ICC
	Session 1	Session 2	Session 1	Session 2	
Total subjects (N = 60)	31.3 ± 19.9	30.5 ± 20.1	0.68 ± 0.39	0.66 ± 0.40	0.97
Subjects with MMSE score of more than 10 points (N = 31)	35.7 ± 19.6	35.7 ± 20.5	0.78 ± 0.36	0.79 ± 0.38	0.98
Subject with MMSE score of 10 points or less (N=29)	26.7 ± 19.5	24.9 ± 18.4	0.56 ± 0.39	0.53 ± 0.39	0.95

Values are mean ± SD
ICC: intraclass correlation coefficient

RELATIONSHIP BETWEEN KNEE EXTENSION STRENGTH AND LOWER EXTREMITY FUNCTION IN PATIENTS WITH DEMENTIA

Methods

Subjects

This part of the study used the same eligibility criteria as described above for testing the **reliability** of knee extension strength measurements. We recruited 54 patients with dementia (13 men, 41 women) from a nursing home. The characteristics of the subjects are presented in Table 3.

Knee Extension Strength

Knee extension strength was measured by the same method as described above for testing of the reliability of knee extension strength measurements.

Activities of Daily Living

The Functional Independence Measure (FIM) tallies 18 activities of daily living, which are

Figure 2. Bland-Altman-Plots of isometric knee extensor strength

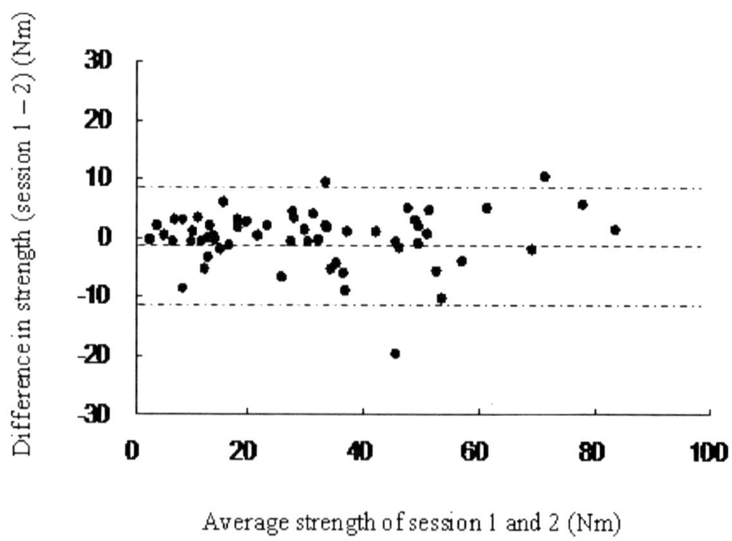

Table 3. Characteristics of patients satisfying eligibility criteria for study of prediction of lower extremity function by knee extension strength

Age (years)	87.0 ± 5.7
Sex(N)	
Female	*41*
Male	*13*
Body Weight (kg)	46.0 ± 9.5
Lower leg length (m)	0.36 ± 0.04
Mini-Mental State Examination	11 (7 −14)
Dementia Behavior Disturbance Scale	19 (12 − 27)

Values are mean ± SD or median (interquartile range).

graded on a 7-point scale: 1 = total assistance; 2 = maximal assistance; 3 = moderate assistance; 4 = minimal contact assistance; 5 = supervision or set-up; 6 = modified independence; and 7 = complete independence (Chino et al., 2003). These activities fall into six categories. Four involve motor functions (FIM-motor) and include self-care (eating, grooming, bathing, dressing the upper body, dressing the lower body and using the toilet), sphincter control (bladder and bowel management), mobility (transferring to a bed/chair/wheelchair, transferring to the toilet and transferring to the tub/shower), and locomotion (walking or wheelchair propulsion and stair climbing). We focused on the activities that reflected lower extremity motor functions, specifically dressing the lower body, using the toilet, transferring to the bed/toilet/shower and walking. We excluded stair climbing from our analysis because nursing home residents with dementia usually use an elevator and not the stairs. The **FIMs** of lower extremity activities were assessed by the nursing home caregiver who had the most regular contact with each subject. In this study, when the FIM activity score for each lower extremity function performed by the subject was 6 points or more, the subject was considered to be independent.

Statistical Analysis

The threshold level for prediction of independence was judged as the point where both negative and positive predictive values were high (Suzuki et al., 2008).

RESULTS

Independence levels for lower extremity functions are presented in Figure 3. Transfer to bed/toilet/shower had a lower independence level than other activities. In contrast, gait performance had the highest independence level. The curve of negative and positive predictive values for the prediction of independence indicated that a threshold level of 0.8 Nm/kg would provide the best balance for dressing the lower body (positive predictive value, 0.74; negative predictive value, 0.77; Figure 3A) and using the toilet (positive predictive value, 0.70; negative predictive value, 0.71; Figure 3B). A threshold level of 1.2 Nm/kg was the best predictor for transferring to the bed/toilet/shower (positive predictive value, 0.83; negative predictive value, 0.71; Figure 3C); and a threshold level of 0.6 Nm/kg was the best predictor for gait performance (positive predictive value, 0.71; negative predictive value, 0.70; Figure 3D).

DISCUSSION

Lower limb strength is essential for the performance of every-day activities. Previous studies have shown that the HHD is a reliable instrument for measuring muscle strength in patients with brain damage (Riddle et al., 1989; Piao et al., 2004), postpolio syndrome (Nollet and Beelen, 1999), and spinal cord injury (May et al., 1997) and in the homebound elderly (Bohannon, 1986; Wikholm and Bohannon, 1991; Schaubert and Bohannon, 2005). However, the reliability of the strength assessment in patients with dementia was

Figure 3. The clinical utility of knee extensor muscles

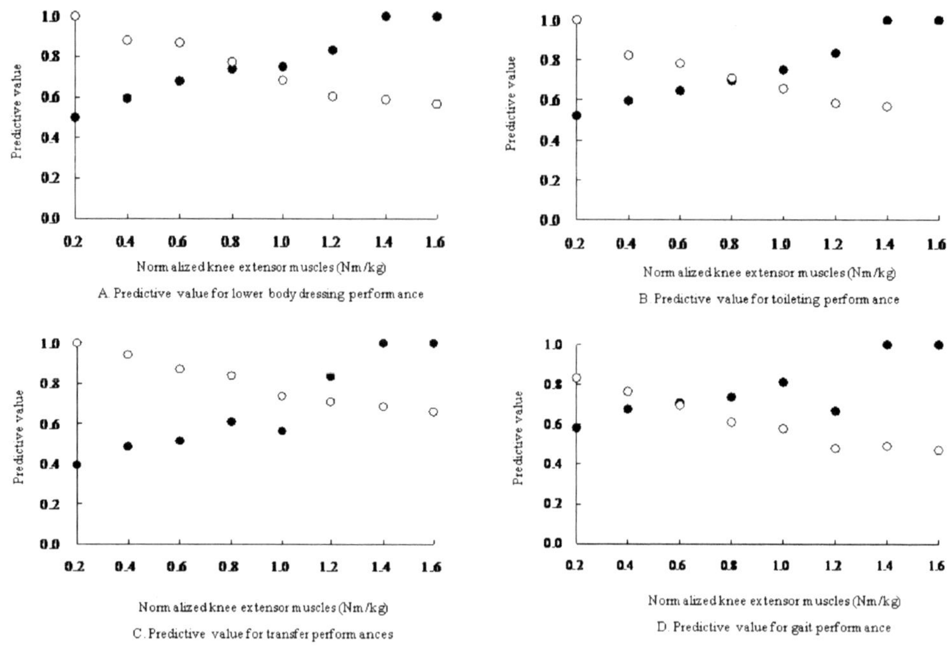

FIGURE 3. The clinical utility of knee extensor muscles.

●: Positive predictive value ○: Negative predictive value

uncertain. In the present study, the test-retest reliability of knee extensor strength measurements with an HHD was found to be excellent.

The present study revealed a relationship between knee extension strength and activities of daily living related to the lower extremities of patients with dementia. Among the lower extremity functions, gait performance required the lowest strength level for knee extension. Approximately 70% of patients with a normalized knee extension strength of ≥0.6 Nm/kg were able to walk independently. However, approximately 70% of patients with a normalized knee extension strength of <0.6 Nm/kg could not walk independently. Dressing the lower body and using the toilet required a moderate strength level for lower extremity function. Approximately 70% of patients with a normalized knee extension strength of ≥0.8 Nm/kg could dress their lower body and use the toilet independently. In contrast, approximately 70 to 80% of patients with a normalized knee extension strength of <0.8 Nm/kg could not perform these tasks independently. Transferring to the bed/toilet/shower required the highest knee extension strength for lower extremity functions. Approximately 80% of patients with a normalized knee extension strength of ≥1.2 Nm/kg were capable of transferring to the bed/toilet/shower independently, whereas approximately 70% of patients with a normalized knee extension strength of <1.2 Nm/kg could not perform this task independently.

In the present study, threshold levels for knee extension strength in patients with dementia who could perform lower extremity activities independently were clearly shown. We believe that these threshold levels could contribute to the prediction of the extent or duration of the loss of lower extremity functions and lower limb weakness. Ultimately, these measurements will lead to an increasingly evidence-based approach for designing resistance training regiments for patients with dementia.

Liu and Latham suggest that performing progressive resistance training two to three times a week in older adults can improve physical function, reduce physical disability, improve some lower extremity functional limitations (i.e., balance, gait speed, timed walk, timed "up-and-go," sit-to-stand ability, and climbing stairs), and improve muscle weakness (Liu & Latham, 2009). Therefore, resistance training appears to be an appropriate intervention for older individuals to improve their performance in simple physical tasks. Despite the well established benefits of exercise training for the improvement of functional capacity in older people (Nelson et al., 2004), comparatively little research has been focused on patients with dementia. Only a few studies have been performed to investigate the feasibility of resistance training for these patients. Thomas and Hageman (Thomas & Hageman, 2003) evaluated the use of a brief resistance-exercise training intervention (three sessions per week over six weeks) to improve neuromuscular strength and function in the lower extremities of community-dwelling dementia patients. They reported some gains in muscle strength and functional performance. Teri et al. (2003) showed that home-based exercise training (performed over a three-month period), combined with teaching behavioral management techniques to caregivers, improved the physical health of and reduced the symptoms of depression in patients with dementia. Rolland et al. (2007) also reported the effectiveness of a simple exercise training program (one hour twice a week) over a one-year period in attenuating the decline in the patients' ability to perform activities of daily living. Recently, Santana-Sosa et al. (2008) showed that a relatively short-term, twelve-week training program combining resistance training with joint mobility and coordination exercises, all of which were performed in a nursing home with inexpensive equipment, significantly improved the overall functional capacity of patients with dementia. Functional improvements were shown in muscle strength, flexibility, agility and coordination while moving. There was also an improvement in the patients' abilities to perform activities of daily living independently (e.g., walking, rising from a chair, transferring from a bed to a chair, bathing, and dressing). Our results suggest that the period required to reach the threshold levels we have established can be estimated during resistance training programs. In addition, preventive training based on normalized knee extensor strength should be implemented for people with normalized knee extensor strengths near the 0.6 Nm/kg to 1.2 Nm/kg threshold.

The results of the present study suggest that threshold levels of knee extensor strength can be used to select individuals likely to require quadriceps strengthening. However, the distribution of test-retest differences in the subjects slightly increased with isometric knee extensor strength. Thus, caution is needed when interpreting the results of strength measurements when testing is carried out on subjects with a high strength level. Furthermore, the positive and negative predictive values for lower extremity functions were only 70% to 80%. Therefore, future studies are needed to investigate the reliability and validity of the HHD for use with multiple muscle groups. Such studies may yield a more comprehensive assessment of total body strength rather than just a single-joint assessment. In addition, further studies should assess whether changes in isometric strength as measured by HHD can reflect the ability of a subject to perform activities of daily life after resistance training.

ACKNOWLEDGMENT

The authors would like to acknowledge Ryosuke Yamamoto, Minako Nishikawa, Yuko Ishiguro,

Masami Suzuki and the staff at the Setagaya Municipal Kitazawa En for their helpful comments and suggestions regarding this study.

REFERENCES

Azegami, M., Ohira, M., Miyoshi, K., Kobayashi, C., Hongo, M., Yanagihashi, R., & Sadoyama, T. (2007). Effect of single and multi-joint lower extremity muscle strength on the functional capacity and ADL/IADL status in Japanese community-dwelling older adults. *Nursing & Health Sciences*, *9*, 168–176. doi:10.1111/j.1442-2018.2007.00317.x

Bartko, J. J. (1966). The intraclass correlation coefficient as a measure of reliability. *Psychological Reports*, *19*, 3–11.

Bennett, D. A., Beckett, L. A., Murray, A. M., Shannon, K. M., Goetz, C. G., Pilgrim, D. M., & Evans, D. A. (1996). Prevalence of parkinsonian signs and associated mortality in a community population of older people. *The New England Journal of Medicine*, *334*, 71–76. doi:10.1056/NEJM199601113340202

Bennett, D. A., Beckett, L. A., Wilson, R. S., Murray, A. M., & Evans, D. A. (1998). Parkinsonian signs and mortality from Alzheimer's disease. *Lancet*, *51*, 16–31.

Bland, J. M., & Altman, D. G. (1986). Statistical methods for assessing agreement between two methods of clinical measurement. *Lancet*, *1*, 307–310.

Bohannon, R. W. (1986). Test-retest reliability of hand-held dynamometry during a single session of strength assessment. *Physical Therapy*, *66*, 206–209.

Bohannon, R. W. (1995). Standing balance, lower extremity muscle strength, and walking performance of patients referred for physical therapy. *Perceptual and Motor Skills*, *80*, 379–385.

Boyle, P. A., Wilson, R. S., Buchman, A. S., Aggarwal, N. T., Tang, Y., & Arvanitakis, Z. (2007). Lower extremity motor function and disability in mild cognitive impairment. *Experimental Aging Research*, *33*, 355–371. doi:10.1080/03610730701319210

Brill, P. A., Drimmer, A. M., Morgan, L. A., & Gordon, N. F. (1995). The feasibility of conducting strength and flexibility programs for elderly nursing home residents with dementia. *The Gerontologist*, *35*, 263–266.

Cheng, P. T., Liaw, M. Y., Wong, M. K., Tang, F. T., Lee, M. Y., & Lin, P. S. (1998). The sit-to-stand movement in stroke patients and its correlation with falling. *Archives of Physical Medicine and Rehabilitation*, *79*, 1043–1046. doi:10.1016/S0003-9993(98)90168-X

Chino, N., Riu, M., Sonoda, S., & Domen, K. (2003). *Nosottyu Kanjya no Kino Hyoka*. Tokyo, Japan: Springer-Verlag.

Corrigan, D., & Bohannon, R. W. (2001). Relationship between knee extension force and stand-up performance in community-dwelling elderly women. *Archives of Physical Medicine and Rehabilitation*, *82*, 1666–1672. doi:10.1053/apmr.2001.26811

Franceschi, C., Bezrukov, V., Blanché, H., Bolund, L., Christensen, K., & de Benedictis, G. (2007). Genetics of healthy aging in Europe: The EU-integrated project GEHA (GEnetics of Healthy Aging). *Annals of the New York Academy of Sciences*, *1100*, 21–45. doi:10.1196/annals.1395.003

Goldman, W. P., Baty, J. D., Buckles, V. D., Sahrmann, S., & Morris, J. C. (1999). Motor dysfunction in mildly demented AD individuals without extrapyramidal signs. *Neurology*, *53*, 956–962.

Janssen, I., Heymsfield, S. B., & Ross, R. (2002). Low relative skeletal muscle mass (sarcopenia) in older persons is associated with functional impairment and physical disability. *Journal of the American Geriatrics Society*, *50*, 889–896. doi:10.1046/j.1532-5415.2002.50216.x

Janssen, I., Heymsfield, S. B., Wang, Z. M., & Ross, R. (2000). Skeletal muscle mass and distribution in 468 men and women aged 18-88 yr. *Journal of Applied Physiology*, *89*, 81–88.

Kinosian, B. P., Stallard, E., Lee, J. H., Woodbury, M. A., & Zbrozek, A. S., Glick, & H. A. (2000). Predicting 10-year care requirements for older people with suspected Alzheimer's disease. *Journal of the American Geriatrics Society*, *48*, 631–638.

Lamoureux, E. L., Sparrow, W. A., Murphy, A., & Newton, R. U. (2002). The relationship between lower body strength and obstructed gait in community-dwelling older adults. *Journal of the American Geriatrics Society*, *50*, 468–473. doi:10.1046/j.1532-5415.2002.50112.x

Lexell, J., Taylor, C. C., & Sjöström, M. (1988). What is the cause of the ageing atrophy? Total number, size and proportion of different fiber types studied in whole vastus lateralis muscle from 15- to 83-year-old men. *Journal of the Neurological Sciences*, *84*, 275–294. doi:10.1016/0022-510X(88)90132-3

Liu, C. J., & Latham, N. K. (2009). Progressive resistance strength training for improving physical function in older adults. *Cochrane Database of Systematic Reviews*, CD002759.

May, L. A., Burnham, R. S., & Steadward, R. D. (1997). Assessment of isokinetic and hand-held dynamometer measures of shoulder rotator strength among individuals with spinal cord injury. *Archives of Physical Medicine and Rehabilitation*, *8*, 251–255. doi:10.1016/S0003-9993(97)90029-0

McKhann, G., Drachman, D., Folstein, M., Katzman, R., Price, D., & Stadlan, E. M. (1984). Clinical diagnosis of Alzheimer's disease: Report of the NINCDS-ADRDA Work Group under the auspices of Department of Health and Human Services Task Force on Alzheimer's Disease. *Neurology*, *34*, 939–944.

Moreland, J. D., Richardson, J. A., Goldsmith, C. H., & Clase, C. M. (2004). Muscle weakness and falls in older adults: a systematic review and meta-analysis. *Journal of the American Geriatrics Society*, *52*, 1121–1129. doi:10.1111/j.1532-5415.2004.52310.x

Nelson, M. E., Layne, J. E., Bernstein, M. J., Nurenberger, A., Castaneda, C., Kaliton, D., … Fiatarone Singh, M. A. (2004). The effects of multidimensional home-based exercise on functional performance in elderly people. *Journals of Gerontology A Biological Sciences and Medical Sciences*, *59*, 154-160.

Nollet, F., & Beelen, A. (1999). Strength assessment in postpolio syndrome: Validity of a hand-held dynamometer in detecting change. *Archives of Physical Medicine and Rehabilitation*, *80*, 1316–1323. doi:10.1016/S0003-9993(99)90036-9

Okamoto, Y. (1992). Health care for the elderly in Japan: Medicine and welfare in an aging society facing a crisis in long term care. *British Medical Journal*, *305*, 403–405. doi:10.1136/bmj.305.6850.403

Ory, M., Kinney Hoffman, K., Hawkins, M., Sanner, B., & Mockenhaupt, R. (2003). Challenging aging stereotypes strategies for creating a more active society. *American Journal of Preventive Medicine*, *25*, 164–171. doi:10.1016/S0749-3797(03)00181-8

Piao, C., Yoshimoto, N., Shitama, H., Makino, K., Wada, F., & Hachisuka, K. (2004). Validity and reliability of the measurement of the quadriceps femoris muscle strength with a hand-held dynamometer on the affected side in hemiplegic patients. *Journal of UOEH*, *26*, 1–11.

Puthoff, M. L., & Nielsen, D. H. (2007). Relationships among impairments in lower-extremity strength and power, functional limitaitons, and disability in older adults. *Physical Therapy*, *87*, 1334–1347. doi:10.2522/ptj.20060176

Riddle, D. L., Finucane, S. D., Rothstein, J. M., & Walker, M. L. (1989). Intrasession and intersession reliability of hand-held dynamometer measurements taken on brain-damaged patients. *Physical Therapy*, *69*, 182–189.

Rolland, Y., Pillard, F., Klapouszczak, A., Reynish, E., Thomas, D., & Andrieu, S. (2007). Exercise program for nursing home residents with Alzheimer's disease: a 1-year randomized, controlled trial. *Journal of the American Geriatrics Society*, *55*, 158–165. doi:10.1111/j.1532-5415.2007.01035.x

Santana-Sosa, E., Barriopedro, M. I., López-Mojares, L. M., Pérez, M., & Lucia, A. (2008). Exercise training is beneficial for Alzheimer's patients. *International Journal of Sports Medicine*, *29*, 845–850. doi:10.1055/s-2008-1038432

Sato, T., Akatsuka, H., Kito, K., Tokoro, Y., Tauchi, H., & Kato, K. (1984). Age changes in size and number of muscle fibers in human minor pectoral muscle. *Mechanisms of Ageing and Development*, *28*, 99–109. doi:10.1016/0047-6374(84)90156-8

Scarmeas, N., Albert, M., Brandt, J., Blacker, D., Hadjigeorgiou, G., & Papadimitriou, A. (2005). Motor signs predict poor outcomes in Alzheimer disease. *Neurology*, *64*, 1696–1703. doi:10.1212/01.WNL.0000162054.15428.E9

Scarmeas, N., Hadjigeorgiou, G. M., Papadimitriou, A., Dubois, B., Sarazin, M., & Brandt, J. (2004). Motor signs during the course of Alzheimer disease. *Neurology*, *63*, 975–982.

Schaubert, K. L., & Bohannon, R. W. (2005). Reliability and validity of three strength measures obtained from community-dwelling elderly persons. *Journal of Strength and Conditioning Research*, *19*, 717–720.

Suomi, R., Surburg, P. R., & Lecius, P. (1993). Reliability of isokinetic and isometric measurement of leg strength on men with mental retardation. *Archives of Physical Medicine and Rehabilitation*, *74*, 848–852. doi:10.1016/0003-9993(93)90012-Y

Suzuki, M., Yamada, S., Inamura, A., Omori, Y., Kirimoto, H., Sugimura, S., & Miyamoto, M. (2009). Reliability and validity of measurements of knee extension strength obtained from nursing home residents with dementia. *American Journal of Physical Medicine & Rehabilitation*, *88*, 924–933. doi:10.1097/PHM.0b013e3181ae1003

Suzuki, M., Yamada, S., Omori, M., Hatakeyama, M., Sugimura, Y., Matsushita, K., & Tagawa, Y. (2008). Development of the upper-body dressing scale for a buttoned shirt: A preliminary correlational study. *American Journal of Physical Medicine & Rehabilitation*, *87*, 740–749. doi:10.1097/PHM.0b013e31818378b0

Taylor, D. H., & Sloan, F. A. (2000). How much do persons with Alzheimer's disease cost Medicare? *Journal of the American Geriatrics Society*, *48*, 639–646.

Teri, L., Gibbons, L. E., McCurry, S. M., Logsdon, R. G., Buchner, D. M., & Barlow, W. E. (2003). Exercise plus behavioral management in patients with Alzheimer disease: A randomized controlled trial. *Journal of the American Medical Association*, *290*, 2015–2022. doi:10.1001/jama.290.15.2015

Thomas, V. S., & Hageman, P. A. (2003). A preliminary study on the reliability of physical performance measures in older day-care center clients with dementia. *International Psychogeriatrics, 14*, 17–23. doi:10.1017/S1041610202008244

Thomas, V. S., & Hageman, P. A. (2003). Can neuromuscular strength and function in people with dementia be rehabilitated using resistance-exercise training? Results from a preliminary intervention study. *Journals of Gerontology A Biological Sciences and Medical Sciences, 58A*, 746-751.

Wikholm, J. B., & Bohannon, R. W. (1991). Hand-held dynamometer measurements: Tester strength makes a difference. *The Journal of Orthopaedic and Sports Physical Therapy, 13*, 191–198.

Wilson, R. S., Bennett, D. A., Gilley, D. W., Beckett, L. A., Schneider, J. A., & Evans, D. A. (2000). Progression of Parkinsonian signs in Alzheimer's disease. *Neurology, 54*, 1284–1289.

Wilson, R. S., Schneider, J. A., Bienias, J. L., Evans, D. A., & Bennett, D. A. (2003). Parkinsonianlike signs and risk of incident Alzheimers disease in older persons. *Archives of Neurology, 60*, 539–544. doi:10.1001/archneur.60.4.539

Wolfson, L., Judge, J., Whipple, R., & King, M. (1995). Strength is a major factor in balance, gait, and the occurrence of falls. *The Journals of Gerontology. Series A, Biological Sciences and Medical Sciences, 50*, 64–67.

KEY TERMS AND DEFINITIONS

Activities of Daily Living: Activities of daily living can be divided into basic activities of daily living and instrumental activities of daily living. Basic activities of daily living are self-maintenance skills such as dressing, using the toilet, transferring, and locomotion. Instrumental activities of daily living involve more complex activities, such as preparing a meal, handling finances, and shopping.

Bland-Altman Plots: Bland-Altman plots of the mean and SD of differences between trials determines the coefficient of repeatability. The plot of differences against the mean allows for the investigation of any possible relationship between the measurement error and the true value. If the mean difference is zero and 95% of the values lie within 2 SDs of the mean difference, the data can indicate that the test has repeatability.

Functional Independence Measure (FIM): FIM tallies 18 activities of daily living that are divided into six categories. Four involve motor functions, including self-care (eating, grooming, bathing, dressing the upper body, dressing the lower body, and using the toilet), sphincter control (bladder management and bowel management), mobility (transferring to a bed/chair/wheelchair, transferring to the toilet, and transferring to the tub/shower), and locomotion (walking or wheelchair propulsion and stair climbing).

Hand-Held Dynamometer (HHD): The HHD is used to quantify maximal strength and may offer several advantages over free weights, including ease of transport, efficiency and low cost.

Muscle Strength: Muscle strength can be defined operationally as the ability of a muscle or muscle group to exert maximal force in a single voluntary effort.

Negative Predictive Value: The negative predictive value represents the proportion of subjects who tested negative and were true negatives. A test with a high negative predictive value will provide a strong estimate of the number of people who do not have the target condition.

Positive Predictive Value: The positive predictive value estimates the likelihood that a person who tests positive actually has the target condition. Positive predictive value represents the proportion of subjects who tested positive and were true positives. Therefore, a test with a high positive predictive value will provide a strong estimate of the actual number of patients who have the target condition.

Reliability: Reliability assessment is used to determine the measurement consistency of an instrument. In a test-retest study, one sample of individuals is subjected to an identical test on two separate occasions while maintaining constant testing conditions.

Chapter 33
Music Therapy for Dementia Patients:
Tuned for Culture Difference

Yuki Tanaka
Tokyo Medical and Dental University, Japan

Hiroki Nogawa
Japan Medical Information Network Association, Japan

Hiroshi Tanaka
Tokyo Medical and Dental University, Japan

ABSTRACT

As the average life expectancy continues to rise, dementia has become a critical health care issue. At this situation, the effective management of dementia requires the development of rehabilitation methods for symptom relief in patients. This chapter hypothesizes that one such method, music therapy, could be improved by taking into account the cultural background of the patient, because musical preference is often dependent upon cultural context. This chapter investigates the effects of Japanese music on the alleviation of dementia symptoms in Japanese patients as compared to the effects of classical music.

The authors collected 87 volunteers including 79 dementia patients, 2 people under 65 years of age, 10 early-stage senior (65-74), and 66 late-stage seniors (>75). The volunteers listened to the following musical selections: two simple melodies of Japanese songs (major/minor with the same tonality) from Edokomoriuta (famous nursery songs in Japan), two songs from Kagomekagome (famous play songs in Japan), Touryanse (children's song widely played in Japan), and two original songs (major/minor) with the same tonality. We prepared two variations of classical musical scales: one in the scale of C major and the other in the scale of C minor. We observed their responses in two ways: the physiological response as determined by Near-Infrared Spectroscopy (NIRS), which measures changes in blood flow, and the subjective response as determined by questionnaires.

DOI: 10.4018/978-1-60960-559-9.ch033

Our results show that dementia patients tend to judge Japanese music as being played in a major key, while healthy subjects judged these songs as being in a minor key. Our results reveal characteristic responses of dementia patients to the Japanese music and provide evidence for the improvement of using music therapy for dementia patients by accounting for their Japanese culture.

INTRODUCTION

A. Research Theme

In this chapter, we discuss two research themes. The first theme is feasibility of music therapy for the precise and appropriate brain rehabilitation of dementia patients. The second theme is measurement of the objective and quantitative effectiveness of music therapy.

These studies are elementary steps toward the goal of our research is to quantify the response of the person when human hear music (see Figure 1), we use music as the input data and human responses as the output data.

B. Background

In recent years, the elderly portion of the population has increased significantly, leading to a related increase in the number of patients with dementia (Japanese Ministry of Health, Labour and Welfare, 2008; United Nations, 2004). This is the reason why prevention, effective rehabilitation and treatment/therapy for dementia are most required in super-aging society. While each of these aspects is equally important, this work focuses on the rehabilitation and treatment/therapy aspects of dementia.

One current method of rehabilitation and treatment/therapy for dementia is music therapy, which

Figure 1. Research aims: The major goal of this work is to objectively quantify both the musical input and the physiological output in response to music therapy

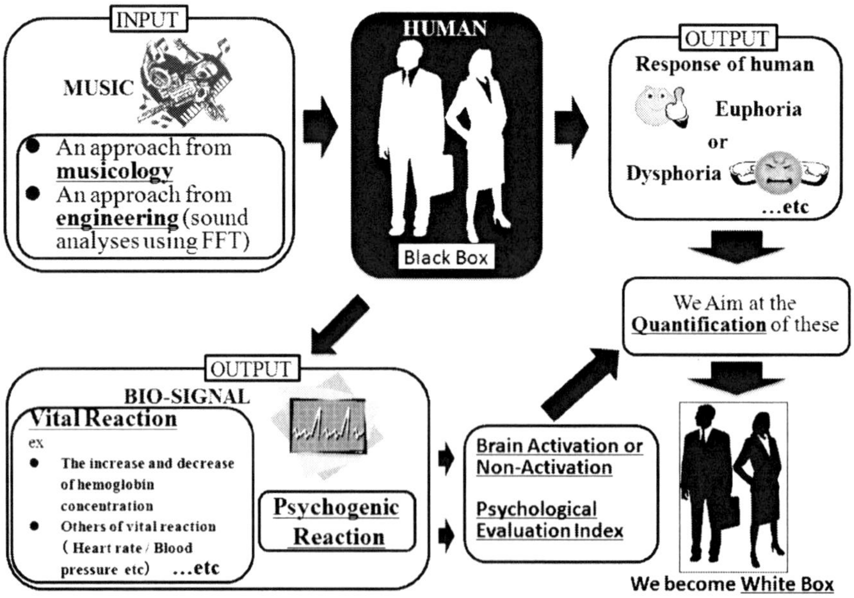

has some serious limitations (see Table 1) (Bando, 2008). Because, (1) The clinical response of the music therapy is thing which only persons who is in the settings realizes, (2) Music therapy is like trial and error, and (3) Music therapy doesn't have objective proof. This situation caused us to believe effectiveness of music therapy is to be proved. And we think music therapy is to be modified to each culture in which the patients live.

C. Conventional Research Details

Various studies have investigated the utility of music therapy in the alleviation of dementia. Several authors have proposed non-pharmaceutical methods for treating dementia (Allen, 1999; Opie, Rosewarne, & O'Connor, 1999), including music therapy for dementia patients (Raglio, & Gianelli, 2009). These reports suggest that dementia cared altered underlying physiologic, psychosocial, and environmental factors. Several empirical studies have reported significant effects of music therapy on dementia patients (Park & Pringle, 2009; Patricia, 1995). Music therapy has been shown to lower the agitation levels of patients. These showed that the music intervention is importance (Park, & Pringle, 2009; Patricia, 1995), facilitate the recollection of long-term memories (Gerdner, 2005), improve the management of verbally disruptive behavior and agitation levels fell significantly in response to both music therapy (Suparna, 2005; J Cohen-Mansfield, & Werner, 1997; Brotons, 1996) and the agitation levels fell using white noise (Burgio, Scilley, Hardin, Hsu, & Yancey, 1996). Studies using music therapy have reported an improvement in language functioning (Brotons, & Koger, 2000), a reduction in depressive symptoms (Ashida, 2000), an increased recognition of music-based exercises (Winckel, 2004), and a sparing of melodic recognition in dementia patients (Cuddy, & Duffin, 2005). The overarching aim of these studies is to reduce the burden of the care staff in charge of these patients. In other words, these studies do not examine music therapy as the brain rehabilitation for the patients. More importantly, these aren't objective but subjective.

Other studies on music therapy for dementia patients focus on the neurological aspects of processing musical input, specifically the role of the temporal lobes. These reports have shown that the auditory cortex influences recognition of pitch and tempo (Liegeois-Chauvel, Peretz, Babai, Laguitton, & Chauvel, 1998; Steinke, Cuddy, & Jakobson, 2001), and that the ability to understand a melody is reduced when the temporal lobe is damaged (Peretz, Kolinsky, Tramo, Labrecque, Hublet, Demeurisse, & Belleville, 1994). In these experiments, the patients had an injury to or excision of the temporal lobe. Other work has examined the relationship between psychological stress and music (Park, & Pringle Specht, 2009; Suda, Morimoto, Obata, Hideaki, & Maki, 2008). The application of music therapy led to a reduction in the levels of salivary cortisol, a stress hormone. In addition, several studies report significant emotional responses to music. Mental fatigue is reduced more by major modernusic than minor modernusic (Suda et al., 2008). In healthy adults, happy and sad moods are mediated by different neural correlates (Habel, Klein, Kellermann, Shah,

Table 1. The problems of Japanese music therapy

	Japan	Sample of other country (USA and UK)
License (Qualification)	Non	Non
System to promote the use and development of music therapy	Non	NCCAM in United States
		RCCM at United Kingdom
Insurance scores	Non	Music therapy can take insurance scores with condition in USA

& Schneider, 2005), and the retrieval of memories with happy or sad affects activates separate areas of the prefrontal and hippocampus (Markowitsch, Vandekerckhove, Lanfermann, & Russ, 2003). However, the mechanisms for musical processing and the generation of emotional responses to music in dementia patients are still unknown.

Several studies using Near-Infrared Spectroscopy (NIRS) (Tsunazawa, Oikawa, Iwamoto, Eda, & Takada, 1996) have been performed (Shimura, Tsunada, Maki, Suzuki, Haida, Kaneko, Yamazaki, Okuyama, Tanaka, Oshiro, Shigemori, Kondou, & Asakawa, 2009; Kono, Matsuo, Tsunashima, Kasai, Takizawa, Rogers, Yamasue, Yano, Taketani, & Kato, 2007; Leon-Carrion, Damas-Lopez, Martin-Rodriguez, Dominguez-Roldan, Murillo-Cabezas, Barroso-Martin, & Dominguez-Morales, 2008; Goto, Noda, Ichikawa, & Fujiwara, 2002). Again, these studies focus mainly on reduction of the burden on care staff, because reduction of nursing staff's burden was the most important in the conventional study. These studies reported the patients' stresses were effectively reduced, but failed to objectively show an increase of brain activity and effectiveness in rehabilitation. Moreover, the music used in these studies was selected without considering effect of each music (music choice is random or trial and error). Also, studies on music therapy for dementia patients were not objective but subjective. Only a few studies on dementia use NIRS; however, a recent trial study used NIRS to measure prefrontal lobe activity in dementia patients in Japan (Shimura et al., 2009). At these situations, we propose to objectively measure the effectiveness of musical therapy on dementia patients using NIRS.

D. Research Aims

In this chapter, we propose two hypotheses on music therapy for dementia. The first hypothesis is that effective brain rehabilitation will be represented by increased activity throughout the pre-frontal lobe after or during music therapy. The second hypothesis is that music therapy with Japanese music will be more effective for Japanese patients than classical music. Validation for our first hypothesis is found in the results of our previous work (Shimura et al., 2009). To support the second hypothesis, we present here a summary of the effects of Japanese music on Japanese patients with dementia.

THEORY

A. Music Therapy

Several definitions for music therapy exist. For the current report we will focus on the definition given by the Japanese Music Therapy Association (JMTA) and the National Association for Music Therapy (NAMT). These organizations define music therapy as a form of healthcare that uses music to address the physical, emotional, cognitive, and social needs of individuals of all ages. Music therapy improves the quality of life (QOL) for all persons and meets the needs of children and adults with disabilities or illnesses (NAMT career leaflet, 1980; Nuki, 1996). In essence, music therapy utilizes the multiple functions of music to address physical, psychological, social, and physiological needs for rehabilitation and healing of disease/ataxia and the improvement of patients' QOL. In clinical medicine, music therapy is one of several Complementary and Alternative Medicines (CAM). Music therapy has two distinct sub-types. The first is active music therapy, in which patients participate by playing a musical instrument, etc. and the second is passive music therapy, in which they only listen music. The other classification of music therapy is dividing into individual therapy and group therapy.

First, we discuss the reason why the music therapy is effective for the dementia patients. The three reasons are proposed for effective music therapy.

1. **Stimulation of memory recall:** Dementia patients often cannot recall recent memories and memories from the near past. However, they easily recall older memories, such as those from childhood under the correct conditions. Music therapy has been shown to stimulate the recollection of older memories.
2. **Stimulation by the rhythm (to have music):** The human body has several life-sustaining rhythms, such as heartbeat, blood pressure, breathing and temperature etc. These rhythms are vital, and as a result, the rhythm in music is shown to be stimulating even before a subject consciously recognizes the music.
3. **Stimulation by individual musical components:** Music has various components, including melody, harmony, and tonality. These components are proposed stimulate brain activity in dementia patients.

Music therapy has been shown to improve the function of both mind and body in dementia patients. This is the reason why music therapy and the process through which it affects patients are gradually attracting attention. (Nuki, 1996)

We give brief description of history of music therapy. Music therapy has demonstrated the close relationship between music and medicine. The use of the music therapy dates back to prehistory. Music has long been closely associated with both religion and medicine and was used as part of the dark arts. There are also records of music therapy in the Ethos theory of ancient Greece. In this theory, music was suggested have both ethical and psychological effects. Originally, the application of music for medical purposes was not systematic; current therapeutic methods developed over time. Modern music therapy began during World War II in a field hospital of the U.S. Army as a way to care for soldiers who suffered from great psychological damage. Music therapy facilitated the mental recovery of soldiers who had not been helped by medical treatment. Thereafter, utilizing a function for the music in a treatment purpose was termed "Music Therapy" in the 1950s.

B. Japanese Music: Comparison between Japanese music and Classical Music

Japanese music is one sub-category of ethnic music (also called as Folk music or World music). Here we define "ethnic music" as a traditional, culture specific musical genre, also referred to as aboriginality music, or developed from aboriginality music. Each country and local ethnicity hand down these music from generation to generation. Historically, ethnic music has included all types of culture specific music that did not originate in Europe. The common music of European (West Europe countries and North America) is referred to as classical music (also called as European art music, European classical music, or Western art music). Generally, "music" is equated with "classical music". Many researchers classify non-classical music based on the theory of classical music. Thus, we characterize Japanese music based on the theory of classical music in this chapter. In addition, we use common "Glossary of musical terms" for words on music.

The history of classical music developed from the 16th century until the early 20th century is classified in 4 stages: the Baroque period, the Classical period, the Romantic period, and the Impressionist period. To qualify as classical music, a musical selection must have four features:

1. The music must consist of the three main elements; rhythm, melody and harmony.
2. The tone (one set of pace class that related to frequency) divides an octave into twelve notes.
3. Classical music is derived from the seven original church modes (Gregorio modes): Lydian, Mixolydian, Aeorian, Locrian, Ionian, Dorian, Phrygian. Classical music consists of major key (Dur) and minor key

(moll), and they are only two survivors from original church mode.

4. The classical music has 30 keys (30 diatonic scale = 15 major scales + 15 minor scales).

Mode (musical mode) is different from scale (musical scale), but these terms are often confused. Scale refers to a group of tones (sounds) organized in an ascending and descending row, which rises or falls according to pitch. Mode is an integrated system made from scale; keeping consistent with other rule. Mode and scale differ on two major points; the limit of the range and the progression of sound.

Japanese music (KISHIBE Shigeo, 1998; Kazusige Chikamori, 2003 (1949); Yuuko Chiba, 2005; Yasuko Tsukahara, Toru Endo, Atsuko Sawada, Haruko Komoda, Hiroko Miura, Yumiko Tanaka, Mika Haikawa, Chie Hukuda, Tsuneko Tsukitani, Susumu Kumada, Hiroko Yamamoto, Rie Kouchi, 2007) is the traditional music developed in Japan, or general term of music that has been used in Japan. The most stringent definition of Japanese music is music formed during the *Edo* era, which lasted until the end of Japanese national isolation in the 19th century, and music from the national style that followed it. A wider definition of Japanese music includes music derived from the Japanese exposure to classical music. In Japan, the more narrow sense of Japanese music is referred to as "*Zyun-Hougaku,*" which means "pure traditional Japanese music," while the wider definition is called "*Shin-Nihon-Ongaku,*" or "new Japanese music". The history of Japanese music begins 1500 years ago, and various opinions on the history of Japanese music exist. Table 2 shows a brief summary of the history of Japanese music.

As noted in Table 2, *Gagaku* is the traditional court music (formal music). *Gagaku* is the oldest form of traditional music performed by an ensemble in the world and is referred to as "the world's oldest orchestra". *Zokugaku* is "popular music", developed among the common people rather than the *Kizoku* (Noble class). The history of these musical traditions is unclear, a systematic description of Japanese music has not been made. But mode of Japanese music is controlled by some not-clear rules (see Figure 2). Japanese music has three types of mode; *Gagaku* mode, *Zokugaku* mode, and *Okinawa* mode. For this study, we focused on *Zokugaku* mode. *Zokugaku* can be divided into *In-Senpou*, *You-Senpou* and *Yonanuki-Senpou*. *In-Senpou* was developed around metropolitan areas, such as *Kyoto*, we call *In-senpou* is Metropolitan mode (It is our notation). Major applications of Metropolitan mode are *Koto* (Japanese harp) and *Syamisen* (Japanese guitar) music. *You-Senpou* was developed in the countryside around Kyoto, we call *You-senpou* is Countryside mode (It is our notation). Countryside mode is used for folk song music, a genre that is rooted in the daily life of people. For example, these songs are used as prayers and thanks for a good harvest, to pray for a good bumper catch or for traditional festival dances (*Bon-odori*), etc. *Yonanuki-senpou* was developed after1800 A.D., we call the Modern mode (It is our notation). Many Japanese children's songs are written in this mode. In fact, many countries in the world use this mode in songs for children, including the folk music of Scotland, Ireland, and China. Table 3 summarizes the different classifications of Japanese music mode.

All Japanese music has seven common features:

1. Japanese music has no specific beat, while classical music has a specific rhythm.
2. Japanese music has no regular harmony, and there are a several discords. Classical music has very specific rules of harmony.
3. Almost Japanese music has minor mode in the meaning of melody in classical music.
4. Few Japanese music define strict tempos; instead the tempo changes in alone music is played.
5. No written scores of traditional Japanese music remain, because Japanese music is

Table 2. History of Japanese music

Period and Substance	Content or Record, etc.
1. **Native Music**	
Until around the 4th or 6th century; Probably consisted of simply music	**Content:** Details concerning this kind of native music are not clear.
	Record:
	Japanese mythology: *The legend of Amanoiwato: Amanouzume, the goddess of entertainment, danced in front of Amanoiwato, the cave made of rocks, to invite out Amaterasu, the sun goddess and the primary god in Japanese mythology, who was imprisoned in the Amanoiwato. Japanese mythology is written in Kojiki and Nihonshoki.*
	The Records of Three Kingdoms (3rd century A.D.): *An official history book of China. In the queendom of Queen Himiko of the third century, the people sang and danced at a funeral services.*
	Excavated artifacts from the remains of the Jomon & Yayoi period and the ancient tomb period. (3rd century B.C. – 7th century A.D.): *Doutaku (Bronze bell-shaped vessel), Ishibue (Stone flute), Tuchibue (Soil flute), Koto, Haniwa (Clay image figure which beats a drum or plays a Koto etc.)*
2. **Transmission of continental music**	
From the end of the Burial Mound age to Asuka & Nara era: 7th century - 9th century (*Gagaku, Seimei, Biwa, Zokugaku*)	**Content:** Entertainment was transmitted from the China Continent; The basics of *Gagaku* had been established.
	Record:
	Taiho Codes (701 A.D.): *Taiho Codes are full-scale legal codes to of Ritsu (Criminal law) and Rei (Civil law / Commercial law). The oldest official Japanese record of music was written in the Taiho Codes. The legal codes of the Gagaku post of the Imperial Court. The Gagaku post was a compilation of foreign music and secular music and used to make Imperial Court music (Gagaku).*
	Kojiki (712 A.D.) and Nihonshoki (740 A.D.): *Kojiki* is the oldest Japanese history book presented to the Emperor. *Nihonshoki* is the oldest official history book for international presentation. The oldest song records of Japanese music are the songs in the *Kojiki* and *Nihonshoki.*
3. **Ethnic music**	
From the *Heian* era to the *Edo* era: 10th century – 19th century (*Heike, Sarugaku,* Soukyoku, *Ziuta, Zyoururi, Nagauta,* etc.)	***Heian* era (10th century-12th century):**
	Import of Chinese cultures had been remarkably discontinued (the stop of envoy to the China Tang Dynasty), which courted the establishment of Japanese native music
	During the period of *Heian*, the Japanese digested, absorbed, followed and learned Chinese music, and established Japanese native music. (*Heian* nationalism)
	The *Kizoku* (Noble class) predominated: *Gagaku* and *Seimei* (*Seimei* is Religious music that added melody to Buddhist Scriptures).
	Zokugaku (Popular music) emerged from commoners.
	***Kamakura & Muromachi* era (12th century- 16th century):**
	The *Kizoku* were ruined.
	Samurai predominated.
	Music was formed to reflect the taste of the Japanese race and climate (Aboriginality).
	Sarugaku, the vanguard of the *Noh. Noh* are the traditional arts of Japan. *Noh* is one of the United Nations Educational, Scientific and Cultural Organization (UNESCO) forms of immaterial cultural heritage. *Heikebiwa:* Chanting of *Heike monogatari.* It was derived from a *biwa* (Japanese lute) of the *Gagaku*
	***Edo* era (16th century-19th century):**
	Samurai predominated.

continued on following page

Table 2. Continued

Period and Substance	Content or Record, etc.
	Sakoku (National isolation) began in fast *Edo* era.
	The culture of *Samurai* and the common citizen became popular.
	Japanese music began to diversify.
	Zyoururi: The accompaniment by a musical instrument is *samisen*, the music that a *tayu* talks about in the literature. *Ziuta*: Music using *samisen* which developed in the upper regions, such as Kyoto and Osaka. *Soukyoku:* Music to play with a Sou=*Kot. Nagauta*: The music that developed in Tokyo.
4. **The introduction of classical music**	
After the Meiji era: late 19th century; Shin-Nihon-Ongaku (New Japanese Music)	The Japanese learned Western classical Music.
	Japanese music and classical music begin to fuse.
	New Japanese music, which partly fuses Japanese native music and Western classical music, emerges.

In this table only summary of Japanese music history is shown.
This Table omits *Okinawa*, because *Okinawa* music has a separate history.

taught primarily through oral instruction and demonstration

6. The basic scale of Japanese music is a pentatonic scale, i.e., songs are comprised of five tones.
7. Japanese music does not necessarily end at the tonal center of a musical mode (Ex. Kimigayo: The national anthem of Japan), in contrast to most classical music pieces.

METHOD

We show 4 experiments. (A) is Analysis of Japanese music, (B) - (1) is Experiment using Questionnaires, (B) - (2) is Experiment using NIRS, and (B) – (3) is Analysis of Japanese music and NIRS Data.

Musical pieces from seven scales were used: five from a Japanese scale and two from a clas-

Figure 2. Mode of Japanese music: (A) In-Senpou (Metropolitan Mode); (B) You-Senpou (Countryside Mode); (C) Major of Yonanuki-Senpou (Major of Modern mode); (D) Minor of Yonanuki-Senpou (Minor of Modern mode); (E) Okinawa. These musical scales are written with a key of C as the root.

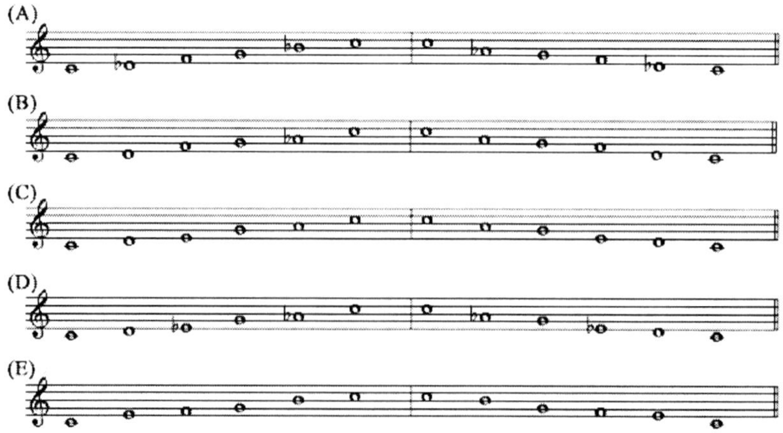

Table 3. Classification of Japanese music mode

	Gagaku	*Zokugaku*				*Okinawa NiRoNuki*-**Senpou**
		In-Senpou	*You-Senpou*	*YoNaNuki-Senpou*		
				major	**minor**	
Scale	Twelve scale ≒Twelve equitempered scale	Pentatonic scale	Pentatonic scale	Pentatonic scale	Pentatonic scale	Pentatonic scale
Mode	minor	minor	minor	Approximate major	Approximate minor	major
History	Old > 1000 yeas	Old > 1000 yeas	Old > 1000 yeas	New 19th: Meiji era. 100 yeas	New 19th: Meiji era. 100 yeas	14th ~15th century
Place	Court	Metropolitan	Countryside	All	All	Only Okinawa
Influenced by	Chinese, but it has developed originally.	Original development	Original development	Classical music	Classical music	Original development
Famous Song	*Kimigayo:* The national anthem of Japan	*Touryanse:* The children's song widely played in Japan from old days	*Kagomekagome:* "Song of the barrier play" during the Edo period	*Edokomoriuta:* The folklore song that is a popular lullaby in Japan	*Edokomoriuta*	*Texinsagunuhana:* song of *Bon* festival dance in Okinawa
Our Notation	*Gagaku*	*Metropolitan Mode*	*Countryside Mode*	*major of Modern mode*	*minor of Modern mode*	*Okinawa*

The score of a famous song refers to Figure 3. (See Figure 3)

sical scale. Of the five music played, three were children's songs and two were original pieces (Table 4). The Japanese scales were presented in Metropolitan mode, Countryside modernajor of Modern moderninor of Modern mode; and *Okinawa* mode. The classical scales included C-dur (major) and c-moll (minor). The children's songs were *Edokomoriuta* (the best known folklore song which is a popular lullaby in Japan) using Modern mode, *Touryanse* (the song of the barrier play from the Edo period) using Metropolitan mode, and *Kagomekagome* (a traditional children's song) using Countryside mode. The two original songs were written in the Modern mode. The use of original music was used to determine the effect of recollection on the subjects' reactions.

The music score was shown Figure 2 and Figure 3.

A. Analysis of Japanese Music

For this analysis, we analyzed the characteristics of Japanese music using by (1) theoretical value and (2) actual values.

A-1. Analysis Using Theoretical Values

The theoretical value of the sound (scale) is found in expression. The theoretical value of the sound (scale) is found in expression. The frequency of an unknown sound is determined in equation (1). In the formula (1), "The frequency of an unknown sound" is Y and "one step smaller than Y sound" is X. The common reference tone is A_4 (440Hz).

$$Y = X \times 2^{\frac{1}{12}}$$

Table 4. Musical pieces

Title	Mood	Summary
Scale	Metropolitan	*m2 M3 M2 m3 M2*
	Countryside	*M2 m3 M2 m3 M2*
	Modern	Using two moods "major scale and minor scale". major: *M2 M2 m3 M2 m3* minor: *M2 m2 M3 m3 M2*
	Okinawa	*M3 m2 M2 M3 m2*
	Classical music	Using two moods "C-dur(major)and c-moll(minor)" major: *M2 M2 m2 M2 M2 M2 m2* minor: *M2 m2 M2 M2 m2 aug2 m2*
Edokomoriuta (lullaby)	Modern	*Edokomoriuta* is the folklore song that is a popular lullaby in Japan.
		This song was composed during the Edo period and was transcribed by *Kousaku Yamada* during the Meiji period.
		The minor song in Modern mode, *Edokomoriuta* is generally sung.
Touryanse	Metropolitan	*Touryanse* is written as "Song of the barrier play" during the Edo period.
		It was arranged by Nagayo Motoori in the Taisho Era.
Kagomekagome	Countryside	*Kagomekagome* is a children's song widely played in Japan from old days.
Original music	Modern	This original music was written in the Modern mode for this experiment by Yuki.T (the author).
		In this experiment, the same original music was transposed to both major and minor mode.
		"Original music" is used to examine whether the subject's reaction depends on the memories of the music played.

* The degree of the music theory. "M" = "major" (For example, M2 is degree of two major), "m" = "minor", "aug" = "augumented".

A-2. Analysis Using Actual Values

This analysis is based on the performance data. An authentic recording of a musical instrument (piano) is played and the signal is processed using FFT. The results are calculated in a power spectrum.

To indicate the results of the long sound data, we deteriorated the sound and the data of the recording. The data included the sampling frequency (44100 Hz to 4000 Hz), and channel (at 2 ch to 1 ch). The sampling period (Δt [s]) and the number of the bits were fixed at 0.00025 [s] and 16 bits, respectively.

B-1. Experiment Using Questionnaires

In this experiment, we used questionnaires to examine the subjective responses to music therapy.

B-1-1. Subjects

Eighty-six volunteers, including seventy-eight dementia patients, were surveyed for this study (Table 5). Dementia patients were grouped by the Degree of Required Care (DRC: Japanese systems), which divides the users of care service into five levels of Required Care (RC) and two Requiring Support (RS). The lightest level is RS1, and the heaviest is RC 5. In this study, 37 participants were RC 1, 22 participants were RC 2, 16 were RC 3, and 2 participants were categorized as RC 4. Each group has a corresponding average mini-mental state examination (MMSE) score, which is listed in Table 5.

Prior to the experiments, subjects were given an explanation of the work, and all volunteers signed consent forms. For patients with dementia, family members signed the consent forms.

Figure 3. Music score: (A) Kimigayo; (B) Touryanse; (C) Kagomekagome; (D) Edokomoriuta (major and minor); (E) Texinsagunuhana; (F) Original Music. Kimigayo is made from Gagaku. Touryanse is made from the Metropolitan mode. Kagomekagome is made from Countryside mode. Edokomoriuta is made from the major or minor Modern mode. Texinsagunuhana (Fork song of Okinawa) is made from Okinasa. The original music for this experiment was written in both the major and minor mode of the Modern mode by Yuki.T (author).

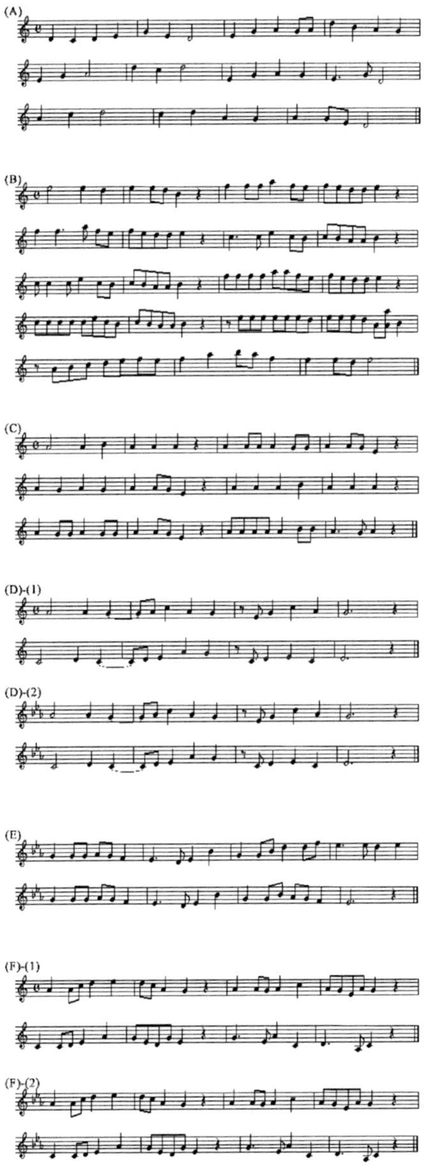

B-1-2. Questionnaires

The questionnaires contained four questions to be answered for each musical piece:

1. Do you know this music? I "know" it or I "do not know" it.
2. Do you like this music? I "like" it or I "do not like" it.
3. How do you think of melody of this music? "Bright" or "Dark".
4. How do you feel when you hear this music? "Happy" or "Sad".

"How do you think of melody of this music?" and "How do you feel when you hear this music?" are equivalent to "rhythm" and "melody" in the three primary elements of classical music, rhythm, melody and harmony. In addition, the questionnaire was done by Japanese language.

B-1-3. Calculation

In the questionnaires, answers on the left ([1] know, [2] like, [3] Bright, [4] Happy) rate as positive, and answers on the right ([1] Do not know, [2] Do not like, [3] Dark, [4] Sad) are negative. The positive rate was found by using equation (2).

$$\text{The positive rate [\%]} = \frac{\text{The number of positive respondents}}{\text{The number of the effective respondents}} \times 100$$

We also calculated the coefficient of correlation for each question.

B-2. Experiment Using NIRS

In this experiment, we used NIRS to measure objective responses to music therapy.

Table 5. the subjects

Degree of Requiring care Lv. (MMSE)	RC 1 (19.7)	RC 2 (17.2)	RC 3 (16.6)	RC 4 (13.0)	Other (-)	Total
Day Service A	18	11	10	1	0	40
Day Service B	19	11	6	1	1 (RS 1)	38
Other (healthy)	0	0	0	0	8	8
Total	37	22	16	2	9	86

B-2-1. Subjects

The six volunteers included an 81-year old RC2 dementia patient, two subjects under 65 years of age, one early-stage senior (65-74), and two late-stage seniors (>75).

B-2-2. Equipment and Measurement Location

The experimental procedure used was the non-invasive monitoring of tissue oxygenation by NIRS. The device is OM-220 that is the product of SHIMADZU CORPORATION. OM-220 has two probes. We measured two locations on the prefrontal lobe (Fp1 and Fp2 of the international ten-twenty electrode system). We focused on the concentration of total hemoglobin ($C_{total-Hb}$), because brain activity is correlated with increases in total blood volume.

The experiment consisted of two repeated tasks: a 90 s dying rest task and the music task. The dying rest task requires subjects to close their eyes and attempt to think about nothing. We took the rest time between the tasks, because we make the brain of subjects take a rest.

B-2-3. Calculation

Figure 4 shows example data from an NIRS time-series on a dementia patient. Using these data, we calculated the $\overline{\Delta C_{total-Hb}}$ (Figure 5), the activated value (AV : $\Delta C_{total-Hb}$), and the activated percent

Figure 4. A sample of NIRS time-series data. (Relax time: subjects close their eyes and rest for 30 s. Music time: one phrase of music)

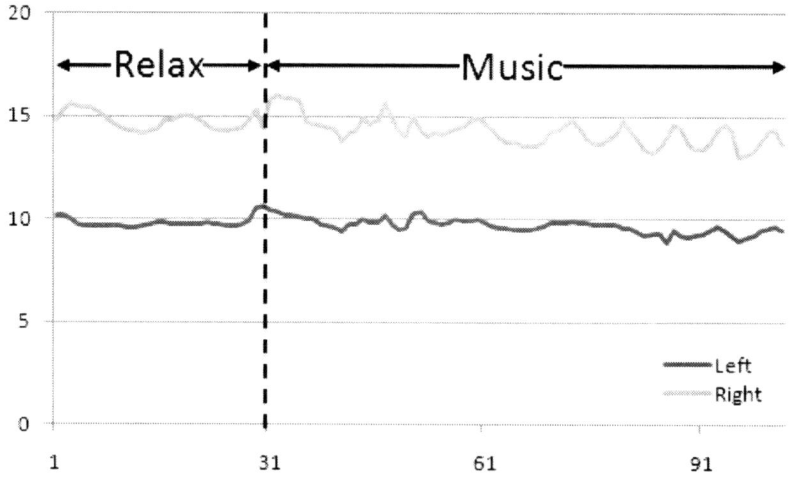

(AP) using equations (3), (4), and (5), respectively (Shimura et al., 2009)

$$\Delta C_{\text{total-Hb}} = C_{\text{total-Hb}}(t_i)_{(\text{music})} - \overline{C_{\text{total-Hb(relax)}}}$$

$$AV = \overline{\Delta C_{\text{total-Hb}}} = \sum \frac{C_{\text{total-Hb}}(t_i)_{(\text{music})} - \overline{C_{\text{total-Hb(relax)}}}}{n}$$

$$AP[\%] = \frac{\overline{\Delta C_{\text{total-Hb}}}}{\Delta C_{\text{total-Hb(relax)}}} \times 100[\%]$$

B-3. Analysis of Japanese Music and NIRS Data

We found linear approximations by the least square method using NIRS data. We compared our previous analysis of Japanese music with these data.

RESULTS

A. Analysis of Japanese Music

A-1. Analysis by Theoretical Values

Figure 6 shows the classification of Japanese modes by the classical theoretical frequency. As a result, we can compare the Countryside mode with the minor of Modern mode, and the Metropolitan mode with major of Modern mode. Our results are similar to those found elsewhere, but this is the first numerical representation of these kinds of data. The pentatonic scale has three degrees, both major and minor. Only the *Okinawa* mode was found to be structurally heterogeneous with the same Japanese scale. The three degrees in the pentatonic scale is distinct from a classical scale because the classical scale is a diatonic scale. The augumented 2 degree (= agrees theoretically with minor 3) which is present in the melodic minor. This could be one of the reasons that the minor key of classical music resembles Japanese music.

Figure 5. Activation calculations for the time-series data. The activation of the time-series data ($\Delta C_{total\text{-}Hb}$) was calculated by subtracting the average data from the relaxing task from the data from music task

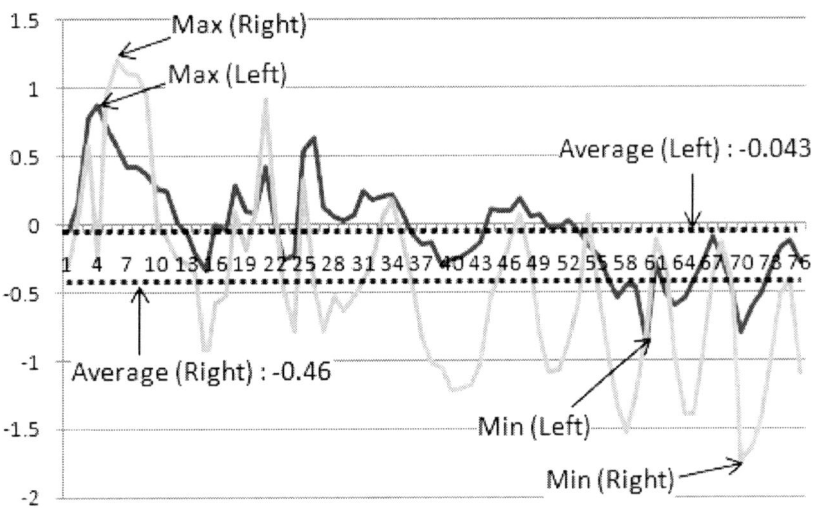

Figure 6. Music classification using the theory frequency. The sign of the figure is the degree of the music theory. Each circle (a solid line, a dashed line, a dotted line) expresses the same degree.

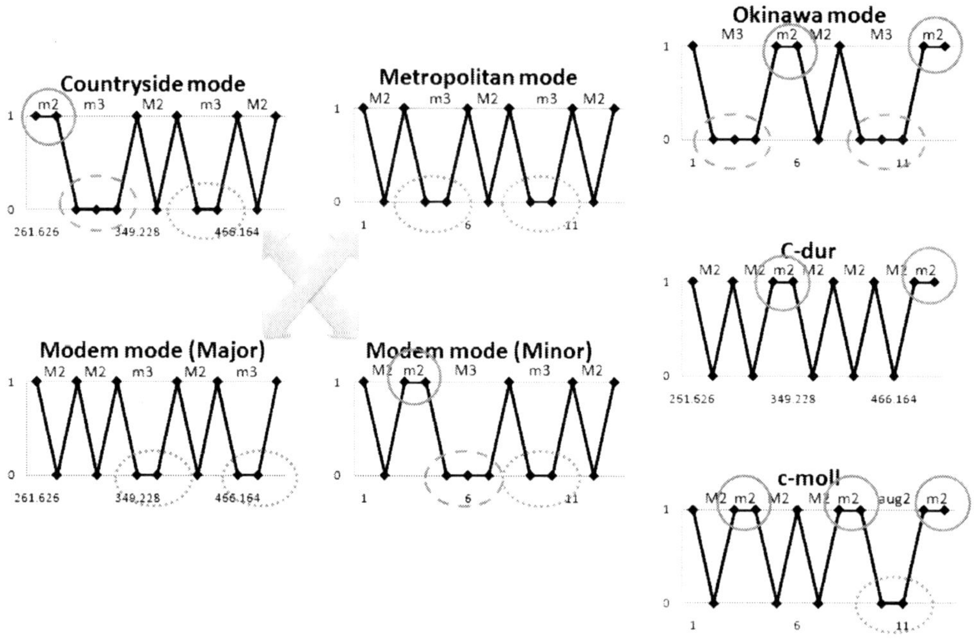

A-2. Analysis by Actual Values

Figure 7 shows an example of a power spectrum. Table 6 shows the analysis of the components of the power spectrum. We found that the maximum spectrum was characteristic: the maximum spectrum in the Countryside mode and the Metropolitan mode was "G", the maximum spectrum in the

Figure 7. A sample spectrum. Basic frequencies of C4 (261.626Hz) - C5 (523.252Hz). Other frequencies are included in harmonic overtones in this experiment

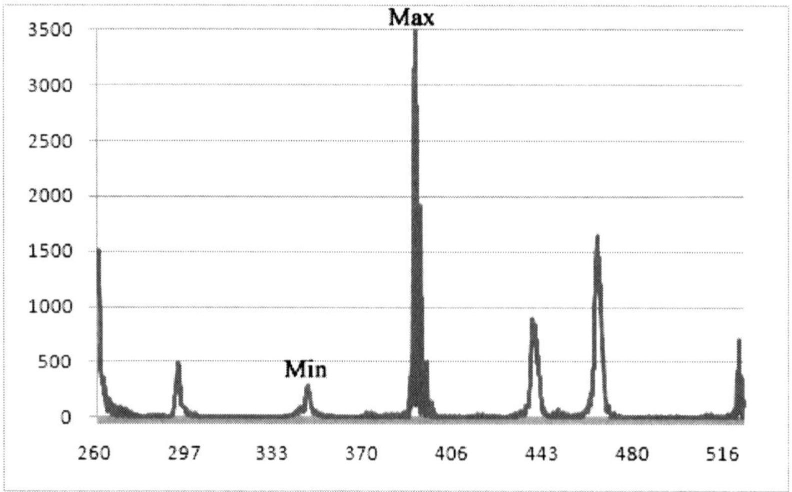

Table 6. A portion of the power spectrum component analysis

	Number	Max	>						Min
Countryside mode	7	390.63 (G)	464.36(Ais)	260.5 (C)	438.23 (A)	521.73 (C)	292.48 (D)		345.95 (F)
Metropolitan mode	7	390.14 (G)	275.15(Cis)	260.01 (C)	413.82 (As)	522.45 (C)	346.19 (F)		463.13 (Ais)
major of Modern mode	6	437.26 (A)	323.73(E)	260.01 (C)	292.97 (D)	521.48 (C)			391.36 (G)
minor of Modern mode	6	412.30 (As)	310.55(Es)	390.87 (G)	260.01 (C)	521.24 (C)			292.24 (D)
Okinawa	6	491.45 (H)	390.87(G)	346.92 (F)	260.01 (C)	328.37 (E)			521.97 (C)
C-dur	8	438.96 (A)	292.97(D)	327.64 (E)	260.01 (C)	348.39 (F)	491.94 (H)	388.18 (G)	521.73 (C)
c-moll	8	413.82 (As)	309.54(Es)	293.21 (D)	260.01 (C)	492.68 (H)	348.14 (F)	385.99 (G)	521.97 (C)
Kagomekagome	1	439.15 (A)							
Touryanse	6	328.61 (E)	439.21(A)	346.68 (F)	293.21 (D)	260.01 (C)			492.19 (H)
major of Modern mode of *Edokomoriuta*	5	260.15 (C)	438.23(A)	292.97 (D)	327.88 (E)				518.07 (C)
minor of Modern mode of *Edokomoriuta*	5	260.15 (C)	309.08(Es)	293.21 (D)	413.33 (As)				518.07 (C)

major of Modern mode and C-dur was "A", and the maximum spectrum in the major of Modern mode and c-moll was "As", and the maximum spectrum in *Okinawa* mode was "H".

Furthermore, we found the correlation of the spectrum for each scale. The correlation of the Countryside mode and the Metropolitan mode was 0.56. The major of Modern mode and C-dur had a correlation of 0.80, and the minor of Modern mode and c-moll had a correlation of 0.75. Other combinations did not yield correlations.

Also, we analyzed the correlation between spectrum melody and scale. As the result, the correlation between the major of Modern mode of *Edokomoriuta* and the major of Modern mode was 0.633. The minor of Modern mode of *Edokomoriuta* and the minor of Modern mode had a correlation of 0.467. As a result, we can quantify how often a sound is used.

We also calculated the basic statistics of the FFT results. We found that a similar nature of scale and melody leads to similar results. The statistic of the *Okinawa* mode is different from the tendency of the statistic of other modes.

B-1. Experiments Using Questionnaires

Figure 8 shows the results of the subjective questionnaires. The results from questions [3] and [4] in the known music are represented in Figure 11. We found that similar responses were given to the original musical pieces; however, in the case of the classical scale, dementia patients were able to differentiate between major and minor keys. In other words, the dementia patients rated the Japanese melodies as consistently positive, but in classical scale, patients were able to identify

Figure 8. Questionnaire results: (A) Touryanse; (B) Kagomekagome; (C) Edokomoriuta (major and minor); (D) Original Music; (E) Classical scales

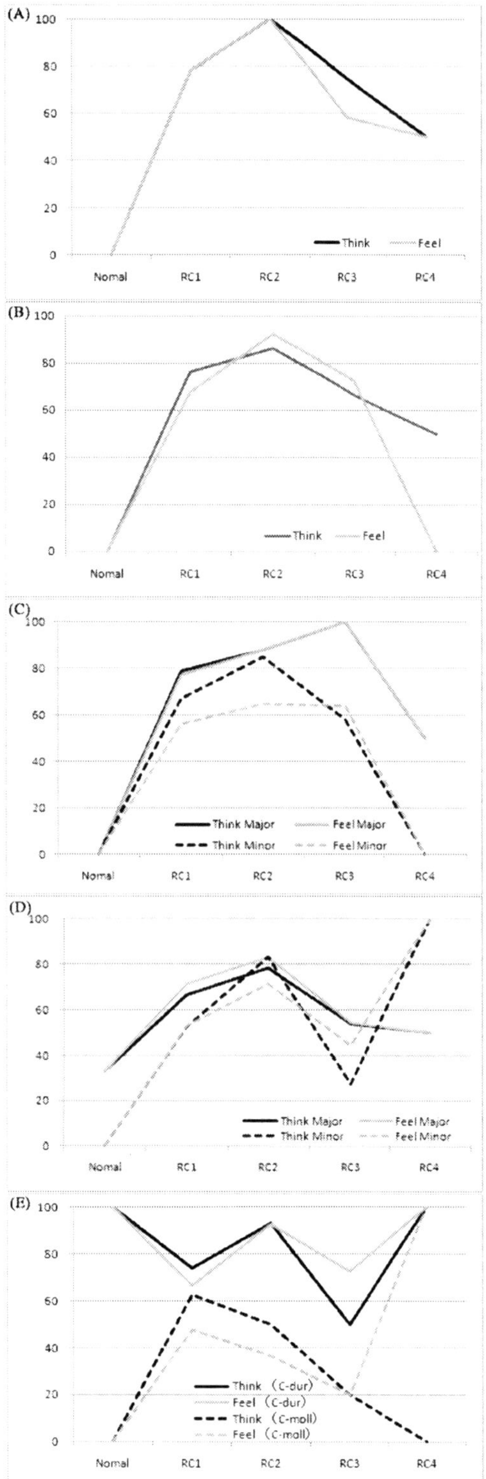

the key. The positive rate was close to 100% in the RC 2 group, a pattern that also carried over to the original music pieces.

We calculated the correlation between FEEL and THINK (Figure 9) in the questionnaires. A positive rate (>0.5) was calculated for 8/8 songs in the RC 1group, 6/8 in RC 2, 7/8 in RC 3, and 0/8 in RC 4. Healthy subjects did not show a positive rate correlation.

B-2. Experiments Using NIRS

The AP_{normal} calculation in dementia patients indicated prefrontal lobe activation in response to the minor of Modern mode of *Edokomoriuta* and c-moll. The prefrontal lobes in non-dementia (healthy) subjects activated in response to the minor of Modern mode of *Edokomoriuta.* We also examined the difference between the APs. ($AP_{difference}$: $AP_{difference}$ is calculated by "$AP_{difference} = AP_{Maximum} - AP_{Minimum}$".) A large $AP_{difference}$ indicated that the subject's brain was activated (up and down) in response to the music. This implied subjects' brain was judging / thinking well. The dementia patient showed a large difference in $AP_{difference}$ in both prefrontal lobes (particularly left brain) in response to all music (particularly *Edokomoriuta* and c-moll). Healthy elderly subjects showed a large difference in the $AP_{difference}$ of the left prefrontal lobe (see Table 7 and Table 8).

B-3. Analysis of Japanese Music and NIRS Data

Figure 10 shows an example of the linear approximations. We compare the analysis of Japanese music (Table 6) with these linear approximations (Table 9). The slope of the linear approximations was positive in the minor of Modern mode of *Edokomoriuta* and c-moll. As can be seen in Table 6, the maximum spectacle was "As (A flat)" both the minor of Modern mode of *Edokomoriuta* and c-moll, although their scale has "Es (E flat)".

Figure 9. The correlation between FEEL and THINK from questionnaires. Positive rate (>0.5) was 8/8 songs for the RC 1 group, 6/8 for RC 2 group, 7/8 for RC 3 group, and 0/8 for RC 4 group. Healthy subjects showed no positive correlations

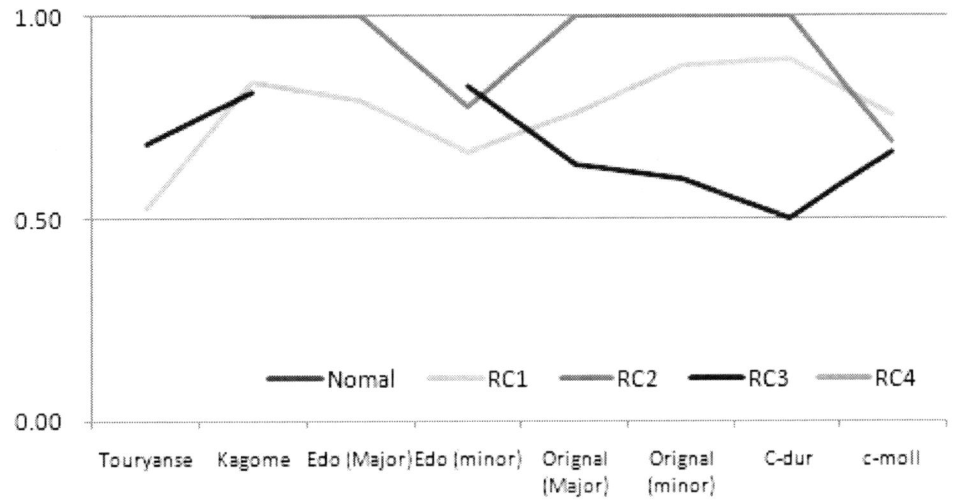

DISCUSSION

We performed Fast Fourier Transform (FFT) for data on Japanese music and scales. We found that scales of the same nature of scales yielded similar results. From this, we inferred that patterning of the music would be possible. Correlations were found between the Countryside mode and the Metropolitan mode, the major of Modern mode and C-dur, and the minor of Modern mode and c-moll. Correlations were not found for other groups. We also calculated the correlation of the spectrum for melody and scale. These results agree

Table 7. Result of $AP_{average}$ by NIRS

			Edokomoriuta **(major)**	*Edokomoriuta* **(minor)**	*Touryanse*	*Kagomekagome*	**Original (major)**	**Original (minor)**	**C-dur**	**c-moll**
Dementia	RC2 81	Left	99.56	96.35	**101.66**	**101.64**	**100.61**	**100.16**	**101.47**	**106.33**
		Right	96.89	99.01	97.66	99.86	98.65	86.78	**102.82**	**109.26**
Healthy	79	Left	97.86	**111.64**	**101.27**	99.66	97.67	**148.96**	**142.18**	**110.84**
		Right	**101.18**	**101.82**	**100.5**	**101.11**	**101.61**	**102.99**	**103.56**	**102.93**
	78	Left	99.25	**101.31**	96.75	**102.08**	99.84	**100.31**	**101.83**	**104.6**
		Right	94.94	96.27	98.04	99.48	98.9	98.75	98.07	95.59
	70	Left	90.79	**149.89**	**100.77**	**113.62**	99.82	**106.87**	84.85	97.69
		Right	98.91	**103.98**	**100.69**	99.42	98.43	99.3	97.64	92.05
	57	Left	98.87	**100.98**	**101.81**	98.19	98.13	96.85	96.24	94.19
		Right	**101.78**	**101.38**	**100.82**	99.64	97.69	**100.43**	99.26	96
	34	Left	96.93	**101.72**	**101.1**	97.82	**100.82**	98.78	98.97	99.11
		Right	**100.96**	**101.97**	**101.46**	**100.19**	**100.68**	**101.09**	99.63	**101.03**

The **Bold Text** represents an average: $AP_{average}$ over 100%

Table 8. Result of $AP_{diffelence}$ *by NIRS*

			Edokomoriuta (major)	*Edokomoriuta* (minor)	*Touryanse*	*Kagomekagome*	Original (major)	Original (minor)	C-dur	c-moll
Demen-tia	RC2 81	Left	**18.12**	**26.97**	8.89	**12.4**	**14.39**	**18.07**	**17.28**	**16.68**
		Right	**19.91**	**26.68**	**15.93**	**13.12**	**13.74**	**50.85**	**27.36**	**52.84**
Healthy	79	Left	**53.63**	**12.39**	**87.46**	**87.31**	**76.67**	**67.6**	**64.09**	**60.06**
		Right	3.51	3.43	3.09	5.24	3.62	3.09	3.52	4.29
	78	Left	8.34	**24.44**	**14.49**	**12.29**	**13.75**	**21.88**	**11.54**	**42.13**
		Right	6.98	**13.44**	**11.24**	7.25	8.91	**10.68**	5.83	**13.4**
	70	Left	**63.75**	**153.62**	**75.45**	**90.34**	**40.68**	**40.84**	**72.85**	**36.34**
		Right	8.28	**10.37**	9.48	8.19	6.52	**11.08**	9.86	**13.32**
	57	Left	2.66	9.48	9.24	8.38	9.59	7.87	7.03	3.43
		Right	2.47	5.33	3.29	8.28	7.88	6.73	5.34	3.99
	34	Left	7.34	6.7	3.22	3.15	4.37	7.41	2.52	5.61
		Right	4.36	2.43	1.67	2.68	3.66	2.88	0.71	2.29

The **Bold Text** represents differences: $AP_{difference}$ over 10%

Table 9. Linear approximations

Music	The right Brain		The left Brain	
	Linear Approximations	Dominant probability	Linear Approximations	Dominant probability
Kagomekagome	y = -0.0067x + 0.36	0.00	y = -0.0046x + 0.13	0.20
Toryanse	y = 0.0003x + 0.14	0.00	y = -0.0094x + 0.04	0.73
major of Modern mode of *Edokomoriuta*	y = -0.0114x + 0.40	0.00	y = -0.0185x + 0.25	0.04
minor of Modern mode of *Edokomoriuta*	y = -0.0067x - 0.06	0.54	y = 0.018x - 0.87	0.00
C-dur	y = -0.0039x + 0.31	0.00	y = -0.0126x + 0.97	0.00
c-moll	y = -0.002x + 0.59	0.00	y = 0.018x + 0.26	0.35

with classical music theory. We can be used to determine how often a sound is used.

"Positive rate (with formula (2))" to the Japanese music made a constant move at THINK and FEEL. In other words, the dementia patients recognize that music in minor key is actually music in major key in Japanese music. But dementia patients were able to distinguish the key of classical scale. So, we could make model that how to catch the key of Japanese music (Figure 11).

Conversely we suspect dementia in elderly people who respond with "a major key" (Bright, Happy etc) to Japanese music. The responses for "FEEL" and "THINK" showed a clear correlation. This shows that dementia patients do not experience a contradiction in connection with the key of the music. However, the true is complete opposite for healthy subjects.

Dementia patients showed elevated brain activity in response to *Edokomoriuta* and c-moll, and responded to songs played in a minor key. Also,

Figure 10. Linear approximations using the least square method: (A) Touryanse; (B) Kagomekagome; (C) Major mode of Edokomoriuta; (D) Minor mode of Edokomoriuta; (E) Scale of C-dur; (F) Scale of c-moll. The degree of leaning of the approximate line shows a positive value for the minor mode of Edokomoriuta and the scale of c-moll. Both the minor mode of Edokomoriuta and the scale of c-moll have a maximum power spectrum of As tone (415.305Hz) and a second power spectrum of Es tone (311.127Hz)

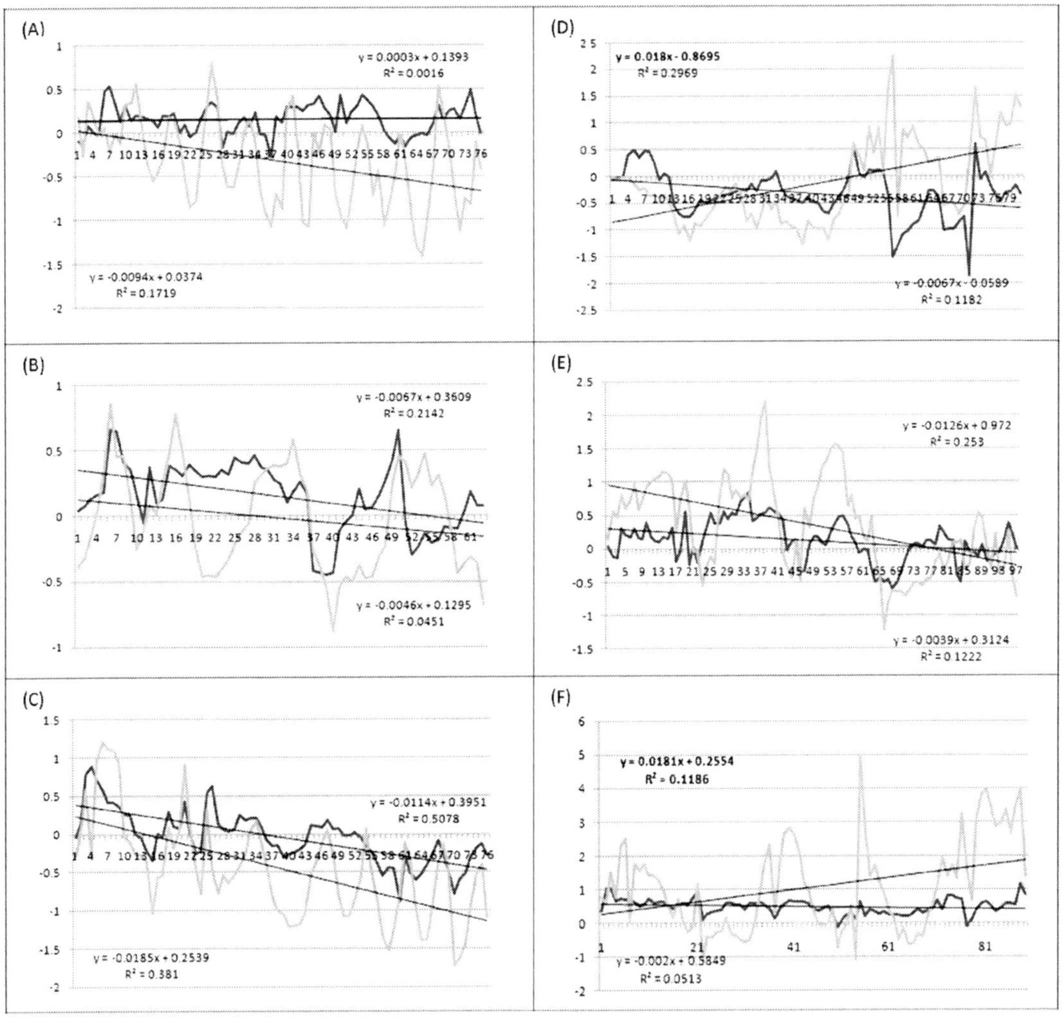

both prefrontal lobes in the dementia patients, particularly the left brain, moved the brain well (increases of concentration of total hemoglobin) in all music. In healthy elderly subjects, the right prefrontal lobe moved the brain well in all music. From this we infer that the subjects' brain was actively judging or thinking. It suggests that the left prefrontal lobe is dominant in recollection for healthy elderly subjects, while the right prefrontal lobe is dominant in recollection for dementia patients.

The slope of linear approximations had positive values in the minor Modern mode of *Edokomoriuta* and c-moll. The maximal spectrum is "As" in both the minor of Modern mode and c-moll, and their scales have Es. This suggests that there is a particular frequency (a tone) that generates a large response in dementia patients.

Figure 11. Proposed model for identifying the key in Japanese music. The dementia patients feel Japanese music with minor mode to be in the major key

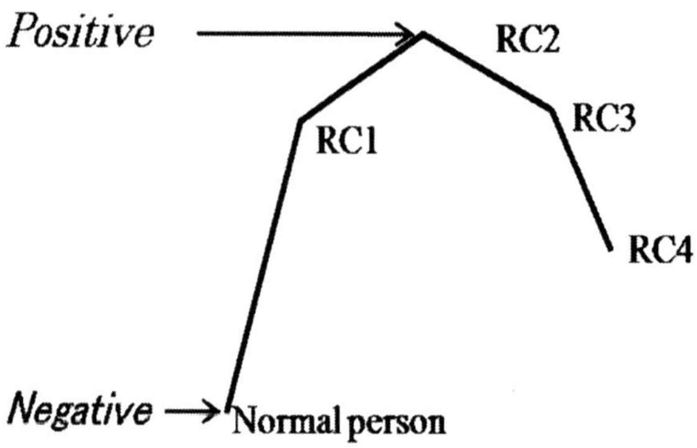

We summarize our results as follows:

1. The patterning of music is possible.
2. The prefrontal lobe is activated by music therapy.
3. Dementia patients recognize that Japanese music (in generally, key of Japanese music is minor) is key of major.
4. For Japanese dementia patients, Japanese music was shown to be effective in music therapy.
5. A specific frequency was found that generates the greatest response in dementia patients (According to this experiment, it's "As" and "Es".)

According to our results, we suggest that music therapy using Japanese music is more effective than the conventional music therapy for Japanese dementia patients.

ACKNOWLEDGMENT

The author is grateful to Ms. Eriko Okuyama and Takaki Shimura, PhD for assistance with experiments. We also wish to thank the staff and patients of Tomizuka park town day service center and Kamijima harmony town service center. We thank Mr. Osamu Fukuda of Industry research institute for the laboratory equipment. Finally we thank all of the volunteers.

REFERENCES

Allen, L. A. (1999). Treating agitation without drugs. *The American Journal of Nursing*, *99*(4), 36–42. doi:10.2307/3472232

Ashida, S. (2000). The effect of reminiscence music therapy sessions on changes in depressive symptoms in elderly persons with dementia. *Journal of Music Therapy*, *37*(3), 170–182.

Bando, H. (2008). Current status of music therapy. *Japanese Journal of Complementary and Alternative Medicine*, *5*(1), 27–36. doi:10.1625/jcam.5.27

Brotons, M. (1996). The effects of music therapy intervention on agitation behaviors of alzheimer's disease patients. *Journal of Music Therapy*, *33*(1), 2–18.

Brotons, M., & Koger, S. M. (2000). The impact of music therapy on language functioning in dementia. *Journal of Music Therapy*, *37*(3), 183–195.

Burgio, L., Scilley, K., Hardin, J. M., Hsu, C., & Yancey, J. (1996). Environmental white noise: An intervention for verbally agitated nursing home residents. *The Journals of Gerontology. Series B, Psychological Sciences and Social Sciences*, *51*(6), 364–373.

Cabinet Office, Government of Japan (Ed.). (2009). *The white paper on aging society in Heisei-era 21*. Oita, Japan: Saiki printing Co. Ltd.

Chiba, Y. (2005). *Nihon-Ongaku ga Wakaru Hon*. Tokyo, Japan: *Ongaku tomo sya corp.*

Chikamori, K. (2003, 1949). *New revised music introduction*. Tokyo, Japan: Ongaku tomo sya corp.

Cohen-Mansfield, J., & Werner, P. (1997). Management of verbally disruptive behaviors in nursing home residents. *The Journals of Gerontology. Series A, Biological Sciences and Medical Sciences*, *52*(6), 369–377.

Cuddy, L. L., & Duffin, J. (2005). Music, memory, and Alzheimer's disease: Is music recognition spared in dementia, and how can it be assessed? *Medical Hypotheses*, *64*, 229–235. doi:10.1016/j.mehy.2004.09.005

Gerdner, L. A. (2005). Use of individualized music by trained staff and family: Translating research into practice. *Journal of Gerontological Nursing*, *31*(6), 22–30.

Goto, Y., Noda, R., Ichikawa, Y., & Fujiwara, M. (2002). Cerebral circulation of consciousness disorder patient using near-infrared spectroscopic topography during brain rehabilitation by music exercise therapy. *International Congress Series*, *1232*, 549–554. doi:10.1016/S0531-5131(01)00689-6

Habel, U., Klein, M., Kellermann, T., Shah, N. J., & Schneider, F. (2005). Same or different? Neural correlates of happy and sad mood in healthy males. *NeuroImage*, *126*(1), 206–214. doi:10.1016/j.neuroimage.2005.01.014

Kono, T., Matsuo, K., Tsunashima, K., Kasai, K., Takizawa, R., & Rogers, M. A. (2007). Multiple-time replicability of near-infrared spectroscopy recording during prefrontal activation task in healthy men. *Neuroscience Research*, *57*(4), 504–512. doi:10.1016/j.neures.2006.12.007

Leon-Carrion, J., Damas-Lopez, J., Martin-Rodriguez, J. F., Dominguez-Roldan, J. M., Murillo-Cabezas, F., Barroso-Martin, J. M., & Dominguez-Morales, M. R. (2008). The hemodynamics of cognitive control: The level of concentration of oxygenated hemoglobin in the superior prefrontal cortex varies as a function of performance in a modified Stroop task. *Behavioural Brain Research*, *193*(2), 248–256. doi:10.1016/j.bbr.2008.06.013

Liegeois-Chauvel, C., Peretz, I., Babai, M., Laguitton, V., & Chauvel, P. (1998). Contribution of different cortical areas in the temporal lobes to music processing. *Brain*, *121*(10), 1853–1867. doi:10.1093/brain/121.10.1853

Markowitsch, H., Vandekerckhove, M., Lanfermann, H., & Russ, M. (2003). Engagement of lateral and medial prefrontal areas in the ecphory of sad and happy autobiographical memories. *Cortex*, *39*(4), 643–665. doi:10.1016/S0010-9452(08)70858-X

NAMT career leaflet. (1980).

Nuki, M. (1996). *Music therapy for the aged*. Tokyo, Japan: Ongaku no tomo sya corp.

Opie, J., Rosewarne, R., & O'Connor, D. W. (1999). The efficacy of psychosocial approaches to behaviour disorders in dementia: A systematic literature review. *The Australian and New Zealand Journal of Psychiatry*, *3*, 789–799. doi:10.1046/j.1440-1614.1999.00652.x

Park, H., & Pringle, P. S. (2009). Effect of individualized music on agitation in individuals with dementia who live at home. *Journal of Gerontological Nursing*, *35*(8), 47–56. doi:10.3928/00989134-20090706-01

Park, H., & Pringle Specht, J. K. (2009). Effect of individualized music on agitation in individuals with dementia who live at home. *Journal of Gerontological Nursing*, *35*(8), 47–55. doi:10.3928/00989134-20090706-01

Patricia, A. T. (1995). Effects of calming music on the level of agitation in cognitively impaired nursing home residents. *American Journal of Alzheimer's Disease and Other Dementias*, *10*(1), 10–15. doi:10.1177/153331759501000105

Peretz, I., Kolinsky, R., Tramo, M., Labrecque, R., Hublet, C., Demeurisse, G., & Belleville, S. (1994). Functional dissociations following bilateral lesions of auditory cortex. *Brain*, *117*(6), 1283–1301. doi:10.1093/brain/117.6.1283

Raglio, A., & Gianelli, M. V. (2009). Music therapy for individuals with dementia: Areas of interventions and research perspectives. *Current Alzheimer Research*, *6*, 293–301. doi:10.2174/156720509788486617

Shigeo, K. (1998). *The traditional music of Japan*. Tokyo, Japan: Ongaku no tomo sya.

Shimura, T., Tsunada, T., Maki, A., Suzuki, T., Haida, M., Kaneko, M., et al. Asakawa, T. (2009). *Prefrontal lobe measurement using near infrared spectroscopy-evaluation of early detection methods and rehabilitation methods of dementia*. Tokyo, Japan: Corona Publishing Co, Ltd.

Steinke, W. R., Cuddy, L. L., & Jakobson, L. S. (2001). Dissociations among functional subsystems governing melody recognition after right-hemisphere damage. *Cognitive Neuropsychology*, *18*(5), 411–437.

Suda, M., Morimoto, K., Obata, A., Koizumi, H., & Maki, A. (2008). Emotional responses to music, towards scientic perspectives on music therapy. *Neuroreport*, *19*(18), 75–78. doi:10.1097/WNR.0b013e3282f3476f

Suparna, M. (2005). Music intervention for disruptive behaviors in long-term care residents with dementia, *Annals of Long-Term Care, 13*.

Tsunazawa, Y., Oikawa, Y., Iwamoto, S., Eda, H., & Takada, M. (1996). Spatially resolved spectroscopy for extracting spectrum of hemoglobin diluted in a highly scattering medium, biomedical optical spectroscopy and diagnostics. In Sevick-Muraca, E., & Benaron, D. (Eds.), *Biomedical optical spectroscopy and diagnostics: Technical digest* (pp. 119–121). Washington, DC: Optical Society of America.

Tukahira, Y., Endo, T., Sawada, A., Komoda, H., Miura, H., & Tanaka, Y. … Kouchi, R. (2007). *A basic glossary of terms of the Japanese music*. Tokyo, Japan: Ongaku tomo sya corp.

United Nations (Ed.). (2004). *World population to 2300*. New York, NY: Bernan Assoc.

Winckel, A. V. (2004). Cognitive and behavioral effects of music-based exercises in patients with dementia. *Clinical Rehabilitation*, *18*(3), 253–260. doi:10.1191/0269215504cr750oa

KEY TERMS AND DEFINITIONS

Brain Rehabilitation: Treatments that are designed to help recover cerebral function. Many researchers think that brain rehabilitation is important because dementia is primarily a disorder of cerebral function.

Classical Music: Classical music refers to art music from Western European countries and North America. The history of classical music developed from the 16th century until the early 20th century. The general term "Music" is usually equated with "Classical music ".

Ethnic Music: "Ethnic music" is culture-specific traditional music handed down by each country and local race. Historically, Ethnic music consists of all culture specific music that did not originate in Europe, while the common music of Western Europe and North America is referred to as classical music (European art music / European classical music / Western art music).

Japanese Music: Japanese music that is subcategory of ethnic music developed in Japan, or more generally, music that has been used in Japan. The basic scale of Japanese music is a pentatonic scale, which means the music is composed of five tones. Japanese music is more than 1500 years old. *Gagaku* is one kind of Japanese music and is the oldest form of traditional music to be performed by an ensemble in the world. It is often referred to as the world's oldest orchestra.

Music Therapy: Music therapy is one form of brain rehabilitation. Music therapy is a healthcare procedure that uses music to address physical, emotional, cognitive, and social needs in individuals of all ages.

NIRS (Near-Infrared Spectroscopy): NIRS is spectrometry measured in the near-infrared light domain. NIRS measurements of brain activity are non-invasive and relatively unrestrictive. They can be used to objectively quantify the effectiveness of brain rehabilitation. The use of NIRS for measuring brain activity in dementia patients is attracting attention. Recently, a trial study of NIRS measurements in the prefrontal lobes of dementia patients was performed in Japan.

Questionnaires: For this method, experimenters distribute answer sheets on which response choices are written and then the answers are analyzed. Questionnaires yield only subjective data. Because the experimenter cannot fully gauge the response of a subject (comfortable or uncomfortable, etc.) by brain measurements alone, the subjective data are essential to developing a complete response profile.

Super-Aging Society: As the average life-span increases, the elderly portion of the population increases, and the number of dementia patients increases accordingly.

Chapter 34
Development of Neurorehabilitation Techniques Using Transcranial Magnetic Stimulation with Voluntary Muscle Contraction

Tetsuo Touge
Health Sciences, School of Nursing, Faculty of Medicine, Kagawa University, Japan

Shin Morita
Division of Rehabilitation, Kagawa University Hospital, Japan

Eiji Yamada
Division of Rehabilitation, Kagawa University Hospital, Japan

Takashi Kusaka
Maternal Perinatal Center, Faculty of Medicine, Kagawa University, Japan

ABSTRACT

The objective of this study was to elucidate the mechanism of transcranial magnetic stimulation (TMS) with maximum voluntary muscle contraction (MVC) (used to facilitate motor neuron function), the effects of magnetic stimulation at the foramen magnum level with MVC were tested by recording motor evoked potentials (MEPs) and the maximum muscle force. In addition, changes in regional cerebral blood flow (rCBF) due to TMS to the motor cortex during MVC were assessed using near infrared spectroscopy (NIRS). Three MEPs in the first dorsal interosseus (FDI) muscle elicited by TMS to the motor cortex or foramen magnum stimulation were recorded before and then at 15 minutes intervals for

DOI: 10.4018/978-1-60960-559-9.ch034

1 hour after 4 MVCs (while subjects maximally pinched a strain-gauge transducer for 2 seconds). Five healthy volunteers received TMS to the left motor cortex while maximally grasping a hand dynamometer for 2 seconds 3 times at 10-second intervals and then repeated TMS with MVC 4 times within 1 hour. Oxy-hemoglobin (Hb) and deoxy-Hb levels were recorded at 24 scalp sites using NIRS while subjects grasped a hand dynamometer with MVC for 5 seconds before and after TMS with MVC. Foramen magnum stimulation with MVC significantly decreased MEP amplitudes after TMS with MVC for 1 hour. Oxy-Hb concentration of the left M1, subtracting the right M1, tended to increase after TMS with MVC. The present results suggest that TMS during MVC induces increased cortical motor neuron excitability. However, further studies are needed to elucidate the mechanism of how TMS with MVC might modulate cortical neuron excitability.

INTRODUCTION

Transcranial magnetic stimulation (TMS) is a non-invasive method that allows the stimulation of cortical neurons; the electrical currents in axons stimulated by TMS activate cortical neuron cell bodies via synaptic transmission (Baker, Jalinous, & Freestone, 1985; Baker, 1991). A single TMS can transiently inhibit cortical neuron excitability for 1-5 ms after stimulation or facilitate excitability for 10-15 ms after stimulation (Kujirai et al., 1993). Further robust effects on cortical neuron excitability are achieved by repetitive stimulation of cortical neurons with TMS (rTMS) (Touge, Gerschlager, Cordivari, Brown, & Rothwell, 2001; Ikeguchi et al., 2005). The effects of rTMS on the brain were confirmed in animal experiments and in human studies by measuring regional cerebral blood flow (rCBF) or metabolism and recording electrical brain potentials or motor evoked potentials (MEPs) in voluntary muscles (Fox et al., 1997; Paus et al., 1997, 1998; Siebner et al., 2000). There has been a great deal of work dedicated to demonstrating the benefits of TMS or rTMS for treating patients with motor disability (Mally, & Stone, 1999; Ikeguchi et al., 2003; Hamada, Ugawa, Tsuji, & The effectiveness of rTMS on Parkinson's disease study group, 2009). However, the effects of TMS and rTMS on patients have been limited to a very short period after the stimulation and have been too weak to induce sufficient clinical outcomes.

A previous study by Urbach, Berth, & Awiszus (2005) reported that giving three single TMSs combined with the maximum voluntary muscle contraction (MVC) to patients with weakness of thigh muscles transiently (but significantly) increased muscle power. However, the effects of TMS with MVC have never been established, and the mechanism is still unknown. In the present study, we report a method of TMS with MVC that was able to induce more prolonged effects on motor neuron function. Furthermore, we evaluated the effects of magnetic brainstem stimulation at the foramen magnum level during MVC on motor evoked potentials (MEPs) and on muscle force in an attempt to explain the mechanism for how TMS with MVC modulates motor neuron function. In addition, we measured rCBF using near-infrared spectroscopy (NIRS) before and after TMS with MVC, to further explore the mechanism of activation of cortical motor neurons. NIRS is a recently developed non-invasive method for measuring oxygenized (oxy) and deoxygenized (deoxy) hemoglobin (Hb) in the cortex (Holper, Biallas, & Wolf, 2009; Nambu, et al., 2009).

The preliminary results of the present study have been reported previously in the International Symposium on Complex Medical Engineering (CME2009), held April 9-11, 2009 in Arizona (Touge, Urai, & Shimamura, 2009).

EXPERIMENT

Subjects and Methods

Nine normal subjects (7 females and 2 males) consented to participate in the study. This study was approved by the local ethics committee of our institution.

Subjects performed MVC for 2 s by using the right thumb and index finger to pinch a button-like strain-gauge transducer 1.5 cm in diameter (9E01-L2, NEC San-ei, Japan) with maximum force. In the initial session, each MVC was repeated 4 times with an interstimulus interval of 10 s.

To induce MEPs in the right first dorsal interosseus (FDI) and the thenar (TH) muscles, either the left motor cortex or the brainstem at the foramen magnum level were stimulated using a single pulse magnetic stimulator (SMN-1200, Nihon-olden, Japan) according to the method described by Ugawa, Uesaka, Terao, Hanajima, & Kanazawa (1994). Magnetic stimulation was delivered 1 s after subjects started MVC, using a round coil for TMS or a figure-8 coil for foramen magnum stimulation (FMS).

Three MEPs and pinching forces during MVC were recorded 5 minutes before and just after the initial 4 MVC session, then every 15 minutes after the trials for 1 hour (test condition). For control conditions, three MEPs were recorded 5 minutes before and 1 hour after the 4 trials of MVC. For the other MEP recordings, sham TMSs were delivered during the 3 MVC trials (Figure 1).

Four normal subjects (2 females and 2 males) consented to participate in a preliminary study for measuring rCBF using NIRS. As a trial of MVC, subjects grasped a hand dynamometer with their right hands for 2 seconds upon verbal cues from an operator, and repeated it 3 times at 10-second intervals. TMS was performed using a single pulse magnetic stimulator (SMN-1200, Nihon-olden, Japan). Subjects received magnetic stimulation to the motor cortex of the right hand with an intensity of 110% of the active motor threshold 1 second after the onset of MVC. Three TMSs with MVC were repeated at intervals of 15 minutes for 1 hour, while MEPs were recorded in the right first dorsal interosseus (FDI) and the thenar (TH) muscles.

Oxy- and deoxy-Hb in the cortex were measured using near infrared spectroscopy (NIRS)

Figure 1. Experimental time schedule

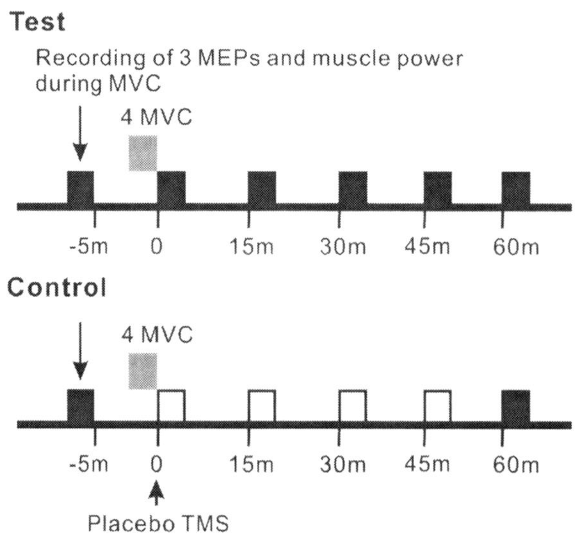

before and after TMS with MVC for 1 hour. Subjects sat in a chair and had a custom-made probe cap attached (which covered the bilateral M1 areas). Using an NIRS station (Shimazu Co, Japan), NIRS was recorded at 24 scalp sites according to the international 10-20 system while subjects grasped a hand dynamometer in their right hands with MVC for 5 seconds; this was repeated three times with 30 second breaks.

Blood oxy-, deoxy- and total Hb concentration were measured during MVC 3 times before and after TMS with MVC in off-line, and the data were averaged. In addition, the data from the left MI area (Ch3) minus the data from the right MI area (Ch17) were examined.

Amplitudes and areas of the three MEPs, as well as the voltages of the pinching force in each recording session were measured and averaged off-line. The data were statistically analyzed using repeated application of analysis of variance (ANOVA) and Tukey's post-hoc analysis.

RESULTS

Changes in the MEP amplitudes or areas in the FDI muscle differed significantly between the test and control conditions ($P<0.02$). Under test conditions, post-hoc analysis showed that MEP amplitudes or areas in the FDI muscle significantly increased 1 hour after TMS with MVC compared to the MEPs measured before TMS ($P<0.01$). The test condition exhibited a significant difference in the pinching muscle force compared to the control condition ($P<0.01$). In the post-hoc analysis, there was no significant change in the pinching muscle force of each condition.

Changes in MEP amplitudes or areas were significantly different between the FMS and control conditions ($P<0.001$). MEP amplitudes in the FDI muscle significantly decreased 1 hour after 4 MVCs ($P<0.05$). The pinching muscle force was not significantly affected by the FMS treatment.

There were no significant changes in the blood oxy-, deoxy-, or total Hb concentrations in the left motor cortex induced by TMS with MVC (Figure 2). However, the difference in the oxy-Hb concentrations of the left motor cortex and the right motor cortex increased after TMS with MVC compared to data taken before TMS with MVC (Figure 3). The hand gripping power tended to decrease 1 hour after TMS with MVC. The MEP amplitudes in the hand muscles did not show any significant changes.

CONCLUSION

The present study showed that TMS to the motor cortex with MVC transiently increased the MEP amplitude. This result corresponds to a previous report, which documented an enhancement of the MVC force and voluntary activation (VA) of the quadriceps femoris muscles using TMS with MVC in normal subjects (Urbach, & Awiszus, 2002). The present study showed the novel finding that foramen magnum stimulation with MVC applied intermittently for 1 hour significantly decreased MEP amplitudes in the FDI muscle, but did not change the pinching muscle force. Therefore, the decreased MEP amplitudes by foramen magnum stimulation with MVC suggest an inhibition of spinal motor neuron excitability and that the effect of TMS with MVC can be ascribed to a supraspinal event.

TMS to the motor cortex with MVC transiently increased the blood oxy-Hb concentration in the motor cortex. Increased blood oxy-Hb concentration appears to reflect increased cortical neuron excitability or synaptic activity in the motor cortex (Holper, Biallas, & Wolf, 2009). However, the present study showed the most robust changes of oxy-Hb concentration when we subtracted the oxy-Hb concentration data in the right motor cortex from the data in the left motor cortex. This result indicates that NIRS data were affected by blood pressure or cerebral blood flow and suggests

Figure 2. Changes in oxy-Hb concentration at the left M1 (CH 3) and the right M1(CH17) before and after TMS with MVC in a subject.

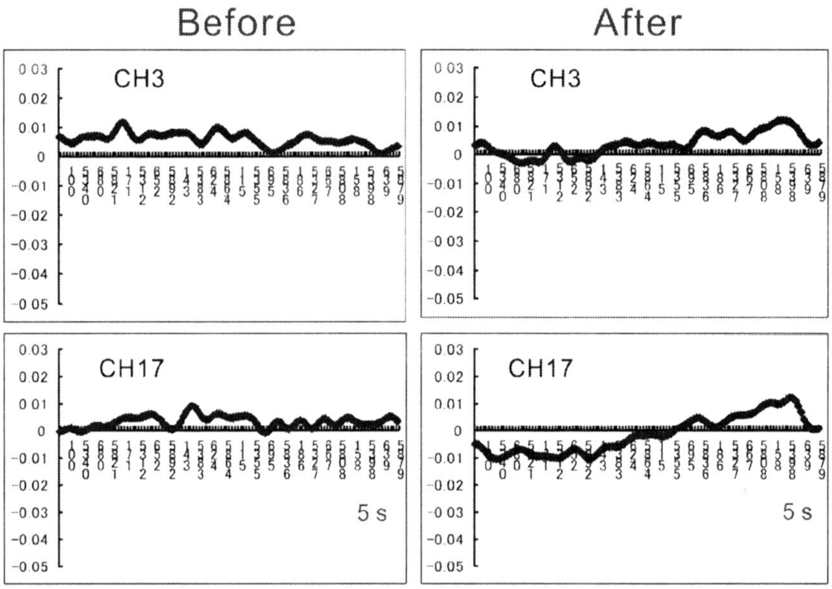

Figure 3. Changes in oxy-Hb concentration at the left M1 (CH3), with right M1 subtracted (CH17), before and after TMS with MVC in a subject.

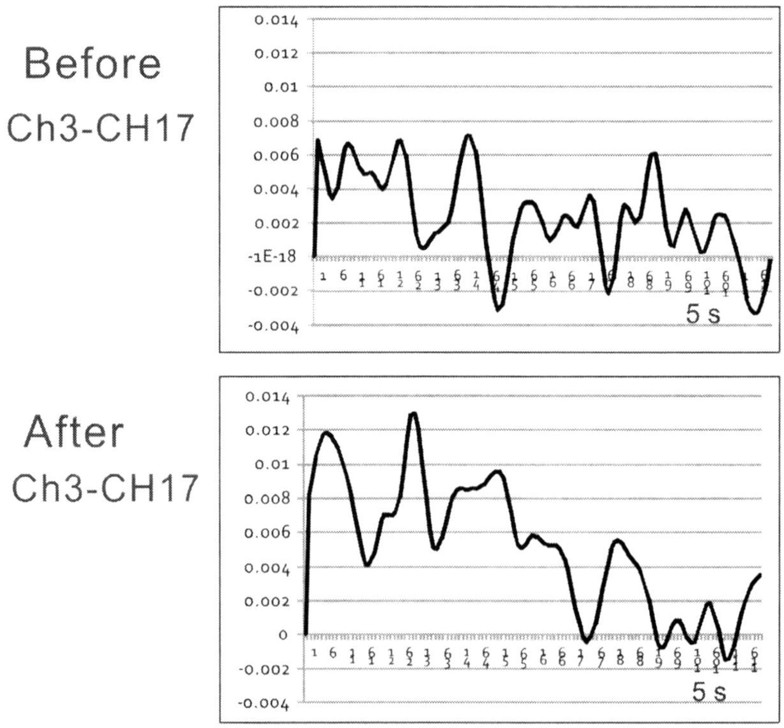

that the recording of NIRS during MVC should consider variations in blood pressure. Subtracting the measurements in the contra-lateral M1 from the measurements in the target M1 seems to be useful for analysis.

We conclude that repeated TMS with MVC is able to facilitate motor neuron excitability at the supraspinal level and is applicable to accelerating functional recovery of motor disability caused by impairments in the central nervous system.

ACKNOWLEDGMENT

This study was partially supported by a Grant-in-Aid for Scientific Research (B), the Japan and AA Science Platform Program from the Japan Society for the Promotion Science.

REFERENCES

Baker, A. T. (1991). An introduction to the basic principles of magnetic nerve stimulation. *Journal of Clinical Neurophysiology*, *8*, 26–37. doi:10.1097/00004691-199101000-00005

Baker, A. T., Jalinous, R., & Freestone, I. L. (1985). Non-invasive magnetic stimulation of the human motor cortex. *Lancet*, *1*, 1106–1107. doi:10.1016/S0140-6736(85)92413-4

Fox, P., Ingham, R., George, M. S., Mayberg, H., Ingham, J., & Roby, J. (1997). Imaging human intra-cerebral connectivity by PET during TMS. *Neuroreport*, *8*, 2787–2791. doi:10.1097/00001756-199708180-00027

Hamada, M., Ugawa, Y., & Tsuji, S. (2009). The effectiveness of rTMS on Parkinson's disease study group. High-frequency rTMS over the supplementary motor area improves bradykinesia in Parkinson's disease: Subanalysis of double-blind sham-controlled study. *Journal of the Neurological Sciences*, *287*, 143–146. doi:10.1016/j.jns.2009.08.007

Holper, L., Biallas, M., & Wolf, M. (2009). Task complexity relates to activation of cortical motor areas during uni- and bimanual performance: A functional NIRS study. *NeuroImage*, *46*, 1105–1113. doi:10.1016/j.neuroimage.2009.03.027

Ikeguchi, M., Touge, T., Kaji, R., Deguchi, K., Sasaki, I., & Tsukaguchi, M. ... Kuriyama, S. (2005). Durable effect of very low- frequency repetitive transcranial magnetic stimulation for modulating cortico-spinal neuron excitability. *Unveiling the mystery of the brain, International Congress Series, 1278*, 272-275.

Ikeguchi, M., Touge, T., Nishiyama, Y., Takeuchi, H., Kuriyama, S., & Ohkawa, M. (2003). Effects of successive repetitive transcranial magnetic stimulation on motor performances and brain perfusion in idiopathic Parkinson's disease. *Journal of the Neurological Sciences*, *209*, 41–46. doi:10.1016/S0022-510X(02)00459-8

Kujirai, T., Caramia, M. D., Rothwell, J. C., Day, B. L., Thompson, P. D., & Ferbert, A. (1993). Corticocortical inhibition in human motor cortex. *The Journal of Physiology*, *471*, 501–519.

Mally, J., & Stone, T. W. (1999). Therapeutic and dose-dependent effect of repetitive micro-electroshock induced by transcranial magnetic stimulation in Parkinson's disease. *Journal of Neuroscience Research*, *57*, 935–940. doi:10.1002/(SICI)1097-4547(19990915)57:6<935::AID-JNR19>3.0.CO;2-8

Nambu, I., Osu, R., Sato, M., Ando, S., Kawato, M., & Naito, E. (2009). Single-trial reconstruction of finger-pinch forces from human motor-cortical activation measured by near-infrared spectroscopy (NIRS). *NeuroImage*, *47*, 628–637. doi:10.1016/j.neuroimage.2009.04.050

Paus, T., Jech, R., Thompson, C. J., Comeau, R., Peters, T., & Evans, A. C. (1997). Transcranial magnetic stimulation during positron emission tomography: a new method for studying connectivity of the human cerebral cortex. *The Journal of Neuroscience*, *17*, 3178–3184.

Paus, T., Jech, R., Thompson, C. J., Comeau, R., Peters, T., & Evans, A. C. (1998). Dose-dependent reduction of cerebral blood flow during rapid-rate transcranial magnetic stimulation of the human sensorimotor cortex. *Journal of Neurophysiology*, *79*, 1102–1107.

Siebner, H. R., Peller, M., Willoch, F., Minoshima, S., Boecker, H., & Auer, C. (2000). Lasting cortical activation after repetitive TMS of the motor cortex. A glucose metabolic study. *Neurology*, *54*, 956–963.

Touge, T., Gerschlager, W., Cordivari, C., Brown, P., & Rothwell, J. C. (2001). Are the after-effects of low–frequency rTMS on motor cortex excitability due to changes in the efficacy of cortical synapses? *Clinical Neurophysiology*, *112*, 2138–2145. doi:10.1016/S1388-2457(01)00651-4

Touge, T., Urai, Y., & Shimamura, Y. (2009). *Excitability changes of corticospinal pathways by magnetic brain stimulation during the maximum voluntary muscle contraction*. CME2009.

Ugawa, Y., Uesaka, Y., Terao, Y., Hanajima, R., & Kanazawa, I. (1994). Magnetic stimulation of corticospinal pathways at the foramen magnum level in humans. *Annals of Neurology*, *36*, 618–624. doi:10.1002/ana.410360410

Urbach, D., & Awiszus, F. (2002). Stimulus strength on maximal voluntary contraction force of human quadriceps femoris muscle. *Experimental Brain Research*, *142*, 25–31. doi:10.1007/s00221-001-0911-x

Urbach, D., Berth, A., & Awiszus, F. (2005). Effect of transcranial magnetic stimulation on voluntary activation in patients with quadriceps weakness. *Muscle & Nerve*, *32*, 164–169. doi:10.1002/mus.20353

KEY TERMS AND DEFINITIONS

Foramen Magnum Stimulation (FMS): Magnetic stimulation of the pyramidal tract at the foramen magnum level.

Maximum Voluntary Muscle Contraction (MVC): Voluntary muscle contraction with maximum force.

Motor Evoked Potentials (MEPs): Muscle responses evoked by TMS.

Near-Infrared Spectroscopy (NIRS): A recently developed method for non-invasive measurement of oxygenized (oxy) and deoxygenized (deoxy) hemoglobin (Hb) in the cortex.

Oxygenized and Deoxygenized Hemoglobin (oxy-Hb and deoxy-Hb): Markers for cerebral blood flow in NIRS.

Regional Cerebral Blood Flow (rCBF): A regional measurement of cerebral blood flow.

Transcranial Magnetic Stimulation (TMS): A non-invasive method to stimulate cortical neurons using coils attached to the scalp.

Chapter 35
Development of Tactile Display Devices using fMRI under High Magnetic Fields

Masayuki Kitazawa
Department of Intelligent Mechanical Engineering, Wakayama National College of Technology, Japan

ABSTRACT

Recently, the physiological function of the human brain has become the subject of several investigations. Several methods have been developed to measure neural functioning. One such method is functional magnetic resonance imaging (fMRI). This approach is utilized under a high magnetic field with an average strength of 1.5T. As a result, special devices are needed to serve as stimuli for subjects in an fMRI study. In particular, devices for the investigation of tactile sense are rare. In this work, the authors report the development of novel tactile display devices. These devices can be used to stimulate the skin of the subject's hand to produces both pressure and movement stimulation. The devices are manipulated with ultrasonic motors that do not have coils and are constructed with non-magnetic materials, such as stainless steel and acrylic acid resin. Therefore, these devices can be used without disturbing the high magnetic field. To quantify the influence of the devices to the magnetic field, signal to noise ratios (SNR) for images generated by MRI were measured. These experiments confirmed that the SNR was altered by 5% when the devices were present; however, this change is within the acceptable range for the quality of an MRI image. From this work, the authors conclude that the developed devices have sufficient performance under high magnetic field conditions.

DOI: 10.4018/978-1-60960-559-9.ch035

INTRODUCTION

Functional magnetic resonance imaging (fMRI) is often used to quantify neural activity when a stimulus is given to a subject. This imaging method, which can identify activation fields in the brain, assesses regional blood flow in response to a stimulus and is conducted under a high magnetic field. Stimulus displays have been developed to test vision and hearing in a high magnetic field, and some have been used in experiments with fMRI. For other senses, however, very few stimulus devices can be used with fMRI. In this report we focus on the tactile sense and the development of tactile displays compatible with fMRI.

A tactile stimulus is produced by a transformation of the skin surface. Though there are several ways to deliver this stimulation, only two methods will be discussed here. The first applies the transformation at one point on the skin and is perceived as pressure. The other transforms a constant area on the skin and is perceived as movement. The developed devices are manipulated by ultrasonic motors and are made with non-magnetic materials. This motor rotates a shaft by using friction instead of a coil. As a result, the ultrasonic motor has minimal influence on the magnetic field. In this paper, we test the proposed devices and confirm their performance through MRI experiments.

TACTILE SENSE

The tactile sense is triggered by the excitation of receptors under the skin. A transformation of the skin's surface causes this excitation. In general, this transformation can be produced by pressure, vibration or movement. Pressure delivers a transformation to a single point on skin, while vibration and movement transform a larger area of skin. Simple motor-driven mechanisms can be used to generate pressure or movement stimulation on skin, such as moving an arm up and down on the skin surface or moving a brush pen along the skin. In this work, we evaluate two kinds of newly designed tactile display devices that can be used to generate sensations of pressure and movement.

TACTILE DISPLAY DEVICES

As mentioned above, two kinds of devices were developed. The first utilizes vertical movement and produces the tactile stimulus by moving the arm of the device up and down with a cam. The shape of the cam is designed to use the weight of the arm to generate a pressure sensation when the tip of the arm touches the surface of the skin. Figure 1a shows the pressure stimulation device, and Figure 1b shows the tip of the arm. The shape of the tip is hemispherical with a diameter of 10 mm. A diameter of less than 10 mm has the

Figure 1. Tactile display device that generates pressure. (a) Body of the device. (b) Tactile portion of the device

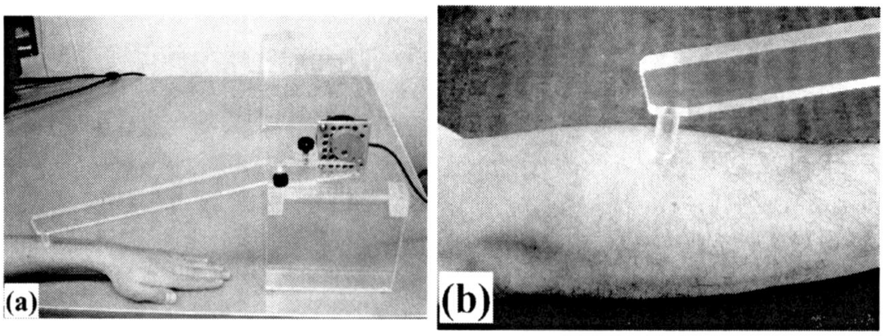

potential to generate not only a tactile sense but also a sense of pain. This device is designed to generate only a tactile stimulus.

The second device utilizes back and forth movements and is constructed with a turning block slider crank mechanism. A brush pen mounted on the slider moves horizontally along the skin to give a tactile stimulus. This device produces a transformation that generates a sense of movement. The speed of the pen movement is important. When the approach speed is fast, subjects are often uncomfortable, thus the speed of this device is set at 0.35 m/s from the reference. Figure 2a shows the movement stimulation device, and Figure 2b shows the brush pen.

These tactile display devices employ ultrasonic motors and non-magnetic materials. The ultrasonic motors rotate the axis with vibration of the piezoelectric elements without a coil. Acrylic acid is as the primary material used in these devices, and the parts of the devices are joined by stainless steel screws. As a result, the influence on the magnetic field is minimized. They are connected to a personal computer (PC) with a 10 m length cable. The number of revolutions for each motor is measured with an encoder. Thus, the motors are able to drive and stop the rotation by receiving an order from the PC. During an fMRI experiment, the PC can control the movement of the device to comply with a set task. Typically, the task for fMRI is composed of repetitions of both a stimulus period and a non-stimulus period.

EXPERIMENT AND RESULTS

Basic experiments were carried out to characterize the two devices. For the device with vertical movement, the movement of the arm was confirmed by analyzing a video of the motion. The speed of the tip was calculated to be 0.012 m/s. The speed of the brush pen for the device with back and forth movement was measured and confirmed to be under 0.35 m/s.

We then analyzed the effects of these devices on the signal to noise ratio (SNR) of an MRI image. Figure3 shows the ultrasonic motor control system. The PC, the converter (UHA-BHU2M) and the driver for the ultrasonic motor were set in the control room beside the MRI room. The developed device with the ultrasonic motor was set on the bed of the MRI (1.5T) as shown in Figure 4a. The imaging object was a cylinder phantom, shown in figure 4b. The phantom is an anthropoid object that was used in place of a human subject.

Images of the phantom are shown in Figure 5. The distance between the device and the magnetic isocenter was 700 mm. Table 1 lists the SNR values with and without the device. An SNR

Figure 2. Tactile display device that generates movement. (a) Body of the device. (b) Tactile portion of the device

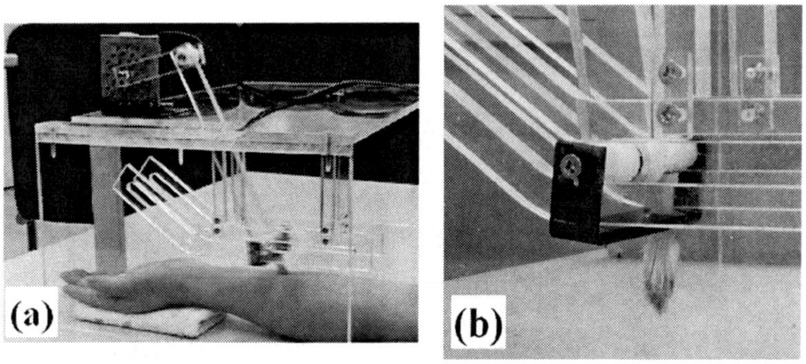

Figure 3. Block diagram of the ultrasonic motor control system

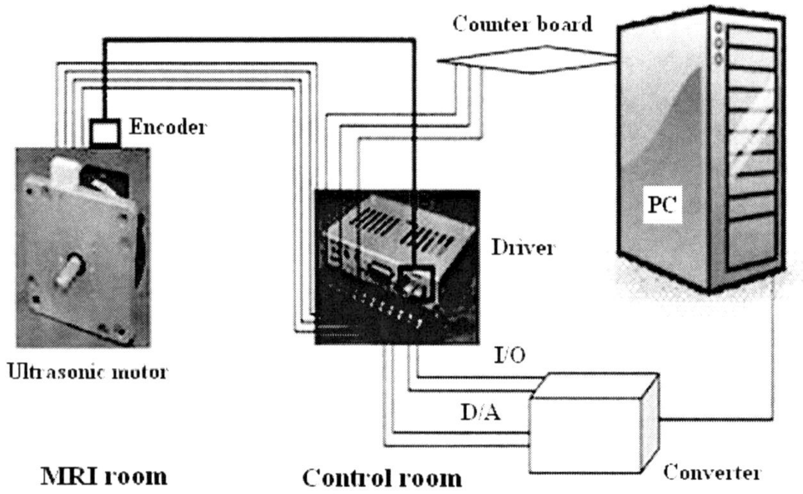

Figure 4. Experimental setup for MRI (SIEMENS MEGNETOM Avanto 1.5T). (a) Tactile display device is set on the MRI table. (b) Phantom

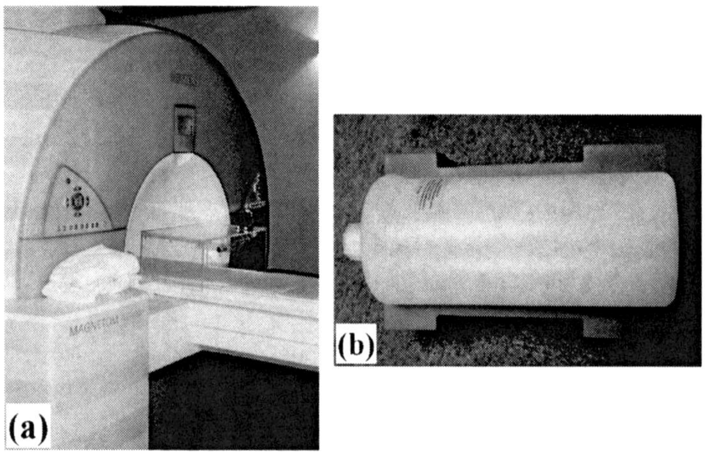

Figure 5. Images of the phantom when (a) the device is not set and (b) the device is moving

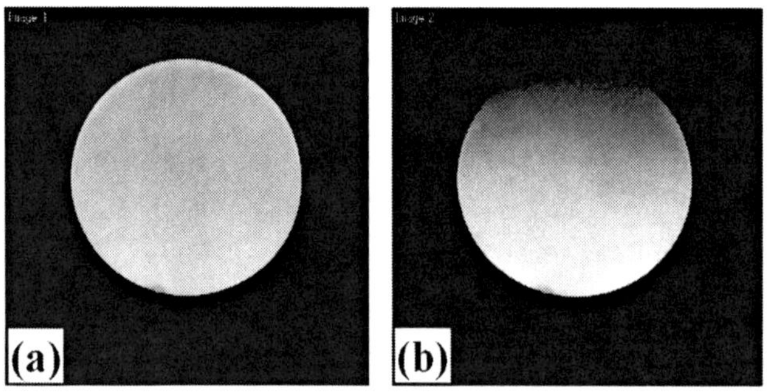

Table 1. Experimental results for SNR

	Phantom	Device (not moving)	Device (moving)
SNR	67.6	65.6	64.2

value is calculated by dividing the average brightness of the phantom image by the standard deviation for the brightness of the background image. The SNR value when imaging the phantom alone is used as a base value. The device was then placed on the MRI table and the phantom was imaged with the device. The SNR value when imaging the phantom with the device was reduced by 3% from the base value. Though the device was not moving, it was plugged into the driver. When the device was moving, the SNR value was reduced by 5% from the base value.

DISCUSSION AND CONCLUSION

Approximately 20 stainless steel screws and one stainless steel plate were used to connect the parts of the developed device. This stainless steel used was austenitic (SUS304) and was neither ferromagnetic nor paramagnetic. It is possible for the steel to be magnetic if it is processed at cold working. As a result, the screws and the plate could be magnetic during processing. This potential magnetization of the stainless steel is thought to be the main source of the SNR reduction when using the devices.

According to the reference, the SNR value was reduced by 6% when the ultrasonic motor was moving during imaging. Our data show that the value of SNR during motor moving is different from the value obtained when the motor is not moving. In previous experiments, the ultrasonic motor was placed 520 mm from the magnetic isocenter. For this work, the motor was set approximately 700 mm from the magnetic isocenter. From these results, the distance between the motor and the magnetic isocenter influences the value of SNR.

In conclusion, the developed devices show a limited influence on the high magnetic field. While the SNR value was decreased by 5%, this change is acceptable. Thus, the proposed device is able deliver tactile stimulation under a high magnetic field.

In future experiments, we plan to investigate materials that do not influence SNR values.

ACKNOWLEDGMENT

The author thanks Dr. Nozomu Takeuchi who belongs to the department of Radiology of Hidaka General Hospital for the use of the MRI machine.

REFERENCES

Chinzei, K., Kikinis, R., & Jolesz, F. A. (1999). MR compatibility of mechatronic devices: Design criteria. *Proceedings of MICCAI'99*, (LNCS 1679), (pp. 1020-1031).

Saito, T., & Ikeda, H. (2005). *Measurement of human pain tolerance to mechanical stimulus of human-collaborative robots*. (NIIS-SRR-No.33), (pp. 15-23)

Yamada, Y., Suita, K., Ikeda, H., Sugimoto, N., Miura, H., & Nakamura, H. (1997). Evaluation of pain tolerance based on a biomechanical method for human-robot coexistence. *Journal of Japan Mechanical Engineers*, *96*(612), 238–243.

KEY TERMS AND DEFINITIONS

fMRI: fMRI is an imaging method which can discover activation fields in the brain using regional blood flow caused by a stimulus. This method differs from MRI.

High Magnetic Field: MRIs with a magnetic strength of 1.5T are used in various medical inspections. For the purposes of this paper, a high magnetic field is over 1.5T.

Phantom: A phantom is typically used to measure the homogeneity of a magnetic field. It is an anthropoid object used in place of a human subject.

SNR: SNR is calculated by dividing a signal by the background noise. In an MRI image, the signal is the average brightness of the subject and the noise is the standard deviation for the brightness of the background.

Tactile Display Device: This device transforms the surface of the skin by using a mechanical stimulus, i.e., pressure, vibration or movement.

Tactile Sense: Tactile sense is generated by the excitation of receptors under the skin. A transformation of the skin surface causes the excitation.

Ultrasonic Motor: This motor rotates a shaft using friction instead of a coil. An ultrasonic vibration generates the friction.

Chapter 36
Development of a Bilateral Assistance and Coordination Rehabilitation Training System

Shuxiang Guo
Faculty of Engineering, Kagawa University, Takamatsu, Japan

Zhibin Song
Graduate School, Kagawa University, Takamatsu, Japan

ABSTRACT

Strokes can lead to lasting neurological impairments. Many researchers are studying this process and have made important discoveries. Researchers are starting to investigate the possibility of neurorehabilitation based on neuroplasticity. On the other hand, robot assisted systems have increasingly been used in rehabilitation. However, studies on bilateral assistance rehabilitation systems have seldom been reported. Industrial robot arms were proposed for rehabilitation in other studies, but the inertia and volume of the system was too large, and the stiffness was hard to change. In this research, the authors proposed a novel bilateral assistance rehabilitation approach to treatment of the upper limbs of stroke patients, and a bilateral coordination rehabilitation approach was also proposed. This system is based on virtual reality, and is composed of two haptic devices (PHANTOM Omni), an advanced inertial sensor (MTx), and a computer. The authors have built some force models, in which one hand can be used to assist the other. Bilateral coordination training can also be performed in rehabilitation. In this system, the virtual reality technique is adopted to provide a virtual force model for rehabilitation training of the upper limbs. Furthermore, it is easy to change the stiffness of the system through changing the parameters of the developed virtual force model. The advantages of high safety, compactness, and bilateral assistance and coordination training make the system suitable for home rehabilitation.

DOI: 10.4018/978-1-60960-559-9.ch036

INTRODUCTION

Stroke can result in neurological impairments. Approximately 700,000 people suffer a first or recurrent stroke each year, according to the American Heart Association [http://www.Americanheart.org/statistics/stroke.htm]. Traditional therapy requires many therapists and increases the health care burden. To solve this problem, robot-mediated rehabilitation systems have been developed (R.F. Boian, M. Bouzit, G.C. Burdea & J.E. Deutsch, 2004).

In 1995, a rehabilitation system named MIT-MANUS was developed at the Massachusetts Institute of Technology, Cambridge (N. Hogan, H. I. Krebs, A. Sharon & J. Charnnarong, 1995; H. I. Krebs, B. T. Volpe, M. L. Aisen & N. Hogan, 2000). The device assisted planar pointing and drawing movements with an impedance controller. Unlike most industrial robots, MIT-MANUS was configured for safe, stable, and compliant operation in close physical contact with humans. This was achieved using impedance control, a key feature of the robot control system that modulates the way the robot reacts to mechanical perturbations from a patient or clinician and ensures gentle, compliant behavior. MIT-MANUS can move, guide, or perturb the movement of a subject's or patient's upper limb, and can record motions and mechanical quantities such as the position, velocity, and applied force. The profile of the system is shown in Figure 1. Several redundant safety features were incorporated into the system.

1. Software cut power to the robot if the error between the commanded and measured angles at the robot's joints exceeded a critical value. This would occur if the robot had encountered an unexpectedly large resistance.
2. A commercially available pneumatic device cut power to the robot when the torque applied to the forearm exceeded a critical value (20 Nm). Straps limited the robot to a safe range of motion.
3. The experimenter always kept an emergency stop button nearby.

Figure 1. MIT-MANUS assisted rehabilitation system

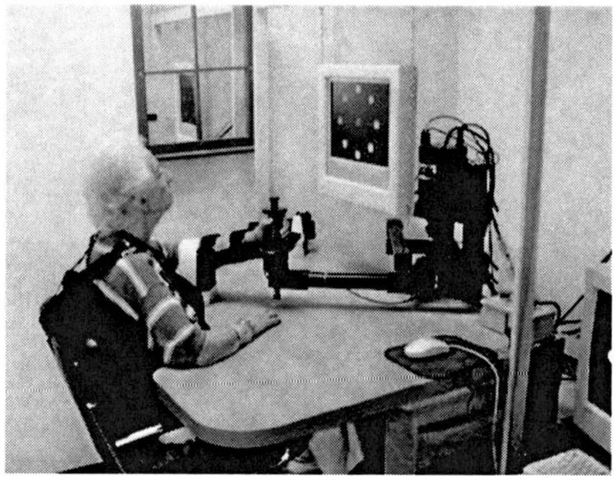

Another typical rehabilitation system, called the MIME assisted rehabilitation system is shown in Figure 2. Preliminary reports of the system were presented in 1999 at the 6th International Conference on Rehabilitation Robotics (ICORR '99), Stanford, CA. The initial version of MIME incorporated two commercial mobile arm supports modified to limit arm movement to the horizontal plane, and a 6-DOF robot arm (PUMA-260) that applied forces and torques to the paretic forearm through one of the arm supports. In the current MIME workstation, the robot is a Puma-560, the paretic limb mobile arm support is eliminated, and a 6-DOF-position digitizer is applied to the system. (R.M. Mahoney, H.F. Machiel Van der Loos, P.S. Lum & C.Burgar, 2003) Redundant hardware and software features assure subject safety while exercising in the MIME.

The ARM Guide (Kahn, L.E., Zygman, M.L, Rymer, W.Z. & Reinkensmeyer,D.J, 2006) is a singly-actuated, four-DOF robotic device that consists of a hand piece attached to an orientable linear track and actuated by a DC servo motor.

Figure 2. MIME assisted rehabilitation system

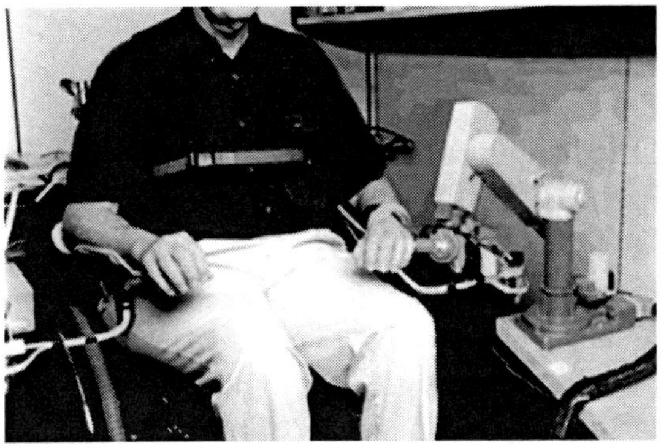

From these three typical assisted rehabilitation systems, we can see that a conventional robot can be used for rehabilitation training, because it can exert large forces and torques. Virtual Reality (VR) technology has also been applied in the MIT-MANUS assisted system. Good rehabilitation effects have been obtained with force feedback and 3-D visual feedback. Both of these systems have been used in hospital settings, but there are still some drawbacks for home rehabilitation. For example, compactness and low impedance (for safety) of the system must be improved. Furthermore, in order to improve the operability and safety of the rehabilitation system, bilateral assistance and coordination is necessary for home rehabilitation. Unfortunately, little research has been performed in this field.

From the perspective of the development of neurorehabilitation, earlier studies have shown that repeated limb movement is effective in the recovery of stroke limbs (Butefisch C, Hummelsheim H, Denzler P & Maurtiz KH, 1995). In the passive rehabilitation approach, the movement trajectory of the robot is predefined, and the patient's limbs move repeatedly with the movement of the robot. The passive rehabilitation approach is effective to some extent for neurological patients, but it is not so obvious in some cases. As a result, the active rehabilitation approach has been introduced into rehabilitation systems, though active rehabilitation is mainly suited to mild stroke patients.

RESEARCH OBJECTIVES

The aim of rehabilitation for stroke patients is to increase the strength, agility, and range of movement (ROM) of the limbs (S.L. Wolf, S. Blanton, H. Baer, J. Breshears & A. J.Butler, 2002). In our study, we assume that the positions of both elbows are unchangeable, but that the forearms can rotate around the elbows in 3 DOF, and we mainly consider rotation of the elbows and wrists. During the rehabilitation process for the elbows and wrists, we suggest that both hands participate in the rehabilitation, instead of only one hand, so that the patient can perform bilateral assistance and coordination rehabilitation (K. A. Danek, R. B. Gillespie, J. W. Aldridge, D. P. Ferrie & J.W. Grizzle, 2005). Our exploration of bilateral assistance and coordination rehabilitation began with the development of a rehabilitation system based on virtual reality (Gang Song & Shuxiang Guo, 2007; Shuxiang Guo & Zhibin Song, 2008). We proposed an original system prototype first, which included two haptic devices and a computer. A task-oriented experiment that includes a randomly moving object was developed. The manipulator's hands could move in 3 dimensions, but only the position in the x-axis is used in the display interface. The next system improved the original system so that manipulators could perform the experiment in three dimensions. Besides the two haptic devices and a computer, a high precision inertial sensor (MTx), equipped on the back of the manipulator's hand, was added to the system. The virtual environment could thus be expanded to 3 dimensions, and could integrate more factors of the upper limb motion. With the help of a bilateral assistance rehabilitation system, a patient can perform training actively rather than be driven to move his limbs passively.

Bilateral assistance rehabilitation is realized when the unimpaired limb guides the impaired limb's motion. Based on its success, we speculate that it might be helpful for subjects to perform bilateral coordination rehabilitation training. Activity in ipsilateral corticospinal pathways is responsible when subjects try to bilaterally move their upper limbs simultaneously. Thus, bilaterally symmetric training after stroke will stimulate ipsilateral corticospinal pathways and enhance recovery [Richard M. Mahoney, H.F. Machiel Van der Loos, Peter S. Lum & Chuck Burgar, 2003]. Bilaterally symmetric training might immerse subjects less than coordination training. Additional evidence for the efficacy of bilateral coordination training comes from structural investigations of the corpus callosum (Johansen-Berg H, Della-Maggiore V, Behrens TE, Smith SM & Paus T, 2007), which report that bilateral coordination training is associated with the integrity of the white matter in the corpus collosum and that such integrity generates interhemispheric pathways to the caudal cingulate motor area and the supplementary motor area (Johansen-Berg H, Della-Maggiore V, Behrens TE, Smith SM & Paus T, 2007). Therefore, we developed another rehabilitation system based on bilateral coordination training (Shuxiang Guo & Zhibin Song, 2009) in which self-assisted rehabilitation is also adopted.

BILATERAL ASSISTANCE AND COORDINATION REHABILITATION SYSTEM

Original Bilateral Assistance Rehabilitation

In the first step, we proposed an original prototype of the rehabilitation system, which included two haptic devices and one computer. The manipulator's hands could move in 3 dimensions, but only the position in x-axis was shown on the display interface. Figure 3 shows the schematic diagram of the original system, with the various available power and information pathways depicted. Through the combined efforts of two hands, the exchange of haptic information between the left hand and the virtual environment and between the right hand and the virtual environment was realized. Based on this mechanism, the system used bilateral assistance rehabilitation and the unimpaired upper limb guided and assisted the impaired upper limb in its corresponding movements. We have designed a virtual force model for the original system, which is shown in Figure 4. The display interface is shown in Figure 5. In the experiment, the virtual object m will track the virtual object m', which moves randomly in the x-axis.

Figure 3. A schematic diagram of the original system

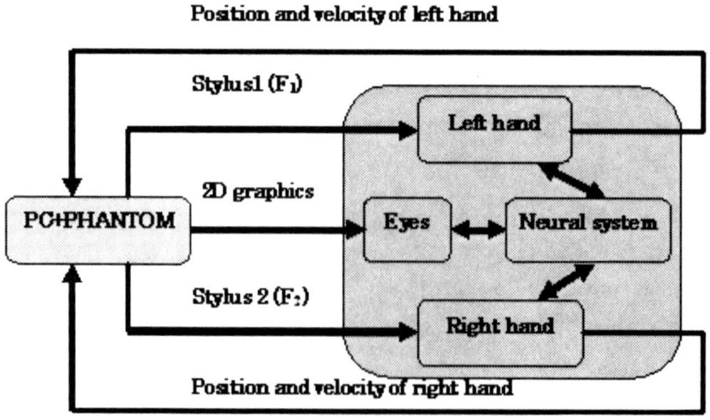

Virtual Force Model

The remarkable character of this system is the realization of the self-assistance function with a proposed virtual force model. In this section, we will analyze the principle of the virtual force model. We have designed a virtual force model for the original system, which is shown in Figure 4. The kinematics equation is shown in (1).

$$m\ddot{x}_m + (b_1 + b_2)\dot{x}_m + (k_1 + k_2 + k)x_m = k_1 x_1 + b_1\dot{x}_1 + k_2 x_2 + b_2\dot{x}_2 \quad (1)$$

Where x_m is the displacement of object m, x_1 and x_2 are the displacement of object 1 and object 2, respectively, $\dot{x}_1$ and $\dot{x}_2$ are the velocity of object 1 and object 2, respectively, k_1, k_2 and k are the stiffness constants of the springs, and b_1 and b_2 are the damping constants of damper 1 and

Figure 4. Virtual force model of the original system

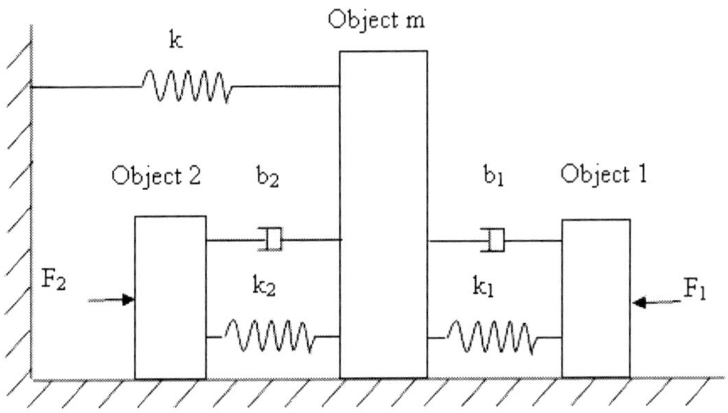

Figure 5. Display interface of the original system

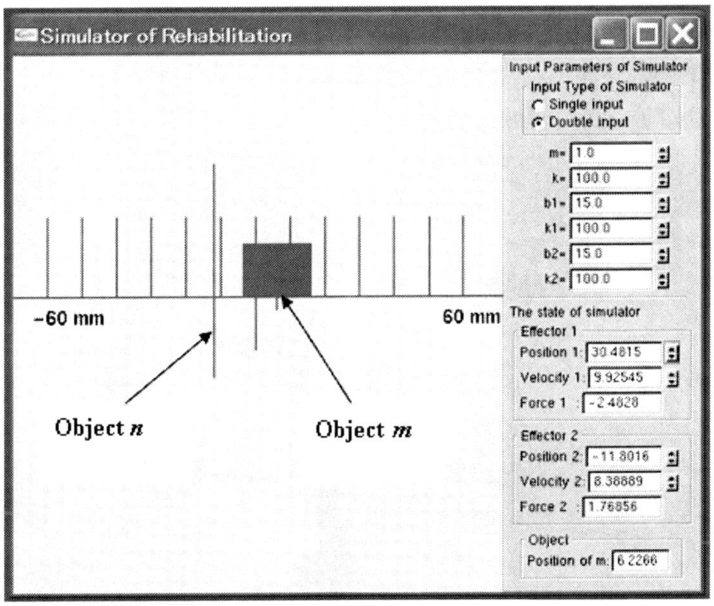

damper 2, respectively. With the scheduler of the haptic devices, the displacement and velocity of the styluses can be sampled by the computer every millisecond, so the displacement, velocity, and acceleration of object m can be calculated with (1).

With the calculated velocity and displacement of object m, the output force on the two effectors can be calculated with (2) and (3). From (1), (2), and (3), we can see that the displacements and velocities of the manipulator's hands determine the output forces on the styluses.

$$F_1 = b_1(\dot{x}_1 - \dot{x}) + k_1(x_1 - x) \tag{2}$$

$$F_2 = b_2(\dot{x}_2 - \dot{x}) + k_2(x_2 - x) \tag{3}$$

The display interface is shown in Figure 5. In the experiment, the virtual object m will track the virtual object m', which moves randomly in the x-axis. In this way, the agility of the manipulator's hands is expected to improve.

Improved Bilateral Assistance Rehabilitation

To improve the performance of the original system, an inertial sensor (MTx) was added [Huiyu Zhou, Huosheng Hu & Yaqin Tao, 2006]. The inertial sensor measured gestures of the manipulator's hand in real-time when equipped on the back of the manipulator's hand. Figure 6 shows the force model of the improved system.

In (4), x_1 and x_2 are the displacement of object 1 and object 2, respectively and $\dot{x}_1$ and $\dot{x}_2$ are the velocity of object 1 and object 2, respectively. The displacement and velocity of the virtual object m can be calculated with (4).

When the hand is not rotated, the exerted forces on the styluses remain in the plane of the x-axis. In (5) and (6), F1 and F2 are the forces that the subject exerts on stylus 1 and stylus 2, respectively, but with the opposite orientation. With these two equations, F1 and F2 can be calculated. F1 and F2 can be changed easily by changing the spring constants and damper constants.

$$\begin{aligned} m\ddot{x}_m &+ (b_1 + b_2)\dot{x}_m + (k_1 + k_2 + k)x_m \\ &= k_1x_1 + b_1\dot{x}_1 + k_2x_2 + b_2\dot{x}_2 - mg\sin^3 \end{aligned} \tag{4}$$

$$F_1 = b_1(\dot{x}_1 - \dot{x}_m) + k_1(x_1 - x_m) \tag{5}$$

$$F_2 = b_2(\dot{x}_2 - \dot{x}_m) + k_2(x_2 - x_m) \tag{6}$$

Figure 6. The force model of the improved system

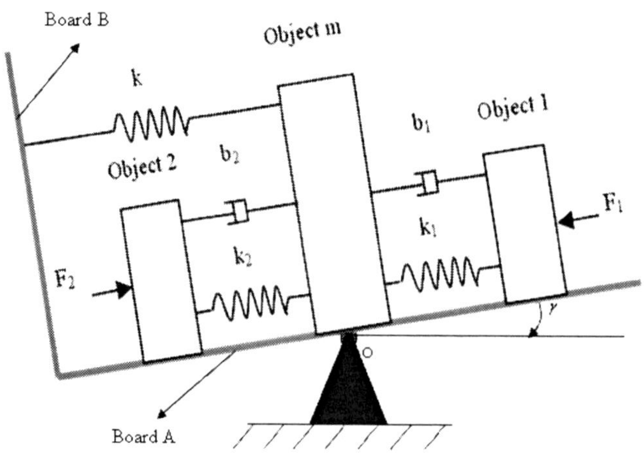

When the MTx sensor is not rotated, the force vector $\overrightarrow{F_1'} = (F1, 0, 0)$, $\overrightarrow{F_2'} = (F2, 0, 0)$. After the rotation, the force vectors become $\overrightarrow{F_1}$ and $\overrightarrow{F_2}$, respectively. We suppose that $\overrightarrow{F_1} = (F1x, F1y, F1z)$ and $\overrightarrow{F_2} = (F2x, F2y, F2z)$. $\overrightarrow{F_1}$ and $\overrightarrow{F_2}$ can be calculated with (7) and (8)

$$\overrightarrow{F_1} = B \times \overrightarrow{F_1'} \quad (7)$$

$$\overrightarrow{F_2} = B \times \overrightarrow{F_2'} \quad (8)$$

and

$$B = \begin{bmatrix} c^3 c\pm - s^3 c^2 s\pm & c^3 s\pm + s^3 c^2 c\pm & s^3 s^2 \\ -s^3 c\pm - c^3 c^2 s\pm & -s^3 s\pm + c^3 c^2 c\pm & c^3 s^2 \\ s^2 s\pm & -s^2 c\pm & c^2 \end{bmatrix}$$

where c and s stand for the cosine and sine functions, respectively.

Figure 7. The interface of path-unlimited training

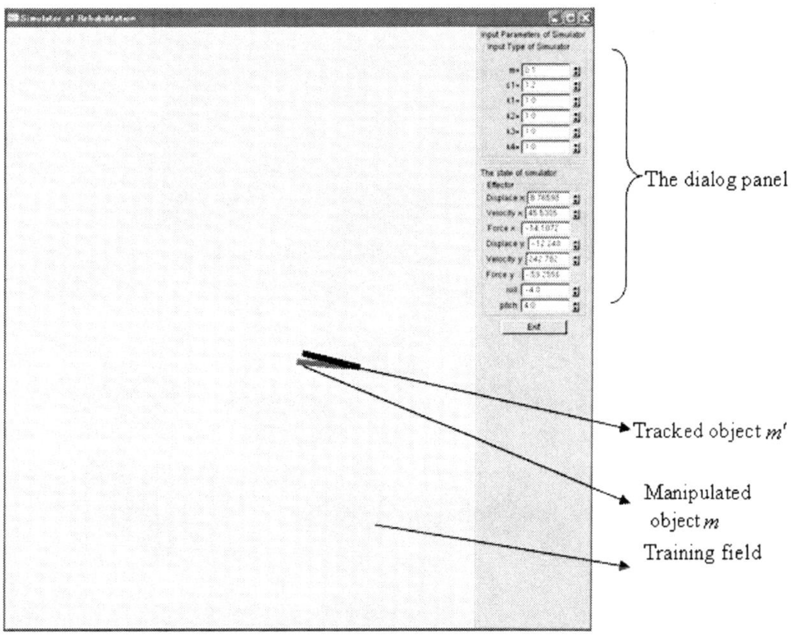

Original Bilateral Coordination Rehabilitation

In a two dimensional virtual environment, a lathy rectangle virtual object (m) is created (Figure 7). In the experiment, subjects manipulate the stylus of the haptic device to control the translation of the virtual object (m) with the dominant hand and rotate the inertial sensor MTx to control the posture of the virtual object (m) with the non-dominant hand. The angle of the virtual object (m) in the manipulation interface is the same as the roll angle of MTx. The other virtual object (m') keeps moving randomly. The shape of m' is the same as that of m, but its color is different. Subjects should track the virtual object (m'), meaning that they manipulate the object m to superpose it onto the other object m', matching both the position and posture.

Similarly to other research on active rehabilitation, impedance is used in this system. A mass-spring-damper force model is used to simulate impedance during the training process. The midpoint of virtual object m is connected separately to A, B, C, and D with springs. The elastic coefficients of the springs can easily be individually set on the dialog panel. The points A, B, C, and D are positioned on the coordinating sides of the rectangle. The force exerted on the stylus of the haptic device is set to 0 when the object m is at the initial position, as shown in Figure 8. On the other hand, a damping force is adopted in the force model. There are four dampers separately linking the virtual object m to four points. The subject manipulates the stylus of the haptic device to control the translation of virtual object m as if he were holding the stylus and moving it in a plane with a spring and viscous damping net. The forces exerted on the stylus of the haptic device are a combination of elastic forces and damping forces. The dynamics formulation is shown in (9).

$$\vec{F} = m\ddot{\vec{p}} + k_1\Delta\overrightarrow{OA} + k_2\Delta\overrightarrow{OB} + k_3\Delta\overrightarrow{OC} + k_4\Delta\overrightarrow{OD} + c_1\dot{\vec{p}}\overrightarrow{OA} + c_1\dot{\vec{p}}\overrightarrow{OB} + c_1\dot{\vec{p}}\overrightarrow{OC} + c_1\dot{\vec{p}}\overrightarrow{OD} \quad (9)$$

where $\vec{F}$ is the force exerted on the stylus of the haptic device, m is the mass of the virtual object, $\ddot{\vec{p}}$ is the acceleration of the midpoint of virtual object m, $\dot{\vec{p}}$ is the velocity of the midpoint of virtual object m, c_1 is the damping coefficient, and k_1, k_2, k_3, and k_4 are the elastic coefficients of the springs. The forces along the x-axis and y-axis are calculated separately in the program.

Improved Bilateral Coordination Rehabilitation

Path-unlimited training based on a mass-spring-damper force model has supplied a large-scale service to subjects. Though the mass-spring-damper force model generates high-fidelity haptic stimuli, there is still not enough scenery to impress subjects. Because of this, we developed path-limited training based on the compound force model. The training interface is made up of two areas of deep blue to impress the patients. A curved path is formed between the boundaries of these two parts, and the boundaries can be felt when the subject controls the object (n), touching it as if he touched a wall. The virtual object (n) is also a lathy rectangle that can be manipulated by the PHANTOM Omni stylus and the MTx inertia sensor. n can not rotate freely in the path,

Figure 8. The mass-spring-damper force model

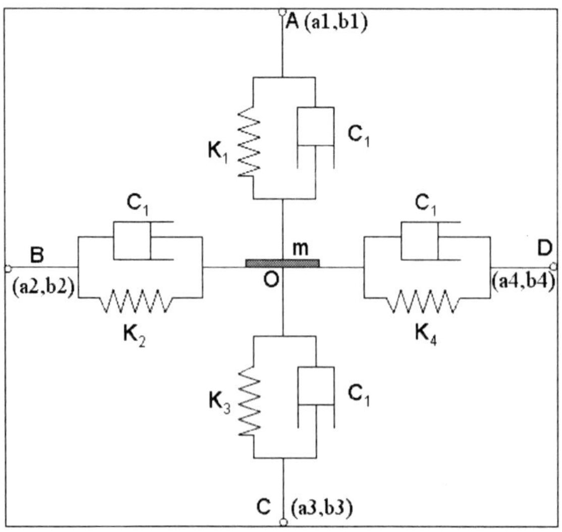

because of the path's finite width. Another object (*n'*) with the same size as *n* has been created in black (as shown in Figure 9). *n'* moves along the predefined path at a variable speed generated by a pseudo-random variable in the program. The task is to manipulate *n* to track *n'*; this task also involves cognitive processing. It is similar to path-unlimited training in that force is still exerted on the stylus of the haptic device. A virtual force model of the system was built after analyzing the kinematic model of the upper limb. Another aspect that is the same as path-unlimited training is that the subject's two hands should be coordinated in performance. It is different from path-unlimited training in that this kind of training offers assistance to subjects by allowing for stroke patients' hemiparesis. To do that, the subject rotates the inertial sensor and adjusts the pitch angle in the reference coordinate. With this system, a patient can use his intact hand to assist his impaired hand. The coordinated manipulation of two hands is beneficial for a patient's neurorehabilitation. There are some parameters that can be changed, such as the width of the predefined path and the coefficients of the dynamics.

The proposed virtual force model is called the compound force model because it has two parts. One part is called the λ-model and is created in order to augment the strength of the upper limbs, The other part is called the γ-model, which mainly simulates the boundary of the curved path.

In the λ-model, the forces exerted on the stylus of the haptic device along the *y*- and *x*-axis are used as impedances to augment the strength of the patients' upper limbs. When the force becomes so strong that a patient cannot move the stylus of the haptic device, assistance is needed and the patient's dominant hand can provide this assistance. We create this force model with the formulation given by (10), (11) and (12). The impedance is stronger in the primary direction of motion. In this model, we hypothesize that the virtual stick has no weight.

$$F_y = k\alpha v_y(|P_y| - a) / (3|\beta| + b) \qquad (10)$$

F_y is the force exerted on the stylus of the haptic device along the *y*-axis in the λ-model, P_y is the coordinate of the midpoint of the virtual object *n* along the *y*-axis, v_y is the velocity of the midpoint of the virtual object *n* along the *y*-axis, α is the roll angle of the MTx sensor, and β is the pitch angle of the MTx sensor. The meaning of *a*

Figure 9. The display interface of the system

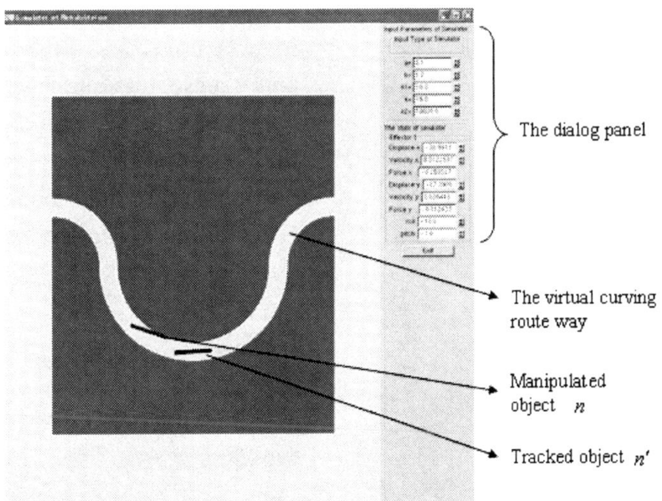

is illustrated in Figure 10. b is used to adjust the force. k is a coefficient that adjusts the stiffness of the system.

When $P_x <= x_1$,

$$F_x = -k_{1'} \mid \alpha \mid v_x (P_x - x_2) / (3 \mid \beta \mid + b) \quad (11)$$

When $P_x >= x_1$,

$$F_x = -k_1' |\alpha| v_x \frac{x_1 - x_2}{x_1 - x_3} (P_x - x_3) / (3|\beta| + b) \quad (12)$$

F_x is the force exerted on the stylus of the haptic device along the x-axis in the λ-model, P_x is the coordinate of the midpoint of the virtual object n along the x axis, v_x is the velocity of the midpoint of the virtual object n along the x-axis, α, β and b are the same as above, x_1, x_2 and x_3 are illustrated in Figure 10, and $k_{1'}$ is a coefficient similar to k.

P_x, P_y, v_x, and v_y can be obtained by the servo loop, and α and β can be obtained by the MTx sensor. The sampling of the MTx sensor is also under the control of the servo loop, and one set of data is recorded every 0.02 seconds. The forces exerted on the stylus of the haptic device are a combination of F_x and F_y when the virtual object n does not touch the boundary of the curved path.

The γ-model is designed to simulate the virtual environment, which provides subjects with the feeling of touching a path boundary. We suppose that the boundary has elasticity, which can be set by changing the elastic coefficient. If the virtual stick does not touch the boundary, the γ-model does nothing. The force against the path boundary is oriented along the normal to the boundary. The times that the boundary is touched are recorded. The resultant of the two force models is exerted in the experiment.

Figure 10. The parameters of the scene

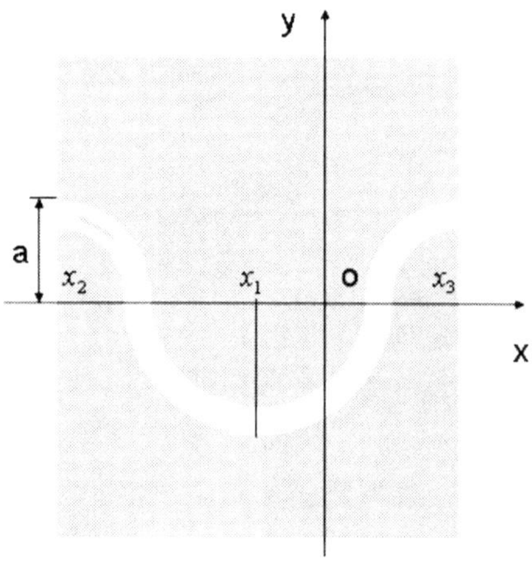

Experimental Subjects

Five healthy subjects participated in the experiments. Two of the subjects were over 50 years old (henceforth referred to as aged) and the other three were under 30 years old (henceforth referred to as young). One was female, the other four were male, and none of them had been previously injured on the upper limbs. Before the recorded experiment, every subject was given five minutes to practice and get familiar with the system. After that, the recorded experiments were performed. All of the subjects participated in the experiments mentioned above, and the aged subjects performed bilateral assistance rehabilitation and bilateral coordination rehabilitation with the path-limited system for two continuous months. With increased age, the agility and strength of the upper limbs decrease. In some sense, this trait is similar to the mild stroke patients, who lost some agility and strength in their upper limbs. Therefore, the two aged subjects participated in the rehabilitation experiment for two continuous months in our initial research.

RESULTS

The tracking performance can be evaluated with the squared error of position and posture between the object being tracked and the object being manipulated. In this paper, only the data from the aged subjects are shown in graphs. The typical position and posture tracking results for the aged subjects are shown in Figure 11 and Figure 12, respectively. The blue curves represent the desired data, and the red curves represent the manipulation results. From Figure 11 and Figure 12, we can see that the tracking performance improved greatly after two months of rehabilitation with the system. From Figure 13 (a) and (b) we can see that, after 2 months' training, the typical squared error of the position tracking experiment decreased from 7.71 mm to 5.13 mm, which means that the upper limb agility of the aged subjects has been greatly improved.

The experimental conditions of bilateral coordination rehabilitation are the same as those of bilateral assistance rehabilitation. Figure 13 shows the position and posture tracking results before and after 2 months of training. The black curves in the four figures below stand for the desired position trajectories or posture curves. We can see the position tracking performance improved greatly after two months of rehabilitation with this system.

CONCLUSION

We have developed a bilateral assistance and coordination rehabilitation system for upper limbs, especially for the wrists and elbows. The stiffness of the system is easy to change by changing the parameters of the virtual force model. Advanced haptic devices and an inertial sensor were used in the system for real-time, accurate acquisition of the position and orientation of the subject's hand, which are significant in the rehabilitation of upper limbs. The performance level of aged subjects improved over two months of training. The system is highly safe, compact, and allows for self-assistance, making the system suitable for home rehabilitation.

The output force on the haptic device is not more than 3.3 N, and the working range of the haptic device does not exceed the upper limb's range of movement, so a high level of safety can be guaranteed. The high level of safety and the compactness of the system make it suitable for home rehabilitation. Because it is an active rehabilitation system, it is only suitable for mild stroke patients. It is also primarily suited to reha-

Figure 11. The position tracking result of one aged subject

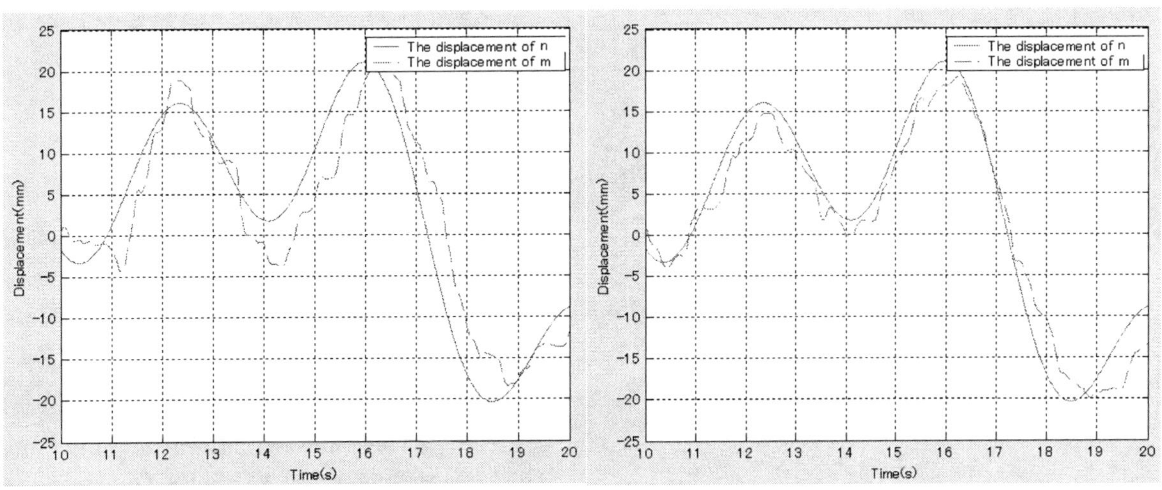

(a) Before the rehabilitation training (δ = 21.49)

(b) After 2 months' rehabilitation training (δ = 7.94)

Figure 12. The orientation tracking result of one aged subject

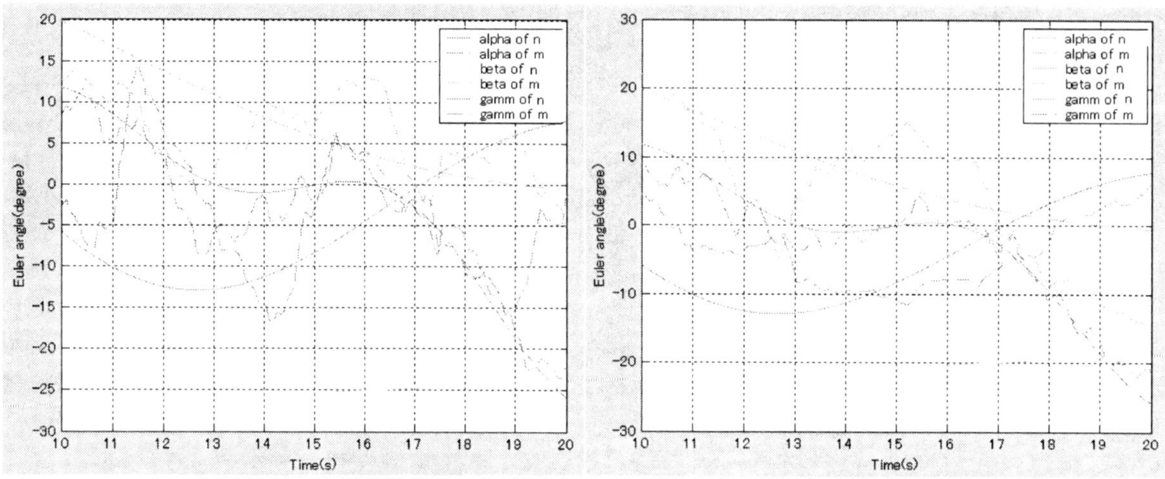

(a) Before rehabilitation training ($\delta_a = 10.40$) (b) After 2 months' rehabilitation training ($\delta_a = 4.95$)

Figure 13. The typical position tracking result for one aged subject

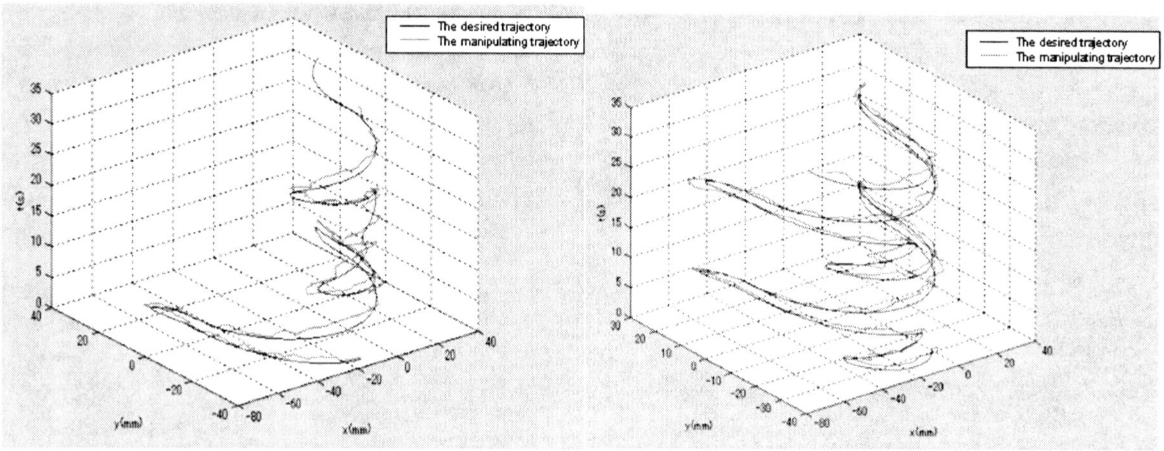

(a) At the start of training. $\delta_p = 7.71\text{mm}$ (b) At the end of training. $\delta_p = 5.13\text{mm}$

bilitation of the elbow and wrist, because of the limited workspace.

ACKNOWLEDGMENT

This research is supported by the Kagawa University Characteristic Prior Research fund 2009.

REFERENCES

American Heart Association. (2010). *American Heart Association stroke statistics*. Retrieved from http://www.Americanheart.org/statistics/stroke.htm

Boian, R. F., Bouzit, M., Burdea, G. C., & Deutsch, J. E. (2004). Dual Stewart platform mobility simulator. *Proceedings of the 26th Annual International Conference of the IEEE EMBS*, (pp. 4848-4851).

Butefisch, C., Hummelsheim, H., Denzler, P., & Mauritz, K. H. (1995). Repetitive training of isolated movements improves the outcome of motor rehabilitation of the centrally paretic hand. *Journal of the Neurological Sciences*, *130*, 59–68. doi:10.1016/0022-510X(95)00003-K

Cauraugh, J. H., Kim, S. B., & Duley, A. (2005). Coupled bilateral movements and active neuromuscular stimulation: Intralimb transfer evidence during bimanual aiming. *Neuroscience Letters*, 39–44. doi:10.1016/j.neulet.2005.02.060

Danek, K. A., Gillespie, R. B., Aldridge, J. W., Ferrie, D. P., & Grizzle, J. W. (2005). *A dual input device for self-assisted control of a virtual pendulum*. 9th International Conference on Rehabilitation Robotics, (pp. 313-318).

Guo, S., & Song, Z. (2009). A novel motor function training assisted system for upper limbs rehabilitation. *Proceeding of the 2009 IEEE International Conference on Intelligent Robots and Systems*, (pp. 1025-1030).

Guo, S., Song, Z., & Ren, C. (2009). *Development of upper limb motor function training and rehabilitation system*. IEEE International Conference on Mechatronics and Automation, (pp. 949-954).

Hogan, N., Krebs, H. I., Sharon, A., & Charnnarong, J. (1995). *Interactive robotic therapist*. (Patent 5466213). Cambridge, MA: Massachusetts Institute of Technology.

Johansen-Berg, H., Della-Maggiore, V., Behrens, T. E., Smith, S. M., & Paus, T. (2007). Integrity of white matter in the corpus callosum correlates with bimanual co-ordination skills. *NeuroImage*, *36*, 16–21. doi:10.1016/j.neuroimage.2007.03.041

Kahn, L. E., Zygman, M. L., Rymer, W. Z., & Reinkensmeyer, D. J. (2006). Robot-assisted reaching exercise promotes arm movement recovery in chronic hemiparetic stroke: A randomized controlled pilot study. *Journal of Neuroengineering and Rehabilitation*, *12*, 1–13.

Krebs, H. I., Volpe, B. T., Aisen, M. L., & Hogan, N. (2000). Increasing productivity and quality of care: Robot-aided neurorehabilitation. *Journal of Rehabilitation Research and Development*, *37*, 639–652.

Mahoney, R. M., Machiel Van der Loos, H. F., Lum, P. S., & Burgar, C. (2003). Robotic stroke therapy assistant. *Robotica*, *21*, 33–44. doi:10.1017/S0263574702004617

Song, G., & Guo, S. (2007). A novel self-assisted rehabilitation system for the upper limbs based on virtual reality. *International Journal of Information Acquisition, 3*.

Wolf, S. L., Blanton, S., Baer, H., Breshears, J., & Butler, A. J. (2002). Contemporary linkages between EMG, kinetics and stroke rehabilitation. *The Neurologist*, *8*, 325–338. doi:10.1097/00127893-200211000-00001

Zhou, H., Hu, H., & Tao, Y. (2006). Inertial measurements of upper limb motion. *International Federation for Medical and Biological Engineering*, *44*, 479–487.

KEY TERMS AND DEFINITIONS

Bilateral Assistance Rehabilitation: In order to improve the recovery of motor function, one limb performs a task with assistance from another limb.

Bilateral Coordination Rehabilitation: An approach to upper limb rehabilitation in which two upper limbs perform some coordinated motion.

Haptic Device: A mechanical device that mediates communication between the user and the computer. It allows users to touch, feel, and manipulate three-dimensional objects in virtual environments and tele-operated systems.

Inertial Sensor: A device to detect and measure acceleration, tilt, shock, vibration, rotation, and multiple degrees-of-freedom (DoF) motion, enabling a wide range of market-differentiating industrial, medical, communications, consumer, and automotive applications.

Neuroplasticity: The brain's natural ability to form new connections to compensate for injury or changes in one's environment.

Neurorehabilitation: A complex medical process that aims to aid recovery from a nervous system injury, and to minimize and/or compensate for any functional alterations resulting from it.

Stroke: A brain attack that happens when the blood supply to the brain is interrupted and the brain does not receive the oxygen it needs. It can potentially cause a great deal of functional disability. In this paper, motor function of the upper limbs is discussed.

Virtual Reality: A computer-simulated environment, whether that environment is a simulation of the real world or an imaginary world. Most current virtual reality environments are primarily visual experiences, displayed either on a computer screen or through special or stereoscopic displays. Some simulations include additional sensory information, such as sound through speakers or headphones.

Chapter 37
The Use of Mesh Glove Neurostimulation for Motor Recovery in Chronic Stroke

Katsuhiro Nishino
Neurosurgical Service Kakunodate City General Hospital, Japan

Suguru Yamaguchi
Neurosurgical Service Kakunodate City General Hospital, Japan

Kousuke Matsuzono
Neurosurgical Service Kakunodate City General Hospital, Japan

Hiroyuki Yamamoto
Neurosurgical Service Kakunodate City General Hospital, Japan

ABSTRACT

In 1994, the whole-hand electrical neural stimulation technique was reported by Dimitijevic to be useful in facilitating the recovery of hand-motor control after spinal cord injury and stroke. The authors of this chapter replicated this work and determined the effectiveness of the technique in restoring fine hand movement in 7 chronic stroke cases.

Prior to treatment with electrical stimulation, all patients received rehabilitation, either for three months (acute cases) or for at least one month (chronic cases), after which no remarkable improvements in hand control were seen. The patient group consisted of 5 females and 2 males. The stroke damage included brain hemorrhage in 5 cases, brain infarct in 1 case, and bled AVM in 1 case. Post-onset duration was between 3 and 44 months, and the ages of patients ranged from 11 to 65 years. The electrical stimulation was carried out according to the protocol previously reported by (Dimitrijevic, 1994).

DOI: 10.4018/978-1-60960-559-9.ch037

The results showed that the range of motion (ROM) was improved in 6 out of 7 cases, while fine movement of the hand was also improved in 4 cases. These improvements were observed a few days after the initiation of whole-hand electrical neural stimulation. In one chronic stroke case, the treatment resulted in an almost full recovery of hand control during the first 30 minutes of sub-threshold sensory stimulation, including pinching and grasping. This dramatic recovery led the authors to hypothesize that the responder would show no lesioning of the motor cortex on CT or MRI images. While more cases are needed to test the limitations of this modality and to determine the relationship between the level of recovery and the topology of CNS lesioning, this work illustrates the utility of this approach for improving motor control of the hand in chronic stroke patients.

I. INTRODUCTION

Restorative neurology is used to improve functional recovery by enhancing neuroplasticity or functional compensation beyond the results obtainable by routine rehabilitation programs (Feeney and Sutton, 1983; Dimitrijevic et al, 1991; Dimitrijevic, 1992; Sunderland et al, 1992). However, motor recovery in patients with upper extremity dysfunction is less likely than recovery from impairments of the lower extremities with orthodox rehabilitation programs. Whole-hand electrical stimulation (Dimitrijevic, 1994) uniquely targets the motor recovery of hand control after stroke. Since our first clinical application in Japan (1995), we have continued to use whole-hand electrical stimulation as a treatment option for cases of stroke and other pathological conditions that are associated with poor recovery of hand control after 3 months of a routine rehabilitation program. Here we describe the clinical results and address factors that could contribute to the level of success attained with this treatment.

II. MATERIALS AND METHODS

Seven patients with no severe muscle atrophy were given whole-hand electrical stimulation. Patient ages ranged from 11 to 65 years old. Post-onset duration was between 3 and 44 months. All cases suffered from spastic hemiparesis or poor hand control that did not show marked improvement with a routine rehabilitation program. Patients with cardiac pacing or epilepsy were not included (Table 1).

After a brief period of neural stimulation with mesh glove electrodes, 4 of the 7 patients showed improved movement, such as grasping and pinching.

A. Stimulating Conditions

A mesh glove electrode (Prizm Med Inc, Norcos, Georgia, USA) was placed on the affected hand after it was moistened with electromist (Pharmaceutical Innovations Inc, Newark, NJ, USA) (Figure 1). Transcutaneous electrical nerve stimulation was conducted below the sensory threshold level for 30 min twice daily for 2 weeks, followed by stimulation at the sensory level for 30 min twice

Table 1. Summary of patient information and the changes in hand control after treatment with whole hand stimulation

Case	Age	Sex	Diag	Post-onset	Results
1	54	m	BI	3y3m	E(R,G,P)
2	61	m	BH	1y4m	E(R,G,P)
3	11	f	AVM	2y	E(R)
4	55	f	BH	3y8m	E(R)
5	60	f	BH	3m	E(R,G,P)
6	59	f	BH	6m	E(R,G,P)
7	57	f	BH	6m	n/E

BI: brain infarction, BH: brain hemorrhage, E: effective, R: range of motor joint, G: grasping, P: pinching.

Figure 1. Setup of electromesh glove whole hand stimulation system. This mesh glove is prototype

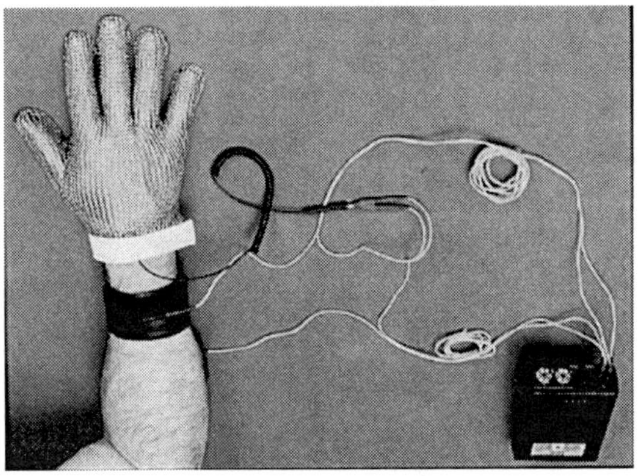

daily for a subsequent 2 weeks. Finally, patients were stimulated with a neurostimulator at motor threshold for 2 weeks (Medtronic model 3128, Respond 2). The stimulatory frequency was 50 c/sec with a pulse width of 300 msec. Square rubber electrodes were placed on the forearm as an anode, and 3 cm distal to the mesh glove as a cathode. This clinical program was performed during admission or as a home task after training the family in our clinic for one week.

Functional improvements of hand control were evaluated by assessing the ROM of the cubital, shoulder, and digital joints as well as the ability to pinch and grasp.

III. RESULTS

Six of seven cases showed improvement in their ROM. Four cases showed improvements in grasping and pinching. Most of these changes began 2-3 days after sub-threshold sensory stimulation and were associated with reductions in muscle spasticity. This level of stimulation facilitated restoration of hand control, as assessed by pinching and grasping. No adverse effects were reported.

The responder is not relevant to post-onset duration.

Represented Cases

Case 1: 54 year-old male, 39 months post-onset of left brain infarct, showed right spastic hemiparesis and was able to walk with a cane. Reduced movement of the right hand was seen. CT on admission found multiple LDA in the left basal ganglia and coronal radiation and right caudate head. A month of a routine rehabilitation program resulted in no restoration of right hemiparesis. Whole-hand stimulation treatment was given. On the second day following the neurostimulation, pinching and grasping were mostly restored.

Case 2: 65 year-old male, 16 months post-onset of ICH, showed right hemiparesis. Physical therapy and occupational therapy programs had been conducted, but fine finger movement had been disturbed. The patient was unable to write, use a spoon, or tie a knot. Soon after beginning whole-hand stimulation, hand control, including pinching and grasping, improved and the spasticity of the upper extremity was reduced.

IV. DISCUSSION

Recovery from motor deficits caused by stroke often follows a characteristic time course: loss of motor function associated with accentuated tendon reflexes and increased resistance on passive extension, followed by a gradual recovery by both reduction of muscle tonus and increase in muscle strength. In general, the probability of upper extremity recovery is lower than that of lower extremity recovery. Only 14% of patients show a full recovery, while 25% show a partial recovery (Wada et al, 1983). In most cases, dysfunctions of the distal muscles and finger joints tend to remain (Dimitrijevic et al, 1996). The time course for recovery differs among treatments (Hewer, 1994). Most motor recovery has occurred within 3 months post-onset. Some cases have reported recovery after a year, but they are very exceptional (Sunderland et al, 1992).

Figure 2. Illustration of spinal premotor center

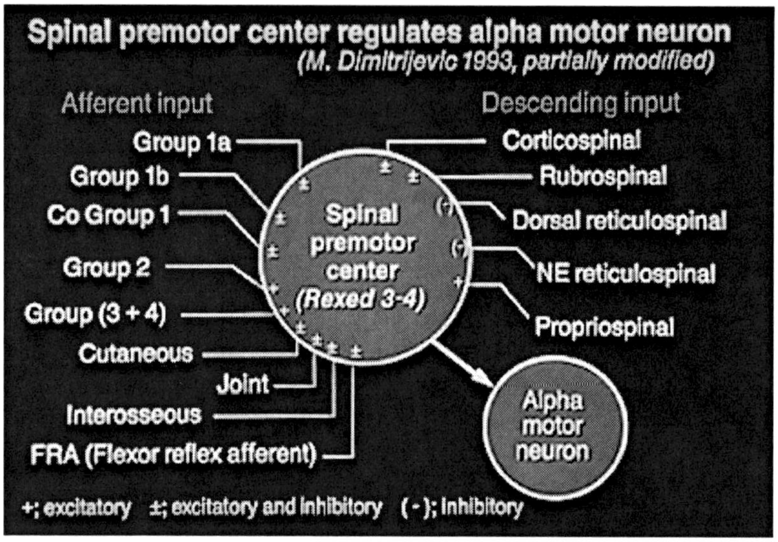

Our results confirm that whole-hand electrical neural stimulation is an effective method for activating the motor recovery process (Dimitrijevic, 1994; Dimitrijevic and Soroker, 1994; Dimitrijevic et al, 1996; Dimitrijevic et al, 2002). To date, the underlying mechanism has not been fully elucidated. Previous studies have suggested that spinal premotor centers and the sensory cortex are involved in this process (Figure 2). Interestingly, spatial hemineglect was diminished in some cases after this procedure. By SEP monitoring, whole-hand electrical stimulation with mesh glove electrodes at 20 mA is similar to recording median nerve neural stimulation (Dimitrijevic & Soroker, 1994). Peurala also reported in 2002 that motor performance, limb sensation, and the configuration of SEP of the paretic limb improved in 59 chronic stroke cases (Peuralas et al, 2002). Preliminary fMRI studies have indicated that the regional blood flow of the cortex is altered after mesh glove whole-hand stimulation at the sub-threshold level (Golaszwski et al, 2004). In this work, we explore the limitations of this mesh glove technique. To the best of our knowledge, this is the first report to do so. We observed motor recovery up to 4 years post-onset of the brain infarct, suggesting that the success of this method is not related to the post-onset duration. Patients that showed the best response to this treatment suffered from spastic paresis, with no localized lesioning of the internal capsule on CT or MRI, and partial preservation of each finger joint. No adverse effects associated with EMG were reported.

V. CONCLUSION

We tentatively conclude that (1) EMG stimulation can be used to facilitate motor recovery. (2) Short durations of EMG stimulation are useful for identifying the primary responders to this treatment. (3) Thus, this method can be used among selected persons before FES is applied.

REFERENCES

Dimitrijevic, M. M. (1992). Development of neuro-physiological aspects of the spinal cord during the past 10 years. *Paraplegia*, *30*, 92–95.

Dimitrijevic, M. M. (1994). Mesh-glove: A method for whole-hand electrical stimulation in upper motor neuron dysfunction. *Scandinavian Journal of Rehabilitative Medicine*, *26*, 183–186.

Dimitrijevic, M. M., Dimitrijevic, M. R., Lissens, M. A., & Makay, W. B. (1991). The present status of neurosurgical poor survival and role of restorative neurology in management of patients. *Neurosurgeons*, *10*, 333–338.

Dimitrijevic, M. M., & Soroker, N. (1994). Modulation of residual upper limb motor control after stroke with whole-hand electric stimulation. *Scandinavian Journal of Rehabilitative Medicine*, *26*, 183–186.

Dimitrijevic, M. M., Soroker, N., & Pollo, E. F. (1996). Mesh glove electrical stimulation. *Science & Medicine*, *3*, 54–63.

Dimitrijevic, M. M., Stokic, S. D., Waero, W. A., & Wun, C.-C. (1996). Modification of motor control of wrist extension by mesh-glove electrical affrent stimulation in stroke patients. *Archives of Physical Medicine and Rehabilitation*, *77*, 252–258. doi:10.1016/S0003-9993(96)90107-0

Feeney, D. M., & Sutton, R. L. (1987). Pharmacotherapy for recovery of function after brain injury. *CRC Critical Review of Neurobiology*, *3*, 135–197.

Golaszwski, S. M., Siedentopf, C. M., Koppelstaetter, F. K., Rhomberg, P., & Guendisch, G. M. (2004). Modulatory effects on human sensorimotor cortex by whole-hand affrent electrical stimulation. *Neurology*, *62*, 2262–2269.

Hewer, R. L. (1994). Rehabilitation after stroke. In Illis, L. S. (Ed.), *Neurological rehabilitation* (pp. 157–168). Oxford, UK: Blackwell Scientific Publications.

Peuralas, S. H., Pitkanen, K., Sivenius, J., & Takka, I. M. (2002). Cutaneous electrical stimulation may enhance sensorimotor recovery in chronic stroke. *Clinical Rehabilitation*, *16*, 709–715. doi:10.1191/0269215502cr543oa

Sunderland, A., Tinson, D. J., Bradely, E. L., Eletcher, D., Langton, H. R., & Wade, D. T. (1992). Enhanced physical therapy improves recovery of arm function after stroke: A randomized controlled trial. *Journal of Neurology, Neurosurgery, and Psychiatry*, *55*, 530–535. doi:10.1136/jnnp.55.7.530

Wade, D. T., Langton, H. R., Woov, V. A., Skilbeck, C. E., & Ismail, H. M. (1983). The hemiplegic arm after stroke: Measurement and recovery. *Journal of Neurology, Neurosurgery, and Psychiatry*, *46*, 521–524. doi:10.1136/jnnp.46.6.521

KEY TERMS AND DEFINITIONS

Mesh Glove (EMG): A silver mesh glove coated in fabric was produced for electric neuronal stimulation. Distal to the wrist joint, only sensory neurons exist. Thus, utilizing the low resistance of silver metal, we were able to use a single electrode to apply the central premotor theory for the restoration of motor deficits.

Motor Recovery: Restoration of a motor deficit after stroke and CNS injury is routinely limited, and thus other techniques are needed to activate motor recovery. All procedures were referred to as restorative neurology.

Pinch and Grasp: Basic motor function of the hand. These tasks were used as the primary assessments for the success of restorative neurology.

Spinal Premotor Center: Located in Rexed 3-4 in the dorsal column and an additional motor center that regulates the activity of spinal secondary motor neurons and receives afferent and efferent projections. Through either the efferent or afferent connections, we can modulate the spinal premotor center and subsequently modulate secondary spinal motor neurons.

Chapter 38
Novel Rehabilitation Devices for Hand Movement Disorders

Akira Gyoten
Graduate School of Natural Science and Technology, Okayama University, Japan

Jinglong Wu
Graduate School of Natural Science and Technology, Okayama University, Japan

Satoshi Takahashi
Graduate School of Natural Science and Technology, Okayama University, Japan

ABSTRACT

Numerous therapeutic rehabilitation devices have been studied. This chapter describes novel rehabilitation devices designed to treat hand movement disorders. Recently, robot-aided rehabilitation using instruments, such as a hand motion robots and a robotic glove, have attracted interest because they help recover motor function in stroke patients. The lack of proper care for at-home patients is a major problem. The authors of this chapter developed a novel portable device, consisting of two grips, that allows the patient to perform exercises at home. While a patient grasps both grips with one hand, the driving grip reciprocates at several speed adjustments. The relative distance between the movable and fixed grip enables the hand to open. In addition, a master-slave system that measures the surface EMG on the healthy arm is proposed for self-controlled rehabilitation therapy. This portable device is not complex and can be used without assistance. Future development will improve the quality of the system, and the recovery effect will be evaluated in clinical trials.

INTRODUCTION

The number of patients with a disability resulting from stroke or bone fracture has increased in proportion with the aging Japanese population. In particular, motor disorders of the hand affect daily activities such as eating, writing, or manipulating objects. Physical rehabilitation is typically performed in hospitals by therapists. However, therapists are in a relative shortage, and it is not always possible for patients to rehabilitate sufficient motor functions from ADL (Activities of Daily Living). There are numerous patients with chronic movement disorders of the hand (Abe,

DOI: 10.4018/978-1-60960-559-9.ch038

Makizako, & Tokuhara, 2005). A rehabilitation device that allows the patient to self-perform exercises would be beneficial.

Mechanical devices that are used for rehabilitation are grouped into two categories. One type is a continuous-passive–motion (CPM) device. During the early stages of hand rehabilitation, a therapist typically performs exercises that repetitively extend and flex finger joints to prevent contracture in a range-of-motion (ROM) exercise. A CPM device performs the ROM exercise in place of the therapist.

Rehabilitation is also performed using robotic devices. Robotic devices accurately and systematically control the applied force and progressively adapt to the ability of the patient. Robot-aided rehabilitation is used to enhance, quantify, and document neurological rehabilitation. Neurological rehabilitation is a complex medical process that aims to aid recovery from a nervous system injury and minimizes and/or compensates for any functional alterations. Whereas classical rehabilitation is limited by the subjective observations of therapists and patients, robotic devices precisely quantify the progress achieved by stroke patients. Robotic arm rehabilitation therapies have been clinically tested (Lum, Burgar, Shor, Majmunda, & Van der Loos, 2002), (Fasoli, Krebs, Stein, Frontera, & Hogan, 2003).

Conversely, hand rehabilitation is somewhat difficult because the hand possesses many degrees of freedom of motion, and the mechanical device would have to be small. There are three joints in each finger, the metacarpophalangeal (MP), proximal interpharangeal (PIP), and distal interphlangeal (DIP) joints. We have previously introduced some rehabilitation devices to be used for hand movement disorders. This chapter describes the development of a novel device that promotes hand rehabilitation at home. A control method is also presented for self-performed exercises.

HAND REHABILITATION DEVICES

CPM Device

Figure 1 shows the CPM device for the hand and wrist (SAKAI Medical Co., Ltd.). Accessories correspond to ROM training of the hand and forearm during the early stages of rehabilitation. Repetitive passive movements are believed to improve joint, muscle and tendon mobility (Hesse, Schulte-Tigges, Konrad, Bardeleben, & Werner, 2003).

Robotic Device

A robotic interface to train opening/closing of the hand and knob manipulation was developed (Dovat, Lambercy, Ruffieux, Chapuis, Gassert, Bleuler, Teo, & Burdet, 2006), (Lambercy, Dovat, Gassert, Burdet, Teo, & Milner, 2007). This DOF device can be used to rehabilitate a complete opening movement, i.e., the movement from a contracted and closed hand to an opened position.

To enhance the quality of life of patients with hand impairments, the Hand Motion Assist Robot was developed (Kawasaki, Ito, Ishigure, Nishimoto, Aoki, Mouri, Sakaeda, & Abe, 2007; Ueki, Nishimoto, Abe, Kawasaki, Ito, Ishigure,

Figure 1. CPM device for joint surgery patients. © 2010 SAKAI Medical Co., Ltd. Used with permission

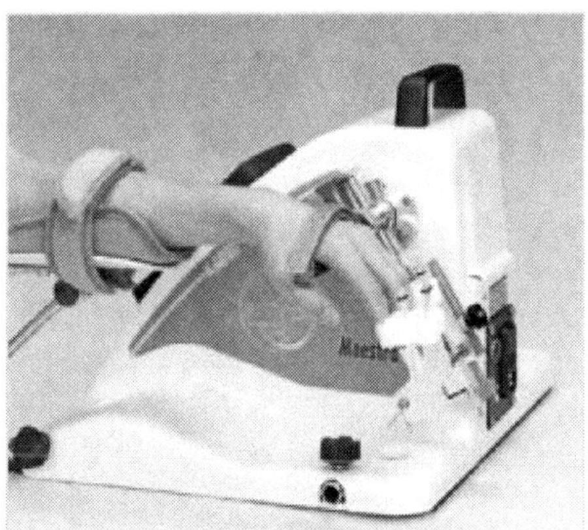

Mizumoto, & Ojika, 2008), as shown in Figure 2. This robot is composed of an exoskeleton with 18 degrees of freedom (DOFs) to assist not only the flexion/extension but also the abduction/adduction motions of each joint of the fingers and thumb independently. This setup is based on a master-slave system; the motion of the healthy hand is recorded with a data glove, and the robot produces an equivalent motion for the affected hand.

Robotic Glove with Pneumatic Actuators

The Rutgers MasterII(Bouzit, Popescu, Burdea, & Boian, 2002) is a robotic glove with pneumatic actuators fixed to the palm that actuate each finger. Experiments with stroke patients showed an increase in the ROM of fingers and force amplitude after training (Jack, Boian, Merians, Tremaine, Burdea, Adamovich, Recce, & Poizner, 2001). A different power-assisted glove has been developed for hand grasping in the ADL of aged or disabled persons, as shown in Figure 3 (Sasaki, Noritsugu, Yamamoto, & Takaiwa, 2006). The glove uses pneumatic artificial rubber muscle that is safe, lightweight, and flexible.

DEVELOPMENT OF A HOME REHABILITATION DEVICE

During severe impairment or when patients undergo an insufficient amount of exercise in the early stages of rehabilitation, the patient may not fully recover motor function. It is possible that these patients may acquire contracture (Abe et al, 2005). Contracture is caused when the joint of an aged person is kept in a rest position too long. At-home care for these patients is difficult. However, it is also difficult to introduce the CPM device and other devices into the home environment because they are heavy, expensive, and difficult to attach the hand. Therefore, we developed a novel device for hand and finger rehabilitation that is to be used at home. Our goal is to prevent contracture and promote recovery of hand function. We initially focused on enabling the patient to open the hand using complex tasks.

Figure 2. Attachment of a disabled hand to the robot. © 2010 Kawasaki and Mouri Laboratory, Graduate School of Engineering, Gifu University. Used with permission

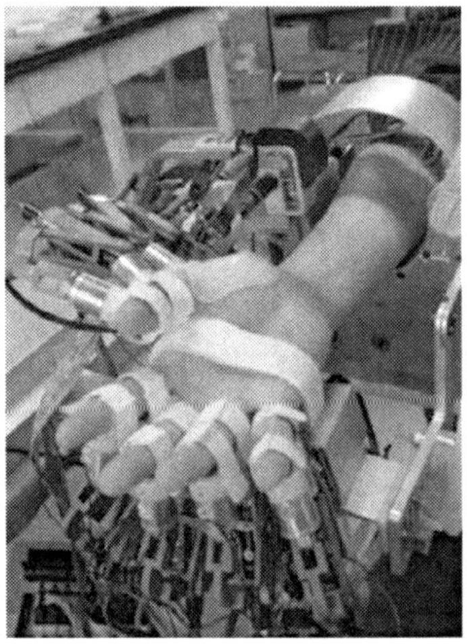

Figure 3. Outlook of the power-assisted glove. © 2010 Intelligent Machine Control Laboratory, Graduate School of Natural Science and Technology, Okayama University. Used with permission

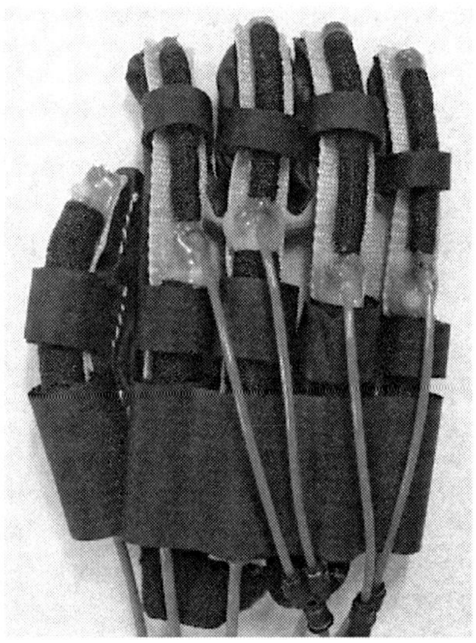

Device Design

Figure 4 shows the rehabilitation device and the passive movement of the device. The device includes two grips. Grip 1 is fixed on a motorized linear slide (Oriental Motor Co., Ltd., EZS 2 EZS3D-K; speed of operation: 0.01-600 mm/s; range resolution: 0.01 mm) controlled by a stepping motor, and Grip 2 is fixed on the table. The motorized liner slide reciprocates Grip 1 at several levels of speed. Grip 2 is used to steady the thumb and wrist. Movement of Grip 1 enables a liner opening of the hand. As shown in Figure 4 (A), the external dimensions of the interface are 30 × 20 × 20 cm^3 and are expected to be reduced in the next generation. The patient grasps both grips with one hand and fixes the wrist using the belt, which is attached to the table [Figure 4 (B)]. When Grip 1 moves toward Grip 2, the hand is extended [Figure 4 (C)] and movement toward the opposite side brings the grip toward the hand. The range of movement is determined by the patient's hand size.

Figure 4. A: Overview of the rehabilitation device. The external dimensions of the interface are 30 × 20 × 20 cm^3. B: The patient grasps both grips with one hand and fixes the wrist. C: The relative motion of Grip 1 enables the fingers to open.

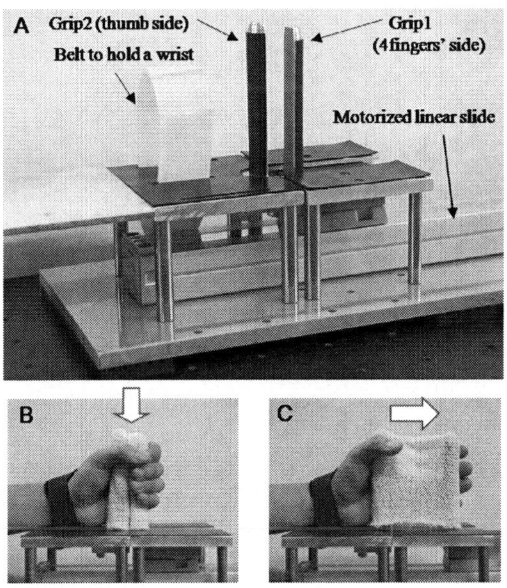

Figure 5 shows an operating system and the signal from limit sensors. To prevent accidents, the fingers and skin of the palm are pinched by the grips and the limit sensor is set on the slide. The limit sensor consists of a photo interrupter. If Grip 1 tends to exceed the range of movement, the motor controllers will automatically stop the movement. However, redundant levels of safety are required to use the device at home. Therefore, features such as an emergency push button switch were incorporated.

Master-Slave System that Measures Surface EMG

In preliminary studies of the rehabilitation device (Lum et al, 2002), (Kawasaki et al, 2007), the master-slave system showed a positive outcome. A master-slave system is used for patients who only have one hand that is impaired. This device causes the disabled hand to produce the same motions produced by the non-disabled hand. We attempted to apply a master-slave system using a different approach.

Figure 6 shows an image of a master-slave system obtained by measuring the surface EMG of the forearm. This control method easily evaluates the state of the non-disabled hand without expensive instruments. Please refer to Funada et al. (2009) for details. The control method will provide the following advantage to hand rehabilitation: Patients can perform training motions for their impaired hand because such motions are generated by their opposite hand. This ability is expected to facilitate the recovery of the disabled function. It has been reported that mirror therapy (Altschuler, Wisdom, Stone, Foster, Galasko, Llewellyn, & Ramachandran, 1999) has a restorative effect. In this method, the patient sees healthy hand motion through a mirror and feels the impaired hand move in concert with the non-disabled hand.

Figure 5. Operating system and the signal from limit sensors. Limit sensors are used for positioning and provide an emergency switch. The range of movement is determined by the size of the patient's hand.

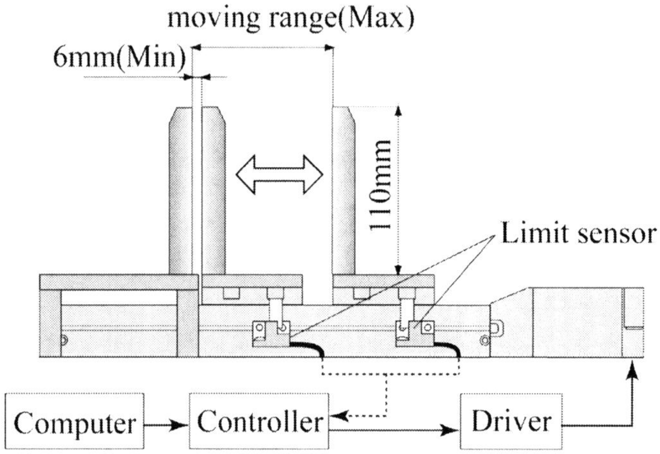

Figure 6. An image of the master-slave system obtained by measuring the surface EMG. This method allows the disabled hand to perform the same motions (opening/grasping) produced by the normal hand.

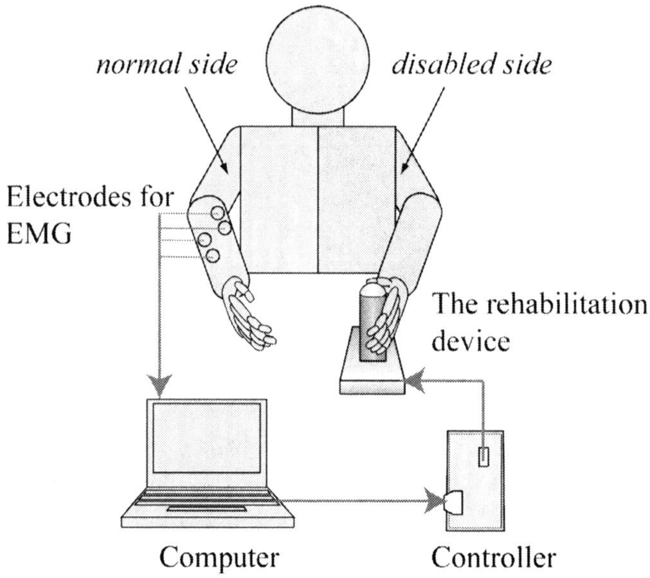

CONCLUSION AND FUTURE WORK

We introduced novel devices to be used for hand rehabilitation. Robot-aided rehabilitation is a recent approach that may enhance and quantify neurological rehabilitation. We particularly focused on the care of the patients at home and have proceeded with the development of novel devices. These portable devices are not complex and are able to be used by the individual without assistance. There are many areas for further improvement, such as:

- Software and hardware emergency systems
- Coordination between the thumb and fingers

- A virtual reality display system for independent rehabilitation therapies at home
- Reduction of the size and weight of the device
- To allow hand rehabilitation at home, this rehabilitation device is being developed using both hardware and software.

ACKNOWLEDGMENT

A portion of this study was supported by a Grant-in-Aid for Scientific Research (B) and the Japan and AA Science Platform Program of the Japan Society for the Promotion Science.

REFERENCES

Abe, T., Makizako, H., & Tokuhara, R. (2005). Assessment and program of the physical activity reflected daily life in the elderly: Target on the prolongation of healthy life span: Report on real image and practice for the object of visiting rehabilitation. *Journal of the Japanese Physical Therapy Association*, *32*(4), 224–226.

Altschuler, E. L., Wisdom, S. B., Stone, L., Foster, C., Galasko, D., Llewellyn, D. M. E., & Ramachandran, V. S. (1999). Rehabilitation of hemiparesis after stroke with a mirror. *Lancet*, *353*(June), 2035–2036. doi:10.1016/S0140-6736(99)00920-4

Bouzit, M., Popescu, G., Burdea, G., & Boian, R. (2002). The Rutgers MasterII-ND Force Feedback Glove. *IEEE/ASME Transactions on Mechatronics*, *7*, 256–263. doi:10.1109/TMECH.2002.1011262

Dovat, L., Lambercy, O., Ruffieux, Y., Chapuis, D., Gassert, R., & Bleuler, H. … Burdet, E. (2006). A haptic knob for rehabilitation of stroke patients. *Proceedings of the 2006 IEEE/RSJ International Conference on Intelligent Robots and Systems*, October 2006, (pp. 977-982).

Fasoli, S. E., Krebs, H. I., Stein, J., Frontera, W. R., & Hogan, N. (2003). Effects of robotic therapy on motor impairment and recovery in chronic stroke. *Archives of Physical Medicine and Rehabilitation*, *84*, 477–482. doi:10.1053/apmr.2003.50110

Funada, K., Takahashi, S., & Wu, J. (2009). A study on motion recognition of hand using surface EMG of forearm for upper-limb rehabilitation. *Proceedings of The 2009 International Symposium on Early Detection and Rehabilitation Technology of Dementia (DRD2009)*, (pp. 175-178).

Hesse, S., Schulte-Tigges, G., Konrad, M., Bardeleben, A., & Werner, C. (2003). Robot-assisted arm trainer for the passive and active practice of bilateral forearm and wrist movements in hemiparetic subjects. *Archives of Physical Medicine and Rehabilitation*, *84*, 915–920. doi:10.1016/S0003-9993(02)04954-7

Jack, D., Boian, R., Merians, A. S., Tremaine, M., Burdea, G. C., & Adamovich, S. V. (2001). Virtual reality-enhanced stroke rehabilitation. *IEEE Transactions on Neural Systems and Rehabilitation Engineering*, *9*(3), 308–318. doi:10.1109/7333.948460

Kawasaki, H., Ito, S., Ishigure, Y., Nishimoto, Y., Aoki, T., & Mouri, T. … Abe, M. (2007). Development of a hand motion assist robot for rehabilitation therapy by patient self-motion control. *Proceedings of the 2007 IEEE 10th International Conference on Rehabilitation Robotics*. June 2007, (pp. 234-240).

Lambercy, O., Dovat, L., Gassert, R., Burdet, E., Teo, C. L., & Milner, T. (2007). A haptic knob for rehabilitation of hand function. *IEEE Transactions on Neural Systems and Rehabilitation Engineering*, *15*, 356–366. doi:10.1109/TNSRE.2007.903913

Lum, P. S., Burgar, C. G., Shor, P. C., Majmundar, M., & Van der Loos, M. (2002). Robot-assisted movement training compared with conventional therapy techniques for the rehabilitation of upper-limb motor function after stroke. *Archives of Physical Medicine and Rehabilitation*, *83*, 952–959. doi:10.1053/apmr.2001.33101

Sakai Medical Co. Ltd. (2010). *CPM Hand and wrist* (Product No.CPM-0050). Retrieved on March 20, 2010, from http://www.sakaimed.co.jp

Sasaki, D., Noritsugu, T., Yamamoto, H., & Takaiwa, M. (2006). Development of power assist glove using pneumatic artificial rubber muscle. *Journal of Robotics Society of Japan*, *24*(5), 640–646.

Ueki, S., Nishimoto, Y., Abe, M., Kawasaki, H., Ito, S., & Ishigure, Y. … Ojika, T. (2008). Development of virtual reality exercise of hand motion assist robot for rehabilitation therapy by patient self-motion control. *Proceedings of the 30th Annual International IEEE EMBS Conference*. August 2008, (pp. 4282-4285).

Young, G. O. (1964). Synthetic structure of industrial plastics. In Peters, J. (Ed.), *Plastics* (2nd ed., pp. 15–64). New York, NY: McGraw-Hill.

KEY TERMS AND DEFINITIONS

Continuous Passive Motion (CPM): In the early stages of hand rehabilitation, a therapist typically performs exercises that extend and flex the joints of the fingers many times to prevent contracture.

Contracture: A condition where the range of motion is decreased.

Master-Slave System: A method in which one hand (slave) undergoes the same motions produced by the other hand (master).

Movement Disorder: When a patient cannot move a certain part of the body.

Robot-Aided Rehabilitation: Therapy that uses a robotic device. Robotic devices can accurately and systematically control the applied force and progressively adapt assistance/resistance to the patient abilities.

Stroke: The general term for a cerebrovascular accident.

Surface EMG: A procedure used to measure muscle activity. It is commonly known that the muscles in the forearm contract during hand movement.

Chapter 39
A Novel Length Display Device for Cognitive Experiments and Rehabilitation

Naotsugu Kitayama
Graduate School of Natural Science and Technology, Okayama University, Japan

Haibo Wang
Graduate School of Natural Science and Technology, Okayama University, Japan

Satoshi Takahashi
Graduate School of Natural Science and Technology, Okayama University, Japan

Jinglong Wu
Graduate School of Natural Science and Technology, Okayama University, Japan

ABSTRACT

The purpose of this study was to develop a finger display device that has a four-degree-of-freedom (4DOF) length. This device was designed for rehabilitation and cognitive experimentation. The device can change the finger span between the thumb and four fingers, and the distance between digits is controlled by four motors. The positions of each unit, including the motor, are self-adjusted. Adjustments are made after recording the motion of the individual's hand and analyzing fingertip movement. Each finger is controlled independently, and rehabilitation is performed on each individual finger. The device can be used for not only rehabilitation but also basic tactile studies. In particular, this device provides a valid method to measure length.

INTRODUCTION

In the aging society, the number of people with disabilities caused by stroke or an accident is increasing. According to the Ministry of Health, Labour and Welfare, there are 1,760,000 crippled people in Japan. This represents the largest fraction of disabled people, more than the number with visual, hearing, and speech impairments or internal impediments. People with upper limb disorders are more numerous than people with lower limb disorders. Physical rehabilitation is

DOI: 10.4018/978-1-60960-559-9.ch039

typically performed by a therapist to recover people's lost abilities and regain the quality of life. However, with the number of patients increasing, satisfactory rehabilitation cannot be administered (Abe, Makizako & Tokuhara, 2005). We aimed to develop a rehabilitation device that is conducive to individual use at home (Tsubahara, 2008). Many devices for lower limb or upper arm rehabilitation have been developed. However, devices that incorporate multi-finger rehabilitation are rare. In particular, it is important to recover finger function and fine motor skills.

Many groups have developed pneumatic rubber muscle (Kobayashi, Ishida & Suzuki, 2004) or tail-arms (Tsukagoshi, Shirato, Ido & Kitagawa, 2004). However, these devices require a change in the linear movement by a linear actuator, and thus, the suit must be large. To solve this problem, the power-assisted glove provides no structure (Sasaki, Noritsugu, Yamamoto & Takaiwa, 2006). Paralysis in stroke patients occurs only in half of the body. Therefore, a master-slave system was developed to provide movement to the disabled side that is dependent on the non-disabled side. The master-slave system allows the impaired hand of a patient to be driven by the healthy hand (Kawasaki, Kimura & Ito, 2006). In this study, a virtual reality training program provided comfortable rehabilitation.

In the field of cognitive science, the environment is very important for remote robot control operation and design of virtual reality technology (Wu & Kawamura, 2000). Tactile senses provide much information (e.g., shapes, length, material, weight), and this information is principally relayed though the hand. Because tactile information is transferred through the hand, remote medical treatments and training of physicians through a virtual device is possible. In previous studies, tactile senses were stimulated with material (Ino & Ifukube, 1997; Lu & Sakai, 2004). The authors evaluated length using three fingers. Wang showed that the thumb and index finger provided more accurate results than the thumb and the middle finger (Wang, Takahashi & Wu, 2009). The experiment showed that the accuracy of the length determined by the thumb and the index finger or the middle finger was the same when evaluating a length range of 10 to 50 mm. However, the results were significantly different when a length in the range of 60 to 70 mm was used. Perception was evaluated when two fingers (index and middle finger) were moved together.

This study describes the development of a four-degree-of-freedom length display device for five fingers. The primary purpose of this device is to provide rehabilitation of finger movement by controlling contact. In addition, we intend for this device to be useful for cognitive research. This device controls four fingers individually and can be customized to an individual's hand this flexibility provides comfort to the individual.

2DOF LENGTH DISPLAY DEVICE

The two-length display device using three fingers is shown in Figure 1. This device is used to determine length perception by the thumb and index finger and the thumb and middle finger. As shown in Figure 1, the electric slider, which is installed vertically, is attached to a wooden board (90×20 cm). The electric slider controller locks onto the wooden board. An acrylic disk, which presents the length stimulus to the fingertips of the index finger and the middle finger, controls the length stimulus between the fingertips by being installed at a fixed distance. An aluminum framework supports the acrylic disk. The pressure sensor, which measures the grip of the fingertip, is installed under the aluminum framework. A portable stand containing two sliders can be used to adjust the distance between three acrylic boards during a continuous presentation of length stimuli.

Figure 1. Two tactile length perception device for three fingers experiments

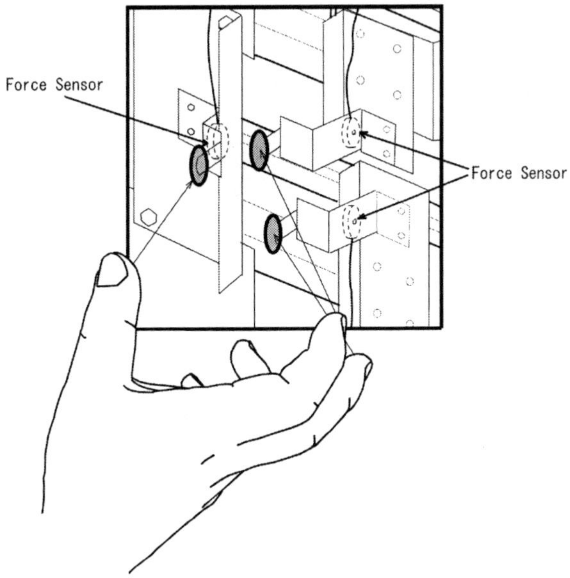

4DOF LENGTH DISPLAY DEVICE

Outline

An overview of the device is shown in Figure 2. Sliders were set up independently for each finger. The contact portion of the thumb was locked. The slider moves linearly and can be customized to the individual. The set position is discussed below. Figure 3 shows a movable contiguous unit. A slider is fixed on the slide screw (NTN corp.), which is fitted to a rail to parallelize the base. The slide screw has chase. The slider moves linearly through the screw spins. Screws had a 24 leads (mm per rotation) and a 8-mm diameter. The slider was able to move from 0 to 70 mm. The contact portion, slider and rail were acrylic. One side of the slide screw was connected to the bearing and the other side was coupled to a stepping motor.

The motor is a five-phase stepping motor holding a torque of 0.24 Newton meters. The drive controller consists of a four-axis controller (CosmoTechs Co., Ltd, USPG-48; universal serial bus interface). During movement, the four axes are able to move at the same time.

As shown in Figure 4, the control system is very simple. The behavior software is Visual Basic 6 (VB6). VB6 calculates and transmits the pulse and operates the stepping motor via the motor driver. The distance and coordinates are displayed on a personal computer. Subjects can stop the device during an emergency at any time.

Configuration of Unit

To fit to the size of an individual's hand and reduce discomfort, the slider was made flexible. Its positioning can be customized to fit finger trajectory.

Fingertip Trajectory

As shown in Figure 5, the fingertip trajectory of the subject's right hand was recorded. However, it is difficult for patients undergoing rehabilitation to open and close their hand. The trajectory positions must be low-impact, and each finger's position is measured at a neutral position. Individuals are asked to put their hands on a plane in a grasping motion. At this time, the fingers are put on a board. After the two-dimensional movement

Figure 2. Four-degree-of-freedom length display device

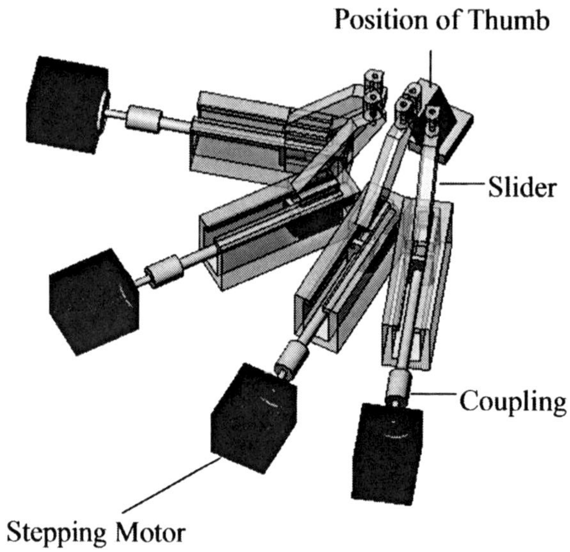

Figure 3. Movable contiguous unit

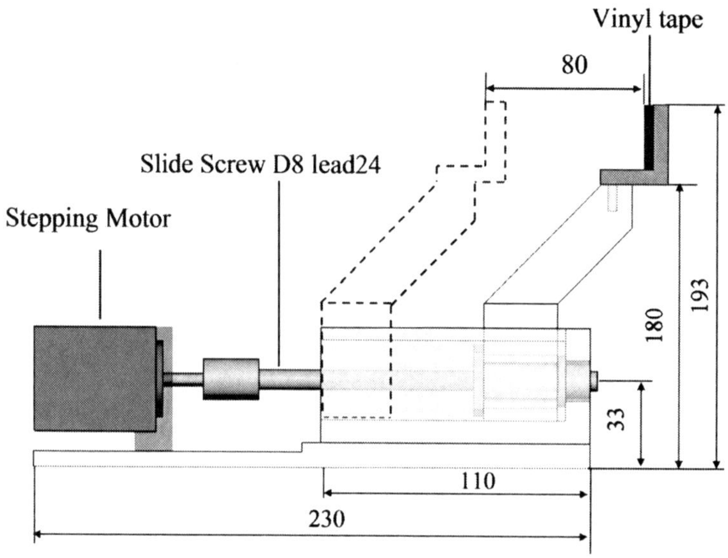

of the fingertips is recorded, the trajectory of each fingertip is analyzed (DITECT Co., Ltd, DIPP Motion XD). The analysis software discriminates color concentration and tracks the trajectory. It is able to track the fingertip trajectory as the hand opens and closes. The coordinate origin (0, 0) was set as the tip of the thumb. Linear approximation was composed from coordinates, and the position of the unit was decided.

Figure 6 illustrates the tracking data of the fingertips of one subject. The X-axis and Y-axis were defined such that the middle finger line was superimposed on a line 30 degrees from the Y-axis. The tracking data of the middle, ring and

Figure 4. Main control system

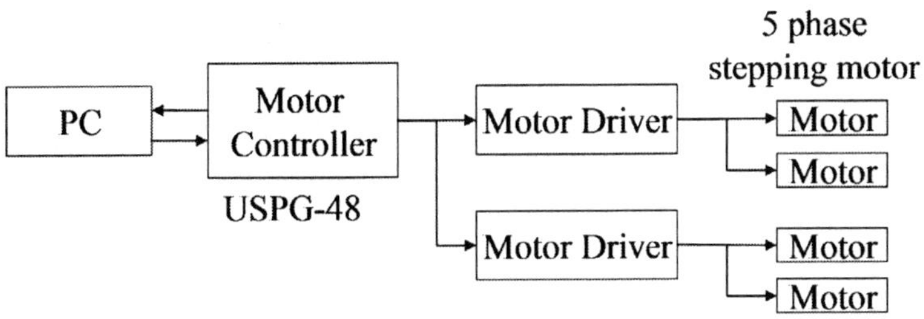

little finger were nearly linear. The data of the index finger were curved. Because we used the middle finger line for the baseline of the coordinates, it was the most linear of the five fingers. Table 1 shows the correlation coefficient of each finger trajectory for approximately 4 subjects. The middle and ring fingers had a high value. As shown in Figure 6 and Table 1, the trajectory of the middle fingertip was a straight line from the origin.

Configuration

The unit placement was observed as the same straight-line approximation of the tracking data. After coordinate transformation, the placement picture is shown in Figure 7.

Figure 5. Trajectory shot image

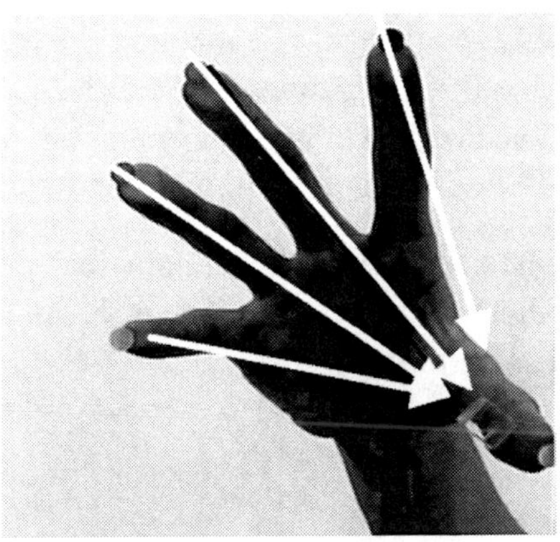

REHABILITATION

In the rehabilitation method that uses this device, the contact portions consist of passive movements of the fingers. The angle and positioning of each slider against the thumb of this device was easy to adjust. Each finger was able to be placed into any position and could not only open and close but also grasp an object. The patient receives rehabilitation. This method was evaluated by the Action Research Arm Test (Stroke center).

CONCLUSION

A novel four-degrees-of-freedom length display device was developed for patient rehabilitation.

Figure 6. An analysis of fingertip trajectory

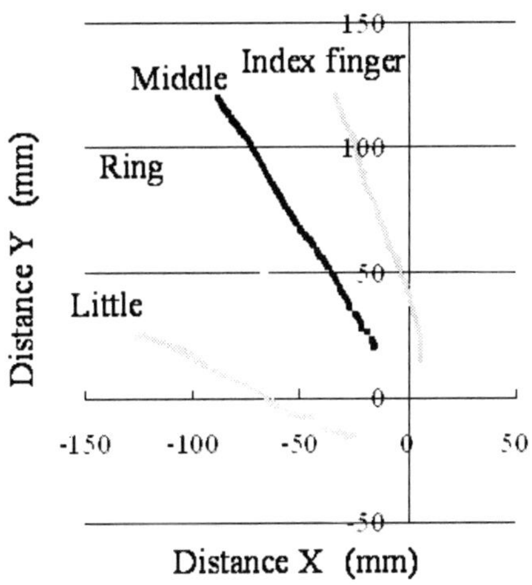

Table 1. Coefficient of correlation of each finger

	Index finger	Middle finger	Ring finger	Little finger
Subject A	0.877	0.987	0.996	0.987
Subject B	0.810	0.956	0.936	0.970
Subject C	0.900	0.997	0.996	0.932
Subject D	0.937	0.998	0.995	0.964
Average	0.881	0.985	0.981	0.963

Whereas many devices have been developed for the lower limb or arm, a device designed for fingers that has many DOFs of motion has not been developed. Our device has the ability to change the distance between the thumb and each finger. The control system provides a simple comparison, and the device is not large. Individuals have hands of different sizes. With this device, the fingertip trajectories were recorded and analyzed during a grasping motion. These results optimized the set position.

In future experiments, we will evaluate the ability of this device to be used for rehabilitation and cognitive science experiments.

Figure 7. Placement image

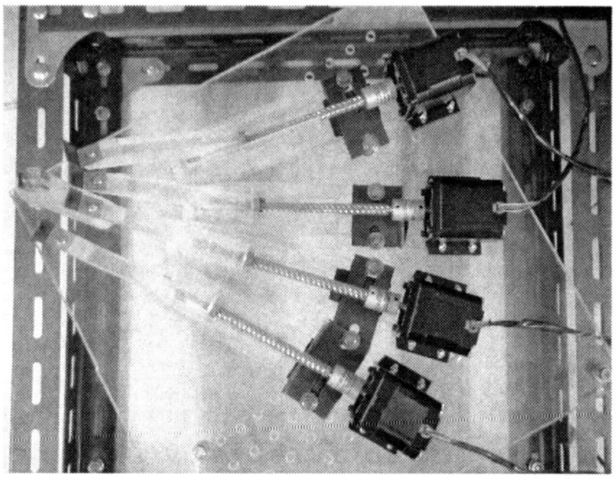

ACKNOWLEDGMENT

A portion of this study was financially supported by the JSPS AA Science Platform Program and a JSPS Grant-in-Aid for Scientific Research (B) (21404002).

REFERENCES

Abe, T., Makizako, H., & Tokuhara, R. (2005). Assessment and program of the physical activity reflected daily life in the elderly: Target on the prolongation of healthy life span: Report on real image and oractice for the object of visiting rehabilitation. *Journal of the Japanese Physical Therapy Association*, *32*(4), 224–226.

Ino, S., & Ifukube, T. (1997). A basic study on a tactile display system for presenting quality of materials. *TIEE Japan, 117*.

Kawasaki, H., Kimura, H., & Ito, S. (2008). Hand rehabilitation support system. *The Japan Society of Mechanical Engineers*, *72*, 228–233.

Kobayashi, H., Ishida, K., & Suzuki, H. (2004). Realization of all motion for the upper kimb by a muscle suit. *Proceedings of the 13th IEEE International Workshop on Robot and Human Interactive Communication RO-MAN2004*, (p. 631).

Lu, S., & Sakai, Y. (2004). Measurement and analysis of the object length perceptive characteristics with visual and tactile information for proposal of three-dimension tactile shape display. *Transactions of the Japan Society of Mechanical Engineers*, 2699–2706.

Sasaki, D., Noritsugu, T., Yamamoto, H., & Takaiwa, M. (2006). Development of power assist glove using pneumatic artificial rubber muscle. *Journal of the Robotics Society of Japan*, *24*, 640–646.

Tsubahara, A. (2008). Technological advance in medical rehabilitation. *Kawasaki Journal of Medical Welfare*, *18*, 7–14.

Tsukagoshi, H., Shirato, K., Ido, M., & Kitagawa, A. (2004). Tail-arm: A wearable unit to stimulate exercise. *Proceedings of the 13th IEEE International Workshop on Robot and Human Interactive Communication RO-MAN2004*, (p. 667).

Wang, H. B., Takahashi, S., & Wu, J. L. (2008). Human characteristics of length perception with three fingers for tactile intelligent interfaces. *Active Media Technology*, 217-225.

Wu, J. L., & Kawamura, S. (2000). Quantitative analysis of human tactile illusory characteristic under visual environment and a haptic device of two-dimensional curved surface. *IEEE Transactions on Robotics and Automation*, *16*, 762–771. doi:10.1109/70.897787

KEY TERMS AND DEFINITIONS

DOF: Is degrees of freedom.

Finger Span: Is the length between the thumb and four fingers.

Fingertip Trajectory: Is line traced by fingertip.

Haptic: Is one of senses of touch.

Length: Is span from one to another point.

Rehabilitation: Is method to improve or heal dissolved body part.

Sensation: Is function of human.

Chapter 40
A Log-Linearized Viscoelastic Model for Measuring Changes in Vascular Impedance

Abdugheni Kutluk
Graduate School of Engineering, Hiroshima University, Japan

Noboru Saeki
Graduate School of Biomedical Sciences, Hiroshima University, Japan

Ryuji Nakamura
Graduate School of Biomedical Sciences, Hiroshima University, Japan

Masao Yoshizumi
Graduate School of Biomedical Sciences, Hiroshima University, Japan

Toshio Tsuji
Graduate School of Engineering, Hiroshima University, Japan

Masashi Kawamoto
Graduate School of Biomedical Sciences, Hiroshima University, Japan

Teiji Ukawa
Nihon Kohden Corporation, Japan

ABSTRACT

This chapter proposes a new nonlinear model, called a log-linearized viscoelastic model, to estimate the dynamic characteristics of human arterial walls. The model employs mechanical impedance factors, including stiffness and viscosity, in beat-to-beat measured from biological signals such as arterial blood pressure and photoplethysmograms. The validity of the proposed method is determined by demonstrating how arterial wall impedance properties change during arm position testing in the vertical direction. The estimated stiffness indices are compared with those of the conventional linear model. Estimated impedance parameters with contribution ratios exceeding 0.97 were used for comparison. The results indicated that stiffness and viscosity decrease when the arm is raised and increase when it is lowered, in the same pattern as mean blood pressure. However, the changes seen in the proposed nonlinear viscoelastic parameter are smaller ($P < 0.05$) than those of the linear model. This result suggests that the proposed nonlinear arterial viscoelastic model is less affected by changes in mean intravascular pressure during arm position changes.

DOI: 10.4018/978-1-60960-559-9.ch040

INTRODUCTION

Blood vessels perform an essential function in human life by supporting the transport of oxygen and nutrients throughout the whole body. They also play a critical role in state changes such as vasoconstriction/vasodilatation blood volume adjustments (Nichols, & O'Rourke, 1998). Vascular state changes can usually be divided into two general categories: organic and functional change. In organic change (arteriosclerosis), the quality of collagen in the arterial wall changes with aging, and the reduced amounts of elastic fiber cause stiffness and poor wall condition (Faber, & Moller-Hou, 1952). Arterial walls demonstrate functional changes such as contraction and relaxation in response to various stimuli and stresses. If the peripheral aspect of a blood vessel becomes stiff due to organic changes, active vascular reactions to external stimuli are deadened, which activates autonomic nerves and in turn reduces circulation. Accordingly, if the dynamic characteristics of arteries could be measured quantitatively without unnatural stimulation, it would be possible to estimate the internal physiological conditions not only during surgical procedures but also during activities common to everyday healthcare, such as physical training and treatment for arteriosclerosis.

Therefore, modeling is useful for interpreting cardiovascular dynamics, and values obtained from cardiovascular signals demonstrate a precise correlation with physiological parameters. As the properties of blood vessels are linked to endothelial and smooth muscle cell function, some researchers have tried to construct detailed descriptions of the characteristics of vascular smooth muscles, whose elasticity can be used as an index of the arterial wall (Greenfield, & Patel, D.J. 1962; Armentano, Simon, Levenson, Chau, Megnien, & Pichel, 1991; Bank, Wilson, Kubo, Holte, Dresing, & Wang, 1995). However, it is quite difficult to use such an invasive approach in healthy individuals because of the ethical problems involved. Some researchers have attempted to describe vascular dynamic characteristics using non-invasive approaches such as arterial wall compliance (Katayama, Shimoda, Maeda, & Takemiya, 1998), but these only addressed stiffness and provided insufficient analysis of vascular characteristics. Accordingly, Sakane et al. modeled the dynamic characteristics of the human arterial wall by employing mechanical impedance factors. This method aimed to estimate changes in the beat-to-beat conditions of blood vessels and ascertain vascular conditions from impedance changes in response to a physician's surgical actions (Sakane, Tsuji, Tanaka, Saeki, & Kawamoto, 2004; Sakane, Tsuji, Saeki, & Kawamoto, 2004). However, the proposed linear model has the limitation of estimated stiffness parameters being dependent upon intravascular blood pressure; it has been experimentally confirmed that the relationship between vascular internal pressure and vascular diameter exhibits nonlinearity (Busse, Bauer, Schabert, Summa, Bumm, & Wetterer, 1979; Hayashi, Handa, Nagasawa, Okumura, & Moritake, 1980). For example, Hayashi et al. confirmed the nonlinearity of the pressure-radius curve through an *in vitro* experiment, and the proposed stiffness parameter was identified as an intravascular pressure-independent elastic modulus (Hayashi, Handa, Nagasawa, Okumura, & Moritake, 1980). However, this index is suitable only for evaluating elasticity and uses only the maximal/minimal values of blood pressure and arterial diameter, making it difficult to estimate the details of arterial dynamics such as viscoelastic properties (Wurzel, Cowper, & McCook, 1969).

In this chapter, we propose a novel log-linearized arterial viscoelastic model that considers the nonlinear relationship between arterial diameter and intravascular pressure (Busse, Bauer, Schabert, Summa, Bumm, & Wetterer, 1979), permitting beat-to-beat evaluation of advanced arterial dynamics such as stiffness and viscosity. In this model, intravascular pressure-independent arterial viscoelastic indices are estimated using the arterial displacement waveform and the logarithmic blood pressure waveform, enabling more precise identification of the vascular changes seen with autonomic nervous system activity than was possible with the conventional method. The chapter explains the proposed method and discusses the results of experiments to validate the vascular viscoelastic index.

LOG-LINEARIZED ARTERIAL VISCOELASTIC MODEL

In this method, the dynamic characteristics of arterial walls are expressed in a viscoelastic model (the Voigt model), and internal pressure dependency is reduced using natural logarithm linearization. To quantify beat-to-beat changes in viscoelastic properties, time series of natural logarithmic blood pressure and radial strain are used for evaluation.

Figure 1 illustrates the proposed impedance model of the arterial wall. This model only represents the characteristics of the arterial wall in the arbitrary radius direction. Considering the relationship (Hayashi et al., 1980) of the exponential function by which the intravascular pressure $P_b(t)$ and strain $\varepsilon(t)$ relate to vascular diameter change in continuous time, arterial dynamic

Figure 1. The arterial wall impedance model

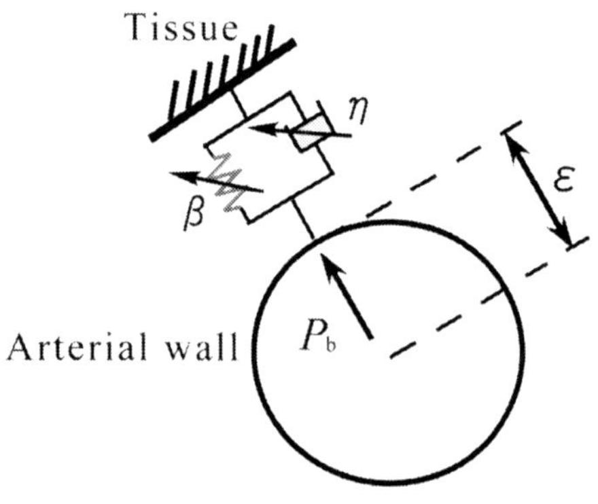

viscoelasticity can be expressed by the following equation:

$$P_b(t) = C \exp\{\beta\varepsilon(t) + \eta\dot{\varepsilon}(t)\} \quad (1)$$

where β and η represent the stiffness and viscosity of vessel walls, respectively, C is a constant of proportion, and $\dot{\varepsilon}(t)$ is strain velocity. A natural logarithm for both sides of Equation (1) gives the following equation:

$$\ln P_b(t) = \beta\varepsilon(t) + \eta\dot{\varepsilon}(t) + \ln C \quad (2)$$

When time t_0 is introduced as the starting time of each heartbeat, the equation becomes:

$$\ln P_b(t_0) = \beta\varepsilon(t_0) + \eta\dot{\varepsilon}(t_0) + \ln C \quad (3)$$

Accordingly, the dynamic characteristics of vessel walls can be expressed as shown below based on Equation (3):

$$\ln P_b(t) - \ln P_b(t_0) = \ln \frac{P_b(t)}{P_b(t_0)}$$
$$= \beta d\varepsilon(t) + \eta d\dot{\varepsilon}(t) \quad (4)$$

where $d\varepsilon(t) = \varepsilon(t) - \varepsilon(t_0)$ and $d\dot{\varepsilon}(t) = \dot{\varepsilon}(t) - \dot{\varepsilon}(t_0)$.

However, direct measurement of vascular strain is quite difficult. For this reason, plethysmogram is utilized instead of strain measurement, as follows (Sakane, Shiba, Tsuji, Saeki, & Kawamoto, 2005):

$$\varepsilon(t) \cong P_l(t) / A_0 \quad (5)$$

where $P_l(t)$ is the measured plethysmogram and A_0 is the mean value of absorbance $A(t)$ in one period

(Sakane et al., 2005). Equation (4) can therefore be described using a plethysmogram:

$$\ln \frac{P_b(t)}{P_b(t_0)} = \tilde{\beta} dP_l(t) + \tilde{\eta} d\dot{P}_l(t) \quad (6)$$

where $dP_l(t) = P_l(t) - P_l(t_0)$, $d\dot{P}_l(t) = \dot{P}_l(t) - \dot{P}_l(t_0)$ and $\dot{P}_l(t)$ is plethysmogram velocity.

$$\tilde{\beta} = \beta / A_0, \; \tilde{\eta} = \eta / A_0 \quad (7)$$

$\tilde{\beta}$ and $\tilde{\eta}$ here correspond to the log-linearized viscoelastic properties of the arterial wall.

The log-linearized viscoelastic parameters $\tilde{\beta}$ (stiffness) and $\tilde{\eta}$ (viscosity) can be estimated on a beat-to-beat basis using the least square method from the measured $P_b(t)$ and $P_l(t)$. The following section describes a validation experiment for this log-linearized arterial viscoelastic model.

METHOD

In this study, the proposed method was used to investigate vascular smooth muscle responses (Bayliss, 1902) induced by changes in intravascular pressure with respect to arm position testing on four patients. Intravascular pressure variations were simulated according to a transmural pressure/vascular smooth muscle response evocation method (Takemiya, Maeda, Suzuki, Nishihira, & Shimoda, 1996) using up-and-down motion of the fingertip artery on the basis of heart position.

The patients lay on an operating table under general anesthesia in a face-up position; the bed was inclined downward and upward on the left side by 10- 15 degrees and was tilted twice alternately. At that time, we estimated the arterial viscoelastic index using arterial blood pressure and photoplethysmogram, and the intravascular pressure dependence was investigated (Figure 2). We used preoperative patients under general anesthesia as study subjects in order to prevent the vasomotor center in the hindbrain from functionalizing the neurogenic vascular regulation mechanism. The degree of dependence on internal-pressure is considered to be reduced if the variation in stiffness values and difference in resting values are decreased. Before starting the study, we obtained approval from our institutional Ethical Review Board and received written informed consent from each patient (Hiroshima University Hospital).

In the experiment, a bedside monitor (BSS-9800, Nihon Kohden Corp., Tokyo, Japan) was used to simultaneously obtain a biomedical signal electrocardiogram (ECG), arterial blood pressure (BP) and a photoplethysmogram (PPG) at 125 Hz. These data were transferred to a computer using Transmission Control Protocol (TCP). BP was measured through a 22-gauge catheter placed in the left radial artery, and PPG was measured from the ipsilateral thumb. As measured biomedical signals are usually affected by a number of factors such as body movement, digital filters were used to regulate the frequency characteristics. The filter properties used in this study included a second-order infinite impulse response (IIR) band-pass filter (14 – 28 Hz) for the electrocardiogram, a second-order IIR low-pass filter with a cutoff frequency of 6 Hz and a first-order IIR high-pass filter with a cutoff frequency of 0.3 Hz for the arterial pressure, and an eighth-order finite impulse response (FIR) low-pass filter with a cutoff frequency of 15 Hz and a first-order IIR high-pass filter with a cutoff frequency of 0.3 Hz for the photoplethysmogram. All $P_b(t)$ and $P_l(t)$ values in the interval between an R wave and the next R wave were considered a data set, and the viscoelastic parameters were estimated by least square fitting using the data set from Equation (6). Also, in the case of estimation, the coefficient of determination (R^2) was established as a contribution ratio for a threshold value. A higher contribution ratio indicates higher estimation ac-

Figure 2. Experimental setup

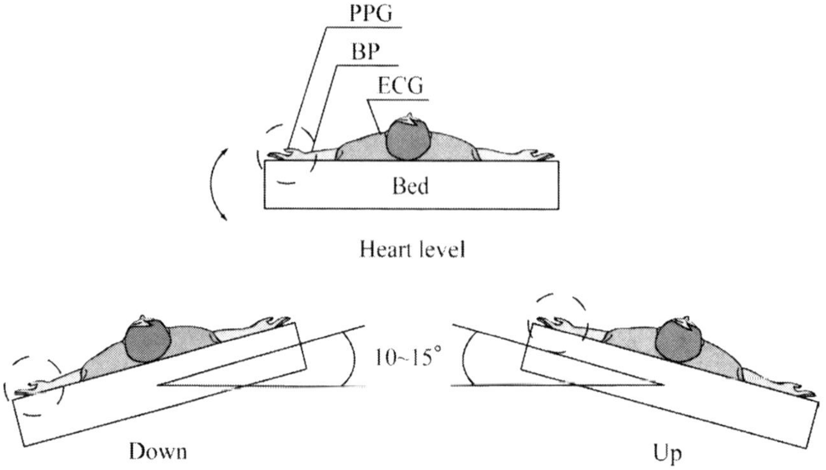

curacy in the proposed model. In this study, the proposed log-linearized model and the stiffness parameter were compared with the estimation accuracy during the arm positioning. The up/down variations for the proposed log-linearized model and the conventional linear model were then compared. Statistical analysis was performed using two-tailed t-test add-in software for Excel 2003, and the significance level was set at $P < 0.05$.

RESULTS

Figure 3 shows an example of the estimated parameters in the arm position test. The estimated viscoelastic indices are compared with those of the conventional linear model (Sakane, Tsuji, Tanaka, Saeki, & Kawamoto, 2004). In order from the top, the figure shows the arm position with the tilting bed (up, heart level, down), the mean blood pressure (*MBP*), the pulse pressure (*PP*), the photoplethysmogram variations (PPG_V), the estimated stiffness parameter $\tilde{K}$ from the linear model, and the estimated stiffness parameter $\tilde{\beta}$ from the proposed log-linearized arterial viscoelastic model. The shaded areas correspond to the time when the arm was lowered, and the estimated impedance parameters are shown only for periods when R^2 was greater than 0.97. This is to remove the decrease in estimation accuracy due to the noise that occurs when the bed is moved. The results indicate that the variations in *MBP* and PPG_V showed remarkable changes when the arm was tilted. However, *PP* demonstrated no remarkable changes. Additionally, there were large changes (increases and decreases) in the stiffness parameter $\tilde{K}$ when the arm was raised and lowered; these changes showed the same tendency as *MBP*. On the other hand, the variations in $\tilde{\beta}$ were smaller than those in $\tilde{K}$.

In order to investigate estimation accuracy, the proposed model (with log-linearized arterial viscoelastic parameters) and stiffness parameter β (Hayashi et al., 1980) were compared with the coefficient of determination. For the arm position test data measured in Patient A, the mean value and standard deviation of R^2 for 20 periods of continuous data (down and up) were calculated from each model. The results are shown in Figure 4, which indicates that the estimation accuracy of our proposed model is significantly better and

Figure 3. Estimated impedance parameters (Patient A)

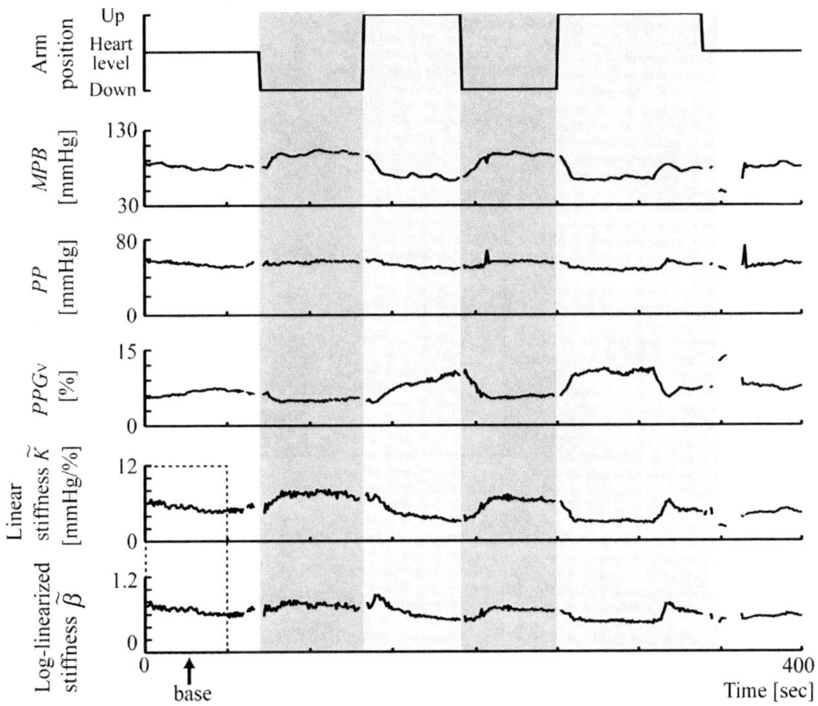

that the standard deviation is smaller. A significant difference ($P < 0.001$) was found between the two models.

Next, the values of $\tilde{K}$ and $\tilde{\beta}$ were normalized with the corresponding mean values for 50 seconds at rest, and the mean values and standard deviations with the up/down arm positions were calculated. A comparison of the results of all trials (Patient A – Patient D) are shown in Figure 5 and indicate that the up/down differences in stiffness values estimated from the log-linearized model are smaller than those of the linearized model. Additionally, by comparing the model parameter variations in the up/down positioning, the up-down ratios were calculated. The calculated mean values and standard deviations in all trials are shown in Figure 6. From these results, we can confirm that the up/down ratio for the log-linearized model is lower than that of the linear model, and that there is a significant difference ($P < 0.05$) between the two models.

DISCUSSION

In this study, we investigated the estimation accuracy of the proposed model (with log-linearized viscoelastic parameters) relative to stiffness parameter β with the coefficient of determination. The results indicate that the estimation accuracy of the proposed model represents a significant improvement on the conventional model (not including viscosity), and that the standard deviation of the coefficients of determination for the proposed model is much smaller than that of the conventional model. We conclude that the proposed model, which includes the viscosity parameter, is useful for precisely estimating the dynamic characteristics of arterial walls, as a significant difference ($P < 0.001$) between the models was observed.

Moreover, the proposed method was used to investigate vascular smooth muscle responses induced by changes in intravascular pressure with

Figure 4. Coefficients of determination (Patient A)

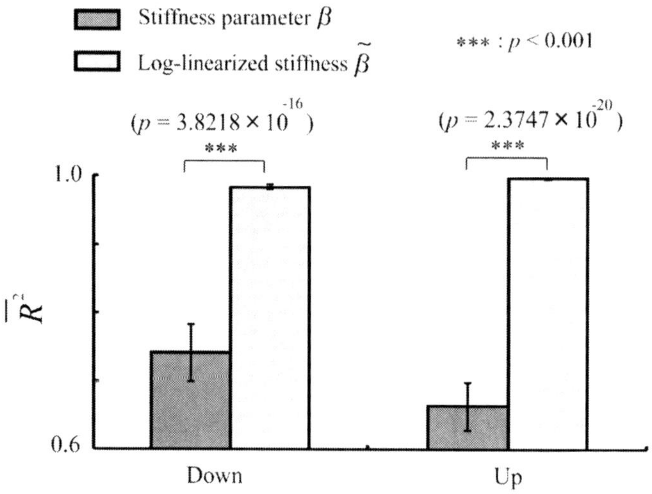

respect to arm position testing. The results confirmed that the value of $\tilde{K}$ fluctuates when the arm position changes and that the variation in $\tilde{\beta}$ is small compared to that of $\tilde{K}$. The values of $\tilde{K}$ and $\tilde{\beta}$ were normalized with the corresponding mean values for 50 seconds at rest, and the mean values and standard deviations with the up/down arm positions were calculated. It appears that the variations in $\tilde{\beta}$ are smaller than those of $\tilde{K}$ in comparison with the up/down differences. Additionally, comparing the ratios of the up/down positioning, the ratio of the log-linearized model was lower than that of the linear model, and a significant difference ($P < 0.05$) was observed for mean values from all trials. As our study was conducted on patients under general anesthesia, it is likely that neurogenic vascular regulation

Figure 5. Normalized stiffness parameters in up/down arm positions

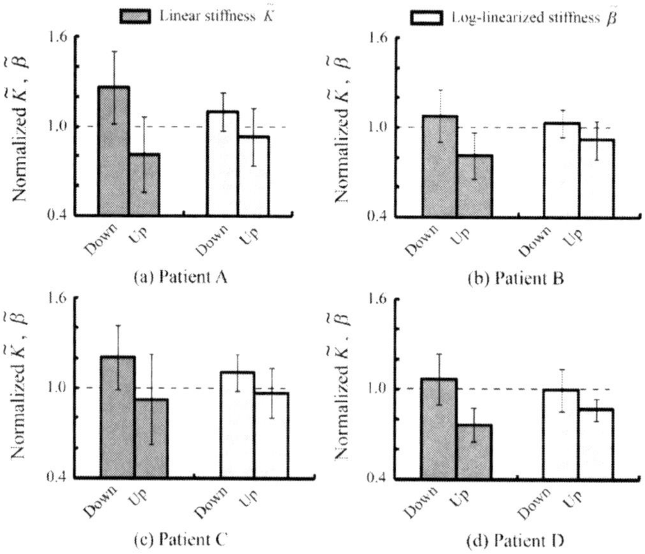

Figure 6. Comparison between ratios of stiffness parameters in the up/down arm positions

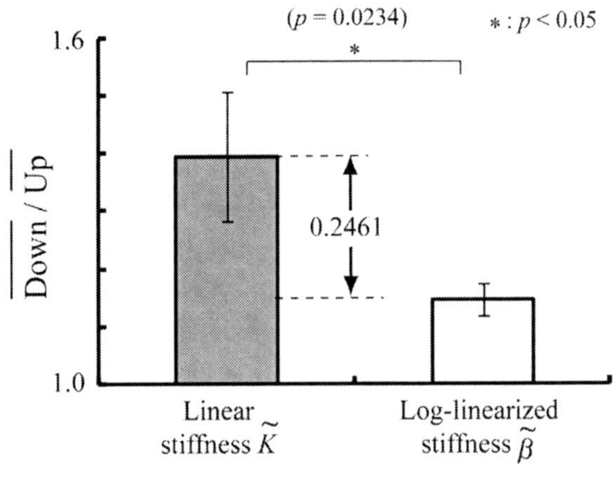

mechanism factors (autochthonous impulses) such as tension were not responsive. Accordingly, we found that the proposed method could reduce the influence of intravascular pressure fluctuation during the arm position test.

CONCLUSION

In future studies, we plan to further consider the relationship between intravascular pressure and the neural vascular regulation mechanism. Additional experiments will be conducted to assess the validity of the proposed method.

ACKNOWLEDGMENT

This work was supported by the Regional Innovation Creating System Enterprise for Ministry of Economy, Trade and Industry (RIETI) of Japan.

REFERENCES

Armentano, R. L., Simon, A., Levenson, J., Chau, N. P., Megnien, J. L., & Pichel, R. (1991). Mechanical pressure versus intrinsic effects of hypertension on large arteries in humans. *Hypertension, 18*(5), 657–664.

Bank, A. J., Wilson, R. F., & Kubo, S. H. (1995). Direct effects of smooth muscle relaxation and contraction on in vivo human brachial artery elastic properties. *Circulation Research, 77*, 1008–1016.

Bayliss, W. M. (1902). On the local reactions of the arterial wall to changes of internal pressure. *The Journal of Physiology, 28*, 220–231.

Busse, R., Bauer, R. D., Schabert, A., Summa, Y., Bumm, P., & Wetterer, E. (1979). The mechanical properties of exposed human common carotid arteries in vivo. *Basic Research in Cardiology, 74*, 545–554. doi:10.1007/BF01907647

Faber, M., & Moller Hou, G. (1952). The human aorta. Part V: Collagen and elastin in the normal and hypertensive aorta. *Acta Pathologica et Microbiologica Scandinavica, 31*, 377–382. doi:10.1111/j.1699-0463.1952.tb00205.x

Greenfield, J. C., & Patel, D. J. (1962). Relation between pressure and diameter in the ascending aorta of man. *Circulation Research, 10*, 778–781.

Hayashi, K., Handa, H., Nagasawa, S., Okumura, A., & Moritake, K. (1980). Stiffness and elastic behavior of human intracranial and extracranial arteries. *Journal of Biomechanics, 13*, 175–184. doi:10.1016/0021-9290(80)90191-8

Katayama, K., Shimoda, M., Maeda, J., & Takemiya, T. (1998). Endurance exercise training increases peripheral vascular response in human fingers. *Japanese Journal of Physiology*, *48*(5), 365–371. doi:10.2170/jjphysiol.48.365

Nichols, W. W., & O'Rourke, M. F. (1998). *McDonald's blood flow in arteries: Theoretical experimental and clinical principles*, 4th ed. London.

Sakane, A., Shiba, K., Tsuji, T., Saeki, N., & Kawamoto, M. (2005). Non-invasive monitoring of arterial wall impedance. *Proceedings of the First International Conference on Complex Medical Engineering*, (pp. 984-989). Takamatsu, May 2005.

Sakane, A., Tsuji, T., Saeki, N., & Kawamoto, M. (2004). Discrimination of vascular conditions using a probabilistic neural network. *Journal of Robotics and Mechatronics*, *16*(2), 138–145.

Sakane, A., Tsuji, T., Tanaka, Y., Saeki, N., & Kawamoto, M. (2004). Monitoring of vascular conditions using plethysmogram. *Journal of the Society of Instrument and Control Engineers*, *40*(12), 1236–1242.

Takemiya, T., Maeda, J., Suzuki, J., Nishihira, Y., & Shimoda, M. (1996). Differential digital photoplethysmographic observations of finger vascular exponential response to the arm position changes in humans. *Advances in Exercise and Sports Physiology*, *2*(2), 83–90.

Wurzel, M., Cowper, G. R., & McCook, J. M. (1969). Smooth muscle contraction and viscoelasticity of arterial wall. *Canadian Journal of Physiology and Pharmacology*, *48*, 510–523.

KEY TERMS AND DEFINITIONS

Arterial Wall Impedance (Vascular Impedance): A relationship between pulsatile pressure and pulsatile flow recorded in an artery feeding a particular vascular bed. Also known as the impediment to flow at the input of a vascular bed where pulsatile flow is involved (aorta and arteries).

Arteriosclerosis: (also known as atherosclerosis) a stiffening of the arteries. Arteriosclerosis is a chronic disease characterized by abnormal thickening and hardening of the arterial walls with resulting loss of elasticity.

Collagen: A protein found in blood vessels that is much stiffer than elastin.

Endothelial Cells: A specialized type of epithelial cell which forms the inner lining of blood vessels.

Intravascular Pressure: The amount of pressure exerted on the walls of blood vessels by the blood.

Mechanical Impedance: A measure of how much a structure resists motion when subjected to a given force. It relates forces with velocities acting on a mechanical system.

Photoplethysmography (PPG): A simple and low-cost optical non-invasive technique that can be used to detect blood volume changes in microvascular tissue beds.

Smooth Muscle: Found in many places; within the tunica media layer of large and small arteries, veins, lymphatic vessels, the urinary bladder, uterus, etc.

Viscoelastic: The property of materials that exhibit both viscous and elastic characteristics when undergoing deformation.

Voigt Model: Consists of a Newtonian damper and Hookean elastic spring connected in parallel.

Chapter 41
Surface EMG and Upper-Limb Rehabilitation

Kazuya Funada
Graduate School of Natural Science and Technology, Okayama University, Japan

Jinglong Wu
Graduate School of Natural Science and Technology, Okayama University, Japan

Satoshi Takahashi
Graduate School of Natural Science and Technology, Okayama University, Japan

ABSTRACT

In rehabilitating hemiplegic patients, purposeful movements such as the opening and closing of hands are reported to be more effective than passive movement with an instrument. The authors of this chapter used surface electromyogram (surface EMG) signals as a way to convey the patient's conscious ability to open and close their hands. The muscles in the forearm contract when the hand is closed or opened, which creates a simple signal that is comparatively easy to measure with surface EMG, a simple measuring device. The action potentials of the muscles involved in the opening-and-closing motions of hands were measured from several points in the forearm when those muscles contracted, and their distribution was analyzed. The purpose of this study is to develop a simple system to recognize the movement of a patient's hand using measurements of EMG signals from only the most characteristic points on the forearm to replace similar, but more complex, research such as multi-channel measurement and wave analysis by FFT. The authors specified the optimum measuring points on the palm and dorsal sides of the forearm for the recognition of hand motion by the experimental system. This system successfully recognized hand motion through the analysis of the surface EMG signals measured from only two optimum points to allow arbitrary control of the rehabilitation device based on the recognition results.

DOI: 10.4018/978-1-60960-559-9.ch041

INTRODUCTION

There are various rehabilitation strategies involving an instrument for patients who suffer from paralysis in a part of their body as a result of disease or injury. For example, hemiplegic patients who cannot open and close their hands caused by a blockage of their nerve pathways due to neurofunctional disorders such as apoplexy can use rehabilitation instruments to assist them in opening and closing their hands. By using such an instrument, however, patients can perform only passive rehabilitation movements. Purposeful movement to open and close their hands has been reported to be more effective than passive movement with an instrument for the rehabilitation of hemiplegic patients (Lum, Burgar, Shor, Majmundar, & Loos, 2002; Lindberg, Schmitz, Forssberg, Engardt, & Borg, 2004; Hogan, Krebs, Rohrer, Palazzolo, & Dipietro, 2006). This active rehabilitation under strong consciousness is believed to greatly contribute to the rebuilding of patient's nerve pathways. Under this form of rehabilitation, the conscious act of opening-and-closing their hands needs to be fed back into a rehabilitation instrument to maintain arbitrary control over the instrument.

The analysis of patient brain-waves is one method for conveying their consciousness to an instrument, but this type of analysis during the purposeful movements of opening-and-closing hands is a large, complex problem and also requires large-scale measuring devices. Instead of brain-waves, surface EMG can be used as a measurement of consciousness for the opening-and-closing of hands because the operation of muscles in the forearm generates a signal that is comparatively easy to measure with simple measuring devices. For example, patients can actively control a rehabilitation instrument by using the action potential of their muscles measured from their forearms on their normal side as a signal of consciousness for opening-and-closing hands (Figure 1). Because this method is a form of active rehabilitation, a high rehabilitation effect can be expected. This method requires measurement of surface EMG from the forearm on the normal side while opening-and-closing the hand and construction of a system that recognizes the motion of the hand from the action potential signal.

The purpose of this study is to develop a simple system to recognize the motion of the hand and support the movement of a patient's hand

Figure 1. Conceptual diagram of the rehabilitation efforts

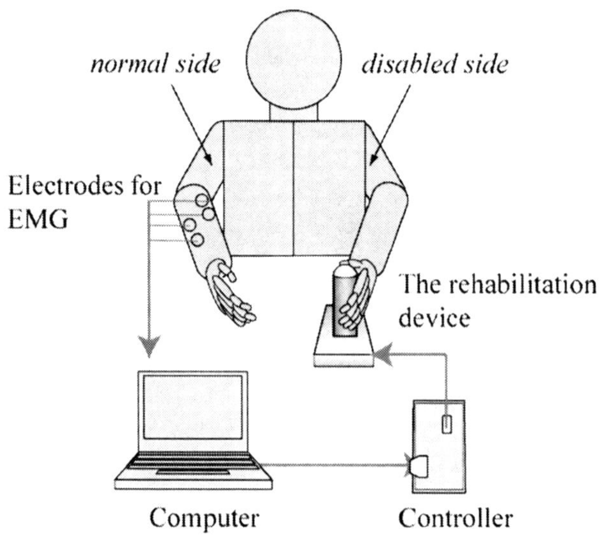

based upon similar research using EMG, such as multi-channel measurement and wave analysis by FFT. Two methods will be used to reduce the complexity of this rehabilitation system: reducing the number of electrodes by specifying the measurement point(s) on the forearm from which the characteristic action potential for the opening-and-closing motion of the hand can be measured and making the recognition program extremely simple.

- **Surface EMG:** Myo-electric potential is an action potential that appears in connection with voluntary or reflective muscle contraction. Surface EMG is a comparatively easy, noninvasive method that records myogenic potential signals using an electromyograph and surface electrodes placed on the skin that cover the target muscles. It is suitable for collecting a wide range of information from muscles for the analysis of physical exertion and can also be useful for detecting involuntary movement in the limbs or face. Surface EMG is often measured with a differential amplifier with configured bipolar electrodes.
- **Prior study on upper limb rehabilitation:** The "Hand Motion Assist Robot" is a device for hand function rehabilitation (Kawasaki, Ito, Ishigure, Nishimoto, Aoki, Mori, Sakaeda, & Abe, 2007). It is an exoskeleton with 18 degrees-of-freedom and assists independent finger motions. This system is based on a master-slave system, which allows the impaired hand of a patient to be driven by his or her healthy hand on the opposite side. The use of this device is limited because it is large, expensive, and complicated to operate.

EXPERIMENT

To simplify the recognition system, the number of electrodes should be reduced as much as possible, which can be accomplished by measuring surface EMG only at an optimum point (Figure 2). Therefore, the optimum point in the forearm that can be used to measure the characteristic action potential created by the opening-and-closing motion of a hand should be determined.

The flexor digitorum superficialis and the flexor digitorum profundus muscles in the palm

Figure 2. Reference points and measuring point

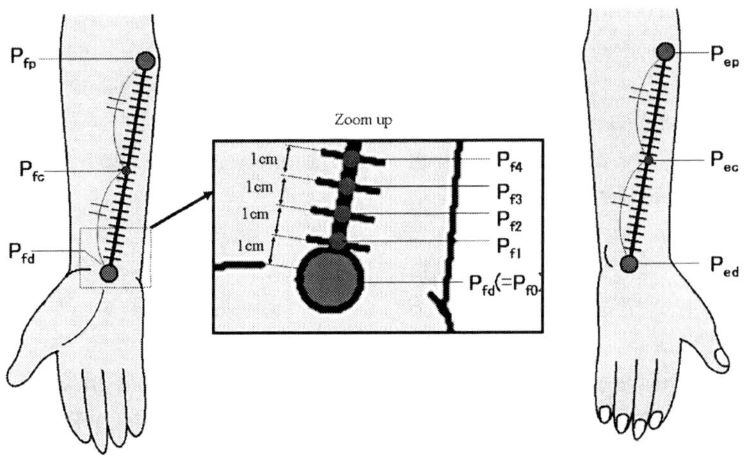

(a) palm side (b) back side

side of the forearm contract when the hand grasps, and the extensor digitorum muscle in the dorsal side of the forearm contracts when the hand opens (Mori, 1969). An action potential of a muscle is generated by its movement upon contraction. Although the anatomical positions of these muscles within the forearm are well known, specifying the optimum point at which the surface EMG is the easiest to measure is difficult.

Surface EMG represents the action potential of a target muscle and is measured by an electrode placed on the skin. Surface EMG is more difficult to measure from abdominal muscles because the distance from the electrode to the target muscle greatly influences surface EMG readings. Moreover, the optimum point for measuring surface EMG may differ from person to person. Thus, determining the optimum point requires several experiments involving the measurement of surface EMG along the forearm using the application of the same load level.

A. Positioning of Reference Points and Measuring Points

A-1. Palm Side of Forearm

- Target muscles: Flexor digitorum superficialis muscle and flexor digitorum profundus muscle
- Action: Bending the second through fifth digits

The flexor digitorum superficialis muscle develops from the joint of the ulna and humerus and passes along the center of the wrist. From there, it is divided into four tendons that reach into the middle phalanx of each finger. Based upon the muscle anatomy, the measuring point, which should be located right above the target muscles to obtain the best quantitative measurements, is limited to the straight line that connects the following two points:.

1. P_{fp}: The proximal reference point···distal ulnar tip of the humerus
2. P_{fd}: The distal reference point···center of the wrist joint

A-2. Dorsal Side of Forearm

- Target muscles: Extensor digitorum muscle
- Action: Extending the second through fifth digits

The extensor digitorum muscle develops from the ulnar epicondyle of the humerus and passes along the center of the wrist. From there, it is divided into four tendons that reach into the middle phalanx of each finger. As above, the measuring point is limited to the straight line that connects the following two points:

1. P_{ep}: The proximal reference point···ulnar epicondyle of the humerus
2. P_{ed}: The distal reference point···center of the wrist joint

B. Experimental Procedure for Specifying the Optimum Points

Surface EMG signals were sampled from P_{fd} (or P_{ed}) and the arbitrary measuring point P_{fn} (or P_{en}) located on the straight line described above. The signal were entered into a computer through an AD translation machine (PowerLab4/25: ADInstruments, Bella Vista NSW, Australia) using an EMG amplifier (EMG021/025: Harada Electronics Industry Ltd, Sapporo-shi, Hokkaido, Japan).

1. The length from P_{fd} to P_{fn} of each subject was measured. The length of P_{fd} - P_{fp} and the length of P_{fd} - P_{fn} was set to L and L_m, respectively.
2. P_{fn} was moved proximally by 1 cm along the straight line from P_{fd} to P_{fp}, and the following experiment was performed at each point.

3. For the measurements on the palm side of the forearm, the subject grasped his or her hand to keep a constant force as much as possible for a few seconds (3~5 seconds) and subsequently relaxed. This motion of grasping-and-relaxing was performed several times (about 10 times) with the grasping power changed each time. Surface EMG signals from P_{fd} and P_{fn} were measured for each motion in the trial. For the measurements of the dorsal side of the forearm, the same series of trials was performed using an opening motion instead of a grasping motion.
4. The Root-Mean-Square amplitude (RMS-amplitude) of the action potentials measured from P_{fd} and P_{fn} were set to V_0 and V, respectively.
5. V_0, V and V/V_0 (ratio of V_0 to V) at grasping (or opening) the hand were calculated.

By this experiment, the distribution of the ease of measuring surface EMG in this section was examined and used to specify the optimum points on each subject.

C. Recognition Program

After determining the locations of the optimum points for measuring surface EMG for this experiment, the measurements of surface EMG taken from those optimum points were applied to the recognition program to evaluate its ability to recognize the motion of a hand. The hand motions were limited to "grasping", "opening", and "relaxing". The recognition program, which was created using general-purpose measurement software (LabVIEW: National Instruments), was designed to recognize the motion of a hand using only the amplitude of the surface EMG reading without using FFT analysis (Tamura, Okumura, & Tanno, 2007). This program consists of an analysis portion to study three states ("Grasp", "Open" and "Relax") and a recognition portion. The program chart for the recognition portion is shown in Figure 3.

RESULTS AND DISCUSSION

An example of the surface EMG signals is shown in Figure 4. Channel 1 is the surface EMG signal from P_{fd}, and channel 2 is the surface EMG signal from P_{fn}. The amplitude of the action potential of channel 1 has a certain correlation with that of channel 2 during the grasping state. Figure 5 and 6 show the experimental results of the distribution of the surface EMG measurements in the forearm. Three healthy male subjects aged 22–28 were used in the experimental trial. Although there were individual differences, the results suggest that the optimum point for measuring surface EMG exists distally from the center of the forearm on both the palm and dorsal sides. We suggest that the measurement of the optimum point be performed using the following equations:

- The optimum point on the palm side: L_p(Distance from P_f)=0.4×L
- The optimum point on the dorsal side: L_b(Distance from P_f)=0.25×L

In this study, we determined the optimum point for measuring surface EMG in the forearm and measured the distribution of surface EMG signals on the forearm on both the palm and dorsal sides. We then evaluated a program that recognizes the motion of a hand using surface EMG measurements taken from the optimum points that were determined earlier. Figure 7 is a picture of the master-slave system running this recognition program, measuring from the optimum points. We successfully designed a rehabilitation device from a master-slave system that can be arbitrarily controlled through the recognition of hand movements based upon surface EMG signals measured in the forearm.

Figure 3. Chart of the recognition program

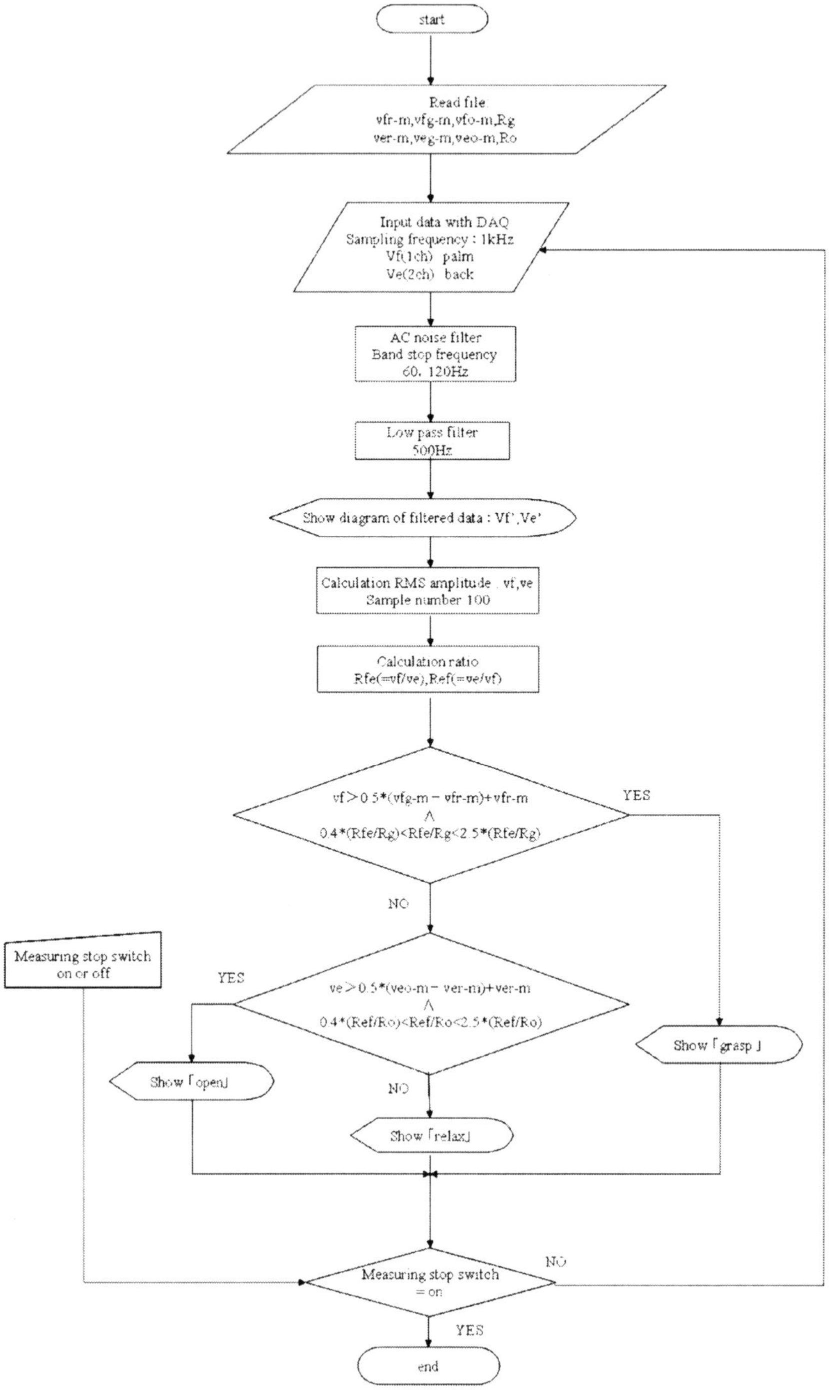

Figure 4. An example of surface EMG signals (Subject C)

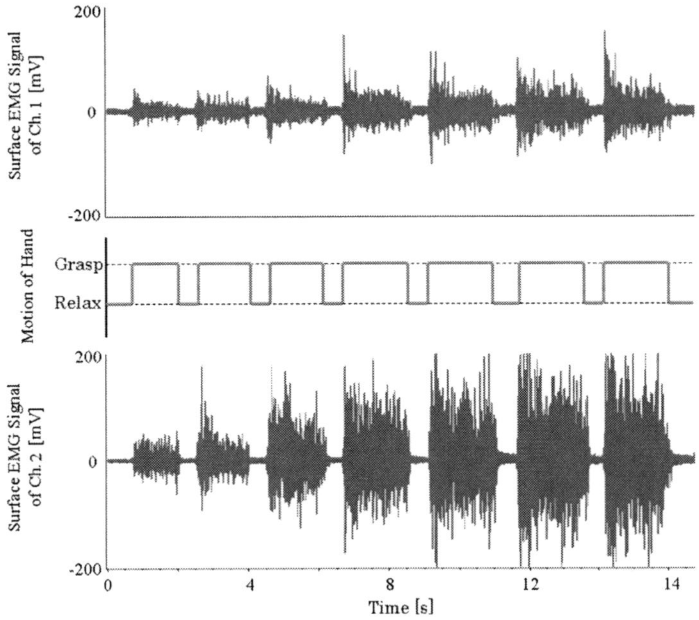

Figure 5. Distribution of the measuring surface EMG on the palm side of the forearm. The vertical and horizontal axes indicate V/V_0 (the mean ratio of V_0 to V) and L_m/L (at P_f: $L_m/L=0$, at P_n: $L_m/L=1$)

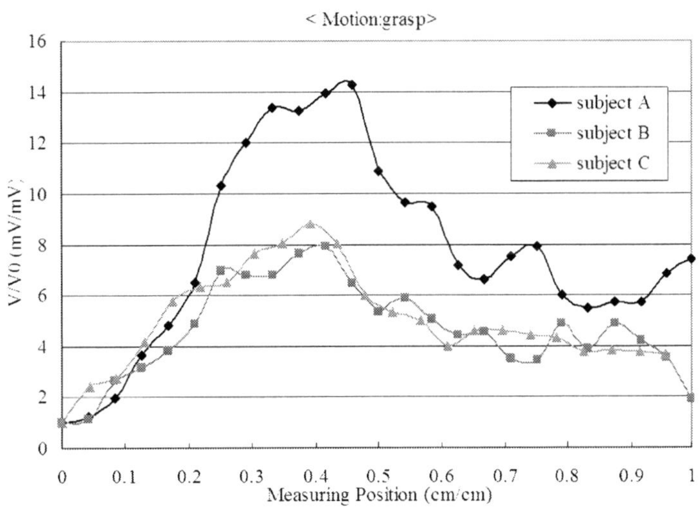

ACKNOWLEDGMENT

A part of this study was financially supported by the JSPS AA Science Platform Program and JSPS Grant-in-Aid for Scientific Research(B) (21404002).

Figure 6. Distribution of the measuring surface EMG on the dorsal side of the forearm

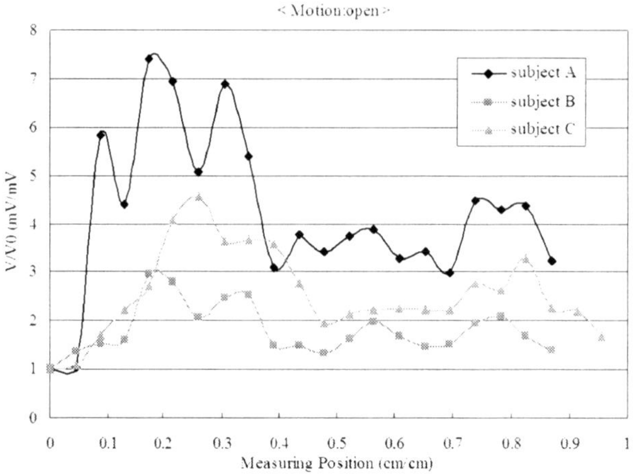

Figure 7. Illustration of the master-slave system that runs the recognition program

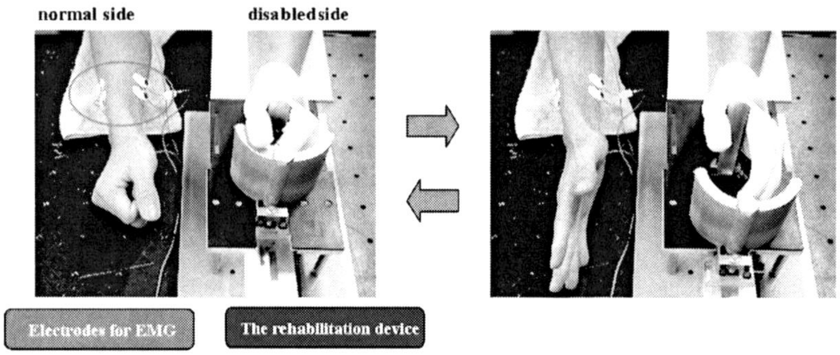

REFERENCES

Hogan, N., Krebs, H. I., Rohrer, B., Palazzolo, J. J., & Dipietro, L. (2006). Motions or muscles? Some behavioral factors underlying robotic assistance of motor recovery. *Journal of Rehabilitation Research and Development*, *43*, 605–618. doi:10.1682/JRRD.2005.06.0103

Kawasaki, H., Ito, S., Ishigure, Y., Nishimoto, Y., Aoki, T., & Mori, T. … Abe, M. (2007). Development of a hand motion assist robot for rehabilitation therapy by patient self-motion control. *Proceedings of the 2007 IEEE 10th International Conference on Rehabilitation Robotics*, June 12-15, (pp. 234-240).

Lindberg, P., Schmitz, C., Forssberg, H., Engardt, M., & Borg, J. (2004). Effects of passive-active movement training on upper limb motor function and cortical activation in chronic patients with stroke: pilot study. *The Japanese Journal of Rehabilitation Medicine*, *36*, 117–123. doi:10.1080/16501970410023434

Lum, P. S., Burgar, C. G., Shor, P. C., Majmundar, M., & Loos, M. V. (2002). Robot-assisted movement training compared with conventional therapy techniques for the rehabilitation of upper-limb motor function after stroke. *Archives of Physical Medicine and Rehabilitation*, *83*, 952–959. doi:10.1053/apmr.2001.33101

Mori, O. (1969). [Kanehara & Co., Ltd.]. *Buntan Kaibougaku, 1*, 346–373.

Tamura, H., Okumura, D., & Tanno, K. (2007). A study of motion recognition without FFT from surface-EMG. *Transactions of the Institute of Electronics, Information and Communication Engineers, J90*, 2652–2655.

KEY TERMS AND DEFINITIONS

Surface Electromyogram (Surface EMG): An electrical potential generated by muscle and measured on the skin.

Rehabilitation: An improvement and recover of their lost function.

Forearm: An upper limb.

Humerus: A bone in the arm from the shoulder to the elbow.

Grasping: Bending the second through fifth digits with power.

Opening: Extending the second through fifth digits with relaxation.

Relaxing: Loosening the power of hand.

Chapter 42
A Method for Eliciting the Support Needs from People with Early-Stage Dementia for Maintaining Social Living

Hirotoshi Yamamoto
Department of Mechanical Engineering and Science, Graduate School of Engineering, Kyoto University, Japan

Yasuyoshi Yokokohji
Department of Mechanical Engineering, Graduate School of Engineering, Kobe University, Japan

Hajime Takechi
Department of Geriatric Medicine, Graduate School of Medicine, Kyoto University, Japan

ABSTRACT

In the area of welfare engineering, various technological research and developmental efforts have been made to support people with dementia. However, it is not clear if these efforts are based on the real needs of these people. When providing support to people with dementia, it is essential to know exactly what their needs are. Nevertheless, it is not easy to obtain appropriate answers from these people by simply asking "How can we help you?" In addition, it is unlikely that answers from those people will cover all of their support needs. In this chapter, a new method based on the "Person-Centered Care" concept is proposed for eliciting the support needs from, and determining their priorities for people with early-stage

DOI: 10.4018/978-1-60960-559-9.ch042

dementia who are eager to maintain their social living despite coping with various difficulties. First, all of the actual and potential tasks of social living in their daily life are determined. Support needs are then extracted systematically from those tasks by paying attention to what factors are bothering these people or are confusing to them rather than directly asking the individuals what type of support they want or need. Finally, the support needs are prioritized by taking the degree of the individuals' confusion and task frequency into consideration. When interviewing people with dementia, special care must be taken to ensure that the individuals who have memory impairment are not overburdened. In the proposed method, visual materials such as cards and boards with illustrations are utilized so that people with dementia can answer questions more easily. Some interviews were conducted based on the proposed method to confirm that support needs can be determined systematically from people with early-stage dementia.

INTRODUCTION

People with early-stage dementia are reported to be eager to maintain their social living by actively contributing to society or continuing to work (Alzheimer's Association, 2008). Over the past five to ten years, many of those people have started to speak out about how deeply they are suffering from dementia (Boden, 1998; Bryden, 2004). Consequently, the support environment for people with dementia is changing, with a new focus on the concept of "Person-Centered Care" (Benson & Kitwood, 2000). In other words, care must be administered with the aim of meeting more of the individuals' expectations than the caregivers' wishes. Of course, holistic support from society at large, including the efforts of government to address dementia care as well as various technological research and developmental efforts, is indispensable. However, it is not clear if the activities in the technological field (Lee & Dey 2008; Hamada, et al. 2008) are aimed at solving the real needs of people with dementia based on the "Person-Centered Care" concept.

How can we determine the real needs of people with early-stage dementia? Generally speaking, it is not easy to obtain appropriate answers from anyone, regardless of whether they are suffering from dementia or not, by simply asking "How can we help you?" People with dementia are even less likely to state their needs because they tend to reduce their wants and needs due to feelings of restraint and/or resignation or the lack of self-awareness of impairment. It is also possible that verbal communication would not be effective for interviewing people with dementia because of their impairment in short term memory. Furthermore, even if these people reply to questions, it is unlikely that the obtained answers will include all of their support needs. Therefore, a solution to these problems must be found to effectively identify the support needs of people with early-stage dementia.

The aim of this research was, first, to identify what kinds of difficulties people with dementia are facing in their social living situations and what kinds of support needs they desire. We then sought to identify which support requirements could be realized effectively by technology. To accomplish these goals, a new interviewing method is proposed for identifying the support needs of people with early-stage dementia. With the proposed method, support needs can be determined by respecting the individuals' needs and wants based on the Person-Centered Care concept along with caregivers' cooperation. This method was carefully designed by considering not only what the individuals cannot do but also what the individuals wish to do, so that their support needs are systematically identified and prioritized from the individuals' point of view. Several interviews of people with dementia were conducted, and the effectiveness as well as the limitations of the proposed method are discussed.

Currently, some tests and evaluation methods have been developed for assessing the competence of older people or grading the cognitive state of patients with dementia (Kaufer et al., 2008). To the best of our knowledge, however, no interview method to determine the support needs of patients themselves has been reported.

A NEW METHOD OF IDENTIFYING SUPPORT NEEDS

Basic Policy to Identify Support Needs

(1) Focusing Individuals' Confusion

Since support needs originate from the requirements of people with dementia who want to obtain help, it is fundamental to hear their voices. Although it does not often work to simply ask "How can I help you?", as mentioned earlier, it would be easier for anyone, for these people in particular, to answer questions like "Is something bothering you?" or "Are you confused about anything?" Hence, support needs can eventually be identified by paying attention to what factors are bothering or confusing these people.

Caregivers, who may provide important information about support needs, can join the interview, but they can give complementary information only after the person with dementia says everything he/she wants to talk about. Such an arrangement is necessary for preventing the interview from leading to an argument between the individual and the caregiver.

(2) Boosting the Degree of Requirement for Support by Inspiring Individuals' Motivation

To identify the true inner feelings of people with dementia who may have feelings of restraint and/or resignation, they are asked to think of an ideal condition where necessary support can be provided anytime before they are asked what to expect.

In case the individuals lack self-awareness of impairment, caregivers can share their observations about the individuals' daily living so that the individuals can become aware of their potential needs from these observations. It should be noted, however, that such arrangements should avoid stress and obtrusion on the individual or allowing the individual to be led purposely by the caregivers when they are sharing their views.

In the proposed method, some discrepancy indices, which will be described in detail later, are introduced during the investigation process. These indices are leveraged to effectively identify support needs.

(3) Visual Material Aids for Promoting Communication

An interview, which relies solely on verbal communication, may place a burden on people with dementia or fail to elicit valuable information from them due to their short term memory impairment. Thus, visual materials, such as cards and boards with illustrations, are present throughout the interview to facilitate communication.

(4) Listing Social Living Tasks

To determine as many support needs as possible from people with dementia, all of the activities of their daily lives (referred to as "tasks") must be identified. To do this, candidate tasks for support were listed based on Lawton's model of the competence of older people (Lawton, 1972). Approximately 130 tasks that belong to the stages "instrumental self-maintenance (IADL)," "intellectual activity," and "social role" in the model were categorized into the following four groups and the instrumental items:

- Domestic affairs such as basic household chores and other duties; 25 items

- Out-of-the-house tasks such as errands, medical treatment, and haircuts; 18 items
- Social activities, such as volunteer work; 12 items
- Hobbies, learning, leisure, and sports; 55 items
- Instrumental items such as transportation and means of communication; 22 items

Each item is represented by a "Task Card" with the title and illustration (see Figure 1).

Outline of the Proposed Method

The proposed method consists of the following four steps:

1. Task Identification
2. Confusion Evaluation
3. Support Requirement Evaluation
4. Support Importance Evaluation.

Step 1. Identification of Social Living Tasks and Their Frequencies

The person with dementia and the caregiver are asked to select task cards that represent the person's daily activities and place them at appropriate positions on the Social Living Task Board (see Figure 2), which represents the task frequency, such as everyday, twice a week, or once a month. The frequency of the task T_i (i=1,2, …, n), where n is the total number of identified tasks, is denoted by F_i, which is either 3 (corresponding to 'done nearly every day'), 2 ('a few times a week'), or 1 ('less frequently'). Note that tasks that the person does not do at present but wishes to do should be included here, and F_i should be identified as the potential frequency at which the person would like to do the task.

Step 2. Evaluation of Confusion

The person is asked to sort the task cards that were selected in Step 1 into three levels by placing them on the Confusion Evaluation Board (see upper half of Figure 3) according to the degree of his/her confusion about the task. The Subjective Confusion Level of T_i is denoted by C_{Si}, which is either 3 ('confused'), 2 ('slightly confused'), or 1 ('no problem').

The interviewer asks the person in detail what makes this task difficult to do (or understand) compared to before and, if possible, what kinds of support he/she would like to get.

The caregiver is then asked to share his/her observations about the tasks that are different from the person's explanations in Step 2-i and to score the "Objective Confusion Level" C_{Oi}, which is either 3 ('looks confused'), 2 ('looks slightly

Figure 1. Task card samples

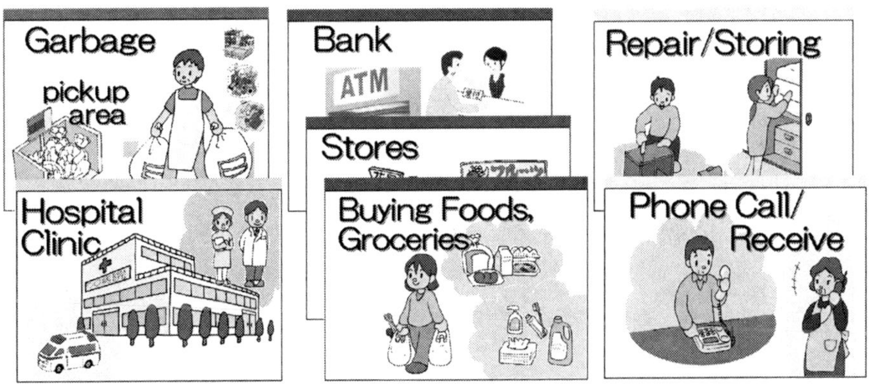

Figure 2. Social living task board

	Nearly Every Day	A Few Times a Week	Less Frequently
a.m. p.m.			
If Possible			

confused'), or 1 ('no problem'), by sorting the task cards on the lower half of the Confusion Evaluation Board. The interviewer asks the caregiver in detail what makes the task difficult for the person to do (or understand) compared to before, and, if possible, what kinds of support should be provided for him/her.

Here, the confusion discrepancy index d_{Ci} of task T_i is defined by the following equation:

$$d_{Ci}=C_{Oi}-C_{Si}. \tag{1}$$

The purpose of this index is described later.

If the confusion discrepancy index is positive ($d_{Ci}\geq 1$) for any task T_i, the interviewer asks the person to score the C_{Si} of the tasks again, taking the caregiver's observation of the tasks into consideration. If he/she feels like changing the C_{Si}, the interviewer lets him/her do so, and d_{Ci} is corrected accordingly.

Step 3. Evaluation of Support Requirements

Once the C_{Si} (Subjective Confusion Level) is clearly identified by the person, the interviewer

Figure 3. Confusion evaluation board

Compared to Before		
Confused	Slightly Confused	No Problem
From the Caregiver's Viewpoint		
Looks Confused	Looks Slightly Confused	Looks No Problem

can identify support requirements from him/her in the following way:

The interviewer shows the person the predicted support requirement $\hat{R}_i$ of T_i, which is obtained by (2) using the final value of C_{Si} obtained in Step 2 - iii, by placing relevant task cards on the corresponding column of the Support Requirement Evaluation Board (see Figure 4).

$$\hat{R}_i = \begin{Bmatrix} C_{Si} \times 1.5 & \text{if } C_{Si} > 1 \\ 0 & \text{if } C_{Si} = 1 \end{Bmatrix} \tag{2}$$

Using $\hat{R}_i$ as a reference, the person is asked to score his/her own support requirement R_i according to five levels (1 through 5) for each task T_i by letting them move the cards on the board as he/she wishes. The interviewer must get rid of the feelings of restraint and/or resignation from the person and motivate him/her to tell his/her true inner feelings. At this time, the interviewer can also ask the person to list new tasks that he/she would like to do. If any, the person is asked to identify the support requirements and frequency of the newly listed tasks by placing such task cards in the appropriate position on the Support Requirement Evaluation Board.

Here, the support requirement discrepancy index d_{Ri} of task T_i is defined by the following equation:

$$d_{Ri} = \hat{R}_i - R_i. \tag{3}$$

The purpose of this index is described later.

Step 4. Evaluation of Subjective Support Importance

In this step, the person is asked to score subjective support importance I_i only for the tasks with $R_i > 0$. The estimated support importance, which is calculated using R_i and F_i, is used as a reference.

The interviewer shows the person the estimated support importance $\hat{I}_i$ of a task T_i by placing the relevant task cards on the corresponding columns of the Support Importance Evaluation Board (see Figure 5). The estimated support importance $\hat{I}_i$ is calculated by the following equation:

$$\hat{I}_i = \left[(R_i \times F_i - 1) / 3\right] + 1 \tag{4}$$

Figure 4. Support requirement evaluation board

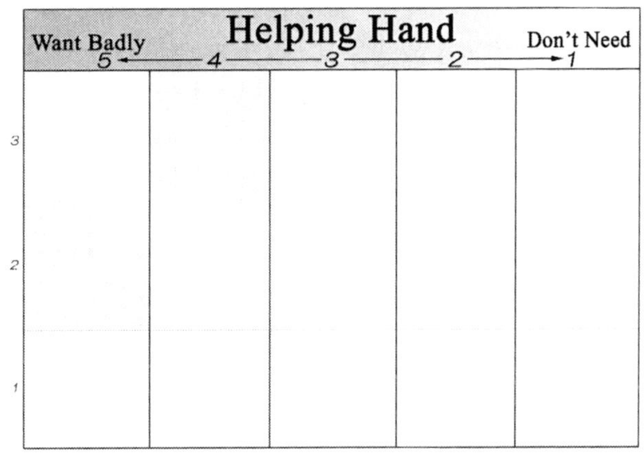

Figure 5. Support importance evaluation board

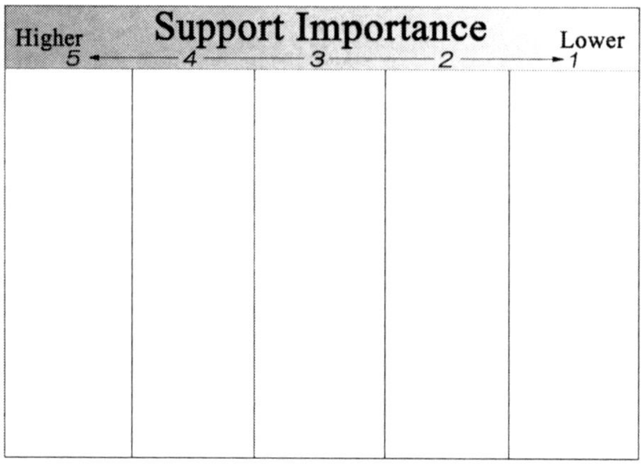

where [•] returns the closest integer of an argument and $\hat{I}_i$ becomes one of the five levels (1 through 5).

The interviewer asks the person if they feel the cards are placed at the right positions and verifies whether $\hat{I}_i$ correctly estimates the importance. If not, the interviewer asks the person to specify his/her subjective support importance I_i according to five levels (1 through 5) by letting them move the cards on the board where he/she wants.

Here, the support importance discrepancy index d_{Ii} of task T_i is defined by the following equation:

$$d_{Ii} = \hat{I}_i - I_i. \tag{5}$$

The purpose of this index is described later. If this index often has a non-zero value, (4) will be reviewed, for example, in terms of the weighting factor of F_i so that $\hat{I}_i$ becomes closer to I_i.

Interview Results from the Proposed Method

After this study was approved by the Ethics Committee of the Graduate School of Medicine at Kyoto University, six participants and their caregivers (see Table 1) were recruited out of ten candidate dyads who were being treated as outpatients at the Kyoto University Hospital.

All of the individuals were in the stage between Mild Cognitive Impairment (MCI) and early-stage dementia, aged 66-79 years. The MMSE in Table 1 indicates the recent Mini-Mental State Examination score of each participant. Interviews were conducted at each person's home (see Figure 6) so that they would feel comfortable, and also so that the interviewer could understand their living environment.

The time required for Steps 1 through 4 of the proposed method was found to be at least two hours. In addition, it was impractical to spend more than two hours for the interview at a time because interviewees tend to have difficulty maintaining concentration due to their tiredness or distractions, such as telephone calls. Thus, the actual interview was focused on getting through all the steps, skipping extra processes such as asking "What kind of support is preferable?" in Step2- i and motivating the person in Step3- ii.

As a result, only the support needs of subject A were properly identified with a single 2-hour interview, whereas for subjects B and C, several tasks remained with a confusion discrepancy and/or a support requirement discrepancy ($d_{Ri} \geq 2$) after the first interview. Second interviews were

Table 1. List of Participant Dyads and Obtained Summary

Support Needs; Extracted	Sub.	Sex	Age	Rel.[a]	MMSE	Total Extracted Tasks	No. of Items by C_{si}/C_{oi}		No. of Items by R_i					No. of Items by I_i				
							3	2	5	4	3	2	1	5	4	3	2	1
From the Person	A	M	68	H/W	23	40	2/2	2/2	2	2		2			2	1	1	2
	B	M	66	H/W	26	50	1/4	9/6	1	3	3	2	2	1		3	3	4
	C	F	69	M/D	23	32	0/3	0/2	5					5				
From the Care-giver	D	M	69	H/W	23	33	0/2	0/4						1[b]		1		
	E	M	79	H/W	25	45	0/0	0/4										
	F	F	67	M/D	23	31	0/0	0/13							1[b]			

[a]Rel. refers to the participant/caregiver relationship, such as, Husband/Wife and Mother/Daughter.
[b]The number of items that the caregiver insisted on including.

Figure 6. A snapshot of an interview with a person with dementia and his wife at their home

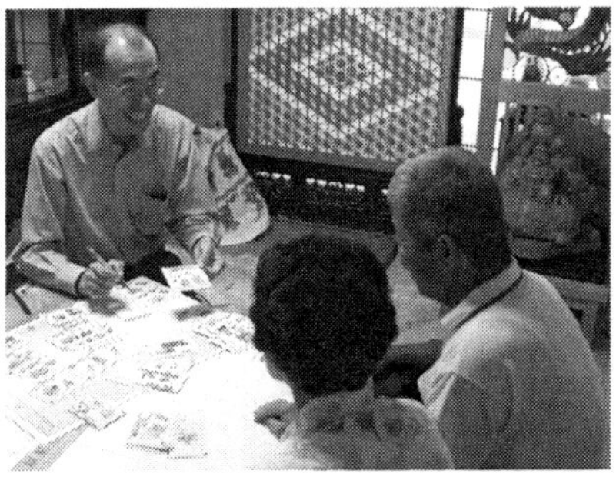

conducted for those subjects. To reduce the discrepancy indices, the following two tactics were successfully employed to identify support needs in the second interview:

1) Reducing the confusion discrepancy

Hypothesis: A strong dependency on a caregiver induces confusion discrepancy.

In other words, the caregiver estimates the person's confusion to be high because he/she always offers help, whereas the person does not feel confusion because help is always available.

Action: Encourage the person to be less dependent on the caregiver.

For example, the interviewer could ask "Is there anything you wish to do on your own so that your wife will be less burdened?"

2) Reducing the support requirement discrepancy

This discrepancy may arise from the individual's feelings of restraint and/or resignation. Therefore, it would be effective to motivate the individual by providing an idea of hopeful or promising support and letting them imagine that such support is always available.

It turned out that the support importance discrepancy was resolved in conjunction with the reduction in the support requirement discrepancy. This implies that the estimation of subjective support importance by (4) is appropriate to some extent. Table 2 shows some examples of the support needs identified.

Table 2. Extracted Support Needs in Detail (Example)

Sub.	Extracted Task	F	C_S	d_C	R	d_R	I	d_I	Support Requirements / Support Measures
A	n = 40 (Total number of tasks)								
1	Buying Foods, Groceries	2[a]	3	0	5	-0.5	4	0	Not confident to buy more than three items at a time. ==> Feels panic.
2	Buying Clothes, Appliances	2[a]	3	0	5	-0.5	4	0	Wants someone who can trigger him to calm down when he is in a panic.
3	Stores (rice, flower, liquor, etc.)	2	2	0	3.5	-0.5	3	0	Tends to forget to pay in a small store (used to pay by credit cards). ==> Has to bring cash in hand.
4	Hospital, Clinic	1	2	0	4	-1	2	0	Loses himself what to do there ("Which hospital am I in ?").
5	Museum, Gallery	1[a]	1	0	2	-2	1	0	Cannot go somewhere distant by changing busses. Doesn't like to bother anyone else by being lost.
6	Concert Hall	1[a]	1	0	2	-2	1	0	==> Useful information such as navigation signs would be appreciated.
B	n = 50								
1	Barrier-free House	3	3	0	5	-0.5	5	0	Steep steps in the house are dangerous. ==>Barrier-free house
2	Gardening	2[a]	2	0	4	-1	3	0	Eager to have his own garden. Wants to do gardening without any concern to others.
3	Hospital, Clinic	2	2	1	2→4	-1	2→3	0	A series of procedures is confusing and overwhelming. ==> Helpful if sequence and order are shown when necessary.
4	Phone Call/Receive	2	2	0	1→3	2→0	1→2.5	-0.5	Not confident in both speaking and listening. ==> Something more convenient than voice recorder
5	Put Garbage to the Pickup Area	2	2	1	3	0	2	0	Meeting with neighbors is bothersome.
6	Visit/Get a Visit	2	2	0	2	1	2	0	Wants to give ride to visitors including his grandchildren. <==He is not allowed to drive.

continues on following page

Table 2. continued

Sub.	Extracted Task	F	C_S	d_C	R	d_R	I	d_I	Support Requirements / Support Measures
7	Procedure (e.g. Bank)	1	2→3	1→0	2→4	2.5→1	1→2	0	Many blanks in application forms are overwhelming. ==> A guiding system with one question at a time
8	Repair/Storing	1	2	1	3	0	1	1	Difficult to perform complicated procedures. ==> Visual guide by video manual
9	Trip	1[a]	2	1	2	1	1	0	Uncomfortable to travel with somebody else. Has to go to the toilet frequently.
10	TV, Radio	3	2	0	1	2	1	0	Hard to hear small voices.
11	Books, Journals	3	2	0	1	2	1	0	Hard to read small letters. Often falls asleep. ==> Rather listens to the radio.

**Arrow* (→) denotes the transition of the score from the 1st interview to the 2nd interview.
[a] Potential Frequency of a Potential Task.

DISCUSSION

Support needs were identified systematically by the proposed method, determining all of the tasks of daily living of the people with dementia first and then paying attention to what factors regarding those tasks are bothering or confusing to the individuals rather than directly asking what type of support they want. Task cards with illustrations were helpful for both the interviewer and the interviewee to share topics, recall activities, and extract associated activities flexibly. Placing the cards on the board was also helpful for the participants to grasp the intention of the interview and make decisions.

Due to the time limitation for a single interview, the individual's potential support requirements (true inner feelings) could not always be determined. In such cases, the confusion discrepancy and support requirement discrepancy, which imply the individual's dependency on the caregiver and feelings of restraint and/or resignation, respectively, were considered in the second interview. The individual's true requirements were then successfully determined by motivating them to resolve the two discrepancies. This indicates that the discrepancy indices described herein seem to play an important role in surveying those needs.

We also found that the success of recruiting people for the interview and identifying needs of the people depended largely on the individuals' personality and their relationship with their caregiver. If the individuals hesitate to participate in the interview at the time of recruiting due to, for example, their refusal to accept the diagnosis, their pride, or unawareness, they would never agree to participate unless the caregiver pushes them. Even if the individual agreed after a strong push from the caregiver, they would not share their true feelings of confusion in the interview. How to determine support requirements from these types of people remains an issue.

CONCLUSION

In this chapter, a new interviewing method was proposed from the Person-Centered viewpoint, in which support needs can be identified systematically from people with early-stage dementia. This is the first step toward providing better support for these people.

This method was applied to six participants and their caregivers, and support needs were successfully identified for three of the individuals. Throughout these interviews, the conditions under which their support needs could be identified by the proposed method were revealed to some extent, such as the person's consciousness of the disease, and the person's relationship with their caregivers.

Future work includes improving the proposed method to identify more support needs from various types of the people, identifying the support items that are technologically feasible, and evaluating the types of support that will actually be provided.

REFERENCES

Alzheimer's Association. (2008). *The emerging voice of Alzheimer's*. Retrieved from http://www.alz.org/townhall/

Benson, S., & Kitwood, T. (2000). *Person centered care*. London, UK: Hawker Publications.

Boden, C. (1998). *Who will I be when I die?* Sydney, Australia: Harper Collins Publishers.

Bryden, C. (2004). *Dancing with dementia*. Sydney, Australia: Jessica Kingsley Publishers.

Hamada, T., Okubo, H., Inoue, K., Maruyama, J., Onari, H., et al. (2008). *Robot therapy as for recreation for elderly people with dementia*. The 17th IEEE International Symposium on Robot and Human Interactive Communication, (pp. 174-179).

Kaufer, D., Williams, C., Braaten, A., Gill, K., Zimmerman, S., & Sloane, P. (2008). Cognitive screening for dementia and mild cognitive impairment in assisted living. *Journal of the American Medical Directors Association, 9*(8), 586–593. doi:10.1016/j.jamda.2008.05.006

Lawton, M. P. (1972). *Assessing the competence of older people* (pp. 122–143). New York, NY: Human Science Press.

Lee, M. L., & Dey, A. K. (2008). Lifelogging memory appliance for people with episodic memory impairment. *Proceedings of UbiComp, 2008*, 44–53. doi:10.1145/1409635.1409643

KEY TERMS AND DEFINITIONS

Early-Stage Dementia: The state where mild cognitive decline is diagnosed. The decline eventually progresses to moderate cognitive decline, and then to severe cognitive decline.

Instrumental Activities of Daily Living (IADL): Consists of the six daily tasks (light housework, preparing meals, taking medications, shopping for groceries or clothes, using the telephone, and managing money) that enable people with disabilities to live independently in their community. These activities rank third highest in Lawton's model of seven stages of competence of older people.

Intellectual Activity: Ranks second highest in Lawton's seven stages of competence of older people.

Lawton's Model of the Competence of Older People: A model composed of seven stages, from the lowest and most basic to the highest functional capacity of older people, which were defined and systemized by Lawton (1972). The stages were, in ascending order of complexity, life maintenance, functional health, perception and cognition, physical self-maintenance, instrumental self-maintenance (IADL), effectance or intellectual activity, and social role.

Mild Cognitive Impairment (MCI): A condition in which a person has problems with memory, language, or another mental function that are severe enough to be noticeable to other people and to show up on tests, but not serious enough to interfere with daily life. It is considered to be the boundary or transitional stage between normal aging and dementia.

Mini-Mental State Examination (MMSE): A quick and simple way to quantify cognitive function and screen for cognitive loss. It tests the individual's orientation, attention, calculation, recall, language and motor skills.

Person-Centered Care: A moral philosophy of care developed by Tom Kitwood and the Bradford Dementia Group in England in the late 1980s.

Short Term Memory: A system for temporarily storing and managing information required to carry out complex cognitive tasks such as learning, reasoning, and comprehension.

Social Role: Ranks highest in the Lawton's model of seven stages of competence of older people.

Chapter 43
The Coimagination Method and its Evaluation via the Conversation Interactivity Measuring Method

Mihoko Otake
Research into Artifacts, Center for Engineering The University of Tokyo, Japan

Motoichiro Kato
Research into Artifacts, Center for Engineering The University of Tokyo, Japan

Toshihisa Takagi
Database Center for Life Science, Research Organization of Information and Systems, Japan

Hajime Asama
Department of Precision Engineering, Graduate School of Engineering, The University of Tokyo, Japan

ABSTRACT

The causes of dementia are divided into genetic factors and cognitive factors. To prevent dementia by reducing the cognitive factors, the authors of this chapter have developed the coimagination method to activate three cognitive functions that decline at an early stage of mild cognitive impairment (MCI): episodic memory, division of attention, and planning function. The coimagination method supports interactive conversation through expressing feelings about images according to a theme. Allocated time periods and turns for each participant are predetermined so that all participants play the roles of both speaker and listener. Measuring the interactivity of conversation qualitatively and quantitatively has been quite difficult, but conversation interactivity may indicate the intensity of cognitive activities. This paper proposes the conversation interactivity measuring method (CIMM) to measure the intensity of cognitive activities employed during conversation using the coimagination method.

DOI: 10.4018/978-1-60960-559-9.ch043

INTRODUCTION

The causes of dementia are divided into genetic factors and cognitive factors. To prevent dementia by reducing the cognitive factors, intellectual activities (Ball., Berch, & Helmers et al., 2000) and the development of a social network (Fratiglioni, Wang, Ericsson, Maytan, & Winblad, 2000; Crooks, Lubben, Petitti, & Chiu, 2008) have been reported to be effective. It is hypothesized that the activation of three cognitive functions that decline in mild cognitive impairment (MCI) is effective for the prevention of dementia (Rentz & Weintraub, 2000; Barberger-Gateau, Fabrigoule, & Rouch et al., 1999). These cognitive functions include episodic memory, division of attention, and planning functions. Interactive communication activates these three functions and intellectual activities and forms the basis of a social network. Reminiscence therapy has been shown to be an effective method for the enhancement of psychological well-being in older adults (Yasuda, Kuwabara, Kuwahara, Abe & Tetsutani, 2009). However, its focus is not on the activation of cognitive functions even though it is based on communication. A novel method known as coimagination has been proposed by the authors of this paper to support interactive communication and activate the three cognitive functions (Otake, Kato, Takagi, & Asama, 2009; Otake, 2009).

To evaluate the intensity of cognitive activities during conversation via the coimagination method, this paper proposes the conversation interactivity measuring method (CIMM).

COIMAGINATION METHOD

The aim of the coimagination method is to support interactive conversation and to activate episodic memory, division of attention, and planning functions, which decline in the early stage of mild cognitive impairment. Figure 1 describes the protocol of the coimagination program, intuitively, for first-time participants. The description of the coimagination method and the cognitive functions that are expected to be activated for each step is given below.

Planning Functions

It is difficult to estimate the internal views or feelings of other people from external observation, but these internal views and feelings are the keys for understanding one another (Figure 1 - 1). To lower such barriers, the coimagination method

Figure 1. Intuitive instruction of the coimagination method for first-time participants

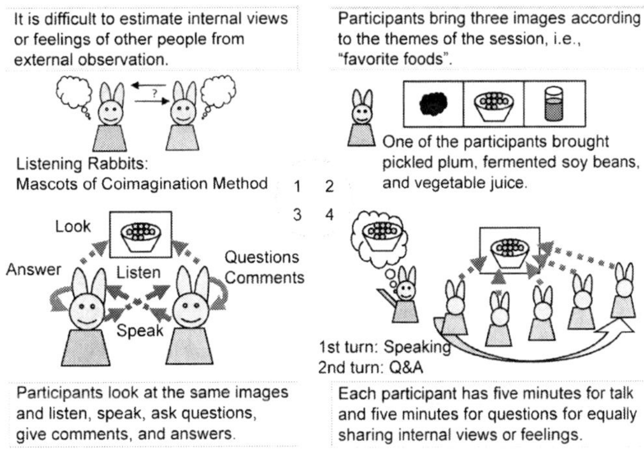

asks participants to bring three images according to the themes of the session to share internal views or feelings and to communicate using the images. To prepare the image topics, participants may ask themselves what they would like to talk about according to the theme and to explore their internal worlds to determine their own topics. Then, participants search images that represent the topics and explore the external world by taking new pictures. Another preparation method is to observe the participants' personal belongings, such as albums and books, and look for familiar things in the external world. Participants recall what they are or where they were located so that they can take note of their original viewpoints, i.e., their internal worlds. In both ways, participants can plan their conversation by moving back and forth between their internal worlds and the external world. The planning functions of the participants are expected to be activated during this process. The themes are arbitrary, but the preferable ones encourage participants to pay attention to the external world, e.g., favorite foods. For instance, one of the participants brought images of pickled plums, fermented soy beans, and vegetable juice for the theme (Figure 1 - 2). All images brought by the participants are registered on the computer by the organizers before the session starts.

Division of Attention

The coimagination method allocates equal time for presentations, questions and comments, with a predefined turn for each participant to engage in interactive communication. This requirement is necessary because interactive communication requires a division of attention for the speakers and listeners. The speakers pay attention to the listeners, listen to questions and comments, understand them, and then answer questions or give comments by speaking. The listeners listen to the speakers, estimate intentions, imagine the stories, ask questions and give comments when the opportunity arises. In addition, both the speakers and listeners look at the images on a screen during the coimagination session. To prevent one-way communication, we define an allotted time for each participant. When the time for the speaker is over, this rule, rather than the listeners, determines the change of the speaker to the next in line. The listeners do not have to say that the speaker has been talking for too long but that it is time for the next speaker. The speaker tries to keep time while speaking, which requires a division of attention. To summarize, the cognitive functions necessary for the division of attention are activated for both the speakers and listeners during an interactive communication that also has images and time limits (Figure 1 - 3).

Episodic Memory

There are two turns during a conversation in the coimagination method. The first turn is for speaking, and the second turn is for the questions and answers (Figure 1 - 4). Each participant has the same amount of time for both turns. This is a very important rule to achieve interactive communication because some people take the initiative in everyday conversations, whereas others do not. In most cases, only a few people who speak a great deal or speak loudly participate in conversations. Other people listen silently or pretend to listen. To avoid such situations, we define the role of the speakers and listeners beforehand. Each speaker takes his or her turn in order. Then, people who are not usually prone to speak out have time to speak, and people who are not good at breaking in to conversations can participate. In this way, all the participants play leading roles in the conversations, one after the other. To present the subject associated with each image, participants express their feelings and thoughts by describing the images. The internal world of each participant is mapped to the external world. The internal views of the participants from their own perspectives are projected onto screens. Other participants look at the same scenes from the same perspective. In this way, the participants can share perspectives that are different from their own. This leads the participants to discover new things in the external world that cannot be discovered from their original viewpoints. The participants can share their subjective experience and extend their viewpoints by sharing the collected views. External worlds originally brought up by one of the participants can then be mapped onto the internal worlds of the other participants. Participation in conversation via the coimagination method may become an episodic memory for each participant. The participants perform a memory task to determine whether the communications themselves formed an episodic memory. The participants then guess the owner and the theme of the collected images after a series of conversation sessions. Episodic memories are assumed to be activated when the topics of the surrounding participants are remembered by each participant.

Definition of Coimagination Method and Typical Coimagination Program

The coimagination method is a method that supports interactive communication through the expression of feelings about images according to a theme. Allocated time periods and turns for each participant are predetermined so that all participants play the roles of both the speaker and listener. We designed the standard coimagination program as follows.

- The program includes five series of sessions. Each session lasts one hour per week. The theme of each session is different.
- There are six participants. There are three images for each participant. The allocated time is five minutes for each participant and for each turn during the first four weeks.
- On the fifth week, the session for the memory task is held. The images from the series of four sessions are displayed one after the other. The participants guess the owner and the theme of the collected images.

CONVERSATION INTERACTIVITY MEASURING METHOD (CIMM)

Invention of the Conversation Interactivity Measuring Method

Previously, the frequency of the comments has been measured to evaluate the interactivity of the conversations. The limitation of this measure is that the flow of the conversations and the quality of the presented topics cannot be measured. Previous studies analyzed conversations based on dictations from tapes, which took several times longer than the conversation periods themselves. It has therefore been difficult to measure both the quality and quantity of conversations in the field. We propose a novel method known as the conversation interactivity measuring method (CIMM) for measuring the interactivity of conversations, which may indicate the intensity of cognitive activities. The method is implemented in three steps. For the first step, diagrams are drawn on sheets of paper during the conversation session by the measurers (Step 1). The second step is that the measurers calculate the scores of each participant for each topic and input them into the computer after the conversation session (Step 2). The third step is that the scores of each participant throughout the session are automatically calculated from the scores of each participant for each topic by spreadsheets (Step 3).

Protocol of the Conversation Interactivity Measuring Method

Drawing of a Conversation State Transition Diagram (Step 1)

The sheet of paper for the conversation state transition diagram is size A4 in landscape orientation.

One form is used for one story. We use 18 sheets for the standard coimagination session attended by six people who each bring three stories with three images. There is an empty oval in the center of the sheets so that the original story presented by each speaker can be written down on each sheet. There are two spreadsheets on both the left and right sides of the sheets for counting. The measurers draw diagrams on the sheets while listening to the series of conversations. On each sheet, the participant who brought the image is a speaker, whereas the other participants are listeners. Verbal expressions are noted as digraphs, and nonverbal expressions are drawn as symbols. Verbal expressions are noted as "conversation digraphs" by the measurers as follows.

One topic presented by an arbitrary participant is expressed as a node. Each edge starts from the node that represents a comment and ends at the node that receives the comment. Each node has a number that represents the participant who made the comment. Each participant has a participant identification (ID) number from 1 to 6. The ID of the first speaker is 1, and that of the last speaker is 6. Participants are seated from left to right according to speaking order in front of the screen. The chains of topics extend from the central oval through the series of comments. The chain is terminated when a totally new topic is presented by a participant. Most edges start from the surrounding area and connect to the center, but some start from the central oval when the topic is switched by the speaker.

Nonverbal expressions such as the laughter and wonder of the other participants that are elicited by each topic represented as a node are drawn as "conversation symbols". A "reaction symbol", which is symbolized as a face with two eyes and a mouth, is drawn when participants say, "Really?", "Wow!", or "Oh!". A "laughter symbol", which is symbolized as a smiling face with two eyes and a mouth with a smile, is drawn when there is a burst of laughter. These symbols are drawn on the lower right side of the nodes that elicited nonverbal reactions.

Calculation of the Scores of Each Participant for Each Topic (Step 2)

Verbal and nonverbal scores are calculated from the conversation digraphs and conversation symbols. Each score is calculated in the following manner.

First, the verbal score for each node is calculated. The verbal score of a node that represents a comment given by participant i of the lth node in the kth chain on the jth topic of speaker i' is expressed as:

$$v(i, j, k, l+1) = v(i, j, k, l) + x. \quad (1)$$

Each node has its original verbal score x, where x=1 when the participant who gave the comment is a speaker ($i=i'$), and x=2 when the participant is a listener ($i \neq i'$). This calculation is applied for all the nodes in the digraphs. All the nodes of the speakers are circled in red for ease of interpretation. The verbal scores are written down on the top right side of each node in red.

Second, the nonverbal score for each node is calculated. The nonverbal score of a node is expressed as:

$$w(i, j, k, l) = y. \quad (2)$$

Each node has its original nonverbal score y, where y=1 when the conversation symbol on the lower right side of the node is a reaction symbol, and y=2 when the conversation symbol is a laughter symbol.

Third, the highest verbal score of each participant on each chain is put on the left spreadsheets for calculating verbal scores. The number of conversation symbols for each participant is put on the right spreadsheets for calculating nonverbal scores. The measurers input both the verbal and nonverbal scores on the left and right spreadsheets into the computer.

Calculation of the Scores of Each Participant Throughout the Session (Step 3)

Four types of scores for each participant throughout the session are calculated automatically using the following algorithm. Scores represent the active or passive and the verbal or nonverbal characteristics of the participation in the series of conversations.

The active verbal score $S_{av}(i)$ of participant *i* is calculated from the verbal scores of the nodes:

$$S_{av}(i) = \sum_{j=1}^{18} \sum_{k=1}^{k_{num}} \max_{l=1}^{l_{num}} v(i, j, k, l). \qquad (3)$$

where k_{num} is the number of chains in the topic *j*, and l_{num} is the number of nodes on the chain *k*. Namely, the active verbal score is a sum of the highest verbal scores of participant *i* for all the chains of all the stories. This score indicates whether the participant actively gave comments or asked questions to other participants' topics.

The active nonverbal score $S_{anv}(i)$ of participant *i* is calculated from the nonverbal scores of the nodes:

$$S_{anv}(i) = \sum_{j=1}^{18} \sum_{k=1}^{k_{num}} \sum_{l=1}^{l_{num}} w(i, j, k, l), \qquad (4)$$

which indicates whether the participant activated the conversations by causing the laughter or wonder of the other participants.

The passive verbal score $S_{pv}(i)$ of participant *i* is calculated from the verbal scores of the nodes:

$$S_{pv}(i) = \sum_{j=3i-2}^{3i} \sum_{k=1}^{k_{num}} v(i, j, k, l_{num}), \qquad (5)$$

which indicates whether the participant involved the surrounding participants in the conversations during the turn. The passive verbal score is obtained by aggregating the highest verbal score of each chain for stories of $j=\{3i\text{-}2,3i\text{-}1,3i\}$, where participant *i* gave them.

The passive nonverbal score $S_{pnv}(i)$ of participant *i* is calculated from the nonverbal scores of the nodes:

$$S_{pnv}(i) = \sum_{i''=1}^{6} \sum_{j=3i-2}^{3i} \sum_{k=1}^{k_{num}} \sum_{l=1}^{l_{num}} w(i'', j, k, l), \qquad (6)$$

which indicates whether the conversations engaged the laughter or wonder of all participants $i''=\{1,2,3,4,5,6\}$ during the turn $j=\{3i\text{-}2,3i\text{-}1,3i\}$ of participant *i*.

Conversation Scores and Exploited Cognitive Functions

Here we discuss which conversation score corresponds to the cognitive functions that are intended to be activated during the conversations. Both the passive verbal score and the passive nonverbal score indicate whether the surrounding participants participated in the conversations initiated by the speaker. These show the number of turns taken, which requires a division of attention for the speaker. Also, they imply the planning function of the speaker who prepared the stories. Both the active verbal score and the active nonverbal score represent the number of interruptions and stimulations by the comments of the participants. These reflect the division of attention of the listeners.

EVALUATION OF THE COIMAGINATION METHOD VIA CIMM

Coimagination Program at a Lifelong Learning Center

We held a coimagination program at a lifelong learning center in Kashiwa, Japan. The participants were elderly people who were interested in the prevention of dementia. There were 18 participants in the program. The participants were divided into three groups, A, B, and C, and each group had six members. The programs were conducted in parallel, containing five series of sessions. Each session lasted one hour per week. The last session provided the memory task, whereas the other four were conversation sessions. The theme of the first session was "favorite things". The second session was "hometown, travel, and neighborhood". The third session was "health and foods". The fourth session was "jokes and mistakes". In this section, we analyze one of the typical groups, group B, which showed a dramatic change in communication during the sessions. Group B contained six normal participants (4 men and 2 women; average age = 70 years). We named the participants B1, B2, B3, B4, B5, and B6. Conversations during the second, third, and fourth sessions were analyzed using the CIMM. The conversation of the first session was excluded because the first session was used to gain familiarity with the method. Below, we refer to the second session as the first session, and the fourth session as the last session.

Intensity of Cognitive Activities During Coimagination as Measured by the Conversation Interactivity Measuring Method

The intensity of cognitive activities during coimagination was measured by the CIMM for group B. Both the verbal and nonverbal characteristics of conversation were measured, and the participation style of each participant was calculated. The active and passive verbal scores of group B are shown in Figure 2. The horizontal axis shows the active verbal score, and the vertical axis shows the passive verbal score of each participant. Both the active and passive verbal scores of participants B2 and B6 increased drastically, whereas those of participant B3 increased slightly over the series of sessions. The active verbal scores of participants B1, B3, and B5 in the last session were greater than those of the first session. The passive verbal score of participant B4 in the last session was greater than that of the first session. The active and passive nonverbal scores of group B are shown in Figure 3. The horizontal axis shows the active nonverbal score and the vertical axis the passive nonverbal score for each participant. Both the active and passive nonverbal scores of all the participants increased. The nonverbal scores of participants B3, B4 and B5 showed a dramatic increase, although their verbal scores either showed only a slight increase or only one of the scores showed an increase in the series of sessions.

Figure 2. Active verbal score (horizontal axis) and passive verbal score (vertical axis) of group B in the series of sessions

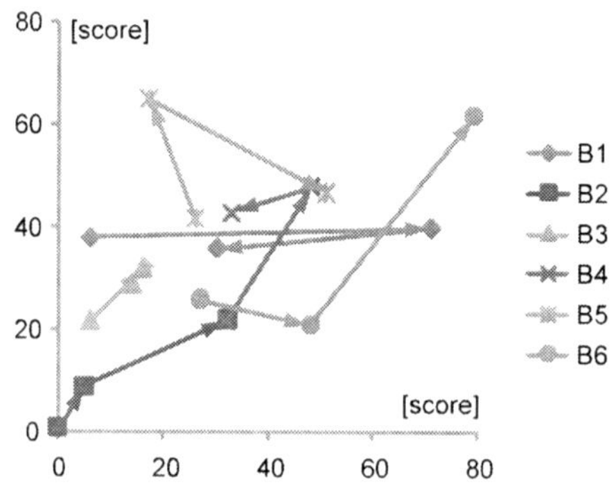

Figure 3. Active nonverbal score (horizontal axis) and passive nonverbal score (vertical axis) of group B in the series of sessions

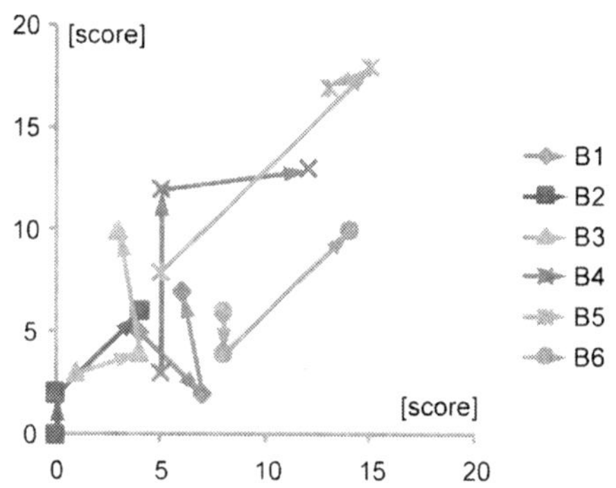

DISCUSSION

First, we will discuss the reason behind the dramatic changes noted in participants B2 and B6. Participant B2 did not participate in the other participants' topics. In the beginning, he kept on speaking during the second turn. He said he was impressed by the instruction given to all participants that it is important to leave some of the contents of the stories for the first turn so that other participants can ask questions and give comments during the second turn. He followed the instruction and experienced interactive conversations after that. Participant B6 talked a lot from the beginning but received fewer comments because his style of speaking did not leave many openings to the other participants. He was impressed by the other participants' stories with punch lines and prepared such stories in the end. These are the presumptive reasons for the dramatic changes.

Second, we will discuss whether the cognitive activities that are effective for the prevention of dementia were employed. Among the participants, participants B2 and B6 gave comments, received comments, asked questions, answered questions, and elicited reactions through their comments. Therefore, their division of attention and planning functions were activated through the series of sessions. The nonverbal scores of all participants increased because the participants became more relaxed and their reactions and laughter improved. We can assume that a social network emerged, and intellectual activities that brought out reactions and laughter between participants were employed.

Third, we will discuss the limitation of the measuring method. The participants who received reactions and laughter scored high during conversation in the CIMM, whereas the participants who reacted and laughed scored low despite the activation of their cognitive functions. The number of reactions and the amount of laughter from each participant should also be scored.

CONCLUSION

In this chapter, we described the coimagination method with three cognitive functions that are expected to be activated for each step: planning, division of attention, and episodic memory. Then, the conversation interactivity measuring method (CIMM) was proposed, and the intensity of cognitive activities during conversation via the coimagination method were measured. The method was validated by providing programs for elderly people at a lifelong learning center in Kashiwa, Japan. The nonverbal scores of each participant increased through the series of sessions. The verbal scores of some of the participants increased dramatically through the series of sessions. These results suggest that the division of the attention and planning functions of the participants were activated, a social network among the participants emerged, and intellectual activities were conducted that brought out reactions and laughter among the participants. Future work should include the development of a method that can quantify the reactions, laughter, and physiological changes of each participant for both short-term and long-term evaluation.

ACKNOWLEDGMENT

This work was supported by a Grant-in-Aid for Scientific Research on priority area Systems Genomics (#014), Mobilligence (#454) and Information Explosion (#456) from the Ministry of Education, Culture, Sports, Science and Technology of Japan (MEXT).

REFERENCES

Ball, K., Berch, D. B., & Helmers, K. F. (2002). Effects of cognitive training intervention with older adults: A randomized controlled trial. *Journal of the American Medical Association, 288*(18), 2271–2281. doi:10.1001/jama.288.18.2271

Barberger-Gateau, P., Fabrigoule, C., & Rouch, I. (1999). Neuropsychological correlates of self-reported performance in instrumental activities of daily living and prediction of dementia. *The Journals of Gerontology. Series B, Psychological Sciences and Social Sciences*, *54*(5), 293–303.

Crooks, V. C., Lubben, J., Petitti, D. B., & Chiu, D. L. V. (2008). Social network, cognitive function, and dementia incidence among elderly women. *American Journal of Public Health*, *98*(7), 1221–1227. doi:10.2105/AJPH.2007.115923

Fratiglioni, L., Wang, H. X., Ericsson, K., Maytan, M., & Winblad, B. (2000). Influence of social network on occurrence of dementia: A community based longitudinal study. *Lancet*, *355*(9212), 1315–1319. doi:10.1016/S0140-6736(00)02113-9

Otake, M. (2009). Coimagination method: Sharing imagination with images and time limit. In. *Proceedings of the International Reminiscence and Life Review Conference*, *2009*, 97–103.

Otake, M., Kato, M., Takagi, T., & Asama, H. (2009). Coimagination method: Communication support system with collected images and its evaluation via memory task. In C. Stephanidis (Ed.), *Universal access in human-computer interaction*, (pp. 403–411). (LNCS 5614), Springer-Verlag.

Rentz, D. M., & Weintraub, S. (2000). Neuropsychological detection of early probable Alzheimer's disease. In Scinto, L. F. M., & Daffner, K. R. (Eds.), *Early diagnosis and treatment of Alzheimer's disease* (pp. 69–189). Totowa, NJ: Humana Press. doi:10.1385/1-59259-005-5:169

Yasuda, K., Kuwabara, K., Kuwahara, N., Abe, S., & Tetsuntani, N. (2009). Effectiveness of personalized reminiscence photo videos for individuals with dementia. *Neuropsychological Rehabilitation*, *19*(4), 603–619. doi:10.1080/09602010802586216

KEY TERMS AND DEFINITIONS

Coimagination Method: A method that supports interactive communication through expressing feelings about images according to a theme. Allocated time periods and turns for each participant are predetermined so that all participants play the roles of both speaker and listener. The method was proposed by one of the authors, Mihoko Otake, in 2006.

Conversation Interactivity Measuring Method (CIMM): A method for measuring the interactivity of conversations that may indicate the intensity of cognitive activities. The method was proposed by one of the authors, Mihoko Otake, in 2008.

Dementia: A medical condition that especially affects old people, causing their memory and other mental abilities to gradually degrade and lead to confusion. The most common form of dementia is Alzheimer's disease.

Division of Attention: To watch, listen to, or think about multiple things and people carefully or with interest.

Episodic Memory: The recollection of information about specific past events that involved the self and occurred at a particular time and place. Semantic and episodic memories together make up the category of declarative memory, which is one of the two major divisions in memory.

Mild Cognitive Impairment (MCI): Transition stage between the cognitive decline of normal aging and the more serious problems caused by Alzheimer's disease.

Planning Function: The act of deciding how to do something.

Chapter 44
An International Investigation of Driver's Licenses for Dementia Patients with Considerations of Their Social Circumstances

Satoshi Takahashi
Graduate School of Natural Science and Technology, Okayama University, Japan

Jinglong Wu
Graduate School of Natural Science and Technology, Okayama University, Japan

ABSTRACT

In recent years, the trend toward the nuclear family and the phenomenon of under-population in rural areas has increased the number of aging people who live alone. Therefore, aging people are more likely to drive themselves to go shopping or to a hospital. However, the elderly person also has a tendency to display reduced abilities of cognition and judgment and, in severe cases, displays dementia.

The brief results of an international investigation of traffic accidents among aging people based on databases published by public institutions are discussed in this chapter. The aging rate and the number of dementia patients increase with the average life expectancy when it is over 70 years. Currently, the number of traffic accidents among aging people is increasing. Policies preventing the renewal of driver's licenses for aging people are implemented in several countries. However, communication with family and neighbors is effective in preventing aging people from being involved in traffic accidents while walking.

DOI: 10.4018/978-1-60960-559-9.ch044

INTRODUCTION

The increasing proportion of young people moving to urban areas associated with economic development brings an increase in the proportion of nuclear families. Therefore, households composed of only aging people are increasing in the depopulated areas. For aging people, an automobile is necessary to go shopping or to a hospital. However, an elderly person may display reduced abilities of judgment and cognition and, in severe cases, may exhibit dementia. As shown in Figure 1, the number of patients with dementia is expected to increase around the world. In Japan, there is a duty for an aging person over the age of 70 to take driver's licenses, and a person who has poor judgment and cognition cannot obtain a driver's license. The loss of a driver's license can make a person's life difficult.

Rapidly changing lifestyles, the policies for living conditions, and security and social infrastructure for aging people differ by country. For instance, European countries have a policy of welfare, but Asian countries have a policy of economic growth. The policies depend not only on the economic growth but also on the convenience of everyday tasks for aging people and their support systems.

In this study, the social infrastructures for aging people regarding driver's licenses and driving in everyday life are investigated for several countries.

EXPERIMENT

Method

Numerical data were collected from the publications and announcements of national organizations.

Results

A. Number of Dementia Patients

The aging rate, which indicates that the proportion of the population over 65 years of age in comparison to the total population (Japan Ministry of International Affairs and Communications, 2009), is plotted against the average life expectancy in

Figure 1. Predicted increase in the prevalence of dementia

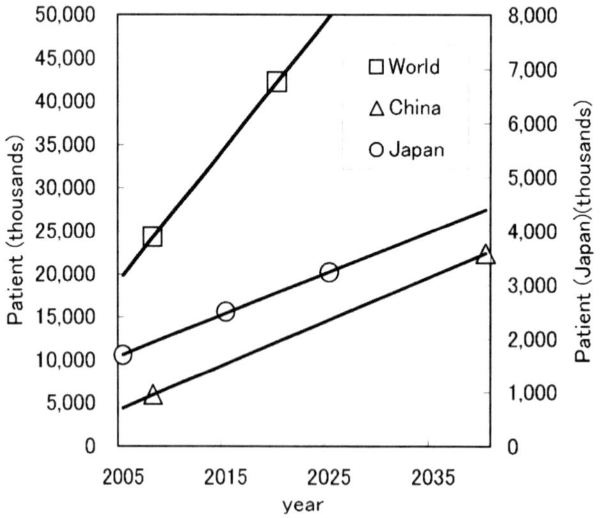

Figure 2. Aging rates of each country as a function of average life expectancy (2008)

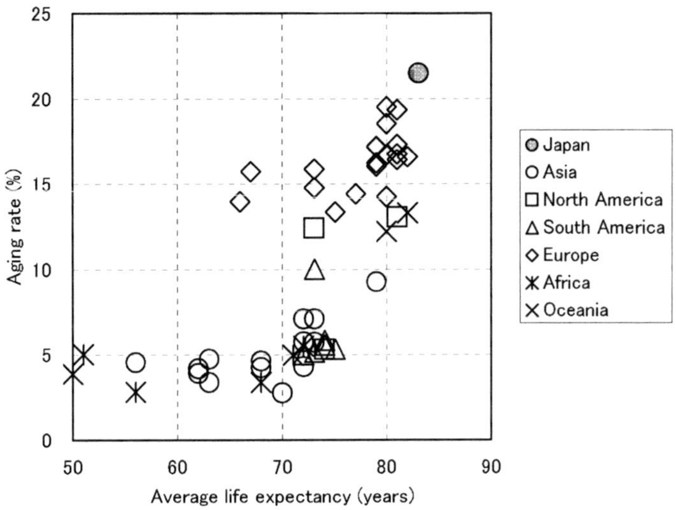

Figure 2. The aging rate and average life expectancy in Japan are the highest of all countries. The average life expectancy in Asia, except for Japan and Korea, has a wide range, from 55 to 85 years old. However, the aging rate in Asia is lower than in other areas, whereas the aging rate in Europe is higher than in other countries. The aging rate has a tendency to increase with the average life expectancy if the average life is over 70 years.

Figure 3 shows the ratio of dementia patients to the total population in each country (Alzheimer's Disease International, 2006, Alzheimer Europe, 2006). In this figure, the ratio in the United States is calculated from the number of patients with Alzheimer's disease. In Japan and Europe, the ratios of dementia patients are over 1%. The number of dementia patients becomes large with the average life expectancy if it is over 70 years. From these results, the average life expectancy may become an indicator for the number of dementia patients.

B. Traffic Accidents for Aging People

The ownership rates for driver's licenses at each age in Japan are shown in Figure 4 (Japan National Police Agency, 2008). The abscissa axis shows the ratio of driver's license ownership to the population. Males are plotted in the left figure, and females are plotted in the right figure. In Japan, the ratio of driver's license ownership for people over 65 is quite high. Half of 80-year-olds have a license. Specifically, more males than females over 65 have a license. This figure shows that many aging people use a car in everyday life. The rates of road user fatalities over 65 years old are shown in Figure 5 (Organization for Economic Co-operation and Development, 2009). Because little information regarding fatalities as a function of age is known, the data, except for Japan and Korea, in Asia are not shown in this figure. The rate for Japan is a lot higher than for the other countries, revealing that about half of the people in road user fatalities are aging people over 65. In many countries, the rate tends to increase with the average life expectancy.

Figure 3. Rates of dementia in each country as a function of average life expectancy (2005)

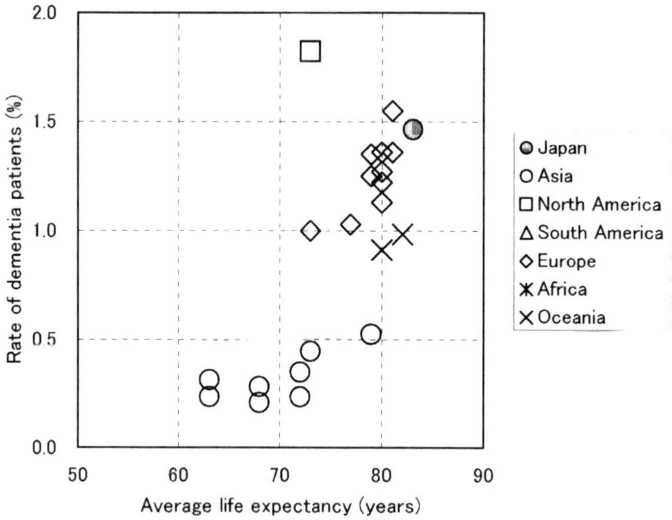

Figure 4. Driver's license ownership ratio by age in Japan (2007)

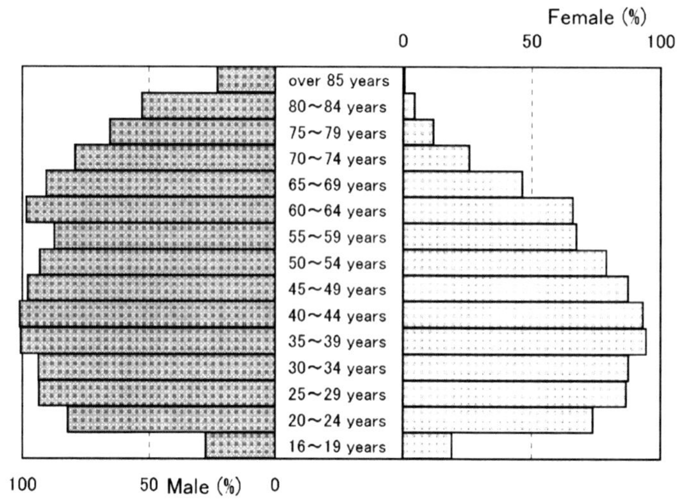

Figure 6 shows the transition of fatalities in driving (Japan National Police Agency, 2008). The number of fatalities in young people under 24 tends to decrease. However, the number of fatalities in aging people does not decrease. This figure shows that new types of social action for traffic safety are required for aging people.

DISCUSSION

To prevent traffic accidents among aging people, two roles that an aging people may find themselves in should be considered: one is as the assailant, and the other is as the victim.

Figure 5. Rates of road user fatalities for those over 65 years old as a function of average life expectancy (2005)

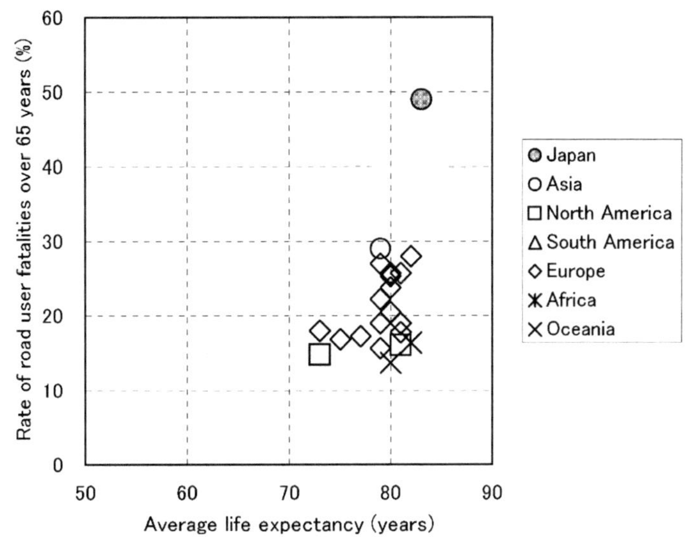

Figure 6. The transition of driving fatalities in Japan

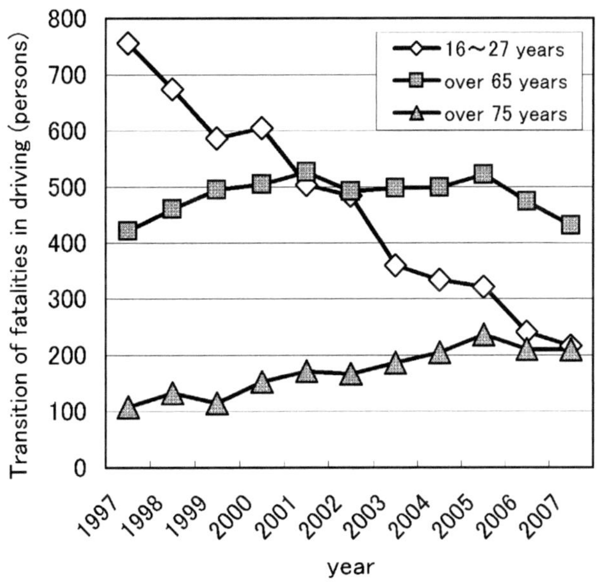

In Japan, everyone over 70 has to be inspected regarding cognitive faculties for the renewal of a driver's license. In the other countries, the renewal of driver's licenses tends to be limited for aging people. In China, people over 70 cannot get a driver's license. However, in the USA, only a vision test is required for aging people in some states. Moreover, for the aging people in depopulated areas, an automobile is essential to go shopping and to a hospital. Public transportation should be constructed not only in urban areas but also in depopulated areas.

The rate of pedestrian accidents among aging people is higher than the rate of driving accidents. Needless to say, it is dangerous for an aging person to walk alone. Walking with a partner or family member is necessary to prevent a traffic accident. Moreover, it may be useful to prevent the pathogeny of dementia.

ACKNOWLEDGMENT

A part of this study was supported by a Grant-in-Aid for Scientific Research (B) and the Japan and AA Science Platform Program of the Japan Society for the Promotion Science.

REFERENCES

Alzheimer's Disease International. (2006). Dementia in the Asia Pacific region. *Access Economics*, 3.

Europe, A. (2006). *Dementia in Europe yearbook* (p. 21).

Japan Ministry of International Affairs and Communications. (2009). *International statistical compendium*. (pp. 43-48, 61-62).

Japan National Police Agency. (2008). *Statistics of driving license* (p. 3).

Japan National Police Agency. (2008). *Report of exploratory committee about support for aging driver*.

Organization for Economic Co-operation and Development. (2009). *International road traffic and accident database*.

KEY TERMS AND DEFINITIONS

Aging Rate: Ratio of the population over 65 years old to the total population.

Average Life Expectancy: Average duration of life at birth in a population.

Dementia: An illness involving a loss of cognitive ability.

Depopulated Area: An area of reduction in a human population.

Driver's License: An official permission to drive an automobile on public roads.

Fatality: The number of deaths.

Nuclear Family: A family group consisting of only a father and mother and their children.

Traffic Accident: An accidental collision of automobiles with each other or with humans.

Compilation of References

Abe, T., Makizako, H., & Tokuhara, R. (2005). Assessment and program of the physical activity reflected daily life in the elderly: Target on the prolongation of healthy life span: Report on real image and practice for the object of visiting rehabilitation. *Journal of the Japanese Physical Therapy Association*, *32*(4), 224–226.

Akaike, H. (1974). A new look at the statistical model identification. *IEEE Transactions on Automatic Control*, *19*(6), 716–723. doi:10.1109/TAC.1974.1100705

Albright, T. D., & Desimone, R. (1987). Local precision of visuotopic organization in the middle temporal area (MT) of the macaque. *Experimental Brain Research*, *65*, 582–592. doi:10.1007/BF00235981

Allen, L. A. (1999). Treating agitation without drugs. *The American Journal of Nursing*, *99*(4), 36–42. doi:10.2307/3472232

Allison, T., Ginter, T. H., & McCarthy, H, G., Nobre, A. C., Puce, A., Luby, M., & Spencer, D. D. (1994). Face-recognition in human extrastriate cortex. *Journal of Neurophysiology*, *71*, 821–825.

Allison, T., Puce, A., Spencer, D. D., & McCarthy, G. (1999). Electrophysiological studies of human face perception. I: Potentials generated in occipitotemporal cortex by face and non-face stimuli. *Cerebral Cortex*, *9*, 415–430. doi:10.1093/cercor/9.5.415

Altschuler, E. L., Wisdom, S. B., Stone, L., Foster, C., Galasko, D., Llewellyn, D. M. E., & Ramachandran, V. S. (1999). Rehabilitation of hemiparesis after stroke with a mirror. *Lancet*, *353*(June), 2035–2036. doi:10.1016/S0140-6736(99)00920-4

Alzheimer's Disease International. (2006). Dementia in the Asia Pacific region. *Access Economics*, 3.

Alzheimer's Association. (2008). *The emerging voice of Alzheimer's*. Retrieved from http://www.alz.org/townhall/

American Heart Association. (2010). *American Heart Association stroke statistics*. Retrieved from http://www.Americanheart.org/statistics/stroke.htm

American Psychiatric Association. (2007). *Practice guideline for the treatment of patients with Alzheimer's disease and other dementias, 2nd ed.* American Psychiatric Association, Inc. Retrieved from http://www.psychiatryonline.com/pracguide/pracguidetopic_3.aspx

Andreasen, N., Vanmechelen, E., Vanderstichele, H., Davidsson, P., & Blennow, K. (2003). Cerebrospinal fluid levels of total-tau, phospho-tau and A beta 42 predicts development of Alzheimer's disease in patients with mild cognitive impairment. *Acta Neurologica Scandinavica*, *179*, 47–51. doi:10.1034/j.1600-0404.107.s179.9.x

Andrew, G. L. (2004). Neuro-opthalmic findings in the visual variant of Alzheimer's disease. *Opthalmology*, *111*, 376–380. doi:10.1016/S0161-6420(03)00732-2

Arakawa, K., Tobimatsu, S., Kato, M., & Kira, J. (1999). Parvocelluar and magnocellular visual processing in spinocerebellar degeneration and Parkinson's disease: An event-related potential study. *Clinical Neurophysiology*, *110*, 1048–1057. doi:10.1016/S1388-2457(99)00049-8

Armentano, R. L., Simon, A., Levenson, J., Chau, N. P., Megnien, J. L., & Pichel, R. (1991). Mechanical pressure versus intrinsic effects of hypertension on large arteries in humans. *Hypertension*, *18*(5), 657–664.

Ashida, S. (2000). The effect of reminiscence music therapy sessions on changes in depressive symptoms in elderly persons with dementia. *Journal of Music Therapy*, *37*(3), 170–182.

Awata, S. (2009). Role of the dementia medical center in the community. *Japanese Journal of Geriatrics, 46*, 203–206. doi:10.3143/geriatrics.46.203

Azegami, M., Ohira, M., Miyoshi, K., Kobayashi, C., Hongo, M., Yanagihashi, R., & Sadoyama, T. (2007). Effect of single and multi-joint lower extremity muscle strength on the functional capacity and ADL/IADL status in Japanese community-dwelling older adults. *Nursing & Health Sciences, 9*, 168–176. doi:10.1111/j.1442-2018.2007.00317.x

Bäckman, L., & Small, B. J. (1998). Influences of cognitive support on episodic remembering: tracing the process of loss from normal aging to Alzheimer's disease. *Psychology and Aging, 13*, 267–276. doi:10.1037/0882-7974.13.2.267

Bäckman, L., & Small, B. J. (2007). Cognitive deficits in preclinical Alzheimer's disease and vascular dementia: Patterns of findings from the Kungsholmen Project. *Physiology & Behavior, 92*, 80–86. doi:10.1016/j.physbeh.2007.05.014

Badgaiyan, R. D., Schacter, D. L., & Alpert, N. M. (1999). Auditory priming within and across modalities: Evidence from positron emission tomography. *Journal of Cognitive Neuroscience, 11*(4), 337–348. doi:10.1162/089892999563463

Baker, A. T. (1991). An introduction to the basic principles of magnetic nerve stimulation. *Journal of Clinical Neurophysiology, 8*, 26–37. doi:10.1097/00004691-199101000-00005

Baker, A. T., Jalinous, R., & Freestone, I. L. (1985). Non-invasive magnetic stimulation of the human motor cortex. *Lancet, 1*, 1106–1107. doi:10.1016/S0140-6736(85)92413-4

Ball, K., Berch, D. B., & Helmers, K. F. (2002). Effects of cognitive training intervention with older adults: A randomized controlled trial. *Journal of the American Medical Association, 288*(18), 2271–2281. doi:10.1001/jama.288.18.2271

Bando, H. (2008). Current status of music therapy. *Japanese Journal of Complementary and Alternative Medicine, 5*(1), 27–36. doi:10.1625/jcam.5.27

Bank, A. J., Wilson, R. F., & Kubo, S. H. (1995). Direct effects of smooth muscle relaxation and contraction on in vivo human brachial artery elastic properties. *Circulation Research, 77*, 1008–1016.

Barberger-Gateau, P., Fabrigoule, C., & Rouch, I. (1999). Neuropsychological correlates of self-reported performance in instrumental activities of daily living and prediction of dementia. *The Journals of Gerontology. Series B, Psychological Sciences and Social Sciences, 54*(5), 293–303.

Bartko, J. J. (1966). The intraclass correlation coefficient as a measure of reliability. *Psychological Reports, 19*, 3–11.

Bayliss, W. M. (1902). On the local reactions of the arterial wall to changes of internal pressure. *The Journal of Physiology, 28*, 220–231.

Bennett, D. A., Schneider, J. A., Bienias, J. L., Evans, D. A., & Wilson, R. S. (2005). Mild cognitive impairment is related to Alzheimer disease pathology and cerebral infarctions. *Neurology, 64*, 834–841.

Bennett, D. A., Beckett, L. A., Murray, A. M., Shannon, K. M., Goetz, C. G., Pilgrim, D. M., & Evans, D. A. (1996). Prevalence of parkinsonian signs and associated mortality in a community population of older people. *The New England Journal of Medicine, 334*, 71–76. doi:10.1056/NEJM199601113340202

Bennett, D. A., Beckett, L. A., Wilson, R. S., Murray, A. M., & Evans, D. A. (1998). Parkinsonian signs and mortality from Alzheimer's disease. *Lancet, 51*, 16–31.

Benson, S., & Kitwood, T. (2000). *Person centered care*. London, UK: Hawker Publications.

Bentin, S., Allison, T., Puce, A., Perez, E., & McCarthy, G. (1996). Electrophysiological studies of face perception in humans. *Journal of Cognitive Neuroscience, 8*, 551–565. doi:10.1162/jocn.1996.8.6.551

Birks, J. S., Melzer, D., & Beppu, H. (2003). Donepezil for mild and moderate Alzheimer's disease. *Cochrane Database of Systematic Reviews*, 3.

Bitan, G., Kirkitadze, M. D., Lomakin, A., Vollers, S. S., Benedek, G. B., & Teplow, D. B. (2003). Amyloid β-protein (Aβ) assembly: Abeta 40 and Abeta 42 oligomerize through distinct pathways. *Proceedings of the National Academy of Sciences of the United States of America, 100*, 330–335. doi:10.1073/pnas.222681699

Bjork, E. L., & Bjork, R. A. (1998). *Memory*. New York, NY: Academic Press.

Bland, J. M., & Altman, D. G. (1986). Statistical methods for assessing agreement between two methods of clinical measurement. *Lancet*, *1*, 307–310.

Boden, C. (1998). *Who will I be when I die?*Sydney, Australia: Harper Collins Publishers.

Bohannon, R. W. (1986). Test-retest reliability of hand-held dynamometry during a single session of strength assessment. *Physical Therapy*, *66*, 206–209.

Bohannon, R. W. (1995). Standing balance, lower extremity muscle strength, and walking performance of patients referred for physical therapy. *Perceptual and Motor Skills*, *80*, 379–385.

Boian, R. F., Bouzit, M., Burdea, G. C., & Deutsch, J. E. (2004). Dual Stewart platform mobility simulator. *Proceedings of the 26th Annual International Conference of the IEEE EMBS*, (pp. 4848-4851).

Booth, J. R., Burman, D. D., Meyer, J. R., Gitelman, D. R., Parrish, T. B., & Mesulam, M. M. (2002). Functional anatomy of intra- and cross-modal lexical tasks. *NeuroImage*, *16*, 7–22. doi:10.1006/nimg.2002.1081

Borroni, B., Alberici, A., Agosti, C., Cosseddu, M., & Padovani, A. (2009). Pattern of behavioral disturbances in corticobasal degeneration syndrome and progressive supranuclear palsy. *International Psychogeriatrics*, *21*, 463–468. doi:10.1017/S1041610209008862

Borroni, B., Garibotto, V., Agosti, C., Brambati, S. M., Bellelli, G., & Gasparotti, R. (2008). White matter changes in corticobasal degeneration syndrome and correlation with limb apraxia. *Archives of Neurology*, *65*, 796–801. doi:10.1001/archneur.65.6.796

Boussaoud, D., Desimone, R., & Ungerleider, L. G. (1992). Subcortical connections of visual areas MST and FST in macaques. *Visual Neuroscience*, *9*, 291–302. doi:10.1017/S0952523800010701

Bouzit, M., Popescu, G., Burdea, G., & Boian, R. (2002). The Rutgers MasterII-ND Force Feedback Glove. *IEEE/ASME Transactions on Mechatronics*, *7*, 256–263. doi:10.1109/TMECH.2002.1011262

Boxer, A. L., Rabinovici, G. D., Kepe, V., Goldman, J., Furst, A. J., & Huang, S. C. (2007). Amyloid imaging in distinguishing atypical prion disease from Alzheimer disease. *Neurology*, *69*, 283–290. doi:10.1212/01.wnl.0000265815.38958.b6

Boyle, P. A., Wilson, R. S., Buchman, A. S., Aggarwal, N. T., Tang, Y., & Arvanitakis, Z. (2007). Lower extremity motor function and disability in mild cognitive impairment. *Experimental Aging Research*, *33*, 355–371. doi:10.1080/03610730701319210

Bozzali, M., & Cherubini, A. (2007). Diffusion tensor MRI to investigate dementias: A brief review. *Magnetic Resonance Imaging*, *25*, 969–977. doi:10.1016/j.mri.2007.03.017

Bozzali, M., Falini, A., Cercignani, M., Baglio, F., Farina, E., & Alberoni, M. (2005). Brain tissue damage in dementia with Lewy bodies: An in vivo diffusion tensor MRI study. *Brain*, *128*, 1595–1604. doi:10.1093/brain/awh493

Bozzali, M., Falini, A., Franceschi, M., Cercignani, M., Franceschi, M., & Schiatti, E. (2002). White matter damage in Alzheimer's disease assessed in vivo using diffusion tensor magnetic resonance imaging. *Journal of Neurology, Neurosurgery, and Psychiatry*, *72*, 742–746. doi:10.1136/jnnp.72.6.742

Bracco, L., Piccini, C., & Amaducci, L. (1998). Rate of progression of mental decline in Alzheimer disease: Summary of European studies. *Alzheimer Disease and Associated Disorders*, *12*, 347–355. doi:10.1097/00002093-199812000-00016

Breteler, M. M. B., Van Swieten, J. C., Bots, M. L., Grobbee, D. E., Claus, J. J., & van den Hout, J. H. (1994). Cerebral white matter lesions, vascular risk factors, and cognitive function in a population-based study: The Rotterdam Study. *Neurology*, *44*, 1246–1252.

Brill, P. A., Drimmer, A. M., Morgan, L. A., & Gordon, N. F. (1995). The feasibility of conducting strength and flexibility programs for elderly nursing home residents with dementia. *The Gerontologist*, *35*, 263–266.

Brotons, M. (1996). The effects of music therapy intervention on agitation behaviors of alzheimer's disease patients. *Journal of Music Therapy*, *33*(1), 2–18.

Brotons, M., & Koger, S. M. (2000). The impact of music therapy on language functioning in dementia. *Journal of Music Therapy*, *37*(3), 183–195.

Brun, A., & Englund, E. (1986). *A white matter disorder in dementia of the Alzheimer type: A pathoanatomical study*. (pp. 253-262).

Bryden, C. (2004). *Dancing with dementia*. Sydney, Australia: Jessica Kingsley Publishers.

Buerger, K., Ewers, M., Andreasen, N., Zinkowski, R., Ishiguro, K., & Vanmechelen, E. (1502-1503). … Hampel, H. (2005). Phosphorylated tau predicts rate of cognitive decline in MCI subjects: A comparative CSF study. *Neurology*, *65*(9).

Buerger, K., Zinkowski, R., Teipel, S. J., Tapiola, T., Arai, H., & Blennow, K. (2002). Differential diagnosis of Alzheimer disease with cerebrospinal fluid levels of tau protein phosphorylated at threonine. *Archives of Neurology*, *59*(8), 1267–1272. doi:10.1001/archneur.59.8.1267

Burgio, L., Scilley, K., Hardin, J. M., Hsu, C., & Yancey, J. (1996). Environmental white noise: An intervention for verbally agitated nursing home residents. *The Journals of Gerontology. Series B, Psychological Sciences and Social Sciences*, *51*(6), 364–373.

Buschke, H., Kuslansky, G., Katz, M., Stewart, W. F., Sliwinski, M. J., & Eckholdt, H. M. (1999). Screening for dementia with the Memory Impairment Screen. *Neurology*, *52*(2), 231–238.

Busse, R., Bauer, R. D., Schabert, A., Summa, Y., Bumm, P., & Wetterer, E. (1979). The mechanical properties of exposed human common carotid arteries in vivo. *Basic Research in Cardiology*, *74*, 545–554. doi:10.1007/BF01907647

Butefisch, C., Hummelsheim, H., Denzler, P., & Mauritz, K. H. (1995). Repetitive training of isolated movements improves the outcome of motor rehabilitation of the centrally paretic hand. *Journal of the Neurological Sciences*, *130*, 59–68. doi:10.1016/0022-510X(95)00003-K

Cabeza, R., & Ohta, N. (1993). Dissociating conceptual priming, perceptual priming and explicit memory. *The European Journal of Cognitive Psychology*, *5*(1), 35–53. doi:10.1080/09541449308406513

Cabinet Office, Government of Japan (Ed.). (2009). *The white paper on aging society in Heisei-era 21*. Oita, Japan: Saiki printing Co. Ltd.

Cagnin, A., Brooks, D. J., Kennedy, A. M., Gunn, R. N., Myers, R., & Turkheimer, F. E. (2001). In-vivo measurement of activated microglia in dementia. *Lancet*, *358*, 461–467. doi:10.1016/S0140-6736(01)05625-2

Capell, A., Steiner, H., Willem, M., Kaiser, H., Meyer, C., & Walter, J. (2000). Maturation and pro-peptide cleavage of beta-secretase. *The Journal of Biological Chemistry*, *275*(40), 30849–30854. doi:10.1074/jbc.M003202200

Carrie, J. S., Reynolds, A., Goodyear, B. G., Ponton, C. W., Dort, J. C., & Eggermont, J. J. (2004). Simultaneous 3-T fMRI and high-density recording of human auditory evoked potentials. *NeuroImage*, *23*, 1129–1142. doi:10.1016/j.neuroimage.2004.07.035

Caughey, B., & Lansbury, P. T. (2003). Protofibrils, pores, fibrils, and neurodegeneration: Separating the responsible protein aggregates from the innocent bystanders. *Annual Review of Neuroscience*, *26*, 267–298. doi:10.1146/annurev.neuro.26.010302.081142

Cauraugh, J. H., Kim, S. B., & Duley, A. (2005). Coupled bilateral movements and active neuromuscular stimulation: Intralimb transfer evidence during bimanual aiming. *Neuroscience Letters*, 39–44. doi:10.1016/j.neulet.2005.02.060

Cheng, P. T., Liaw, M. Y., Wong, M. K., Tang, F. T., Lee, M. Y., & Lin, P. S. (1998). The sit-to-stand movement in stroke patients and its correlation with falling. *Archives of Physical Medicine and Rehabilitation*, *79*, 1043–1046. doi:10.1016/S0003-9993(98)90168-X

Chiba, Y. (2005). *Nihon-Ongaku ga Wakaru Hon*. Tokyo, Japan: *Ongaku tomo sya corp*.

Chikamori, K. (2003, 1949). *New revised music introduction*. Tokyo, Japan: Ongaku tomo sya corp.

Chino, N., Riu, M., Sonoda, S., & Domen, K. (2003). *Nosottyu Kanjya no Kino Hyoka*. Tokyo, Japan: Springer-Verlag.

Chinzei, K., Kikinis, R., & Jolesz, F. A. (1999). MR compatibility of mechatronic devices: Design criteria. *Proceedings of MICCAI'99*, (LNCS 1679), (pp. 1020-1031).

Cho, J., Kato, S., & Itoh, H. (2009). *Comparison of sensibilities of Japanese and Koreans in recognizing emotions from speech by using Bayesian Networks*. In IEEE International Conference on Systems, Man, and Cybernetics, (pp. 2945-2950).

Choi, S. J., Lim, K. O., Monteiro, I., & Reisberg, B. (2005). Diffusion tensor imaging of frontal white matter microstructure in early Alzheimer's disease: A preliminary study. *Journal of Geriatric Psychiatry and Neurology*, *18*, 12–19. doi:10.1177/0891988704271763

Ciccarelli, O., Toosy, A. T., Parker, G. J., Wheeler-Kingshott, C. A., Barker, G. J., Miller, D. H., & Thompson, A. J. (2003). Diffusion tractography based group mapping of major white-matter pathways in the human brain. *NeuroImage*, *19*, 1545–1555. doi:10.1016/S1053-8119(03)00190-3

Cockburn, J. (1995). Task interruption in prospective memory: A frontal lobe function? *Cortex*, *31*, 87–97.

Cohen-Mansfield, J., & Werner, P. (1997). Management of verbally disruptive behaviors in nursing home residents. *The Journals of Gerontology. Series A, Biological Sciences and Medical Sciences*, *52*(6), 369–377.

Corbetta, M., Miezin, F. M., Shulman, G. L., & Petersen, S. E. (1993). A PET study of visuospatial attention. *The Journal of Neuroscience*, *13*(3), 1202–1226.

Corrigan, D., & Bohannon, R. W. (2001). Relationship between knee extension force and stand-up performance in community-dwelling elderly women. *Archives of Physical Medicine and Rehabilitation*, *82*, 1666–1672. doi:10.1053/apmr.2001.26811

Coull, J. T., & Frith, C. D. (2000). Orienting attention in time: Behavioural and neuroanatomical distinction between exogenous and endogenous shifts. *Neuropsychologia*, *38*(6), 808–819. doi:10.1016/S0028-3932(99)00132-3

Coull, J. T., & Nobre, A. C. (1998). Where and when to pay attention: The neural systems for directing attention to spatial locations and to time intervals as revealed by both PET and fMRI. *The Journal of Neuroscience*, *18*(18), 7426–7435.

Cowie, R., Douglas-Cowie, E., Tsapatsoulis, N., Votsis, G., Kollias, S., & Fellenz, W. (2001). Emotion recognition in human-computer interaction. *IEEE Signal Processing Magazine*, *18*(1), 32–80. doi:10.1109/79.911197

Craik, F. I. M. (1986). A functional account of age differences in memory. In Clix, F., & Hangendorf, H. (Eds.), *Human memory and cognitive capabilities: Mechanisms and performances* (pp. 409–422). Amsterdam, The Netherlands: Elsevier.

Crooks, V. C., Lubben, J., Petitti, D. B., & Chiu, D. L. V. (2008). Social network, cognitive function, and dementia incidence among elderly women. *American Journal of Public Health*, *98*(7), 1221–1227. doi:10.2105/AJPH.2007.115923

Crutch, S. J., Rossor, M. N., & Warrington, E. K. (2007a). A novel technique for the quantitative assessment of apraxic deficits: Application to individuals with mild cognitive impairment. *Journal of Neuropsychology*, *1*, 237–257. doi:10.1348/174866407X209943

Crutch, S. J., Rossor, M. N., & Warrington, E. K. (2007b). The quantitative assessment of apraxic deficits in Alzheimer's disease. *Cortex*, *43*, 976–986. doi:10.1016/S0010-9452(08)70695-6

Cuddy, L. L., & Duffin, J. (2005). Music, memory, and Alzheimer's disease: Is music recognition spared in dementia, and how can it be assessed? *Medical Hypotheses*, *64*, 229–235. doi:10.1016/j.mehy.2004.09.005

Cummings, J. L., McRae, T., & Zhang, R. (2006). Effects of donepezil on neuropsychiatric symptoms in patients with dementia and severe behavioral disorders. *The American Journal of Geriatric Psychiatry*, *14*(7), 605–612. doi:10.1097/01.JGP.0000221293.91312.d3

Dale, A. M., Liu, A. K., Fischi, B. R., Buckner, R. L., Belliveau, J. W., Lewine, J. D., & Halgren, E. (2000). Dynamic statistical parametric mapping: Combining fMRI and MEG for high-resolution imaging of cortical activity. *Neuron*, *26*, 55–67. doi:10.1016/S0896-6273(00)81138-1

Danek, K. A., Gillespie, R. B., Aldridge, J. W., Ferrie, D. P., & Grizzle, J. W. (2005). *A dual input device for self-assisted control of a virtual pendulum*. 9th International Conference on Rehabilitation Robotics, (pp. 313-318).

David, B. H. (1993). *Visual fields* (p. 2). Oxford Medical Publishers.

de Groot, J. C., de Leeuw, F. E., Oudkerk, M., van Gijn, J., Hofman, A., Jolles, J., & Breteler, M. M. (2000). Cerebral white matter lesions and cognitive function: The Rotterdam scan study. *Annals of Neurology*, *47*, 145–151. doi:10.1002/1531-8249(200002)47:2<145::AID-ANA3>3.0.CO;2-P

Degerman, A., & Rinne, T. (2006). Selective attention to sound location or pitch studied with fMRI. *Brain Research*, *1077*(1), 123–134. doi:10.1016/j.brainres.2006.01.025

Delbeuck, X., Van der Linden, M., & Collette, F. (2003). Alzheimer' disease as a disconnection syndrome? *Neuropsychology Review*, *13*, 79–92. doi:10.1023/A:1023832305702

Denk, W., Strickler, J. H., & Webb, W. W. (1990). Two-photon laser scanning fluorescence microscopy. *Science*, *248*, 73–76. doi:10.1126/science.2321027

Di Fede, G., Catania, M., Morbin, M., Rossi, G., Suardi, S., & Mazzoleni, G. (2009). A recessive mutation in the APP gene withdominant-negative effect on amyloidogenesis. *Science*, *323*, 1473–1477. doi:10.1126/science.1168979

Dimitrijevic, M. M. (1992). Development of neurophysiological aspects of the spinal cord during the past 10 years. *Paraplegia*, *30*, 92–95.

Dimitrijevic, M. M. (1994). Mesh-glove: A method for whole-hand electrical stimulation in upper motor neuron dysfunction. *Scandinavian Journal of Rehabilitative Medicine*, *26*, 183–186.

Dimitrijevic, M. M., Dimitrijevic, M. R., Lissens, M. A., & Makay, W. B. (1991). The present status of neurosurgical poor survival and role of restorative neurology in management of patients. *Neurosurgeons*, *10*, 333–338.

Dimitrijevic, M. M., & Soroker, N. (1994). Modulation of residual upper limb motor control after stroke with whole-hand electric stimulation. *Scandinavian Journal of Rehabilitative Medicine*, *26*, 183–186.

Dimitrijevic, M. M., Soroker, N., & Pollo, E. F. (1996). Mesh glove electrical stimulation. *Science & Medicine*, *3*, 54–63.

Dimitrijevic, M. M., Stokic, S. D., Waero, W. A., & Wun, C.-C. (1996). Modification of motor control of wrist extension by mesh-glove electrical affrent stimulation in stroke patients. *Archives of Physical Medicine and Rehabilitation*, *77*, 252–258. doi:10.1016/S0003-9993(96)90107-0

Diordjevic, J., Zatorre, R. J., Petrides, M., Boyle, J. A., & Jones-Gotman, M. (2005). Functional neuroimaging of odor imagery. *NeuroImage*, *24*, 791–801. doi:10.1016/j.neuroimage.2004.09.035

Doty, R. L. (2007). Olfaction in Parkinson's disease. *Parkinsonism & Related Disorders*, *13*(3), S225–S228. doi:10.1016/S1353-8020(08)70006-3

Doty, R. L., Shaman, P., Kimmelman, C. P., & Dann, M. S. (1984). University of Pennsylvania smell identification test: A rapid quantitative olfactory function test for the clinic. *The Laryngoscope*, *94*, 176–178. doi:10.1288/00005537-198402000-00004

Dovat, L., Lambercy, O., Ruffieux, Y., Chapuis, D., Gassert, R., & Bleuler, H. ... Burdet, E. (2006). A haptic knob for rehabilitation of stroke patients. *Proceedings of the 2006 IEEE/RSJ International Conference on Intelligent Robots and Systems*, October 2006, (pp. 977-982).

Draper, N., & Smith, H. (1998). *Applied regression analysis* (3rd ed.). John Wiley & Sons.

Dubowitz, D. J., Chen, D. Y., Atkinson, D. J., Grieve, K. L., Gillikin, B., Bradley, W. G. Jr, & Andersen, R. A. (1998). Functional magnetic resonance imaging in macaque cortex. *Neuroreport*, *9*, 2213–2218. doi:10.1097/00001756-199807130-00012

Duffy, C. J., & Wurtz, R. H. (1991b). Sensitivity of MST neurons to optic flow stimuli. I. A continuum of response selectivity to large-field stimuli. *Journal of Neurophysiology*, *65*, 1329–1345.

Dukelow, S. P., DeSouza, J. F. X., Culham, J. C., van den Berg, A. V., Menon, R. S., & Vilis, T. (2001). Distinguishing subregions of the human MT+ complex using visual fields and pursuit eye movements. *Journal of Neurophysiology*, *86*, 1991–2000.

Eimer, M., & Schroger, E. (1998). ERP effects of intermodal attention and cross-modal links in spatial attention. *Psychophysiology*, *35*(3), 313–327. doi:10.1017/S004857729897086X

Einstein, G. O., & McDaniel, M. A. (1990). Normal aging and prospective memory. *Journal of Experimental Psychology. Learning, Memory, and Cognition*, *16*, 717–726. doi:10.1037/0278-7393.16.4.717

Endres, C., Bencherif, B., Hilton, J., Madar, I., & Frost, J. (2003). Quantification of brain mu-opioid receptors with 11C carfentanil: Reference-tissue methods. *Nuclear Medicine and Biology*, *30*(2), 177–186. doi:10.1016/S0969-8051(02)00411-0

Endres, C., & Carson, R. (1998). Assessment of dynamic neurotransmitter changes with bolus or infusion delivery of neuro-receptor ligands. *Journal of Cerebral Blood Flow and Metabolism*, *18*(11), 1196–1210. doi:10.1097/00004647-199811000-00006

Endres, C., Kolachana, B., Saunders, R., Su, T., Weinberger, D., & Breier, A. (1997). Kinetic modeling of 11C raclopride: Combined PET-microdialysis studies. *Journal of Cerebral Blood Flow and Metabolism*, *17*(9), 932–942. doi:10.1097/00004647-199709000-00002

Europe, A. (2006). *Dementia in Europe yearbook* (p. 21).

Evans, J. G., Wilcock, G., & Birks, J. (2004). Evidence-based pharmacotherapy of Alzheimer's disease. *The International Journal of Neuropsychopharmacology*, *7*, 351–369. doi:10.1017/S1461145704004444

Ewers, M., Buerger, K., Teipel, S. J., Scheltens, P., Schroeder, J., Zinkowski, R., … Hampel, H. (2007). *Multicenter assessment of CSF-phosphorylated tau for the prediction of conversion of MCI.*

Faber, M., & Moller Hou, G. (1952). The human aorta. Part V: Collagen and elastin in the normal and hypertensive aorta. *Acta Pathologica et Microbiologica Scandinavica*, *31*, 377–382. doi:10.1111/j.1699-0463.1952.tb00205.x

Farlow, M. R., & Cummings, J. L. (2007). Effective pharmacologic management of Alzheimer's disease. *The American Journal of Medicine*, *120*, 388–397. doi:10.1016/j.amjmed.2006.08.036

Farrer, L. A., Cupples, L. A., Haines, J. L., Hyman, B., Kukull, W. A., & Mayeux, R. (1997). Effects of age, sex, and ethnicity on the association between apolipoprotein E genotype and Alzheimer disease. A meta-analysis. [APOE and Alzheimer Disease Meta Analysis Consortium]. *Journal of the American Medical Association*, *278*(16), 1349–1356. doi:10.1001/jama.278.16.1349

Fasoli, S. E., Krebs, H. I., Stein, J., Frontera, W. R., & Hogan, N. (2003). Effects of robotic therapy on motor impairment and recovery in chronic stroke. *Archives of Physical Medicine and Rehabilitation*, *84*, 477–482. doi:10.1053/apmr.2003.50110

Feeney, D. M., & Sutton, R. L. (1987). Pharmacotherapy for recovery of function after brain injury. *CRC Critical Review of Neurobiology*, *3*, 135–197.

Fernández, A., Arrazola, J., Maestú, F., Amo, C., Gil-Gregorio, P., Wienbruch, C., & Ortiz, T. (2003). Correlations of hippocampal atrophy and focal low-frequency magnetic activity in Alzheimer disease: Volumetric MR imaging-magnetoencephalographic study. *AJNR. American Journal of Neuroradiology*, *24*, 481–487.

Ferri, C. P., Prince, M., Brayne, C., Brodaty, H., Fratiglioni, L., & Ganguli, M. (2005). Global prevalence of dementia: A Delphi consensus study. *Lancet*, *366*, 2112–2117. doi:10.1016/S0140-6736(05)67889-0

Fischer, F. W., & Schmidt, Y. H. (1998). 40year's of the perimetry. *Klinische Monatsblatter fur Augenheilkunde*, *193*, 237–242. doi:10.1055/s-2008-1050251

Fodero-Tavoletti, M. T., Mulligan, R. S., Okamura, N., Furumoto, S., Rowe, C. C., & Kudo, Y. (2009). In vitro characterisation of BF227 binding to alpha-synuclein/Lewy bodies. *European Journal of Pharmacology*, *617*, 54–58. doi:10.1016/j.ejphar.2009.06.042

Folstein, M. F., Folstein, S. E., & McHugh, P. R. (1975). Mini-mental state: A practical method for grading the cognitive state of patients for the clinician. *Journal of Psychiatric Research*, *12*(3), 189–198. doi:10.1016/0022-3956(75)90026-6

Fort, A., Delpuech, C., Pernier, J., & Giard, M.-H. (2002). Early auditory-visual interactions in human cortex during nonredundant target identification. *Brain Research. Cognitive Brain Research*, *14*(1), 20–30. doi:10.1016/S0926-6410(02)00058-7

Fox, P., Ingham, R., George, M. S., Mayberg, H., Ingham, J., & Roby, J. (1997). Imaging human intra-cerebral connectivity by PET during TMS. *Neuroreport*, *8*, 2787–2791. doi:10.1097/00001756-199708180-00027

Frackowiak, R. S., Lenzi, G. L., Jones, T., & Heather, J. D. (1980). Quantitative measurement of regional cerebral blood flow and oxygen metabolism in man using 15o and positron emission tomography: Theory, procedure, and normal values. *Journal of Computer Assisted Tomography*, *4*(6), 727–736. doi:10.1097/00004728-198012000-00001

Frackowiak, R. S. J., Friston, K. J., Frith, C. D., Dolan, R. J., Price, C. J., & Zeki, S. … Penny, W. (2003). *Human brain function*, 2nd ed. Amsterdam, The Netherlands: Elsevier Academic Press.

Franceschi, C., Bezrukov, V., Blanché, H., Bolund, L., Christensen, K., & de Benedictis, G. (2007). Genetics of healthy aging in Europe: The EU-integrated project GEHA (GEnetics of Healthy Aging). *Annals of the New York Academy of Sciences*, *1100*, 21–45. doi:10.1196/annals.1395.003

Frank, R. A., Galasko, D., Hampel, H., Hardy, J., de Leon, M. J., & Mehta, P. D. (2003). Biological markers for therapeutic trials in Alzheimer's disease. *Neurobiology of Aging*, *24*(4), 521–536. doi:10.1016/S0197-4580(03)00002-2

Fraser, P. E., Darabie, A. A., & McLaurin, J. (2001). Amyloid-β interactions with chondroitin sulfate-derived monosaccharides and disaccharides: Implications for drug development. *The Journal of Biological Chemistry*, *276*, 6412–6419. doi:10.1074/jbc.M008128200

Fratiglioni, L., Wang, H. X., Ericsson, K., Maytan, M., & Winblad, B. (2000). Influence of social network on occurrence of dementia: A community based longitudinal study. *Lancet*, *355*(9212), 1315–1319. doi:10.1016/S0140-6736(00)02113-9

Friston, K. J., Frith, C. D., Liddle, P. F., & Frackowiak, R. S. (1991). Comparing functional (PET) images: The assessment of significant change. *Journal of Cerebral Blood Flow and Metabolism*, *11*, 690–699.

Fukumoto, H., Cheung, B. S., Hyman, B. T., & Irizarry, M. C. (2002). Beta-secretase protein and activity are increased in the neocortex in Alzheimer disease. *Archives of Neurology*, *59*(9), 1381–1389. doi:10.1001/archneur.59.9.1381

Fukuyama, H., Ogawa, M., Yamauchi, H., Yamaguchi, S., Kimura, J., Yonekura, Y., & Konishi, J. (1994). Altered cerebral energy metabolism in Alzheimer's disease: A PET study. *Journal of Nuclear Medicine*, *35*, 1–6.

Fukuyama, H. (2009). Is (123)I-MIBG cardiac scintigraphy a surrogate marker for Parkinson's disease? *European Journal of Nuclear Medicine and Molecular Imaging.*

Funada, K., Takahashi, S., & Wu, J. (2009). A study on motion recognition of hand using surface EMG of forearm for upper-limb rehabilitation. *Proceedings of The 2009 International Symposium on Early Detection and Rehabilitation Technology of Dementia (DRD2009)*, (pp. 175-178).

Furukawa, K., Okamura, N., Tashiro, M., Waragai, M., Furumoto, S., & Iwata, R. (2009). Amyloid PET in mild cognitive impairment and Alzheimer's disease with BF-227: Comparison to FDG-PET. *Journal of Neurology*, *257*, 721–727. doi:10.1007/s00415-009-5396-8

Furukawa K., Okamura, N., Tashiro, M., Waragai, M., Furumoto, S., Iwata, R., … Arai, H. (2010). Amyloid PET in mild cognitive impairment and Alzheimer's disease with BF-227: Comparison to FDG-PET. *Journal of Neurology*.

Furumoto, S., Okamura, N., Iwata, R., Yanai, K., Arai, H., & Kudo, Y. (2007). Recent advances in the development of amyloid imaging agents. *Current Topics in Medicinal Chemistry*, *7*, 1773–1789. doi:10.2174/156802607782507402

Gabrieli, J. D., Poldrack, R. A., & Desmond, J. E. (1998). The role of left prefrontal cortex in language and memory. *Proceedings of the National Academy of Sciences of the United States of America*, *95*, 906–913. doi:10.1073/pnas.95.3.906

Gardner, E. P., & Kandel, E. R. (2000). Touch. In Kandel, E. R. (Eds.), *Principles of neural science* (pp. 451–471). New York, NY: McGraw-Hill.

Gatta, L. B., Albertini, A., Ravid, R., & Finazzi, D. (2002). Levels of beta-secretase BACE and alpha-secretase ADAM10 mRNAs in Alzheimer hippocampus. *Neuroreport*, *13*(16), 2031–2033. doi:10.1097/00001756-200211150-00008

Gazzaniga, M. S., Ivry, R. B., & Mangun, G. R. (2002). *Cognitive neuroscience*.

Gellermann, G. P., Byrnes, H., Striebinger, A., Ullrich, K., Mueller, R., Hillen, H., & Barghorn, S. (2008). Abeta-globulomers are formed independently of the fibril pathway. *Neurobiological Disorders*, *30*, 212–220. doi:10.1016/j.nbd.2008.01.010

Gerdner, L. A. (2005). Use of individualized music by trained staff and family: Translating research into practice. *Journal of Gerontological Nursing*, *31*(6), 22–30.

Gilkey, R. H., & Good, M. D. (1996). Effects of frequency on free-field masking. *Human Factors*, *37*(4), 835–843. doi:10.1518/001872095778995580

Gjedde, A. (1981). High-and low-affinity transport of D-glucose from blood to brain. *Journal of Neurochemistry*, *36*(4), 1463–1471. doi:10.1111/j.1471-4159.1981.tb00587.x

Golaszwski, S. M., Siedentopf, C. M., Koppelstaetter, F. K., Rhomberg, P., & Guendisch, G. M. (2004). Modulatory effects on human sensorimotor cortex by whole-hand affrent electrical stimulation. *Neurology*, *62*, 2262–2269.

Goldenberg, G. (2009). Apraxia and the parietal lobes. *Neuropsychologia*, *47*, 1449–1459. doi:10.1016/j.neuropsychologia.2008.07.014

Goldman, W. P., Baty, J. D., Buckles, V. D., Sahrmann, S., & Morris, J. C. (1999). Motor dysfunction in mildly demented AD individuals without extrapyramidal signs. *Neurology*, *53*, 956–962.

Gomperts, S. N., Rentz, D. M., Moran, E., Becker, J. A., Locascio, J. J., & Klunk, W. E. (2008). Imaging amyloid deposition in Lewy body diseases. *Neurology*, *71*, 903–910. doi:10.1212/01.wnl.0000326146.60732.d6

Goto, Y., Noda, R., Ichikawa, Y., & Fujiwara, M. (2002). Cerebral circulation of consciousness disorder patient using near-infrared spectroscopic topography during brain rehabilitation by music exercise therapy. *International Congress Series*, *1232*, 549–554. doi:10.1016/S0531-5131(01)00689-6

Graff-Radford, N. R., Crook, J. E., Lucas, J., Boeve, B. F., Knopman, D. S., & Ivnik, R. J. (2007). Association of low plasma Abeta42/Abeta40 ratios with increased imminent risk for mild cognitive impairment and Alzheimer disease. *Archives of Neurology*, *64*(3), 354–362. doi:10.1001/archneur.64.3.354

Greenfield, J. C., & Patel, D. J. (1962). Relation between pressure and diameter in the ascending aorta of man. *Circulation Research*, *10*, 778–781.

Gross, R. G., & Grossman, M. (2008). Update on apraxia. *Current Neurology and Neuroscience Reports*, *8*, 490–496. doi:10.1007/s11910-008-0078-y

Guo, S., & Song, Z. (2009). A novel motor function training assisted system for upper limbs rehabilitation. *Proceeding of the 2009 IEEE International Conference on Intelligent Robots and Systems*, (pp. 1025-1030).

Guo, S., Song, Z., & Ren, C. (2009). *Development of upper limb motor function training and rehabilitation system*. IEEE International Conference on Mechatronics and Automation, (pp. 949-954).

Habel, U., Klein, M., Kellermann, T., Shah, N. J., & Schneider, F. (2005). Same or different? Neural correlates of happy and sad mood in healthy males. *NeuroImage*, *126*(1), 206–214. doi:10.1016/j.neuroimage.2005.01.014

Hachinski, V. C., Potter, P., & Merskey, H. (1987). Leukoaraiosis. *Archives of Neurology*, *44*, 21–23.

Hamada, M., Ugawa, Y., & Tsuji, S. (2009). The effectiveness of rTMS on Parkinson's disease study group. High-frequency rTMS over the supplementary motor area improves bradykinesia in Parkinson's disease: Subanalysis of double-blind sham-controlled study. *Journal of the Neurological Sciences*, *287*, 143–146. doi:10.1016/j.jns.2009.08.007

Hamada, T., Okubo, H., Inoue, K., Maruyama, J., Onari, H., et al. (2008). *Robot therapy as for recreation for elderly people with dementia*. The 17th IEEE International Symposium on Robot and Human Interactive Communication, (pp. 174-179).

Hämäläinen, M., Hari, R., Ilmoniemi, R. J., Knuutila, J., & Lounasmaa, O. V. (1993). Magnetoencephalograph-theory, instrumentation, and applications to noninvasive studies of the working human brain. *Reviews of Modern Physics*, *65*, 413–497. doi:10.1103/RevModPhys.65.413

Hampel, H., Teipel, S. J., Fuchsberger, T., Andreasen, N., Wiltfang, J., & Otto, M. (2004, Jul). Value of CSF beta-amyloid1-42 and tau as predictors of Alzheimer's disease in patients with mild cognitive impairment. *Molecular Psychiatry*, *9*(7), 705–710.

Han, L., Cole, M., Bellavance, F., McCusker, J., & Primeau, F. (2000). Tracking cognitive decline in Alzheimer's disease using the miniMini-mentalMental stateState examinationExamination: A meta-analysis. *International Psychogeriatrics*, *12*, 231–247. doi:10.1017/S1041610200006359

Handel, B., Lutzenberger, W., Thier, P., & Haarmeier, T. (2007). Opposite dependencies on visual motion coherence in human area MT+ and early visual cortex. *Cerebral Cortex*, *17*, 1542–1549. doi:10.1093/cercor/bhl063

Haniu, M., Denis, P., Young, Y., Mendiaz, E. A., Fuller, J., & Hui, J. O. (2000). Characterization of Alzheimer's beta -secretase protein BACE. A pepsin family member with unusual properties. *The Journal of Biological Chemistry*, *275*(28), 21099–21106. doi:10.1074/jbc.M002095200

Hanson, R. L., Looker, H. C., Ma, L., Muller, Y. L., Baier, L. J., & Knowler, W. C. (2006). Design and analysis of genetic association studies to finely map a locus identified by linkage analysis: Sample size and power calculations. *Annals of Human Genetics*, *70*(3), 332–349. doi:10.1111/j.1529-8817.2005.00230.x

Hanyu, H., Sakurai, H., Iwamoto, T., Takasaki, M., Shindo, H., & Abe, K. (1998). Diffusion-weighted MR imaging of the hippocampus and temporal white matter in Alzheimer's disease. *Journal of the Neurological Sciences*, *156*, 195–200. doi:10.1016/S0022-510X(98)00043-4

Hardy, J. A., & Allsop, D. (1991). Amyloid deposition as the central event in the aetiology of Alzheimer's disease. *Trends in Pharmacological Sciences*, *12*, 383–388. doi:10.1016/0165-6147(91)90609-V

Hardy, J. A., & Higgins, G. A. (1992). Alzheimer's disease: The amyloid cascade hypothesis. *Science*, *256*, 184–185. doi:10.1126/science.1566067

Harvey, L. O. (1986). Efficient estimation of sensory thresholds. *Behavior Research Methods, Instruments, & Computers*, *18*, 623–632. doi:10.3758/BF03201438

Hashimoto, S. (2003). The dynamic perimetry program by using an automatic perimeter. *Kinki University Medical Journal*, *28*, 207–221.

Hayashi, K., Handa, H., Nagasawa, S., Okumura, A., & Moritake, K. (1980). Stiffness and elastic behavior of human intracranial and extracranial arteries. *Journal of Biomechanics*, *13*, 175–184. doi:10.1016/0021-9290(80)90191-8

Henderson, V. W., Mack, W., & Williams, B. W. (1989). Spatial disorientation in Alzheimer's disease. *Archives of Neurology*, *46*, 391–394.

Henson, R. N., Rylands, A., Ross, E., Vuilleumeir, P., & Rugg, M. D. (2004). The effect of repetition lag on electrophysiological and haemodynamic correlates of visual object priming. *NeuroImage*, *21*, 1674–1689. doi:10.1016/j.neuroimage.2003.12.020

Herukka, S. K., Hallikainen, M., Soininen, H., & Pirttila, T. (2005). CSF Abeta42 and tau or phosphorylated tau and prediction of progressive mild cognitive impairment. *Neurology*, *64*(7), 1294–1297.

Hesse, S., Schulte-Tigges, G., Konrad, M., Bardeleben, A., & Werner, C. (2003). Robot-assisted arm trainer for the passive and active practice of bilateral forearm and wrist movements in hemiparetic subjects. *Archives of Physical Medicine and Rehabilitation*, *84*, 915–920. doi:10.1016/S0003-9993(02)04954-7

Hewer, R. L. (1994). Rehabilitation after stroke. In Illis, L. S. (Ed.), *Neurological rehabilitation* (pp. 157–168). Oxford, UK: Blackwell Scientific Publications.

Hirata, Y., Matsuda, H., Nemoto, K., Ohnishi, T., Hirao, K., & Yamashita, F. (2005). Voxel-based morphometry to discriminate early Alzheimer's disease from controls. *Neuroscience Letters*, *382*, 269–274. doi:10.1016/j.neulet.2005.03.038

Hirata, Y. (2001). A study of the effective way to release scent to maintain alertness. *JSAE Review*, *22*, 331–336. doi:10.1016/S0389-4304(01)00105-9

Hodges, J. R., & Patterson, K. (1995). Is semantic memory consistently impaired early in the course of Alzheimer's disease? Neuroanatomical and diagnostic implications. *Neuropsychologia*, *33*, 441–459. doi:10.1016/0028-3932(94)00127-B

Hodl, A. K., Hodl, E., Otti, D. V., Herranhof, B., Ille, R., & Bonelli, R. M. (2008). Ideomotor limb apraxia in Huntington's disease: A case-control study. *Journal of Neurology*, *255*, 331–339.

Hogan, N., Krebs, H. I., Rohrer, B., Palazzolo, J. J., & Dipietro, L. (2006). Motions or muscles? Some behavioral factors underlying robotic assistance of motor recovery. *Journal of Rehabilitation Research and Development*, *43*, 605–618. doi:10.1682/JRRD.2005.06.0103

Hogan, N., Krebs, H. I., Sharon, A., & Charnnarong, J. (1995). *Interactive robotic therapist*. (Patent 5466213). Cambridge, MA: Massachusetts Institute of Technology.

Holper, L., Biallas, M., & Wolf, M. (2009). Task complexity relates to activation of cortical motor areas during uni- and bimanual performance: A functional NIRS study. *NeuroImage*, *46*, 1105–1113. doi:10.1016/j.neuroimage.2009.03.027

Holsinger, R. M., Lee, J. S., Boyd, A., Masters, C. L., & Collins, S. J. (2006). CSF BACE1 activity is increased in CJD and Alzheimer disease versus other dementias. *Neurology*, *67*(4), 710–712. doi:10.1212/01.wnl.0000229925.52203.4c

Holsinger, R. M., McLean, C. A., Beyreuther, K., Masters, C. L., & Evin, G. (2002). Increased expression of the amyloid precursor beta-secretase in Alzheimer's disease. *Annals of Neurology*, *51*(6), 783–786. doi:10.1002/ana.10208

Hoshi, M., Sato, M., Matsumoto, S., Noguchi, A., Yasutake, K., Yoshida, N., & Sato, K. (2003). Spherical aggregates of beta-amyloid (amylospheroid) show high neurotoxicity and activate tau protein kinase I/glycogen synthase kinase-3β. *Proceedings of the National Academy of Sciences of the United States of America*, *100*, 6370–6375. doi:10.1073/pnas.1237107100

Hoshi, Y., & Tamura, M. (1993). Dynamic multichannel near-infrared optical imaging of human brain activity. *Journal of Applied Physiology*, *75*, 1842–1846.

Hosomi, A., Nagakane, Y., Yamada, K., Kuriyama, N., Mizuno, T., Nishimura, T., & Nakagawa, M. (2009). Assessment of arcuate fasciculus with diffusion-tensor tractography may predict the prognosis of aphasia in patients with left middle cerebral artery infarcts. *Neuroradiology*, *51*, 549–555. doi:10.1007/s00234-009-0534-7

Hoyte, K., Brownell, H., & Wingfield, A. (2009). Components of speech prosody and their use in detection of syntactic structure by older adults. *Experimental Aging Research*, *35*(1), 129–151. doi:10.1080/03610730802565091

Huk, A. C., Dougherty, R. F., & Heeger, D. J. (2002). Retinotopy and functional subdivision of human areas MT and MST. *The Journal of Neuroscience*, *22*, 7195–7205.

Hummel, T., Damm, M., Vent, J., Schmidt, M., Theissen, P., Larsson, M., & Klussmann, J. P. (2003). Depth of olfactory sulcus and olfactory function. *Brain Research*, *975*, 85–89. doi:10.1016/S0006-8993(03)02589-7

Huppert, F. A., & Beardsall, L. (1993). Prospective memory impairment as an early indicator of dementia. *Journal of Clinical and Experimental Neuropsychology*, *15*, 805–821. doi:10.1080/01688639308402597

Huse, J. T., & Doms, R. W. (2000). Closing in on the amyloid cascade: recent insights into the cell biology of Alzheimer's disease. *Molecular Neurobiology*, *22*(1-3), 81–98.

Iadecola, C. (2004). Neurovascular regulation in the normal brain and in Alzheimer's disease. *Nature Reviews. Neuroscience*, *5*, 347–360. doi:10.1038/nrn1387

Ikeguchi, M., Touge, T., Nishiyama, Y., Takeuchi, H., Kuriyama, S., & Ohkawa, M. (2003). Effects of successive repetitive transcranial magnetic stimulation on motor performances and brain perfusion in idiopathic Parkinson's disease. *Journal of the Neurological Sciences*, *209*, 41–46. doi:10.1016/S0022-510X(02)00459-8

Ikeguchi, M., Touge, T., Kaji, R., Deguchi, K., Sasaki, I., & Tsukaguchi, M. … Kuriyama, S. (2005). Durable effect of very low- frequency repetitive transcranial magnetic stimulation for modulating cortico-spinal neuron excitability. *Unveiling the mystery of the brain, International Congress Series, 1278*, 272-275.

Ikoma, Y., Watabe, H., Hayashi, T., Miyake, Y., Teramoto, N., & Minato, K. (2009). Quantitative evaluation of changes in binding porential with a simplified reference tissue model and multiple injections of 11c raclopride. *NeuroImage*, *47*(4), 1639–1648. doi:10.1016/j.neuroimage.2009.05.099

Ikoma, Y., Watabe, H., Hayashi, T., Miyake, Y., Teramoto, N., & Minato, K. (2010). Measurement of density and affinity for dopamine d(2) receptors by a single positron emission tomography scan with multiple injections of (11)c raclopride. *Journal of Cerebral Blood Flow and Metabolism*, *30*, 663–667. doi:10.1038/jcbfm.2009.239

Ikonomovic, M. D., Klunk, W. E., Abrahamson, E. E., Mathis, C. A., Price, J. C., & Tsopelas, N. D. (2008). Post-mortem correlates of in vivo PIB-PET amyloid imaging in a typical case of Alzheimer's disease. *Brain*, *131*, 1630–1645. doi:10.1093/brain/awn016

Imanishi, A., & Oyama-Higa, M. (2006). *The relation between observers' psychophysiological conditions and human errors during monitoring task*. 2006 IEEE Conference on Systems, Man, and Cybernetics, Taipei, Taiwan, (pp. 2035–2039).

Innami, Y., Kobayashi, T., Jung, J., Ohashi, S., Hamada, S., & Nagamine, T. (2004). An fMRI-MEG integrative method for dynamic imaging of multiple cortical activities [in Japanese]. *Transactions of the Japanese Society For Medical Biological Engineering*, *44*, 777–784.

Ino, S., & Ifukube, T. (1997). A basic study on a tactile display system for presenting quality of materials. *TIEE Japan*, *117*.

Inzitari, D., Giordano, G. P., Ancona, A. L., Pracucci, G., Mascalchi, M., & Amaducci, L. (1990). Leukoaraiosis, intracerebral hemorrhage, and arterial hypertension. *Stroke*, *21*, 1419–1423.

Ishii, H., Ishikawa, H., Meguro, K., Tashiro, M., & Yamaguchi, S. (2009). Decreased cortical glucose metabolism in converters from CDR 0.5 to Alzheimer's disease in a community: The Osaki-Tajiri Project. *International Psychogeriatrics*, *21*, 148–156. doi:10.1017/S1041610208008132

Ito, E., Hatta, T., Yasuhiro, I., Kosuge, T., & Watanabe, H. (2004). Performance of verbal fluency tasks in Japanese healthy adults: Effect of gender, age and education on the performance. *Japanese Journal of Neuropsychology*, *20*, 254–263.

Jack, C. R. Jr, Petersen, R. C., Xu, Y. C., O'Brien, P. C., Smith, G. E., & Ivnik, R. J. (1999). Prediction of AD with MRI-based hippocampal volume in mild cognitive impairment. *Neurology*, *52*(7), 1397–1403.

Jack, D., Boian, R., Merians, A. S., Tremaine, M., Burdea, G. C., & Adamovich, S. V. (2001). Virtual reality-enhanced stroke rehabilitation. *IEEE Transactions on Neural Systems and Rehabilitation Engineering*, *9*(3), 308–318. doi:10.1109/7333.948460

James, W. (1890). *Principles of psychology*. New York, NY: Holt. doi:10.1037/10538-000

Janssen, I., Heymsfield, S. B., & Ross, R. (2002). Low relative skeletal muscle mass (sarcopenia) in older persons is associated with functional impairment and physical disability. *Journal of the American Geriatrics Society*, *50*, 889–896. doi:10.1046/j.1532-5415.2002.50216.x

Janssen, I., Heymsfield, S. B., Wang, Z. M., & Ross, R. (2000). Skeletal muscle mass and distribution in 468 men and women aged 18-88 yr. *Journal of Applied Physiology*, *89*, 81–88.

Japan Ministry of International Affairs and Communications. (2009). *International statistical compendium*. (pp. 43-48, 61-62).

Japan National Police Agency. (2008). *Statistics of driving license* (p. 3).

Japan National Police Agency. (2008). *Report of exploratory committee about support for aging driver*.

Jiang, Y., & Wang, S. (2007). The human visual recognition ability for incomplete letters. *International Journal of Innovative Computing. Information and Control*, *3*, 1183–1192.

Jiang, Y., & Wang, S. (2008). Measurement and quantitative analysis of human visual interpolation ability for partially erased objects. *ICIC Express Letters*, *2*, 7–13.

Jobard, G., Crivello, F., & Tzourio-Mazoyer, N. (2003). Evaluation of the dual route theory of reading: A metanalysis of 35 neuroimaging studies. *NeuroImage*, *20*, 693–712. doi:10.1016/S1053-8119(03)00343-4

Johansen, K. K., White, L. R., Sando, S. B., & Aasly, J. O. (2010). Biomarkers: Parkinson disease with dementia and dementia with lewy bodies. *Parkinsonism & Related Disorders*, *16*(5), 307–315. doi:10.1016/j.parkreldis.2010.02.015

Johansen-Berg, H., Della-Maggiore, V., Behrens, T. E., Smith, S. M., & Paus, T. (2007). Integrity of white matter in the corpus callosum correlates with bimanual coordination skills. *NeuroImage*, *36*, 16–21. doi:10.1016/j.neuroimage.2007.03.041

Johnson, J. A., & Zatorre, R. J. (2005). Attention to simultaneous unrelated auditory and visual events: behavioral and neural correlates. *Cerebral Cortex*, *15*(10), 1609–1620. doi:10.1093/cercor/bhi039

Johnson, J. A., & Zatorre, R. J. (2006). Neural substrates for dividing and focusing attention between simultaneous auditory and visual events. *NeuroImage*, *31*(4), 1673–1681. doi:10.1016/j.neuroimage.2006.02.026

Jones, S., Small, B. J., Fratiglioni, L., & Backman, L. (2002). Predictors of cognitive change from preclinical to clinical Alzheimer's disease. *Brain and Cognition*, *49*(2), 210–213.

Jonkman, E. J., Poortvliet, D. C., Veering, M. M., De Weerd, A. W., & John, E. R. (1985). The use of neurometrics in the study of patients with cerebral ischaemia. *Electroencephalography and Clinical Neurophysiology*, *61*, 333–341. doi:10.1016/0013-4694(85)91023-5

Kahn, L. E., Zygman, M. L., Rymer, W. Z., & Reinkensmeyer, D. J. (2006). Robot-assisted reaching exercise promotes arm movement recovery in chronic hemiparetic stroke: A randomized controlled pilot study. *Journal of Neuroengineering and Rehabilitation*, *12*, 1–13.

Kaji, H., & Isobe, T. (2006). Large-scale analysis of glycoproteins by LC-MS method. *Trends in Glycoscience and Glycotechnology*, *18*, 313–332.

Kaneko, M. (1990). Dementia and frontal lobe function. *Higher Brain Function Research*, *10*, 127–131. doi:10.2496/apr.10.127

Katayama, K., Shimoda, M., Maeda, J., & Takemiya, T. (1998). Endurance exercise training increases peripheral vascular response in human fingers. *Japanese Journal of Physiology*, *48*(5), 365–371. doi:10.2170/jjphysiol.48.365

Katoh, S., Simogaki, H., Onodera, A., Ueda, H., Oikawa, K., & Ikeda, K. (1991). Development of the revised version of Hasegawa's Dementia Scale (HDS-R). *Japanese Journal of Geriatric Psychiatry*, *2*(11), 1339–1347.

Kaufer, D., Williams, C., Braaten, A., Gill, K., Zimmerman, S., & Sloane, P. (2008). Cognitive screening for dementia and mild cognitive impairment in assisted living. *Journal of the American Medical Directors Association*, *9*(8), 586–593. doi:10.1016/j.jamda.2008.05.006

Kawahira, K., Noma, T., Iiyama, J., Etoh, S., Ogata, A., & Shimodozono, M. (2009). Improvements in limb kinetic apraxia by repetition of a newly designed facilitation exercise in a patient with corticobasal degeneration. *International Journal of Rehabilitation Research. Internationale Zeitschrift fur Rehabilitationsforschung. Revue Internationale de Recherches de Readaptation*, *32*, 178–183. doi:10.1097/MRR.0b013e32831e4546

Kawakami, Y., & Fukushima, S. (2002). *The development of the Alzheimer's disease diagnosis system by using ocular movement.* (pp. 63-67). (Technological University of Nagaoka Report 24).

Kawasaki, H., Kimura, H., & Ito, S. (2008). Hand rehabilitation support system. *The Japan Society of Mechanical Engineers*, *72*, 228–233.

Kawasaki, H., Ito, S., Ishigure, Y., Nishimoto, Y., Aoki, T., & Mouri, T. … Abe, M. (2007). Development of a hand motion assist robot for rehabilitation therapy by patient self-motion control. *Proceedings of the 2007 IEEE 10th International Conference on Rehabilitation Robotics*. June 2007, (pp. 234-240).

Kawashima, R., & Imaizumi, S. (1999). Selective visual and auditory attention toward utterances-a PET study. *NeuroImage*, *10*(2), 209–215. doi:10.1006/nimg.1999.0452

Kayed, R., Head, E., Thompson, J. L., McIntire, T. M., Milton, S. C., Cotman, C. W., & Glabe, C. G. (2003). Common structure of soluble amyloid oligomers implies common mechanism of pathogenesis. *Science*, *300*, 486–489. doi:10.1126/science.1079469

Kelley, W. M., Miezin, F. M., McDermott, K. B., Buckner, R. L., Raichle, M. E., & Chohen, N. J. (1998). Hemispheric specialization in human dorsal frontal cortex and medial temporal lobe for verbal and nonverbal memory encoding. *Neuron*, *20*, 927–936. doi:10.1016/S0896-6273(00)80474-2

Kertesz, A., & McMonagle, P. (2010). Behavior and cognition in corticobasal degeneration and progressive supranuclear palsy. *Journal of the Neurological Sciences*, *89*(1-2), 138–143. doi:10.1016/j.jns.2009.08.036

Kikuchi, A., Takeda, A., Okamura, N., Tashiro, M., Hasegawa, T., & Furumoto, S. (2010). In vivo visualization of α-synuclein deposition by carbon-11-labeled 2-(2-[2-dimethylaminothiazol-5-yl]ethenyl)-6-(2-[fluoro]ethoxy)benzoxazole positron emission tomography in multiple system atrophy. *Brain*, *133*, 1772–1778. doi:10.1093/brain/awq091

Kim, J., & Jeong, Y. (2009). *Measurement of vascular function in mice brain using two-photon laser scanning microscopy*. Presented at the 4th Asian Pacific Symposium on BioPhotonics 2009.

Kinoshita, M., Yamada, K., Hashimoto, N., Kato, A., Izumoto, S., & Baba, T. (2005). Fiber-tracking does not accurately estimate size of fiber bundle in pathological condition: Initial neurosurgical experience using neuronavigation and subcortical white matter stimulation. *NeuroImage*, *25*, 424–429. doi:10.1016/j.neuroimage.2004.07.076

Kinosian, B. P., Stallard, E., Lee, J. H., Woodbury, M. A., & Zbrozek, A. S., Glick, & H. A. (2000). Predicting 10-year care requirements for older people with suspected Alzheimer's disease. *Journal of the American Geriatrics Society*, *48*, 631–638.

Kiyo, A. (1980). *Appear frequency of Japanese words* (pp. 42–87). Doushisya University Press.

Kiyosawa, M., Bosley, T. M., Chawluk, J., Jamieson, D., Schatz, N. J., & Savino, P. J. (1989). Alzheimer's disease with prominent visual symptoms clinical and metabolic evaluation. *Ophthalmology*, *96*, 1077–1086.

Klunk, W. E., Engler, H., Nordberg, A., Wang, Y., Blomqvist, G., & Holt, D. P. (2004). Imaging brain amyloid in Alzheimer's disease with Pittsburgh Compound-B. *Annals of Neurology*, *55*, 306–319. doi:10.1002/ana.20009

Klunk, W. E., Mathis, C. A., Price, J. C., Lopresti, B. J., & DeKosky, S. T. (2006). Two-year follow-up of amyloid deposition in patients with Alzheimer's disease. *Brain*, *129*, 2805–2807. doi:10.1093/brain/awl281

Klunk, W. E., Bacskai, B. J., Mathis, C. A., Kajdasz, S. T., McLellan, M. E., & Frosch, M. P. (2002). Imaging Abeta plaques in living transgenic mice with multiphoton microscopy and methoxy-X04, a systemically administered Congo red derivative. *Journal of Neuropathology and Experimental Neurology*, *61*, 797–805.

Kobayashi, T. (2009). Basics and applications of functional MRI [in Japanese]. *Human Interface*, *11*, 39–44.

Kobayashi, T., Ozaki, I., & Nagata, K. (Eds.). (2009). *Brain topography and multimodal imaging*. Kyoto, Japan: Kyoto University Press.

Kobayashi, E., Kusaka, T., Karaki, M., Kobayashi, R., Ito, S., & Mori, N. (2007). Functional optical hemodynamic imaging of the olfactory cortex. *The Laryngoscope*, *117*, 541–546. doi:10.1097/MLG.0b013e31802ffe2a

Kobayashi, E. (2007). Functional optical hemodynamic imaging of the olfactory cortex. *The Laryngoscope*, *117*, 1–6. doi:10.1097/MLG.0b013e31802ffe2a

Kobayashi, H., Ishida, K., & Suzuki, H. (2004). Realization of all motion for the upper kimb by a muscle suit. *Proceedings of the 13th IEEE International Workshop on Robot and Human Interactive Communication RO-MAN2004*, (p. 631).

Koizuka, I., Yano, H., Nagahara, M., Mochizuki, R., Seo, R., & Shimada, K. (1994). Functional imaging of the human olfactory cortex by magnetic resonance imaging. *Journal of Oto-Rhino-Laryngology*, *56*, 273–275.

Kominis, I. K., Kornak, T. W., Allred, J. C., & Romalis, M. V. (2003). A subfemtotesla multichannel atomic magnetometer. *Nature*, *422*, 596–599. doi:10.1038/nature01484

Kondo, H., Matsuda, T., Hashiba, M., & Baba, S. (1998). A study of the relationship between the T&T olfactometer and the University of Pennsylvania Smell Identification Test in a Japanese population. *American Journal of Rhinology*, *12*, 353–358. doi:10.2500/105065898780182390

Konishi, J., Yamada, K., Kizu, O., Ito, H., Sugimura, K., & Yoshikawa, K. (2005). MR tractography for the evaluation of functional recovery from lenticulostriate infarcts. *Neurology*, *64*, 108–113.

Kono, T., Matsuo, K., Tsunashima, K., Kasai, K., Takizawa, R., & Rogers, M. A. (2007). Multiple-time replicability of near-infrared spectroscopy recording during prefrontal activation task in healthy men. *Neuroscience Research*, *57*(4), 504–512. doi:10.1016/j.neures.2006.12.007

Koriat, A., Ben-Zur, H., & Nussbaum, A. (1990). Encoding information for future action; Memory for to-be-performed tasks versus memory for to-be-recalled tasks. *Memory & Cognition*, *18*, 568–578. doi:10.3758/BF03197099

Kosaka, K. (1990). Diffuse Lewy body disease in Japan. *Journal of Neurology*, *237*, 197–204. doi:10.1007/BF00314594

Kostopolous, P., Albanese, M. C., & Petrides, M. (2007). Ventrolateral prefrontal cortex and tactile memory disambiguation in the human brain. *Proceedings of the National Academy of Sciences of the United States of America*, *104*(24), 10223–10228. doi:10.1073/pnas.0700253104

Kranick, S. M., & Duda, J. E. (2008). Olfactory dysfunction in Parkinson's disease. *Neuro-Signals*, *16*(1), 35–40. doi:10.1159/000109757

Krebs, H. I., Volpe, B. T., Aisen, M. L., & Hogan, N. (2000). Increasing productivity and quality of care: Robot-aided neurorehabilitation. *Journal of Rehabilitation Research and Development*, *37*, 639–652.

Kuchibhotla, K. V., Lattarulo, C. R., Hyman, B. T., & Bacskai, B. J. (2009). Synchronous hyperactivity and intercellular calcium waves in astrocytes in Alzheimer mice. *Science*, *323*, 1211–1215. doi:10.1126/science.1169096

Kudo, Y., Okamura, N., Furumoto, S., Tashiro, M., Furukawa, K., & Maruyama, M. (2007). 2-(2-(2-dimethylaminothiazol-5-yl)ethenyl)-6-(2-(fluoro)ethoxy) benzoxazole: A novel pet agent for in vivo detection of dense amyloid plaques in Alzheimer's disease patients. *Journal of Nuclear Medicine*, *48*(4), 553–561. doi:10.2967/jnumed.106.037556

Kudomi, N., Hayashi, T., Teramoto, N., Watabe, H., Kawachi, N., & Ohta, Y. (2005). Rapid quantitative measurement of CMRO(2) and CBF by dual administration of (15)O-labeled oxygen and water during a single PET scan-a validation study and error analysis in anesthetized monkeys. *Journal of Cerebral Blood Flow and Metabolism*, *25*, 1209–1224. doi:10.1038/sj.jcbfm.9600118

Kujirai, T., Caramia, M. D., Rothwell, J. C., Day, B. L., Thompson, P. D., & Ferbert, A. (1993). Corticocortical inhibition in human motor cortex. *The Journal of Physiology*, *471*, 501–519.

Kumakura, Y., Gjedde, A., Danielsen, E., Christensen, S., & Cumming, P. (2006). Dopamine storage capacity in caudate and putamen of patients with early Parkinson's disease: Correlation with asymmetry of motor symptoms. *Journal of Cerebral Blood Flow and Metabolism*, *26*(3), 358–370. doi:10.1038/sj.jcbfm.9600202

Kuo, W. J., Yeh, T. C., Duann, J. R., Wu, Y. T., Ho, L. T., & Huang, D. (2001). A left-lateralized network for reading Chinese words: A 3T fMRI study. *Neuroreport*, *12*, 3997–4001. doi:10.1097/00001756-200112210-00029

Kuo, W. J., Yeh, T. C., Lee, J. R., Chen, L. F., Lee, P. L., & Chen, S. S. (2004). Orthographic and phonological processing of Chinese characters: An fMRI study. *NeuroImage*, *21*, 1721–1731. doi:10.1016/j.neuroimage.2003.12.007

Kuo, W.-J., Yeh, T.-C., Lee, J.-R., Chen, L.-F., Lee, P.-L., & Chen, S.-S. (2004). Orthographic and phonological processing of Chinese characters: An fMRI study. *NeuroImage*, *21*, 1721–1731. doi:10.1016/j.neuroimage.2003.12.007

Kurylo, D. D., Corkin, S., Allard, T., Zatorre, R. J., & Growdon, J. H. (1993). Auditory function in Alzheimer's disease. *Neurology*, *43*(10), 1893–1899.

Kusaka, T., Kawada, K., Okubo, K., Nagano, K., Namba, M., & Okada, H. (2004). Noninvasive optical imaging in the visual cortex in young infants. *Human Brain Mapping*, *22*, 122–132. doi:10.1002/hbm.20020

Lambercy, O., Dovat, L., Gassert, R., Burdet, E., Teo, C. L., & Milner, T. (2007). A haptic knob for rehabilitation of hand function. *IEEE Transactions on Neural Systems and Rehabilitation Engineering*, *15*, 356–366. doi:10.1109/TNSRE.2007.903913

Lambert, M. P., Barlow, A. K., Chromy, B. A., Edwards, C., Freed, R., & Liosatos, M. … Klein, W. L. (1998). Diffusible, nonfibrillar ligands derived from Aβ1-42 are potent central nervous system neurotoxins. *Proceedings of the National Academy of Sciences USA*, *95*, 6448–6453.

Lammertsma, A., & Hume, S. (1996). Simplified reference tissue model for pet receptor studies. *NeuroImage*, *4*(3 Pt 1), 153–158. doi:10.1006/nimg.1996.0066

Lamoureux, E. L., Sparrow, W. A., Murphy, A., & Newton, R. U. (2002). The relationship between lower body strength and obstructed gait in community-dwelling older adults. *Journal of the American Geriatrics Society*, *50*, 468–473. doi:10.1046/j.1532-5415.2002.50112.x

Laurienti, P. J., Burdette, J. H., Wallace, M. T., Yen, Y. F., Field, A. S., & Stein, B. E. (2002). Deactivation of sensory-specific cortex by cross-modal stimuli. *Journal of Cognitive Neuroscience*, *14*(3), 420–429. doi:10.1162/089892902317361930

Lawton, M. P. (1972). *Assessing the competence of older people* (pp. 122–143). New York, NY: Human Science Press.

Lee, M. S., Kao, S. C., Lemere, C. A., Xia, W., Tseng, H. C., & Zhou, Y. (2003). APP processing is regulated by cytoplasmic phosphorylation. *The Journal of Cell Biology*, *163*(1), 83–95. doi:10.1083/jcb.200301115

Lee, M., Sparatore, A., Del Soldato, P., McGeer, E., & McGeer, P. L. (2009). Hydrogen sulfide-releasing NSAIDs attenuate neuroinflammation induced by microglial and astrocytic activation. *Glia*, *58*, 103–113. doi:10.1002/glia.20905

Lee, M. L., & Dey, A. K. (2008). Lifelogging memory appliance for people with episodic memory impairment. *Proceedings of UbiComp*, *2008*, 44–53. doi:10.1145/1409635.1409643

Lehmann, D., & Skrandies, W. (1980). Reference-free identification of components of checkerboard-evoked multichannel potential fields. *Electroencephalography and Clinical Neurophysiology*, *48*, 609–621. doi:10.1016/0013-4694(80)90419-8

Leon-Carrion, J., Damas-Lopez, J., Martin-Rodriguez, J. F., Dominguez-Roldan, J. M., Murillo-Cabezas, F., Barroso-Martin, J. M., & Dominguez-Morales, M. R. (2008). The hemodynamics of cognitive control: The level of concentration of oxygenated hemoglobin in the superior prefrontal cortex varies as a function of performance in a modified Stroop task. *Behavioural Brain Research*, *193*(2), 248–256. doi:10.1016/j.bbr.2008.06.013

Lesne, S., Koh, M. T., Kotilinek, L., Kayed, R., Glabe, C. G., & Yang, A. (2006). A specific amyloid-β protein assembly in the brain impairs memory. *Nature*, *440*, 352–357. doi:10.1038/nature04533

Levy, R. (1994). Aging -associated cognitive decline. *International Psychogeriatrics*, *6*, 63–68. doi:10.1017/S1041610294001626

Lexell, J., Taylor, C. C., & Sjöström, M. (1988). What is the cause of the ageing atrophy? Total number, size and proportion of different fiber types studied in whole vastus lateralis muscle from 15- to 83-year-old men. *Journal of the Neurological Sciences*, *84*, 275–294. doi:10.1016/0022-510X(88)90132-3

Lezak, M. D. (1995). *Neuropsychological assessment* (3rd ed.). New York, NY: Oxford University Press.

Liegeois-Chauvel, C., Peretz, I., Babai, M., Laguitton, V., & Chauvel, P. (1998). Contribution of different cortical areas in the temporal lobes to music processing. *Brain*, *121*(10), 1853–1867. doi:10.1093/brain/121.10.1853

Lin, X., Koelsch, G., Wu, S., Downs, D., Dashti, A., & Tang, J. (2000). Human aspartic protease memapsin 2 cleaves the beta-secretase site of betaamyloid precursor protein. *Proceedings of the National Academy of Sciences of the United States of America*, *97*(4), 1456–1460. doi:10.1073/pnas.97.4.1456

Lin, C. P., Tseng, W. Y., Cheng, H. C., & Chen, J. H. (2001). Validation of diffusion tensor magnetic resonance axonal fiber imaging with registered manganese-enhanced optic tracts. *NeuroImage*, *14*, 1035–1047. doi:10.1006/nimg.2001.0882

Lindberg, P., Schmitz, C., Forssberg, H., Engardt, M., & Borg, J. (2004). Effects of passive-active movement training on upper limb motor function and cortical activation in chronic patients with stroke: pilot study. *The Japanese Journal of Rehabilitation Medicine*, *36*, 117–123. doi:10.1080/16501970410023434

Lippert, M. T., Takagaki, K., Xu, W., Huang, X., & Wu, J. Y. (2007). Methods for voltage-sensitive dye imaging of rat cortical activity with high signal-to-noise ratio. *Journal of Neurophysiology*, *98*, 502–512. doi:10.1152/jn.01169.2006

Liu, T., & Chui, D. H. (2008). Role of lipids and lipid-associated proteins in Alzheimer s disease. *Nervous Diseases and Mental Health*, *8*(5), 329–334.

Liu, C. J., & Latham, N. K. (2009). Progressive resistance strength training for improving physical function in older adults. *Cochrane Database of Systematic Reviews*, CD002759.

Livingstone, M., & Hubel, D. (1998). Segregation of form, color, movement, and depth: Anatomy, physiology, and perception. *Science*, *240*, 740–749. doi:10.1126/science.3283936

Logan, J., Fowler, J. S., Volkow, N. D., Wang, G. J., Ding, Y. S., & Alexoff, D. L. (1996). Distribution volume ratios without blood sampling from graphical analysis of PET data. *Journal of Cerebral Blood Flow and Metabolism*, *16*, 834–840. doi:10.1097/00004647-199609000-00008

Logan, J., Fowler, J. S., Volkow, N. D., Wolf, A. P., Dewey, S. L., & Schlyer, D. J. (1990). Graphical analysis of reversible radioligand binding from time-activity measurements applied to [N-11C-methyl]-(-)-cocaine PET studies in human subjects. *Journal of Cerebral Blood Flow and Metabolism*, *10*, 740–747.

Lopresti, B. J., Klunk, W. E., Mathis, C. A., Hoge, J. A., Ziolko, S. K., & Lu, X. (2005). Simplified quantification of Pittsburgh Compound B amyloid imaging PET studies: A comparative analysis. *Journal of Nuclear Medicine*, *46*, 1959–1972.

Lu, S., & Sakai, Y. (2004). Measurement and analysis of the object length perceptive characteristics with visual and tactile information for proposal of three-dimension tactile shape display. *Transactions of the Japan Society of Mechanical Engineers*, 2699–2706.

Lum, P. S., Burgar, C. G., Shor, P. C., Majmundar, M., & Van der Loos, M. (2002). Robot-assisted movement training compared with conventional therapy techniques for the rehabilitation of upper-limb motor function after stroke. *Archives of Physical Medicine and Rehabilitation*, *83*, 952–959. doi:10.1053/apmr.2001.33101

Maeshima, S., Tanemura, J., Osawa, A., Kawarada, M., & Yamada, Y. (2006). Prospective memory in the Elderly: The difference between presence and contents of intentions to remember. *Japanese Journal of Rehabilitation Medicine*, *43*, 446–453. doi:10.2490/jjrm1963.43.446

Mahieux-Laurent, F., Fabre, C., Galbrun, E., Dubrulle, A., & Moroni, C. (2009). Validation of a brief screening scale evaluating praxic abilities for use in memory clinics. Evaluation in 419 controls, 127 mild cognitive impairment and 320 demented patients. *Revue Neurologique*, *165*, 560–567. doi:10.1016/j.neurol.2008.11.016

Mahoney, R. M., Machiel Van der Loos, H. F., Lum, P. S., & Burgar, C. (2003). Robotic stroke therapy assistant. *Robotica*, *21*, 33–44. doi:10.1017/S0263574702004617

Mally, J., & Stone, T. W. (1999). Therapeutic and dose-dependent effect of repetitive microelectroshock induced by transcranial magnetic stimulation in Parkinson's disease. *Journal of Neuroscience Research*, *57*, 935–940. doi:10.1002/(SICI)1097-4547(19990915)57:6<935::AID-JNR19>3.0.CO;2-8

Mapstone, M., Teresa, M., Steffenella, M., & Duffy, C. J. (2003). A visuospatial variant of mild cognitive impairment. Getting lost between aging and AD. *Neurology*, *60*, 802–808.

Markowitsch, H., Vandekerckhove, M., Lanfermann, H., & Russ, M. (2003). Engagement of lateral and medial prefrontal areas in the ecphory of sad and happy autobiographical memories. *Cortex*, *39*(4), 643–665. doi:10.1016/S0010-9452(08)70858-X

Maruyama, M., Matsui, T., Tanji, H., Nemoto, M., Tomita, N., & Ootsuki, M. (2004). Cerebrospinal fluid tau protein and periventricular white matter lesions in patients with mild cognitive impairment: Implications for 2 major pathways. *Archives of Neurology*, *61*(5), 716–720. doi:10.1001/archneur.61.5.716

Massy, W. F. (1965). Principal components regression in exploratory statistical research. *Journal of the American Statistical Association*, *60*(309), 234–256. doi:10.2307/2283149

Matsubara, K., Watabe, H., Hayashi, T., Minato, K., & Iida, H. (2010). Evaluation of bias of the influx constant estimated by patlak analysis for (18F) FDOPA PET: Influence of metabolites for (18F) FDOPA (Japanese). *Transactions of the Japanese Society for Medical and Biological Engineering*, *48*(1), 66–74.

Matsuo, K., Mizuno, T., Yamada, K., Akazawa, K., Kasai, T., & Kondo, M. (2008). Cerebral white matter damage in frontotemporal dementia assessed by diffusion tensor tractography. *Neuroradiology*, *50*, 605–611. doi:10.1007/s00234-008-0379-5

Mattia, D., Babiloni, F., Romigi, A., Cincotti, F., Bianchi, L., & Sperli, F. (2003). Quantitative EEG and dynamic susceptibility contrast MRI in Alzheimer's disease: A correlative study. *Clinical Neurophysiology*, *114*, 1210–1216. doi:10.1016/S1388-2457(03)00085-3

May, L. A., Burnham, R. S., & Steadward, R. D. (1997). Assessment of isokinetic and hand-held dynamometer measures of shoulder rotator strength among individuals with spinal cord injury. *Archives of Physical Medicine and Rehabilitation*, *8*, 251–255. doi:10.1016/S0003-9993(97)90029-0

McGurk, H., & MacDonald, J. (1976). Hearing lips and seeing voices. *Nature*, *264*(5588), 746–748. doi:10.1038/264746a0

McKhann, G., Drachman, D., Folstein, M., Katzman, R., Price, D., & Stadlan, E. M. (1984). Clinical diagnosis of Alzheimer's disease: Report of the NINCDS-ADRDA Work Group under the auspices of Department of Health and Human Services Task Force on Alzheimer's Disease. *Neurology*, *34*, 939–944.

Meltzer, C. C., Kinahan, P. E., Greer, P. J., Nichols, T. E., Comtat, C., & Cantwell, M. N. (1999). Comparative evaluation of MR-based partial-volume correction schemes for PET. *Journal of Nuclear Medicine*, *40*, 2053–2065.

Meyer-Luehmann, M., Spires-Jones, T. L., Prada, C., Garcia-Alloza, M., de Calignon, A., & Rozkalne, A. (2008). Rapid appearance and local toxicity of amyloid-beta plaques in a mouse model of Alzheimer's disease. *Nature*, *451*, 720–724. doi:10.1038/nature06616

Miao, T., Shimoyama, O., & Oyama-Higa, M. (2006). *Modelling plethysmogram dynamics based on baroreflex under higher cerebral influences*. 2006 IEEE Conference on Systems, Man, and Cybernetics, Taipei, Taiwan, (pp. 2868–2873).

Michotte, A., Thines, G., & Crabbe, G. (1964/1991). Amodal completion of perceptual structures. In Thines, G., Costall, A., & Butterworth, G. (Eds.), *Michotte's experimental phenomenology of perception*. Hillsdale, NJ: Lawrence Erlbaum Associates.

Miller, J. (1982). Divided attention: Evidence for coactivation with redundant signals. *Cognitive Psychology*, *14*(2), 247–279. doi:10.1016/0010-0285(82)90010-X

Miller, J. (1986). Timecourse of coactivation in bimodal divided attention. *Perception & Psychophysics*, *40*(5), 331–343. doi:10.3758/BF03203025

Min, B.-C. (2003). Analysis of mutual information content for EEG responses to odor stimulation for subjects classified by occupation. *Chemical Senses*, *28*(9), 741–749. doi:10.1093/chemse/bjg066

Min, K.-Y., Chung, S.-C., & Min, B.-C. (2005). Physiological evaluation on emotional change induced by imagination. *Applied Psychophysiology and Biofeedback*, *30*(2). doi:10.1007/s10484-005-4310-0

Minoshima, S., Foster, N. L., & Kuhl, D. E. (1994). Posterior cingulate cortex in Alzheimer's disease. *Lancet*, *344*, 895. doi:10.1016/S0140-6736(94)92871-1

Minoshima, S., Frey, K. A., Koeppe, R. A., Foster, N. L., & Kuhl, D. E. (1995). A diagnostic approach in Alzheimer's disease using three-dimensional stereotactic surface projections of fluorine-18-FDG PET. *Journal of Nuclear Medicine*, *36*, 1238–1248.

Mintun, M., Raichle, M., Martin, W., & Herscovitch, P. (1984). Brain oxygen utilization measured with O-15 radiotracers and positron emission tomography. *Journal of Nuclear Medicine*, *25*(2), 177–187.

Mintun, M. A. (2005). Utilizing advanced imaging and surrogate markers across the spectrum of Alzheimer's disease. *CNS Spectrums*, *10*, 13–16.

Molholm, S., Ritter, W., Murray, M. M., Javitt, D. C., Schroeder, C. E., & Foxe, J. J. (2002). Multisensory auditory-visual interactions during early sensory processing in humans: a high-density electrical mapping study. *Brain Research. Cognitive Brain Research*, *14*(1), 115–128. doi:10.1016/S0926-6410(02)00066-6

Moody, D. M., Thore, C. R., Anstrom, J. A., Challa, V. R., Langefeld, C. D., & Brown, W. R. (2004). Quantification of afferent vessels shows reduced brain vascular density in subjects with leukoaraiosis. *Radiology, 233*, 883–890. doi:10.1148/radiol.2333020981

Moreland, J. D., Richardson, J. A., Goldsmith, C. H., & Clase, C. M. (2004). Muscle weakness and falls in older adults: a systematic review and meta-analysis. *Journal of the American Geriatrics Society, 52*, 1121–1129. doi:10.1111/j.1532-5415.2004.52310.x

Mori, E., Mitani, Y., & Yamadori, A. (1985). Usefulness of a Japanese version of the mini-mental state test in neurological patients. *Japanese Journal of Neuropsychology, 1*, 82–90.

Mori, S., Crain, B. J., Chacko, V. P., & van Zijl, P. C. (1999). Three-dimensional tracking of axonal projections in the brain by magnetic resonance imaging. *Annals of Neurology, 45*, 265–269. doi:10.1002/1531-8249(199902)45:2<265::AID-ANA21>3.0.CO;2-3

Mori, O. (1969). [Kanehara & Co., Ltd.]. *Buntan Kaibougaku, 1*, 346–373.

Morimoto, A., Irie, K., Murakami, K., Masuda, Y., Ohigashi, H., & Nagao, M. (2004). Analysis of thesecondary structure of β-amyloid (Aβ42) fibrils by systematic prolinere placement. *The Journal of Biological Chemistry, 279*, 52781–52788. doi:10.1074/jbc.M406262200

Morris, J. C. (1993). The Clinical Dementia Rating (CDR): Current version and scoring rules. *Neurology, 43*(11), 2412–2414.

Morrone, M. C., Tosetti, M., Montanaro, D., Fiorentini, A., Cioni, G., & Burr, D. C. (2000). A cortical area that responds specifically to optic flow, revealed by fMRI. *Nature Neuroscience, 12*, 1322–1328. doi:10.1038/81860

Mozolic, J. L., Hugenschmidt, C. E., Peiffer, A. M., & Laurienti, P. J. (2008). Modality-specific selective attention attenuates multisensory integration. *Experimental Brain Research, 184*(1), 39–52. doi:10.1007/s00221-007-1080-3

Munsat, S. (1966). *The concept of memory*. New York, NY: Random House.

Murakami, A., Morimoto, M., Yamada, K., Kizu, O., Nishimura, A., Nishimura, T., & Sugimoto, T. (2008). Fiber-tracking techniques can predict the degree of neurologic impairment for periventricular leukomalacia. *Pediatrics, 122*, 500–506. doi:10.1542/peds.2007-2816

Nagakane, Y., Yamada, K., Ohara, T., Yoshikawa, K., Kuriyama, N., & Takayasu, N. (2008). Acute lenticulostriate infarction presenting with skip lesions may reflect the selective vulnerability of gray and white matter. *Stroke, 39*, 494–496. doi:10.1161/STROKEAHA.107.484337

Nagayama, S., Zeng, S., Xiong, W., Fletcher, M. L., Masurkar, A. V., & Davis, D. J. (2007). In vivo simultaneous tracing and Ca(2+) imaging of local neuronal circuits. *Neuron, 53*, 789–803. doi:10.1016/j.neuron.2007.02.018

Nakamura, S. (2004). A guideline for the treatment of dementia in Japan. *Internal Medicine (Tokyo, Japan), 43*, 18–29. doi:10.2169/internalmedicine.43.18

Nakano, S., Asada, T., Matsuda, H., Uno, M., & Takasaki, M. (2001). Donepezil hydrochloride preserves regional cerebral blood flow in patients with Alzheimer's disease. *Journal of Nuclear Medicine, 42*, 1441–1445.

Nakashima, T., Goto, Y., Abe, T., Kaneko, K., Saito, T., Makinouchi, A., & Tobimatsu, S. (2008). Electrophysiological evidence for sequential discrimination of positive and negative facial expressions. *Clinical Neurophysiology, 119*, 1803–1811. doi:10.1016/j.clinph.2008.04.014

Nakashima, T., Kaneko, K., Goto, Y., Abe, T., Mitsudo, T., & Ogata, K. (2008). Early ERP components differentially extract facial features: Evidence for spatial frequency-and-contrast detectors. *Neuroscience Research, 62*, 225–235. doi:10.1016/j.neures.2008.08.009

Nambu, I., Osu, R., Sato, M., Ando, S., Kawato, M., & Naito, E. (2009). Single-trial reconstruction of finger-pinch forces from human motor-cortical activation measured by near-infrared spectroscopy (NIRS). *NeuroImage, 47*, 628–637. doi:10.1016/j.neuroimage.2009.04.050

NAMT career leaflet. (1980).

Nelson, M. E., Layne, J. E., Bernstein, M. J., Nurenberger, A., Castaneda, C., Kaliton, D., … Fiatarone Singh, M. A. (2004). The effects of multidimensional home-based exercise on functional performance in elderly people. *Journals of Gerontology A Biological Sciences and Medical Sciences, 59*, 154-160.

Newsome, W. T., & Paré, E. B. (1988). A selective impairment of motion perception following lesions of the middle temporal area (MT). *The Journal of Neuroscience*, *8*, 2201–2211.

Nichols, W. W., & O'Rourke, M. F. (1998). *McDonald's blood flow in arteries: Theoretical experimental and clinical principles*, 4th ed. London.

Niedeggen, M., & Wist, E. R. (1999). Characteristics of visual evoked potentials generated by motion coherence onset. *Brain Research. Cognitive Brain Research*, *8*, 95–105. doi:10.1016/S0926-6410(99)00009-9

Nimsky, C., Ganslandt, O., Merhof, D., Sorensen, A. G., & Fahlbusch, R. (2006). Intraoperative visualization of the pyramidal tract by diffusion-tensor-imaging-based fiber tracking. *NeuroImage*, *30*, 1219–1229. doi:10.1016/j.neuroimage.2005.11.001

Nobre, A. C., & Gitelman, D. R. (2000). Covert visual spatial orienting and saccades: Overlapping neural systems. *NeuroImage*, *11*(3), 210–216. doi:10.1006/nimg.2000.0539

Nollet, F., & Beelen, A. (1999). Strength assessment in postpolio syndrome: Validity of a hand-held dynamometer in detecting change. *Archives of Physical Medicine and Rehabilitation*, *80*, 1316–1323. doi:10.1016/S0003-9993(99)90036-9

Nordberg, A. (2004). PET imaging of amyloid in Alzheimer's disease. *The Lancet Neurology*, *3*, 519–527. doi:10.1016/S1474-4422(04)00853-1

Nowomiejsk, K. (2005). Comparison between semiautomated kinetic oerimetry and conventional Goldmann manual kinetic perimetry in advanced visual field loss. *Ophthalmology*, *112*, 1343–1354. doi:10.1016/j.ophtha.2004.12.047

Nuki, M. (1996). *Music therapy for the aged*. Tokyo, Japan: Ongaku no tomo sya corp.

Obayashi, C., Nakashima, T., Onitsuka, T., Maekawa, T., Hirano, Y., & Hirano, S. (2009). Decreased spatial frequency sensitivities for processing faces in male patients with chronic schizophrenia. *Clinical Neurophysiology*, *120*, 1525–1533. doi:10.1016/j.clinph.2009.06.016

Ohashi, Y., Innami, Y., Jung, J., Hamada, S., & Kobayashi, T. (2006). A study on the application of a linearly-constrained adaptive beamformer to fMRI-MEG integrative analysis [in Japanese]. *Transactions of the Japanese Society for Medical and Biological Engineering*, *44*, 722–727.

Okada, Y., Ohashi, S., Jung, J., Hamada, S., & Kobayashi, T. (2007). An fMRI-MEG integrative neuroimaging method: Improvements of its accuracy and robustness by suppression of fMRI-invisible coherent activities [in Japanese]. *Transactions of the Japanese Society for Medical and Biological Engineering*, *45*, 275–284.

Okada, T., Mikuni, N., Miki, Y., Kikuta, K., Urayama, S., & Hanakawa, T. (2006). Corticospinal tract localization: integration of diffusion-tensor tractography at 3-T MR imaging with intraoperative white matter stimulation mapping-preliminary results. *Radiology*, *240*, 849–857. doi:10.1148/radiol.2403050916

Okamoto, M., Dan, H., Shimizu, K., Takeo, K., Amita, T., & Oda, I. (2004). Multimodal assessment of cortical activations during apple peeling by NIRS and fMRI0. *NeuroImage*, *21*, 1275–1288. doi:10.1016/j.neuroimage.2003.12.003

Okamoto, Y. (1992). Health care for the elderly in Japan: Medicine and welfare in an aging society facing a crisis in long term care. *British Medical Journal*, *305*, 403–405. doi:10.1136/bmj.305.6850.403

Okamura, N., Fodero-Tavoletti, M. T., Kudo, Y., Rowe, C. C., Furumoto, S., & Arai, H. (2009). Advances in molecular imaging for the diagnosis of dementia. *Expert Opinion on Medical Diagnostics*, *3*, 705–716. doi:10.1517/17530050903133790

Okamura, N., Furumoto, S., Arai, H., Iwata, R., Yanai, K., & Kudo, Y. (2008). Imaging amyloid pathology in the living brain. *Current Medical Imaging Reviews*, *4*, 56–62. doi:10.2174/157340508783502840

Okamura, N., Suemoto, T., Furumoto, S., Suzuki, M., Shimadzu, H., & Akatsu, H. (2005). Quinoline and benzimidazole derivatives: Candidate probes for in vivo imaging of tau pathology in Alzheimer's disease. *The Journal of Neuroscience*, *25*, 10857–10862. doi:10.1523/JNEUROSCI.1738-05.2005

Okamura, N., Suemoto, T., Shimadzu, H., Suzuki, M., Shiomitsu, T., & Akatsu, H. (2004). Styrylbenzoxazole derivatives for in vivo imaging of amyloid plaques in the brain. *The Journal of Neuroscience*, *24*, 2535–2541. doi:10.1523/JNEUROSCI.4456-03.2004

Okamura, N., Shiga, Y., Furumoto, S., Tashiro, M., Tsuboi, Y., Furukawa, K., … Doh-Ura, K. (2010). In vivo detection of prion amyloid plaques using [^{11}C]BF-227 PET. *European Journal of Nuclear Medicine and Molecular Imaging*.

Opie, J., Rosewarne, R., & O'Connor, D. W. (1999). The efficacy of psychosocial approaches to behaviour disorders in dementia: A systematic literature review. *The Australian and New Zealand Journal of Psychiatry*, *3*, 789–799. doi:10.1046/j.1440-1614.1999.00652.x

Organization for Economic Co-operation and Development. (2009). *International road traffic and accident database*.

Orimo, S., Amino, T., Itoh, Y., Takahashi, A., Kojo, T., & Uchihara, T. (2005). Cardiac sympathetic denervation precedes neuronal loss in the sympathetic ganglia in Lewy body disease. *Acta Neuropathologica*, *109*, 583–588. doi:10.1007/s00401-005-0995-7

Ory, M., Kinney Hoffman, K., Hawkins, M., Sanner, B., & Mockenhaupt, R. (2003). Challenging aging stereotypes strategies for creating a more active society. *American Journal of Preventive Medicine*, *25*, 164–171. doi:10.1016/S0749-3797(03)00181-8

Otake, M. (2009). Coimagination method: Sharing imagination with images and time limit. In. *Proceedings of the International Reminiscence and Life Review Conference, 2009*, 97–103.

Otake, M., Kato, M., Takagi, T., & Asama, H. (2009). Coimagination method: Communication support system with collected images and its evaluation via memory task. In C. Stephanidis (Ed.), *Universal access in human-computer interaction*, (pp. 403–411). (LNCS 5614), Springer-Verlag.

Oyama-Higa, M., & Miao, T. (2006). *Discovery and application of new index for cognitive psychology*. 2006 IEEE Conference on Systems, Man, and Cybernetics, Taipei, Taiwan, (pp. 2040–2044).

Oyama-Higa, M., Miao, T., & Mizuno-Matsumoto, Y. (2006). *Analysis of dementia in aged subjects through chaos analysis of fingertip pulse waves*. 2006 IEEE Conference on Systems, Man, & Cybernetics, Taipei, Taiwan, 2863–2867.

Palmer, E. D., Rosen, H. J., Ojemann, J. G., Buckner, R. L., Kelley, W. M., & Petersen, S. E. (2001). An event-related fMRI study of overt and covert word stem completion. *NeuroImage*, *14*, 182–193. doi:10.1006/nimg.2001.0779

Park, K., Yasuda, N., Toyonaga, S., Yamada, S. M., Nakabayashi, H., & Nakasato, M. (2007). Significant association between leukoaraiosis and metabolic syndrome in healthy subjects. *Neurology*, *69*, 974–978. doi:10.1212/01.wnl.0000266562.54684.bf

Park, H., & Pringle Specht, J. K. (2009). Effect of individualized music on agitation in individuals with dementia who live at home. *Journal of Gerontological Nursing*, *35*(8), 47–55. doi:10.3928/00989134-20090706-01

Parker, G. J., Stephan, K. E., Barker, G. J., Rowe, J. B., MacManus, D. G., & Wheeler-Kingshott, C. A. (2002). Initial demonstration of in vivo tracing of axonal projections in the macaque brain and comparison with the human brain using diffusion tensor imaging and fast marching tractography. *NeuroImage*, *15*, 797–809. doi:10.1006/nimg.2001.0994

Pascual-Marqui, R. D., Esslen, M., Kochi, K., & Lehmann, D. (2002). Functional imaging with low-resolution brain electromagnetic tomography (LORETA): A review. *Methods and Findings in Experimental and Clinical Pharmacology*, *24*, 91–95.

Patlak, C., Blasberg, R., & Fenstermacher, J. (1983). Graphical evaluation of blood-to-brain transfer constants from multiple-time uptake data. *Journal of Cerebral Blood Flow and Metabolism*, *3*(1), 1–7.

Patricia, A. T. (1995). Effects of calming music on the level of agitation in cognitively impaired nursing home residents. *American Journal of Alzheimer's Disease and Other Dementias*, *10*(1), 10–15. doi:10.1177/153331759501000105

Paus, T., Jech, R., Thompson, C. J., Comeau, R., Peters, T., & Evans, A. C. (1997). Transcranial magnetic stimulation during positron emission tomography: a new method for studying connectivity of the human cerebral cortex. *The Journal of Neuroscience*, *17*, 3178–3184.

Paus, T., Jech, R., Thompson, C. J., Comeau, R., Peters, T., & Evans, A. C. (1998). Dose-dependent reduction of cerebral blood flow during rapid-rate transcranial magnetic stimulation of the human sensorimotor cortex. *Journal of Neurophysiology*, *79*, 1102–1107.

Pelli, D. G., Burns, C. W., Farell, B., & Moore, D. C. (2006). Feature detection and letter identification. *Vision Research*, *46*, 4646–4674. doi:10.1016/j.visres.2006.04.023

Peretz, I., Kolinsky, R., Tramo, M., Labrecque, R., Hublet, C., Demeurisse, G., & Belleville, S. (1994). Functional dissociations following bilateral lesions of auditory cortex. *Brain*, *117*(6), 1283–1301. doi:10.1093/brain/117.6.1283

Petersen, R. C., Smith, G. E., Waring, S. C., Ivnik, R. J., Tangalos, E. G., & Kokmen, E. (1999). Mild cognitive impairment; clinical characterization and outcome. *Archives of Neurology*, *56*, 303–308. doi:10.1001/archneur.56.3.303

Petersen, R. C., Smith, G. E., Waring, S. C., Ivnik, R. J., Tangalos, E. G., & Kokmen, E. (1999). Mild cognitive impairment: clinical characterization and outcome. *Archives of Neurology*, *56*, 303–308. doi:10.1001/archneur.56.3.303

Petersson, K. M., Reis, A., Askelof, S., Castro-Caldas, A., & Ingvar, M. (2000). Language processing modulated by literacy: A network analysis of verbal repetition in literate and illiterate subjects. *Journal of Cognitive Neuroscience*, *12*, 364–382. doi:10.1162/089892900562147

Petersson, K. M., Reis, A., & Ingvar, M. (2001). Cognitive processing in literate and illiterate subjects: A review of some recent behavioral and functional neuroimaging data. *Scandinavian Journal of Psychology*, *42*, 251–267. doi:10.1111/1467-9450.00235

Peticolas, W. L., Goldsborough, J. P., & Rieckhoff, K. E. (1963). Double photon excitation in organic crystals. *Physical Review Letters*, *10*, 43–45. doi:10.1103/PhysRevLett.10.43

Peuralas, S. H., Pitkanen, K., Sivenius, J., & Takka, I. M. (2002). Cutaneous electrical stimulation may enhance sensorimotor recovery in chronic stroke. *Clinical Rehabilitation*, *16*, 709–715. doi:10.1191/0269215502cr543oa

Piao, C., Yoshimoto, N., Shitama, H., Makino, K., Wada, F., & Hachisuka, K. (2004). Validity and reliability of the measurement of the quadriceps femoris muscle strength with a hand-held dynamometer on the affected side in hemiplegic patients. *Journal of UOEH*, *26*, 1–11.

Pietrini, P., Alexander, G. E., Furey, M. L., Dani, A., Mentis, M. J., & Horwitz, B. (2000). Cerebral metabolic response to passive audiovisual stimulation in patients with Alzheimer's disease and healthy volunteers assessed by PET. *Journal of Nuclear Medicine*, *41*(4), 575–583.

Ponton, M. O., Satz, P., Herrera, L., Ortiz, F., Urrutia, C. P., & Young, R. (1996). Normative data stratified by age and education for the Neuropsychological Screening Battery for Hispanics (NeSBHIS): Initial report. *Journal of the International Neuropsychological Society*, *2*, 96–104. doi:10.1017/S1355617700000941

Price, J. C., Klunk, W. E., Lopresti, B. J., Lu, X., Hoge, J. A., & Ziolko, S. K. (2005). Kinetic modeling of amyloid binding in humans using PET imaging and Pittsburgh Compound-B. *Journal of Cerebral Blood Flow and Metabolism*, *25*, 1528–1547. doi:10.1038/sj.jcbfm.9600146

Puthoff, M. L., & Nielsen, D. H. (2007). Relationships among impairments in lower-extremity strength and power, functional limitaitons, and disability in older adults. *Physical Therapy*, *87*, 1334–1347. doi:10.2522/ptj.20060176

Qazi, A. A., Radmanesh, A., O'Donnell, L., Kindlmann, G., Peled, S., & Whalen, S. (2009). Resolving crossings in the corticospinal tract by two-tensor streamline tractography: Method and clinical assessment using fMRI. *NeuroImage*, *47*(2), T98–T106. doi:10.1016/j.neuroimage.2008.06.034

Raglio, A., & Gianelli, M. V. (2009). Music therapy for individuals with dementia: Areas of interventions and research perspectives. *Current Alzheimer Research*, *6*, 293–301. doi:10.2174/156720509788486617

Raina, P., Santaguida, P., Ismaila, A., Patterson, C., Cowan, D., & Levine, M. (2008). Effectiveness of cholinesterase inhibitors and memantine for treating dementia: Evidence review for a clinical practice guideline. *Annals of Internal Medicine*, *148*(5), 379–397.

Raven, J. C. (1976). *Colored progressive matrices. London, UK*. Lewis: Oxford Psychologists Press.

Rentz, D. M., & Weintraub, S. (2000). Neuropsychological detection of early probable Alzheimer's disease. In Scinto, L. F. M., & Daffner, K. R. (Eds.), *Early diagnosis and treatment of Alzheimer's disease* (pp. 69–189). Totowa, NJ: Humana Press. doi:10.1385/1-59259-005-5:169

Rey, A. (1964). *L'examen clinique en psychogie*. Paris, France: Presses Universitaires de France.

Richie, K., Artero, S., & Touchon, J. (2001). Classification criteria for mild cognitive impairment: A population based validation study. *Neurology*, *56*, 37–42.

Riddle, D. L., Finucane, S. D., Rothstein, J. M., & Walker, M. L. (1989). Intrasession and intersession reliability of hand-held dynamometer measurements taken on brain-damaged patients. *Physical Therapy*, *69*, 182–189.

Ritchie, C. W. (2004). Meta-analysis of randomised trials of the efficacy and safety of donepezil, galantamine and rivastigmine for the treatment of Alzheimer's disease. *The American Journal of Geriatric Psychiatry*, *12*, 358–369.

Rizzolatti, G., & Matelli, M. (2003). Two different streams from the dorsal visual system: Anatomy and functions. *Experimental Brain Research*, *153*, 146–157. doi:10.1007/s00221-003-1588-0

Rolland, Y., Pillard, F., Klapouszczak, A., Reynish, E., Thomas, D., & Andrieu, S. (2007). Exercise program for nursing home residents with Alzheimer's disease: a 1-year randomized, controlled trial. *Journal of the American Geriatrics Society*, *55*, 158–165. doi:10.1111/j.1532-5415.2007.01035.x

Ross, G. W., Petrovitch, H., Abbott, R. D., Tanner, C. M., Popper, J., & Masaki, K. (2008). Association of olfactory dysfunction with risk for future Parkinson's disease. *Annals of Neurology*, *63*(2), 167–173. doi:10.1002/ana.21291

Roychaudhuri, R., Yang, M., Hoshi, M. M., & Teplow, D. B. (2009). Amyloid-protein assembly and Alzheimer disease. *The Journal of Biological Chemistry*, *284*, 4749–4753. doi:10.1074/jbc.R800036200

Saito, H., Kato, M., Kashima, H., Asai, M., & Hosaki, H. (1992). Effects of disinhibition on performance of the Word Fluency Test in patients with frontal lesions. *Higher Brain Function Research*, *12*, 223–231. doi:10.2496/apr.12.223

Saito, T., & Ikeda, H. (2005). *Measurement of human pain tolerance to mechanical stimulus of human-collaborative robots*. (NIIS-SRR-No.33), (pp. 15-23)

Sakai Medical Co. Ltd. (2010). *CPM Hand and wrist* (Product No.CPM-0050). Retrieved on March 20, 2010, from http://www.sakaimed.co.jp

Sakane, A., Tsuji, T., Saeki, N., & Kawamoto, M. (2004). Discrimination of vascular conditions using a probabilistic neural network. *Journal of Robotics and Mechatronics*, *16*(2), 138–145.

Sakane, A., Tsuji, T., Tanaka, Y., Saeki, N., & Kawamoto, M. (2004). Monitoring of vascular conditions using plethysmogram. *Journal of the Society of Instrument and Control Engineers*, *40*(12), 1236–1242.

Sakane, A., Shiba, K., Tsuji, T., Saeki, N., & Kawamoto, M. (2005). Non-invasive monitoring of arterial wall impedance. *Proceedings of the First International Conference on Complex Medical Engineering*, (pp. 984-989). Takamatsu, May 2005.

Sano, M., & Sawada, Y. (1985). Measurement of the Lyapunov spectrum from a chaotic time series. *Physical Review Letters*, *55*, 1082. doi:10.1103/PhysRevLett.55.1082

Santana-Sosa, E., Barriopedro, M. I., López-Mojares, L. M., Pérez, M., & Lucia, A. (2008). Exercise training is beneficial for Alzheimer's patients. *International Journal of Sports Medicine*, *29*, 845–850. doi:10.1055/s-2008-1038432

Sarvas, J. (1987). Basic mathematical and electromagnetic concepts of the biomagnetic inverse problem. *Physics in Medicine and Biology*, *32*(1), 11–22. doi:10.1088/0031-9155/32/1/004

Sasaki, D., Noritsugu, T., Yamamoto, H., & Takaiwa, M. (2006). Development of power assist glove using pneumatic artificial rubber muscle. *Journal of the Robotics Society of Japan*, *24*, 640–646.

Sato, T., Akatsuka, H., Kito, K., Tokoro, Y., Tauchi, H., & Kato, K. (1984). Age changes in size and number of muscle fibers in human minor pectoral muscle. *Mechanisms of Ageing and Development*, *28*, 99–109. doi:10.1016/0047-6374(84)90156-8

Savic, B. (2004). Imaging of olfaction and gestation. *Nutrition Reviews*, *62*, 224–241.

Sawamoto, N., Honda, M., Hanakawa, T., Fukuyama, H., & Shibasaki, H. (n.d.). Cognitive slowing in Parkinson's disease: A behavioral evaluation independent of motor slowing. *The Journal of Neuroscience*, *22*, 5198–5203.

Scarmeas, N., Albert, M., Brandt, J., Blacker, D., Hadjigeorgiou, G., & Papadimitriou, A. (2005). Motor signs predict poor outcomes in Alzheimer disease. *Neurology*, *64*, 1696–1703. doi:10.1212/01.WNL.0000162054.15428.E9

Scarmeas, N., Hadjigeorgiou, G. M., Papadimitriou, A., Dubois, B., Sarazin, M., & Brandt, J. (2004). Motor signs during the course of Alzheimer disease. *Neurology*, *63*, 975–982.

Schacter, D. L., Badgaiyan, R. D., & Alpert, N. M. (1999). Visual word stem completion priming within and across modalities: A PET study. *Neuroreport*, *10*, 2061–2065. doi:10.1097/00001756-199907130-00013

Schaubert, K. L., & Bohannon, R. W. (2005). Reliability and validity of three strength measures obtained from community-dwelling elderly persons. *Journal of Strength and Conditioning Research*, *19*, 717–720.

Scherer, K. R., Johnstone, T., & Klasmeyer, G. (2003). Vocal expression of emotion. In Davidson, R. J., Goldsmith, H., & Scherer, K. R. (Eds.), *Handbook of the affective sciences* (pp. 433–456). Oxford University Press.

Schmidt, M. L., & Trojanowski, J. Q. (1985). Immunoblot analysis of horseradish peroxidase conjugates of wheat germ agglutinin before and after retrograde transport in the rat peripheral nervous system. *The Journal of Neuroscience*, *5*, 2779–2785.

Schubotz, R. I., & von Cramon, D. Y. (2003). Auditory what, where, and when: A sensory somatotopy in lateral premotor cortex. *NeuroImage*, *20*(1), 173–185. doi:10.1016/S1053-8119(03)00218-0

Schulz, M., Chau, W., Graham, S. J., McIntosh, A. R., Ross, B., Ishii, R., & Pantev, C. (2004). An integrative MEG-fMRI study of the primary somatosensory cortex using cross-modal correspondence analysis. *NeuroImage*, *22*, 120–133. doi:10.1016/j.neuroimage.2003.10.049

Schwarz, G. E. (1978). Estimating the dimension of a model. *Annals of Statistics*, *6*(2), 461–464. doi:10.1214/aos/1176344136

Sekuler, R., & Blake, R. (2002). *Perception* (4th ed.). Boston, MA: McGraw-Hill Higher Education.

Selkoe, D. J. (2002). Alzheimer's disease is a synaptic failure. *Science*, *298*, 789–791. doi:10.1126/science.1074069

Shallice, T., & Burgress, P. W. (1991). Higher order cognitive impairments and frontal lobe lesions in man. In Levin, H. S., Eisenberg, H. M., & Benton, A. L. (Eds.), *Frontal lobe function and dysfunction* (pp. 125–138). New York, NY: Oxford University Press.

Sheth, S., Nemoto, M., Guiou, M., Walker, M., Pouratian, N., & Toga, A. W. (2003). Evaluation of coupling between optical intrinsic signals and neuronal activity in rat somatosensory cortex. *NeuroImage*, *19*, 884–894. doi:10.1016/S1053-8119(03)00086-7

Shiga, K., Yamada, K., Yoshikawa, K., Mizuno, T., Nishimura, T., & Nakagawa, M. (2005). Local tissue anisotropy decreases in cerebellopetal fibers and pyramidal tract in multiple system atrophy. *Journal of Neurology*, *252*, 589–596. doi:10.1007/s00415-005-0708-0

Shigeo, K. (1998). *The traditional music of Japan*. Tokyo, Japan: Ongaku no tomo sya.

Shimura, T., Tsunada, T., Maki, A., Suzuki, T., Haida, M., Kaneko, M., et al. Asakawa, T. (2009). *Prefrontal lobe measurement using near infrared spectroscopy-evaluation of early detection methods and rehabilitation methods of dementia*. Tokyo, Japan: Corona Publishing Co, Ltd.

Shoghi-Jadid, K., Small, G. W., Agdeppa, E. D., Kepe, V., Ercoli, L. M., & Siddarth, P. (2002). Localization of neurofibrillary tangles and beta-amyloid plaques in the brains of living patients with Alzheimer disease. *The American Journal of Geriatric Psychiatry*, *10*, 24–35.

Siebner, H. R., Peller, M., Willoch, F., Minoshima, S., Boecker, H., & Auer, C. (2000). Lasting cortical activation after repetitive TMS of the motor cortex. A glucose metabolic study. *Neurology*, *54*, 956–963.

Singer, H. W., & Gray, C. M. (1995). Visual feature integration and the temporal correlation hypothesis. *Annual Review of Neuroscience*, *18*, 555–586. doi:10.1146/annurev.ne.18.030195.003011

Sinha, S., Anderson, J. P., Barbour, R., Basi, G. S., Caccavello, R., & Davis, D. (1999). Purification and cloning of amyloid precursor protein beta-secretase from human brain. *Nature*, *402*(6761), 537–540. doi:10.1038/990114

Sioka, C., Fotopoulos, A., & Kyritsis, A. P. (2010). Recent advances in PET imaging for evaluation of Parkinson's disease. *European Journal of Nuclear Medicine and Molecular Imaging*.

Skoog, I., Davidsson, P., Aevarsson, O., Vanderstichele, H., Vanmechelen, E., & Blennow, K. (2003). Cerebrospinal fluid beta-amyloid 42 is reduced before the onset of sporadic dementia: A population-based study in 85-year-olds. *Dementia and Geriatric Cognitive Disorders*, *15*(3), 169–176. doi:10.1159/000068478

Smith, A. T., Wall, M. B., Williams, A. L., & Singh, K. D. (2006). Sensitivity to optic flow in human cortical areas MT and MST. *The European Journal of Neuroscience*, *23*, 561–569. doi:10.1111/j.1460-9568.2005.04526.x

Snowden, R. J., Treue, S., Erickson, R. G., & Andersen, R. A. (1991). The response of area MT and V1 neurons to transparent motion. *The Journal of Neuroscience*, *11*, 2768–2785.

Sobel, N., Prabhakaran, V., Desmond, J. E., Glover, G. H., Goode, R. L., & Sullivan, E. V. (1998). Sniffing and smelling: Separate subsystems in the human olfactory cortex. *Nature*, *392*, 282–286. doi:10.1038/32654

Solfrizzi, V., Panza, F., Colacicco, A. M., D'Introno, A., Capurso, C., & Torres, F. (2004). Vascular risk factors, incidence of MCI, and rates of progression to dementia. *Neurology*, *63*(10), 1882–1891.

Song, G., & Guo, S. (2007). A novel self-assisted rehabilitation system for the upper limbs based on virtual reality. *International Journal of Information Acquisition, 3*.

Spires, T. L., Meyer-Luehmann, M., Stern, E. A., McLean, P. J., Skoch, J., & Nguyen, P. T. (2005). Dendritic spine abnormalities in amyloid precursor protein transgenic mice demonstrated by gene transfer and intravital multiphoton microscopy. *The Journal of Neuroscience*, *25*, 7278–7287. doi:10.1523/JNEUROSCI.1879-05.2005

Steinke, W. R., Cuddy, L. L., & Jakobson, L. S. (2001). Dissociations among functional subsystems governing melody recognition after right-hemisphere damage. *Cognitive Neuropsychology*, *18*(5), 411–437.

Stosiek, C., Garaschuk, O., Holthoff, K., & Konnerth, A. (2003). In vivo two-photon calcium imaging of neuronal networks. *Proceedings of the National Academy of Sciences of the United States of America*, *100*, 7319–7324. doi:10.1073/pnas.1232232100

Strayer, D. L., & Drews, F. A. (2006). A comparison of the cell phone driver and the drunk driver. *Human Factors: The Journal of the Human Factors and Ergonomics Society*, *48*(2), 381–391. doi:10.1518/001872006777724471

Subramanyam, R., Alpert, N. M., Hoop, B., Brownell, G. L., & Taveras, J. M. (1978). A model for regional cerebral oxygen distribution during continuous inhalation of 15O2, C15O, and C15O2. *Journal of Nuclear Medicine*, *19*(1), 48–53.

Suda, M., Morimoto, K., Obata, A., Koizumi, H., & Maki, A. (2008). Emotional responses to music, towards scientic perspectives on music therapy. *Neuroreport*, *19*(18), 75–78. doi:10.1097/WNR.0b013e3282f3476f

Sugishita, M., & Yamazaki, K. (1993). *Japanese raven's coloured progressive matrices*. Tokyo, Japan: Nihonbunnkakagakusya.

Suh, G. H., Ju, Y. S., Yeon, B. K., & Shah, A. (2004). A longitudinal study of Alzheimer's disease: Rates of cognitive and functional decline. *International Journal of Geriatric Psychiatry*, *19*(9), 817–824. doi:10.1002/gps.1168

Sunderland, A., Tinson, D. J., Bradely, E. L., Eletcher, D., Langton, H. R., & Wade, D. T. (1992). Enhanced physical therapy improves recovery of arm function after stroke: A randomized controlled trial. *Journal of Neurology, Neurosurgery, and Psychiatry*, *55*, 530–535. doi:10.1136/jnnp.55.7.530

Suomi, R., Surburg, P. R., & Lecius, P. (1993). Reliability of isokinetic and isometric measurement of leg strength on men with mental retardation. *Archives of Physical Medicine and Rehabilitation*, *74*, 848–852. doi:10.1016/0003-9993(93)90012-Y

Suparna, M. (2005). Music intervention for disruptive behaviors in long-term care residents with dementia, *Annals of Long-Term Care, 13*.

Suzuki, M., Yamada, S., Inamura, A., Omori, Y., Kirimoto, H., Sugimura, S., & Miyamoto, M. (2009). Reliability and validity of measurements of knee extension strength obtained from nursing home residents with dementia. *American Journal of Physical Medicine & Rehabilitation, 88*, 924–933. doi:10.1097/PHM.0b013e3181ae1003

Suzuki, M., Yamada, S., Omori, M., Hatakeyama, M., Sugimura, Y., Matsushita, K., & Tagawa, Y. (2008). Development of the upper-body dressing scale for a buttoned shirt: A preliminary correlational study. *American Journal of Physical Medicine & Rehabilitation, 87*, 740–749. doi:10.1097/PHM.0b013e31818378b0

Szelies, B., Grond, M., Herholz, K., Kessler, J., Wullen, T., & Heiss, W. D. (1992). Quantitative EEG mapping and PET in Alzheimer's disease. *Journal of the Neurological Sciences, 110*, 46–56. doi:10.1016/0022-510X(92)90008-9

Takahashi, S., Yonezawa, H., Takahashi, J., Kudo, M., Inoue, T., & Tohgi, H. (2002). Selective reduction of diffusion anisotropy in white matter of Alzheimer disease brains measured by 3.0 Tesla magnetic resonance imaging. *Neuroscience Letters, 332*, 45–48. doi:10.1016/S0304-3940(02)00914-X

Takayama, Y. (2003). Conditions necessary for the screening tests to detect early stage of dementia. *Japanese Journal of Geriatric Psychiatry, 14*, 13–19.

Takemiya, T., Maeda, J., Suzuki, J., Nishihira, Y., & Shimoda, M. (1996). Differential digital photoplethysmographic observations of finger vascular exponential response to the arm position changes in humans. *Advances in Exercise and Sports Physiology, 2*(2), 83–90.

Takens, F. (1985). *Dynamical systems and bifurcations* (Braaksma, B. L. J., Broer, H. W., & Takens, F., eds). (LNM 1125). Heidelberg, Germany: Springer.

Takeuchi, Y., Matsumoto, Y., Miki, T., Yokoyama, T., Warita, K., & Wang, Z. Y. (2009). Anterograde synaptic transport of neuronal tracer enzyme (WGA-HRP): Further studies with Rab3A-siRNA in the rat. *Biomedical Research, 20*, 149–154. doi:10.4103/0970-938X.54832

Talbot, P. S., & Laruelle, M. (2002). The role of in vivo molecular imaging with PET and SPECT in the elucidation of psychiatric drug action and new drug development. *European Neuropsychopharmacology, 12*(6), 503–511. doi:10.1016/S0924-977X(02)00099-8

Taler, V., Baum, S. R., Chertkow, H., & Saumier, D. (2008). Comprehension of grammatical and emotional prosody is impaired in Alzheimer's disease. *Neuropsychology, 22*(2), 188–195. doi:10.1037/0894-4105.22.2.188

Taler, V., & Phillips, N. (2007). Language performance in Alzheimer's disease and mild cognitive impairment: A comparative review. *Journal of Clinical and Experimental Neuropsychology, 30*(5), 501–556. doi:10.1080/13803390701550128

Talsma, D., Doty, T. J., & Woldorff, M. G. (2007). Selective attention and audiovisual integration: Is attending to both modalities a prerequisite for early integration? *Cerebral Cortex, 17*(3), 679–690. doi:10.1093/cercor/bhk016

Talsma, D., & Woldorff, M. G. (2005). Selective attention and multisensory integration: multiple phases of effects on the evoked brain activity. *Journal of Cognitive Neuroscience, 17*(7), 1098–1114. doi:10.1162/0898929054475172

Tamura, H., Okumura, D., & Tanno, K. (2007). A study of motion recognition without FFT from surface-EMG. *Transactions of the Institute of Electronics, Information and Communication Engineers, J90*, 2652–2655.

Tan, L. H., Chan, A. H. D., Kay, P., Khong, P. L., Yip, L. K. C., & Luke, K. K. (2008). Language affects patterns of brain activation associated with perceptual decision. *Proceedings of the National Academy of Sciences of the United States of America, 105*, 4004–4009. doi:10.1073/pnas.0800055105

Tan, L. H., Liu, H. L., Perfetti, C. A., Spinks, J. A., Fox, P. T., & Gao, J. H. (2001). The neural system underlying Chinese logograph reading. *NeuroImage, 12*, 836–846. doi:10.1006/nimg.2001.0749

Tan, L. H., Spinks, J. A., Feng, C. M., Siok, W. T., Perfetti, C. A., & Xiong, J. (2003). Neural systems of second language reading are shaped by native language. *Human Brain Mapping, 18*, 158–166. doi:10.1002/hbm.10089

Tan, L. H., Spinks, J. A., Gao, J. H., Liu, H. L., Perfetti, C. A., & Xiong, J. H. (2000). Brain activation in the processing of Chinese characters and words: A functional MRI study. *Human Brain Mapping*, *10*, 16–27. doi:10.1002/(SICI)1097-0193(200005)10:1<16::AID-HBM30>3.0.CO;2-M

Taoka, T., Iwasaki, S., Sakamoto, M., Nakagawa, H., Fukusumi, A., & Myochin, K. (2006). Diffusion anisotropy and diffusivity of white matter tracts within the temporal stem in Alzheimer disease: Evaluation of the tract of interest by diffusion tensor tractography. *AJNR. American Journal of Neuroradiology*, *27*, 1040–1045.

Tashiro, M., Itoh, M., Fujimoto, T., Masud, M. M., Watanuki, S., & Yanai, K. (2008). Application of positron emission tomography to neuroimaging in sports sciences. *Methods (San Diego, Calif.)*, *45*, 300–306. doi:10.1016/j.ymeth.2008.05.001

Tashiro, M., Miyake, M., Masud, M. M., Ogura, M., Watanuki, S., & Yanai, K. (2010). Nano-bio-imaging with radiopharmaceuticals and its application to health sciences. *Annals of nanoBME, 3*, 73-87.

Taue, S., Ichihara, S., Sugihara, Y., Ishikawa, K., Sugioka, H., & Mizutani, N. … Kobayashi, T. (2008). Measurement of biomagnetic fields in small animals by use of an optical pumping atomic magnetometer. In R. Kakigi, et al (Eds.), *Biomagnetism*. (pp. 9-11). Hokkaido University Press.

Taylor, D. H., & Sloan, F. A. (2000). How much do persons with Alzheimer's disease cost Medicare? *Journal of the American Geriatrics Society*, *48*, 639–646.

Teder-Salejarvi, W. A., Di Russo, F., McDonald, J. J., & Hillyard, S. A. (2005). Effects of spatial congruity on audio-visual multimodal integration. *Journal of Cognitive Neuroscience*, *17*(9), 1396–1409. doi:10.1162/0898929054985383

Teder-Salejarvi, W. A., McDonald, J. J., Di Russo, F., & Hillyard, S. A. (2002). An analysis of audio-visual crossmodal integration by means of event-related potential (ERP) recordings. *Brain Research. Cognitive Brain Research*, *14*(1), 106–114. doi:10.1016/S0926-6410(02)00065-4

Teri, L., Gibbons, L. E., McCurry, S. M., Logsdon, R. G., Buchner, D. M., & Barlow, W. E. (2003). Exercise plus behavioral management in patients with Alzheimer disease: A randomized controlled trial. *Journal of the American Medical Association*, *290*, 2015–2022. doi:10.1001/jama.290.15.2015

Thomas, V. S., & Hageman, P. A. (2003). A preliminary study on the reliability of physical performance measures in older day-care center clients with dementia. *International Psychogeriatrics*, *14*, 17–23. doi:10.1017/S1041610202008244

Thomas, V. S., & Hageman, P. A. (2003). Can neuromuscular strength and function in people with dementia be rehabilitated using resistance-exercise training? Results from a preliminary intervention study. *Journals of Gerontology A Biological Sciences and Medical Sciences, 58A*, 746-751.

Tobimatsu, S. (2002). Neurophysiologic tools to explore visual cognition. *Electroencephalography and Clinical Neurophysiology*, *S54*, 261–265. doi:10.1016/S1567-424X(09)70459-3

Tobimatsu, S., & Celesia, G. G. (2006). Studies of human visual pathophysiology with visual evoked potentials. *Clinical Neurophysiology*, *117*, 1414–1433. doi:10.1016/j.clinph.2006.01.004

Tobimatsu, S., Celesia, G. G., Haug, B. A., Onofrj, M., Sartucci, F., & Porciatti, V. (2000). Recent advances in clinical neurophysiology of vision. *Electroencephalography and Clinical Neurophysiology*, *S53*, 312–322. doi:10.1016/S1567-424X(09)70174-6

Tobimatsu, S., Goto, Y., Yamasaki, T., Tsurusawa, R., & Taniwaki, T. (2006). An integrated approach to face and motion perception in humans. *Clinical Neurophysiology*, *S59*, 41–46.

Tobimatsu, S., & Kato, M. (1998). Multimodality visual evoked potentials in evaluating visual dysfunction in optic neuritis. *Neurology*, *50*, 715–718.

Tobimatsu, S., Shigeto, H., Arakawa, K., & Kato, M. (1999). Electrophysiological studies of parallel visual processing in humans. *Electroencephalography and Clinical Neurophysiology*, *S49*, 103–107.

Tobimatsu, S., Tomoda, H., & Kato, M. (1995). Parvocellular and magnocellular contributions to visual evoked potentials in humans: Stimulation with chromatic and achromatic gratings and apparent motion. *Journal of the Neurological Sciences*, *34*, 73–82. doi:10.1016/0022-510X(95)00222-X

Tobimatsu, S., & Celesia, G. G. (2006). Studies of human visual pathophysiology with visual evoked potentials. *Clinical Neurophysiology*, *117*, 1414–1433. doi:10.1016/j.clinph.2006.01.004

Tobimatsu, S., Goto, Y., Yamasaki, T., Nakashima, T., Tomoda, Y., & Mitsudome, A. (2008). Visual ERPs and cortical function in Progress in epileptic disorders vol. 5, Event-related potentials in patients with epilepsy: From current state to future prospects. (A. Ikeda A and Y. Inoue, Eds). (pp. 37-48). Paris, France: John Libbey Eurotext.

Tomiyama, T., Nagata, T., Shimada, H., Teraoka, R., Fukushima, A., & Kanemitsu, H. (2008). A new Amyloid β variant favoring oligomerization in Alzheimer's-type dementia. *Annals of Neurology*, *63*, 377–387. doi:10.1002/ana.21321

Tootell, R. B., Reppas, J. B., Kwong, K. K., Malach, R., Born, R. T., & Brady, T. J. (1995). Functional analysis of human MT and related visual cortical areas using magnetic resonance imaging. *The Journal of Neuroscience*, *15*, 3215–3230.

Toshiyoki, K., Masashi, S., & Makoto, T. (2002). Sound localization with the speakers in the front vertical plane. (IEICE technical report). *ME and Bio Cybernetics*, *101*(733), 103–107.

Touge, T., Gerschlager, W., Cordivari, C., Brown, P., & Rothwell, J. C. (2001). Are the after-effects of low–frequency rTMS on motor cortex excitability due to changes in the efficacy of cortical synapses? *Clinical Neurophysiology*, *112*, 2138–2145. doi:10.1016/S1388-2457(01)00651-4

Touge, T., Urai, Y., & Shimamura, Y. (2009). *Excitability changes of corticospinal pathways by magnetic brain stimulation during the maximum voluntary muscle contraction*. CME2009.

Trick, G. L., Trick, L. R., Morris, P., & Wolf, W. (1995). Visual field loss in senile dementia of the Alzheimer's type. *Neurology*, *45*, 68–74.

Troyer, A. K. (2000). Normative data for clustering and switching on verbal fluency tasks. *Journal of Clinical and Experimental Neuropsychology*, *22*, 370–378. doi:10.1076/1380-3395(200006)22:3;1-V;FT370

Troyer, A. K., & Murphy, J. K. (2007). Memory for intentions in amnestic mild cognitive impairment; Time- and event-based prospective memory. *Journal of the International Neuropsychological Society*, *13*, 365–369. doi:10.1017/S1355617707070452

Tsubahara, A. (2008). Technological advance in medical rehabilitation. *Kawasaki Journal of Medical Welfare*, *18*, 7–14.

Tsuda, I., Tahara, T., & Iwanaga, I. (1992). Chaotic pulsation in capillary vessels and its dependence on mental and physical conditions. *International Journal of Bifurcation and Chaos in Applied Sciences and Engineering*, *2*, 313–324. doi:10.1142/S0218127492000318

Tsuguo, O. (1972). *Appear frequency of Japanese words* (pp. 1–62). Doushisya University Press.

Tsukagoshi, H., Shirato, K., Ido, M., & Kitagawa, A. (2004). Tail-arm: A wearable unit to stimulate exercise. *Proceedings of the 13th IEEE International Workshop on Robot and Human Interactive Communication RO-MAN2004*, (p. 667).

Tsunazawa, Y., Oikawa, Y., Iwamoto, S., Eda, H., & Takada, M. (1996). Spatially resolved spectroscopy for extracting spectrum of hemoglobin diluted in a highly scattering medium, biomedical optical spectroscopy and diagnostics. In Sevick-Muraca, E., & Benaron, D. (Eds.), *Biomedical optical spectroscopy and diagnostics: Technical digest* (pp. 119–121). Washington, DC: Optical Society of America.

Tukahira, Y., Endo, T., Sawada, A., Komoda, H., Miura, H., & Tanaka, Y. … Kouchi, R. (2007). *A basic glossary of terms of the Japanese music*. Tokyo, Japan: Ongaku tomo sya corp.

Ueki, S., Nishimoto, Y., Abe, M., Kawasaki, H., Ito, S., & Ishigure, Y. … Ojika, T. (2008). Development of virtual reality exercise of hand motion assist robot for rehabilitation therapy by patient self-motion control. *Proceedings of the 30th Annual International IEEE EMBS Conference*. August 2008, (pp. 4282-4285).

Ugawa, Y., Uesaka, Y., Terao, Y., Hanajima, R., & Kanazawa, I. (1994). Magnetic stimulation of corticospinal pathways at the foramen magnum level in humans. *Annals of Neurology*, *36*, 618–624. doi:10.1002/ana.410360410

Umeda, S. (2004). Prospective memory impairment in elderly. *Japanese Journal of Geriatric Psychiatry*, *15*, 725–730.

Umeda, S., & Koyazu, T. (1998). Prospective memory and its theoretical consideration. *Shinrigaku Kenkyu*, *69*, 317–333.

United Nations (Ed.). (2004). *World population to 2300*. New York, NY: Bernan Assoc.

Urbach, D., & Awiszus, F. (2002). Stimulus strength on maximal voluntary contraction force of human quadriceps femoris muscle. *Experimental Brain Research*, *142*, 25–31. doi:10.1007/s00221-001-0911-x

Urbach, D., Berth, A., & Awiszus, F. (2005). Effect of transcranial magnetic stimulation on voluntary activation in patients with quadriceps weakness. *Muscle & Nerve*, *32*, 164–169. doi:10.1002/mus.20353

Vanbellingen, T., Kersten, B., Van Hemelrijk, B., Van de Winckel, A., Bertschi, M., & Muri, R. (2010). Comprehensive assessment of gesture production: A new test of upper kimb apraxia (TULIA). *European Journal of Neurology*, *17*(1), 59–66. doi:10.1111/j.1468-1331.2009.02741.x

Vassar, R., Bennett, B. D., Babu-Khan, S., Kahn, S., Mendiaz, E. A., & Denis, P. (1999). Beta-secretase cleavage of Alzheimer's amyloid precursor protein by the transmembrane aspartic protease BACE. *Science*, *286*(5440), 735–741. doi:10.1126/science.286.5440.735

Verheijen, J. H., Huisman, L. G., van Lent, N., Neumann, U., Paganetti, P., & Hack, C. E. (2006). Detection of a soluble form of BACE-1 in human cerebrospinal fluid by a sensitive activity assay. *Clinical Chemistry*, *52*(6), 1168–1174. doi:10.1373/clinchem.2006.066720

Verhoeff, N. P., Wilson, A. A., Takeshita, S., Trop, L., Hussey, D., & Singh, K. (2004). In-vivo imaging of Alzheimer disease beta-amyloid with [11C]SB-13 PET. *The American Journal of Geriatric Psychiatry*, *12*, 584–595.

Vickers, J. C., Dickson, T. C., Adlard, P. A., Saunders, H. L., King, C. E., & McCormack, G. (2000). The cause of neuronal degeneration in Alzheimer's disease. *Progress in Neurobiology*, *60*, 139–165. doi:10.1016/S0301-0082(99)00023-4

Vidal, J., Giard, M. H., Roux, S., Barthelemy, C., & Bruneau, N. (2008). Cross-modal processing of auditory-visual stimuli in a no-task paradigm: a topographic event-related potential study. *Clinical Neurophysiology*, *119*(4), 763–771. doi:10.1016/j.clinph.2007.11.178

Villemagne, V. L., McLean, C. A., Reardon, K., Boyd, A., Lewis, V., & Klug, G. (2009). ^{11}C-PiB PET studies in typical sporadic Creutzfeldt-Jakob disease. *Journal of Neurology, Neurosurgery, and Psychiatry*, *80*, 998–1001. doi:10.1136/jnnp.2008.171496

Voisin, J., Benoit, G., & Chapman, C. E. (2002). Haptic discrimination of object shape in humans: Two-dimensional (2-D) angle discrimination. *Experimental Brain Research*, *145*, 239–250. doi:10.1007/s00221-002-1117-6

Voisin, J., Lamarre, Y., & Capman, C. E. (2002). Haptic discrimination of object shape in humans: Contribution of cutaneous and proprioceptive inputs. *Experimental Brain Research*, *145*, 251–260. doi:10.1007/s00221-002-1118-5

von Bartheld, C. S. (2004). Axonal transport and neuronal transcytosis of trophic factors, tracers, and pathogens. *Journal of Neurobiology*, *58*, 295–314. doi:10.1002/neu.10315

Vroomen, J., & de Gelder, B. (2000). *Sound enhances visual perception: Cross-modal effects of auditory organization on vision*. Washington, DC: ETATS-UNIS, American Psychological Association.

Vuilleumier, P., Armony, J. L., Driver, J., & Dolna, R. J. (2003). Distinct spatial frequency sensitivities for processing faces and emotional expressions. *Nature Neuroscience*, *6*, 624–631. doi:10.1038/nn1057

Wade, D. T., Langton, H. R., Woov, V. A., Skilbeck, C. E., & Ismail, H. M. (1983). The hemiplegic arm after stroke: Measurement and recovery. *Journal of Neurology, Neurosurgery, and Psychiatry*, *46*, 521–524. doi:10.1136/jnnp.46.6.521

Wakamatsu, N., Anamizu, S., & Kato, M. (2003). Rey Auditory Verbal Learning Test (RAVLT). *Japanese Journal of Clinical Medicine*, *61*(9), 279–284.

Walsh, D. M., Klyubin, I., Fadeeva, J. V., Cullen, W. K., Anwyl, R., & Wolfe, M. S. (2002). Naturally secreted oligomers of amyloid β protein potently inhibit hippocampal long-term potentiation in vivo. *Nature*, *416*, 535–539. doi:10.1038/416535a

Walsh, D. M., Lomakin, A., Benedek, G. B., Condron, M. M., & Teplow, D. B. (1997). Amyloid beta-protein fibrillogenesis. Detection of a protofibrillar intermediate. *The Journal of Biological Chemistry*, *272*, 22364–22372. doi:10.1074/jbc.272.35.22364

Wang, H. B., Takahashi, S., & Wu, J. L. (2008). Human characteristics of length perception with three fingers for tactile intelligent interfaces. *Active Media Technology*, 217-225.

Waragai, M., Okamura, N., Furukawa, K., Tashiro, M., Furumoto, S., & Funaki, Y. (2009). Comparison study of amyloid PET and voxel-based morphometry analysis in mild cognitive impairment and Alzheimer's disease. *Journal of the Neurological Sciences*, *285*, 100–108. doi:10.1016/j.jns.2009.06.005

Waragai, M., Okamura, N., Furukawa, K., Tashiro, M., Furumoto, S., & Funaki, Y. (2009). Comparison study of amyloid PET and voxel-based morphometry analysis in mild cognitive impairment and Alzheimer's disease. *Journal of the Neurological Sciences*, *285*, 100–108. doi:10.1016/j.jns.2009.06.005

Warkentin, S., Risberg, J., & Nilsson, A. (1991). Cortical activity during speech production; A study of regional blood flow in normal subjects performing a word fluency task. *Neuropsychiatry, Neuropsychology, and Behavioral Neurology*, *4*, 305–316.

Warren, W. H., & Hannon, D. J. (1988). Direction of self-motion is perceived from optic flow. *Nature*, *336*, 162–163. doi:10.1038/336162a0

Watabe, H., Endres, C., Breier, A., Schmall, B., Eckelman, W., & Carson, R. (2000). Measurement of dopamine release with continuous infusion of (11C) raclopride: Optimization and signal-to-noise considerations. *Journal of Nuclear Medicine*, *41*(3), 522–530.

Watabe, H., Ikoma, Y., Kimura, Y., Naganawa, M., & Shidahara, M. (2006). PET kinetic analysis–compartmental model. *Annals of Nuclear Medicine*, *20*(9), 583–589. doi:10.1007/BF02984655

Watamori, T., Hara, H., Miyamori, T., & Eto, F. (2002). *The Japanese version of the Rivermead Behavioural Memory Test*. Tokyo, Japan: Chiba Test Center.

Westlind-Danielsson, A., & Arnerup, G. (2001). Spontaneous in vitro formation of supramolecular β-amyloid structures, βamyballs, by β- amyloid 1-40 peptide. *Biochemistry*, *40*, 14736–14743. doi:10.1021/bi010375c

Wheaton, L. A., & Hallett, M. (2007). Ideomotor apraxia: A review. *Journal of the Neurological Sciences*, *260*, 1–10. doi:10.1016/j.jns.2007.04.014

Wiegell, M. R., Larsson, H. B., & Wedeen, V. J. (2000). Fiber crossing in human brain depicted with diffusion tensor MR imaging. *Radiology*, *217*, 897–903.

Wikholm, J. B., & Bohannon, R. W. (1991). Hand-held dynamometer measurements: Tester strength makes a difference. *The Journal of Orthopaedic and Sports Physical Therapy*, *13*, 191–198.

Wikipedia. (2010). *Language*. http://en.wikipedia.org/wiki/Language.

Wilson, B. A., Cockburn, J. M., & Baddeley, A. D. (1985). *The Rivermead Behavioral Memory Test. Bury St.* Edmunds, England: Thames Valley Test Company.

Wilson, R. S., Bennett, D. A., Gilley, D. W., Beckett, L. A., Schneider, J. A., & Evans, D. A. (2000). Progression of Parkinsonian signs in Alzheimer's disease. *Neurology*, *54*, 1284–1289.

Wilson, R. S., Schneider, J. A., Bienias, J. L., Evans, D. A., & Bennett, D. A. (2003). Parkinsonianlike signs and risk of incident Alzheimers disease in older persons. *Archives of Neurology*, *60*, 539–544. doi:10.1001/archneur.60.4.539

Winckel, A. V. (2004). Cognitive and behavioral effects of music-based exercises in patients with dementia. *Clinical Rehabilitation*, *18*(3), 253–260. doi:10.1191/0269215504cr750oa

Witwer, B. P., Moftakhar, R., Hasan, K. M., Deshmukh, P., Haughton, V., & Field, A. (2002). Diffusion-tensor imaging of white matter tracts in patients with cerebral neoplasm. *Journal of Neurosurgery*, *97*, 568–575. doi:10.3171/jns.2002.97.3.0568

Wolf, S. L., Blanton, S., Baer, H., Breshears, J., & Butler, A. J. (2002). Contemporary linkages between EMG, kinetics and stroke rehabilitation. *The Neurologist*, *8*, 325–338. doi:10.1097/00127893-200211000-00001

Wolfson, L., Judge, J., Whipple, R., & King, M. (1995). Strength is a major factor in balance, gait, and the occurrence of falls. *The Journals of Gerontology. Series A, Biological Sciences and Medical Sciences*, *50*, 64–67.

Woo, S., Watabe, H., Choi, Y., Kim, K., Park, C., & Bloomfield, P. (2004). Sinogram-based motion correction of PET images using optical motion tracking system and list-mode data acquisition. *IEEE Transactions on Nuclear Science*, *51*(3), 782–788. doi:10.1109/TNS.2004.829786

Wu, J. L., & Kawamura, S. (2000). Quantitative analysis of human tactile illusory characteristic under visual environment and a haptic device of two-dimensional curved surface. *IEEE Transactions on Robotics and Automation*, *16*, 762–771. doi:10.1109/70.897787

Wurzel, M., Cowper, G. R., & McCook, J. M. (1969). Smooth muscle contraction and viscoelasticity of arterial wall. *Canadian Journal of Physiology and Pharmacology*, *48*, 510–523.

Xian, X., Liu, T., Yu, J., Wang, Y., Miao, Y., & Zhang, J. (2009). Presynaptic defects underlying impaired learning and memory function in lipoprotein lipase deficient mice. *The Journal of Neuroscience*, *29*(14), 4681–4685. doi:10.1523/JNEUROSCI.0297-09.2009

Yamada, K. (2009). Diffusion tensor tractography should be used with caution. *Proceedings of the National Academy of Sciences of the United States of America*, *106*, E14. doi:10.1073/pnas.0812352106

Yamada, K., Ito, H., Nakamura, H., Akada, W., Kubota, T., & Goto, M. (2004). Stroke patients' evolving symptoms assessed by tractography. *Journal of Magnetic Resonance Imaging*, *20*, 923–929. doi:10.1002/jmri.20215

Yamada, K., Kizu, O., Ito, H., & Nishimura, T. (2004). Tractography for an arteriovenous malformation. *Neurology*, *62*, 669.

Yamada, K., Kizu, O., Kubota, T., Ito, H., Matsushima, S., Oouchi, H., & Nishimura, T. (2007). The pyramidal tract has a predictable course through centrum semiovale: A diffusion-tensor based tractography study. *Journal of Magnetic Resonance Imaging*, *26*, 519–524. doi:10.1002/jmri.21006

Yamada, K., Kizu, O., Mori, S., Ito, H., Nakamura, H., & Yuen, S. (2003). Clinically feasible diffusion-tensor imaging for fiber tracking. *Radiology*, *227*, 295–301. doi:10.1148/radiol.2271020313

Yamada, K., Mori, S., Nakamura, H., Ito, H., Kizu, O., & Shiga, K. (2003). Fiber-tracking method reveals sensorimotor pathway involvement in stroke patients. *Stroke*, *34*, E159–E162. doi:10.1161/01.STR.0000085827.54986.89

Yamada, K., Nagakane, Y., Yoshikawa, K., Kizu, O., Ito, H., & Kubota, T. (2007). Somatotopic organization of thalamocortical projection fibers as assessed by MR tractography-initial observations. *Radiology*, *242*, 840–845. doi:10.1148/radiol.2423060297

Yamada, K., Shiga, K., Kizu, O., Ito, H., Akiyama, K., Nakagawa, M., & Nishimura, T. (2006). Oculomotor nerve palsy evaluated by diffusion-tensor tractography. *Neuroradiology*, *48*, 434–437. doi:10.1007/s00234-006-0070-7

Yamada, Y., Suita, K., Ikeda, H., Sugimoto, N., Miura, H., & Nakamura, H. (1997). Evaluation of pain tolerance based on a biomechanical method for human-robot coexistence. *Journal of Japan Mechanical Engineers*, *96*(612), 238–243.

Yamamoto, T., Yamada, K., Nishimura, T., & Kinoshita, S. (2005). Tractography to depict three layers of visual field trajectories to the calcarine gyri. *American Journal of Ophthalmology*, *140*, 781–785. doi:10.1016/j.ajo.2005.05.018

Yamasaki, T., Fujita, T., Kamio, Y., & Tobimatsu, S. (2009). Visual motion processing in autism spectrum disorder. *Clinical EEG (Electroencephalography)*, *51*, 463–469.

Yamasaki, T., Goto, Y., & Tobimatsu, S. (2006). Evoked potentials related to motion perception and face recognition. *Clinical EEG (Electroencephalography)*, *48*, 413–418.

Yan, Y., Jin, F., & Wu, J. (2009). *Correlated size variations measured in human visual cortex V1/V2/V3 with functional MRI. (LNAI 5819)* (pp. 36–44). Berlin/ Heidelberg, Germany: Brain Informatics/Springer-Verlag.

Yan, R., Bienkowski, M. J., Shuck, M. E., Miao, H., Tory, M. C., & Pauley, A. M. (1999). Membraneanchored aspartyl protease with Alzheimer's disease beta-secretase activity. *Nature*, *402*(6761), 533–537. doi:10.1038/990107

Yanai, K., & Tashiro, M. (2007). The physiological and pathophysiological roles of neuronal histamine: An insight from human positron emission tomography studies. *Pharmacology & Therapeutics*, *113*, 1–15. doi:10.1016/j.pharmthera.2006.06.008

Yang, L. B., Lindholm, K., Yan, R., Citron, M., Xia, W., & Yang, X. L. (2003). Elevated beta-secretase expression and enzymatic activity detected in sporadic Alzheimer disease. *Nature Medicine*, *9*(1), 3–4. doi:10.1038/nm0103-3

Yankner, B. A., Dawes, L. R., Fisher, S., Villa-Komaroff, L., Oster-Granite, M. L., & Neve, R. L. (1989). Neurotoxicity of a fragment of the amyloid precursor associated with Alzheimer's disease. *Science*, *245*, 417–420. doi:10.1126/science.2474201

Yasmin, H., Nakata, Y., Aoki, S., Abe, O., Sato, N., & Nemoto, K. (2008). Diffusion abnormalities of the uncinate fasciculus in Alzheimer's disease: Diffusion tensor tract-specific analysis using a new method to measure the core of the tract. *Neuroradiology*, *50*, 293–299. doi:10.1007/s00234-007-0353-7

Yasuda, K., Kuwabara, K., Kuwahara, N., Abe, S., & Tetsuntani, N. (2009). Effectiveness of personalized reminiscence photo videos for individuals with dementia. *Neuropsychological Rehabilitation*, *19*(4), 603–619. doi:10.1080/09602010802586216

Yoshida, T., Shiga, K., Yoshikawa, K., Yamada, K., & Nakagawa, M. (2004). White matter loss in the splenium of the corpus callosum in a case of posterior cortical atrophy: A diffusion tensor imaging study. *European Neurology*, *52*, 77–81. doi:10.1159/000079750

Yoshihara, Y. (2002). Visualizing selective neural pathways with WGA transgene: Combination of neuroanatomy with gene technology. *Neuroscience Research*, *44*, 133–140. doi:10.1016/S0168-0102(02)00130-X

Yoshikawa, K., Nakata, Y., Yamada, K., & Nakagawa, M. (2004). Early pathological changes in the Parkinsonian brain demonstrated by diffusion tensor MRI. *Journal of Neurology, Neurosurgery, and Psychiatry*, *75*, 481–484. doi:10.1136/jnnp.2003.021873

Yoshiura, T., Mihara, F., & Koga, H. (2006). Mapping of subcortical white matter abnormality in Alzheimer's disease using diffusion-weighted magnetic resonance imaging. *Academic Radiology*, *13*, 1460–1464. doi:10.1016/j.acra.2006.09.042

Young, G. O. (1964). Synthetic structure of industrial plastics. In Peters, J. (Ed.), *Plastics* (2nd ed., pp. 15–64). New York, NY: McGraw-Hill.

Zadikoff, C., & Lang, A. E. (2005). Apraxia in movement disorders. *Brain*, *128*, 1480–1497. doi:10.1093/brain/awh560

Zarei, M., Damoiseaux, J. S., Morgese, C., Beckmann, C. F., Smith, S. M., & Matthews, P. M. (2009). Regional white matter integrity differentiates between vascular dementia and Alzheimer disease. *Stroke*, *40*, 773–779. doi:10.1161/STROKEAHA.108.530832

Zatorre, R. J., & Mondor, T. A. (1999). Auditory attention to space and frequency activates similar cerebral systems. *NeuroImage*, *10*(5), 544–554. doi:10.1006/nimg.1999.0491

Zhong, Z., Ewers, M., Teipel, S., Burger, K., Wallin, A., & Blennow, K. (2007). Levels of beta-secretase (BACE1) in cerebrospinal fluid as a predictor of risk in mild cognitive impairment. *Archives of General Psychiatry*, *64*(6), 718–726. doi:10.1001/archpsyc.64.6.718

Zhou, H., Hu, H., & Tao, Y. (2006). Inertial measurements of upper limb motion. *International Federation for Medical and Biological Engineering*, *44*, 479–487.

About the Contributors

Jinglong Wu was born in Jiutai, China, on August 8, 1958. He received a BS from Jilin Vocational Teachers College, China, and MS from Kyoto University, Japan, both in electrical engineering, in 1984 and 1991, respectively. He received his PhD in electric engineering from Kyoto University, Japan, in 1994. He was an assistant professor at Ritsumeikan University, Japan, from 1994 to 1997, a lecturer in the Department of Mechanical Engineering, Faculty of Engineering, Yamaguchi University, from 1997 to 1999. From 1999, he was an associate professor, and from 2002, he was a full professor in the Department of Intelligent Mechanical Systems, Faculty of Engineering, Kagawa University, Japan. Since 2008, he has been Professor and Laboratory Head, Biomedical Engineering Laboratory, Graduate School of Natural Science and Technology, Okayama University, Japan. His current research interests are biomedical engineering, cognitive neuroscience, ergonomics and human science. Dr. Wu received the Best Paper Award of the IEEE Joint International Conference on Neural Network in 1993 and the SICE Best Paper Award in 2000. In 2003, he received the Gennai Grand Prize, Ozaki Foundation, Japan.

* * *

Koji Abe is 53 years old and is currently Professor and Chairman of Neurology at Okayama University Medical School in Japan. He graduated from Tohoku University School of Medicine (M.D.) in Sendai (Japan) and then received a PhD from Tohoku University. Professor Koji Abe has published more than 400 papers on clinical neurology, translational stroke research, and the discovery of many genes involved in neurological diseases (e.g., Alzheimer's, amyotrophic lateral sclerosis, and Parkinson's diseases), all of which are deeply related to dementia. His research interests cover many important fields of neurology, with particular focuses on the mechanism of ischemic brain damage, gene and stem cell therapy, and neuroimaging. He is currently serving as the President of the International Society of Cerebral Blood Flow and Metabolism and as the Executive Director of the Japanese Societies of Neurology and Stroke.

Kentaro Akazawa received his MD degree from KPUM, Japan, in 2001. He received his PhD from KPUM in 2008. He is currently a faculty member of the Radiology Department at KPUM.

Kosuke Akiyama was born on January 21, 1978 in Japan. He graduated from Kagawa Medical University on March 31, 2002 and received a PhD from Kagawa Medical University in March 2008. He was an Otolaryngologist at Kagawa Medical University from May 2002 to March 2004 and at Sakaide City Hospital from April 2004 to March 2005. He attended the Postgraduate School of the Faculty of Medicine, Kagawa University beginning in April 2005 and graduated on March 31, 2009. He has been an Otolaryngologist at Kagawa Medical University since April 2009. His current research interest is ion transport systems of the endolymphatic sac.

Hiroyuki Arai was born in Maebashi, Gunma, Japan on June 15, 1955. He received an MD from Tohoku University, Japan, in 1980 and a Doctorate in Neuroscience from Tohoku University, Japan in 1986. He was an Assistant Professor at Tohoku University, Japan, from April 1994 to January 1999 and an Associate Professor in the Department of Geriatrics and Gerontology, Faculty of Medicine, Tohoku University from February 1999 to September 2003. From October 2003 to December 2007, he was a Professor in the Department of Complementary and Alternative Medicine, Faculty of Medicine, Tohoku University. Since January 2008, he has been a Professor in the Department of Geriatrics and Gerontology, Institute of Development, Aging and Cancer, Tohoku University. His current research interests include clinical research on dementia, Alzheimer's disease, and related disorders. Dr. Arai received the 1995 Gold Award from the Tohoku University School of Medicine in 1995 and the Best Paper Award from the Japanese Society of Geriatric Medicine, 1997.

Hajime Asama is a Professor in the Department of Precision Engineering, Graduate School of Engineering, The University of Tokyo. He was a Research Associate at RIKEN (The Institute of Physical and Chemical Research) since 1986, a Senior Scientist at RIKEN since 1998, a Professor of RACE (Research into Artifacts, Center for Engineering) at The University of Tokyo since 2002, and a Professor in the Department of Precision Engineering, Graduate School of Engineering, The University of Tokyo since 2009. His main work includes "Distributed Task Processing by a Multiple Autonomous Robot System Using an Intelligent Data Carrier System," Intelligent Automation and Soft Computing, An International Journal, vol. 6, no. 3, pp. 215-224, (2000). He is a member of the Institute of Electrical and Electronics Engineers, Inc. (IEEE), the Japan Society of Mechanical Engineers (JSME), the Robotics Society of Japan (RSJ), and the Japanese Society of Instrumentation and Control Engineers (SICE).

Zheng Chen is President of the Beijing Geriatric Hospital and the Director of the Division of Tuberculosis. He received MBA training at York University Business School in Toronto in 2002, DRG training at the Public Health School of Johns Hopkins University in 2006, and social gerontology training at the UN international Institute on Aging in Malta in 2008. He is Vice Chairman of the Geriatric Committee of Gerontological Society of China and serves on the editorial board of Clinical Medicine of China. He has spent more than 20 years on research and clinical work in tuberculosis and geriatrics, especially senile fall and dementia.

Dehua Chui, MD, PhD is a professor who does research on brain aging and cognitive impairment in the Neuroscience Research Institute of Peking University Health Science Center. He is also the Chief Scientist in the Neurology Department of Peking University Third Hospital, Director-General of the Scientific Committee of Aging and Anti-Aging for the China Gerontological Society, a council member of Professional Committee of Chinese Pharmacological Society for Anti-Aging and Alzheimer's disease, Chief Editor of The Neurological Diseases and Mental Health magazine, and Associate Editor of the Journal of Alzheimer's Disease. Prof. Chui has been researching the molecular-neurobiological mechanisms of neurodegenerating diseases and Alzheimer's disease for more than 20 years at the Japan National Center of Neurology and Psychiatry and Japan RIKEN and has published more than 60 academic articles in Nature Medicine, Proceedings of the National Academy of Sciences, USA, Journal of Neuroscience, Journal of Alzheimer's Disease, Human Molecular Genetics, Journal of Biological Chemistry, FASEB Journal, Journal of Neurochemistry, and American Journal of Pathology. His major research fields are neurobiological mechanisms of neurodegenerative diseases, the connection between cognitive impairment and aging-related factors, brain molecular imaging and biomarkers of neurodegenerative diseases, especially Alzheimer's disease, and the development of new anti-aging and anti-dementia drugs, including immune therapy, synthetic compounds, and traditional Chinese medicine.

Shun'ichi Doi was born in 1947. He received his MS and PhD degrees in Mechanical Engineering from Nagoya Institute of Technology in 1972 and 1994, respectively. In 1972, he joined Toyota Central R&D Labs, Inc. He has been a Professor of the Faculty of Engineering, Kagawa University, Japan, since 2004. His current research interests include vehicle dynamics and active safety technology. Dr. Doi is a member of the Society of Automotive Engineers of Japan, the Japanese Society of Mechanical Engineers, and the Society of Instrument and Control Engineers.

Dongsheng Fan is Vice President and Director of Neurology, Research Fellow, Chief Physician, Professor and Doctoral Tutor of Peking University Third Hospital. He received his MD from the Medical University of Japan Graduate School of Autonomy in 1996 and spent two years in Japan Medical self-completed post-doctoral research home. His main research areas cover neurodegenerative disease, neuromuscular disease, and cerebrovascular disease. He has published more than 240 articles and won first prize in scientific and technological progress from the Ministry of Education, Ministry of Science and Technology Progress Award 1, third prize in Chinese medical science, the Outstanding Youth Award for Chinese Medicine, Beijing Municipal Education innovation model, Peking University Health Science Education Teaching Achievement Award, Peking University Teaching Achievement Award, Peking University Yang Fuqing Yang Yuan Academy Award for Outstanding Teaching and Research, Peking University Excellent Communist Model, and Peking University Outstanding Teacher title, and the Ministry of Education selected him for the New Century Excellent Project Support Personnel Development Plans.

Katsutoshi Furukawa was born in Nagoya, Japan, on December 1, 1960. He received an MD from Yamagata University, Japan, in 1988 and a PhD in Neurological Science from Tohoku University, Japan in 1992. He was an Assistant Professor at the Department of Neurophysiology, Tohoku University, Japan, from July 1992 to February 1994, a Postdoctoral Fellow at the Center on Aging, University of Kentucky, USA from February 1994 to September 1997, an Instructor in the Department of Medicine, University of Washington, Seattle, USA from September 1997 to December 1998, an Assistant Professor in the Department of Neurology, Tohoku University from December 1998 to May 2001, a tenure track Investigator at the Laboratory of Neurosciences, National Institute on Aging, USA from May 2001 to May 2005, an Associate Professor in the Department of Geriatric and Complementary Medicine, Tohoku University from June 2005 to March 2008, and an Associate Professor in the Department of Geriatrics and Gerontology, Tohoku University since April 2008. His current research interests are clinical neurology and geriatric medicine, as well as pathological mechanisms, molecular imaging, and clinical intervention of dementia, with a focus on Alzheimer's disease. Dr. Furukawa received the American Federation for Aging Research Award, USA in 1996, the Ellison Medical Foundation Scholar Award, USA in 1998, and the Novartis Foundation for Gerontological Research, Japan, in 2009.

Hidenao Fukuyama was born on Aug. 13, 1949 in Japan. He received a B.M. degree from Kyoto University, Japan, in 1975 and a PhD from Kyoto University Graduate School of Medicine in 1981. He was an Assistant Professor at Kyoto University from April 1986 until 1991 and a Lecturer in the Department of Neurology, Faculty of Medicine, Kyoto University, from 1991 to March 1995. From April 1995 until 2000, he was an Associate Professor of the Department of Brain Pathophysiology, Kyoto University Faculty of Medicine. He was then appointed as the professor of the functional brain imaging of human brain research center, Kyoto University Graduate School of Medicine. His current research interests are focused on brain imaging and functional neuroscience using MRI.

Kazuya Funada was born in Okayama, Japan, in 1981. He received a Bachelor of Engineering degree and Master of Engineering degree, both from the Graduate School of Natural Science and Technology, Okayama University, Okayama, Japan, in 2008 and 2010, respectively. He majored in Mechanical Engineering and Biomedical Engineering under the guidance of Professor Wu at the Biomedical Engineering Laboratory. He researched motion recognition of hands using surface EMG of the forearms for the application of controlling an upper-limb rehabilitation device. He succeeded in recognizing the motion of hands by analyzing only the surface EMG signals measured from two optimum points specified with the experiment and was able to control the rehabilitation device arbitrarily, depending on the recognition results. At present, he is an engineer at West Japan Railway Technos, Hyogo, Japan. He is mainly focused on the design of railway vehicles.

Yoshihito Funaki was born in Sendai, Japan on April 29, 1968. He received BS and MS degrees in Pharmaceutical Science from Tohoku University, Japan in 1991 and 1993, respectively, and a Doctorate in Medicine from Tohoku University, Japan in 2004. He was a Research Assistant at Tohoku University, Japan from April 1993 to March 2007. Since April 2007, he has been an Assistant Professor in the Department of Radiopharmaceuticals, Cyclotron and Radioisotope Center, Tohoku University. His current research interests are the synthesis of radiopharmaceuticals and their biological evaluation.

Katsutoshi Furukawa was born in Nagoya, Japan, on December 1, 1960. He received an MD from Yamagata University, Japan, and a PhD in Neurological Science from Tohoku University, Japan in 1988 and 1992, respectively. He was an Assistant Professor in the Department of Neurophysiology, Tohoku University, Japan, from July 1992 to February 1994, a Postdoctoral Fellow at the Center on Aging, University of Kentucky, USA from February 1994 to September 1997, an Instructor in the Department of Medicine, University of Washington, Seattle, USA from September 1997 to December 1998, an Assistant Professor in the Department of Neurology, Tohoku University from December 1998 to May 2001, a tenure track Investigator at the Laboratory of Neurosciences, National Institute on Aging, USA from May 2001 to May 2005, an Associate Professor in the Department of Geriatric and Complementary Medicine, Tohoku University from June 2005 to March 2008, and an Associate Professor in the Department of Geriatrics and Gerontology, Tohoku University from April 2008 to present. His current research interests are clinical neurology and geriatric medicine, as well as pathological mechanisms, molecular imaging, and clinical intervention of dementia, with a particular focus on Alzheimer's disease. Dr. Furukawa received the American Federation for Aging Research Award, USA in 1996, the Ellison Medical Foundation Scholar Award, USA in 1998, and the Novartis Foundation Award for Gerontological Research, Japan, in 2009.

Shozo Furumoto majored in Pharmaceutical Science at Tohoku University and received his BS degree in 1997. He then studied Radiopharmaceutical Science under the direction of Prof. T. Ido at the Graduate School of Pharmaceutical Science, Tohoku University and earned his PhD degree in Pharmaceutical Science in 2002. He conducted 2 years of postdoctoral work in Radiochemistry at Tohoku University, going on to become an Assistant Professor in May 2004 and then a Senior Assistant Professor in April 2009 in Radiochemistry at Tohoku University. In March 2010, he became an Associate Professor of the Graduate School of Medicine, Tohoku University. His research includes radiopharmaceutical chemistry for positron emission tomography.

Qiyong Guo was born on May 24, 1958 in China. He received Bachelor's and Master's degrees from China Medical University, Shenyang, China in 1983 and 1988, respectively. He received an MD from Japan Nara Medical University, Japan in 1993 and worked as a Resident at No.3 Affiliated Hospital of China Medical University from 1983 to 1986. He was an Assistant Professor at the Second Clinical College of China Medical University from 1993 to 1995 and has been a Professor there since 1995. His social duties and achievements include serving as the President of the China Society of Radiology, the President of Shengjing Hospital of China Medical University, being named a national notable expert in abdominal imaging diagnosis and interventional therapy, serving as the Chief Editor of more than ten national journals (including the Chinese Journal of Radiology and the Journal of China Clinic Medical Imaging), and serving as the Chief Editor of four textbooks, including "Interventional Radiology" and "Practical Radiology."

Gao Maolong was born in Shanxi Province, China, on April 7, 1980. He received a Bachelor's of Science in preventive medicine from Shanxi Medical University, China, in 2004, and a Master's of Science in epidemiology and health statistics from Shanxi Medical University, China in 2007. He is an Associate Researcher in Beijing Geriatrics Hospital. His current research interests focus on generalized estimating equations (GEE).

Shuxiang Guo (S'93-M'95-SM'03 for IEEE) received his PhD in mechano-informatics and systems from Nagoya University, Nagoya, Japan, in 1995. Currently, he is a professor in the Department of Intelligent Mechanical System Engineering at Kagawa University. He has published approximately 220 refereed journal and conference papers. His current research interests include micro-robotics and mechatronics, microrobotics systems for minimally invasive surgery, micro-catheter systems, micropumps, and smart material (SMA, ICPF) based on actuators. Dr. Guo received research awards from the Tokai Section of the Japan Society of Mechanical Engineers (JSME), the Tokai Science and Technology Foundation, the Best Paper Award at the IS International Conference, Best Paper award at the 2003 International Conference on Control Science and Technology, Best Conference Paper Award at IEEE ROBIO2004 and Best Conference Paper Award at IEEE ICAL 2008, in 1997, 1998, 2000, 2003, 2004, and 2008, respectively. He is the founding chair of the IEEE International Conference on Mechatronics and Automation.

Akira Gyoten received a Master's degree in Mechanical Engineering from Okayama University, Okayama, Japan, in 2010. He majored in ergonomics and studied the human-machine interface. His research focused on the development of a rehabilitation device for hand movement disorders. Providing home care for patients is a major problem in hand rehabilitation. In order to prevent contracture and promote recovery of motor function, he developed a home rehabilitation device that is portable, features simple mechanics, and enables patients to perform self-controlled exercise. He proposed a master-slave system to measure surface EMG on the healthy arm for self-controlled exercise. He presented his research at the 2009 International Symposium on Early Detection and Rehabilitation Technology of Dementia (DRD2009). He is currently working at Terumo Corporation, Japan where he is participating in the development of medical products.

Mark Hallett obtained his MD at Harvard University and trained in Neurology at Massachusetts General Hospital. He had fellowships in Neurophysiology at the National Institutes of Health and at the Institute of Psychiatry in London. From 1976 to 1984, Dr. Hallett was the Chief of the Clinical Neurophysiology Laboratory at the Brigham and Women's Hospital and Associate Professor of Neurology at Harvard Medical School. From 1984, he has been at the National Institute of Neurological Disorders and Stroke where he serves as Chief of the Human Motor Control Section and pursues research on the physiology of human movement disorders and other problems of motor control. He also served as Clinical Director of NINDS until July 2000. He is past President of the American Association of Electrodiagnostic Medicine and the Movement Disorder Society. He also served as Vice-President of the American Academy of Neurology. He is an Associate Editor of *Brain* and Editor in Chief of *World Neurology.* Currently, he also serves on the editorial boards of *Clinical Neurophysiology, Acta Neurologica Scandinavica, Journal of Clinical Neurophysiology, Medical Problems of Performing Artists, Annals of Neurology, The Cerebellum, NeuroTherapeutics,* and *European Neurology*. The main work of his group focuses on the physiology and pathophysiology of movement. Dr. Hallett's interests in motor control are wide-ranging, and include brain plasticity and its relevance to neurological disorders and the pathophysiology of dystonia, Parkinsonism, and myoclonus. Recently he has become interested in disorders of volition, including tic and psychogenic movement disorders.

Hongbin Han was born in June 1971. Dr. Han received a B.M. in clinical medicine and a M.M. in radiology from Dalian Medical University in 1988 and 1996, respectively, and a MD and PhD in radiology from Peking University Health Science Center in 1999. Dr. Han is now Chief Physician and Professor, Radiology Department, Peking University Third Hospital, and Deputy Director of the Scientific Research Department of Peking University Health Science Center. His main research fields include "Diagnosis and therapy of ischemic stroke in preclinical and clinical research" and "Development and clinical application of novel imaging techniques". More than 60 of his papers have been published in such journals as *Journal of Physical Chemistry B Condensed Matter, Neuroscience Letters, Neuroradiology, Journal of Neuroscience Method* and *Chinese Journal of Radiology*. Dr. Han is the chief editor of the book *MRI Sequence Design and Clinical Application* and the chief editor for the translation of *Sectional Anatomy by MRI and CT* (3rd Edition).

Sachio Hanya was born in Nagoya, Japan on July 15, 1984. He received BS and MS degrees in Information from Nagoya Institute of Technology, Japan in 2008 and 2010, respectively. His current research interests are acoustic signal analysis, statics, and Bayesian networks.

Hidenori Hiraki was born in Matsuyama, Ehime Prefecture, Japan in 1985. He received a Bachelor of Engineering degree and a Master's degree in Biomedical Engineering from the Graduate School of Natural Science and Technology, Okayama University, Okayama, Japan in 2008 and 2010, respectively. In this book, he writes about kinetic visual fields, which are visual fields that measure which moving targets subjects can find. Previous studies have not measured kinetic visual fields with changing background brightness and contrast ratios between targets and background brightness. Therefore, this study measured kinetic visual fields with changing background brightness and contrast ratios using an improved Goldmann perimeter. At present, he is an Engineer at the JFE Steel Company, 2-2-3, Uchisaiwaicho, Chiyoda-ku, Tokyo, Japan, where he is focusing on improving the iron manufacturing process.

Yoko Hirohashi was born in Tokyo, Japan, on November 24, 1950. She received B.S. from St. Luke's College of Nursing, Japan, in nursing and M.S. from Bukkyo University, Japan, in social welfare in 1973 and 2006, respectively. She was an assistant professor at Seisen Junior College, Japan, from April 2002 to March 2006 and at Hagoromo University from April 2006 to March 2008, a lecturer in the Department of Nursing Care Studies, Osaka International College, from April 2008 to March 2010, and a lecturer in the Department of Child Care Studies. Since April 2010, she has been an assistant professor in the Department of Nursing, Faculty of Health and Welfare Science, Nayoro City University. Her current research interests are quality of care for the elderly and care management.

Akira Homma, MD was born in Japan on December 28, 1948. He received a BM degree in Medicine from Tokyo Jikeikai University, Japan, in 1973 and an MD in Psychiatry from St. Marianna University, Japan in 1981. He was a Lecturer in the Department of Psychiatry at St. Marianna University, Japan from April 1981 to December 1984 and the Department Director of Psychiatry, Tokyo Metropolitan Institute of Gerontology from January 1985 to March 2009. He is currently serving as the Director of the Center for Dementia Care Research in Tokyo, a post he has held since June 2009. His current research interest is geriatric psychiatry. He has served as the Treasurer and the Secretary of the International Psychogeriatric Association and as the President of the Japanese Psychogeriatric Society. He is currently serving as the President of the Japanese Society for Dementia Care.

Yoko Ikoma was born in Hyogo, Japan, on May 17, 1975. She received a BS and MS from Waseda University, Japan, both in electronics and communications, in 1998 and 2000, respectively, and a doctorate in electronics and communications from Waseda University in 2003. She was an assistant at Waseda University, Japan, from April 2001 to March 2003, a postdoctoral research fellow at the National Institute of Radiological Sciences from April 2003 to April 2007, and a research associate at the Graduate School of Information Science, Nara Institute of Science and Technology, from May 2007 to March 2009. Since May 2009, she has been a visiting researcher in the Department of Clinical Neuroscience, Karolinska Institute, Sweden. Her current research interest is focused on neuroreceptor imaging with positron emission tomography.

Atsushi Imamura was born in Ibaraki, Japan on October 9, 1966. He became a licensed Physical Therapist in 1989 and received a BS degree from the Open University of Japan in 2002. He was a Physical Therapist in the Department of Rehabilitation Medicine, Yokohama General Hospital, Japan, from

April 1989 to February 2001. Since February 2001, he has worked in the Department of Health Support, Setagaya Municipal Kitazawa En.

Hidenori Itoh completed the doctoral program in Electrical and Electronic Engineering at Nagoya University, Japan in 1974 and received a D.Eng. degree. From 1974 to 1985, he worked at Nippon Telephone and Telegraph Laboratories. From 1985 to 1989, he developed knowledge-based systems at the Institute for New Generation Computer Technology. He has been a Professor at Nagoya Institute of Technology since 1989 and is now affiliated with the Department of Computer Science and Engineering. He has been engaged in R&D in the fields of the mathematical theory of language, computer network communications, operating systems, knowledge databases, and artificial intelligence. He received the Japanese Society of Kansei Engineering Best Technical Paper Award in 2006.He is a member of the Information Processing Society of Japan, the Institute of Electronics, Information, and Communication Engineers, the Japanese Society for Artificial Intelligence, the Society for Science on Form, Japan, the Robotics Society of Japan, and the IEEE computer society.

Ren Iwata was born in Toyama, Japan on April 17, 1949. He received BS and MS degrees in Chemistry from the University of Tokyo, Japan in 1972 and 1974, respectively, and a Doctorate in Chemistry from the University of Tokyo, Japan in 1984. He was a Research Chemist at the National Institute of Radiological Sciences, Japan from April 1974 to March 1981, an Assistant Professor at the Cyclotron and Radioisotope Center (CYRIC), Tohoku University, Japan from April 1981 to July 1993, and an Associate Professor in CYRIC and the Graduate School of Engineering, Tohoku University from August 1993 to June 2002. Since July 2002, he has been a Professor at CYRIC, Tohoku University. His current research fields are radiochemistry with a focus on PET probes and engineering in microfluidic radiosynthesis. Dr. Iwata received the 20th Award of the Japanese Society of Nuclear Medicine in 1982. He has been a Board Member of the Directors of the Society of Radiopharmaceutical Sciences since 2007.

Yong Jeong was born in 1966 in Gwangjoo, Korea. He received an MD degree from Yonsei University, Korea, an MS degree and a PhD in neurophysiology from the same University in 1993 and 1997, respectively. He was certified by the Neurology board after he finished his residency at Severance Hospital in 2002. He finished a clinical and research fellowship at Samsung Medical Center and at the University of Florida in dementia and neuropsychology with Dr. Duk L. Na and Dr. Kenneth M. Heilman, respectively. He has been an associate Professor in the Department of Bio and Brain Engineering at KAIST since 2008. His research fields are cognitive neuroscience, clinical neurology (degenerative disease, vascular disease), functional neuroimaging, and bioengineering (bio-signals). His interest is the fundamental architecture of cognitive function. He wants to develop restoration, augmentation and modulation systems for patients with brain dysfunctions using bioengineering techniques. He also serves as a neurologist at the Samsung Medical Center.

Yinlai Jiang was born in Liaoning, China on July 27, 1979. He received BE and ME degrees in Computer Science from Northeastern University, China in 2002 and 2005, respectively, and a Doctorate in Engineering from Kochi University of Technology, Japan in 2008. He has been an Assistant Professor in the Department of Intelligent Mechanical Systems Engineering at Kochi University of Technology,

Japan since April 2008. His current research interests are visual cognition, medical and biological engineering, and computational intelligence.

Masayuki Karaki was born on August 21, 1965 in Japan. He graduated from Kagawa Medical University on March 31, 1993 and received a DMSc degree from Kagawa Medical University in June 2005. He was a Medical Doctor from May 1993 to June 1996 in the Department of Otolaryngology, Kagawa Medical University (now referred to as the Department of Otolaryngology, Head, and Neck Surgery, Faculty of Medicine, Kagawa University). He moved to Eikou Hospital as a Medical Doctor in July 1996 and then to the Department of Otolaryngology, Head, and Neck Surgery, Faculty of Medicine, Kagawa University as a Medical Doctor in May 1997, where he has been an Assistant Professor since September 2005. His current research interests are functional optical hemodynamic imaging of the olfactory cortex using NIRS, and the study of the anatomic relationship between the paranasal structures and orbital contents for endoscopic endonasal transethmoidal approach to the orbit.

Shohei Kato was born in Nagoya, Japan on May 31, 1970. He received BS, MS, and Ph.D degrees in Engineering from Nagoya Institute of Technology, Japan, in 1993, 1995, and 1998, respectively. He joined the Department of Electrical and Electronic Engineering at Toyota National College of Technology as a Research Associate from 1998 to 1999 and as a Lecturer from 1999 to 2002. He was an Assistant Professor in the Department of Computer Science and Engineering at Nagoya Institute of Technology from 2002 to 2003 and has been an Associate Professor there since 2003. His current research interests include computational intelligence in robotics, artificial life, reasoning under uncertainty, and Kansei engineering. He received the Japanese Society of Kansei Engineering Best Technical Paper Award in 2006. He is a member of the Information Processing Society of Japan, the Institute of Electronics, Information, and Communication Engineers, the Japanese Society for Artificial Intelligence, the Robotics Society of Japan, the Japanese Society of Kansei Engineering, and the IEEE.

Motoichiro Kato is an Associate Professor in the Department of Neuropsychiatry, Keio University School of Medicine. He became an Instructor in Neuropsychiatry at Keio University in 1980. He was an Associate Professor and Director of Neuropsychiatry at Tokyo Dental College since 1993 and an Associate Professor in the Department of Neuropsychiatry, Keio University School of Medicine since 2002. His main work includes "Dissociative contributions of the medial temporal region and frontal cortex to prospective remembering," Reviews in the Neurosciences, 17, pp. 267-278, (2006). He is a member of the American Academy of Neurology (AAN), the International Neuropsychological Society (INS), and the Cognitive Neuroscience Society (CNS).

Masashi Kawamoto, MD PhD, was born in Hiroshima, Japan. He received his Japanese Medical license and his PhD from the Hiroshima University Faculty of Medicine in 1989. He has served as an Instructor, an Assistant Professor, and an Associate Professor at Hiroshima University, Japan, and since April 2007, he has been a Professor in the Department of Anesthesiology and Critical Care, Division of Clinical Medical Science, Graduate School of Biomedical Sciences, Hiroshima University. His current research interests concern the autonomic nervous system and clinical anesthesia.

Miho Kawarada is from Aomori, Japan. She completed a Clinical Psychology program in 1999 and received an MA in Clinical Psychology in 2001 from the Department of Clinical Psychology, Kawasaki University of Medical Welfare, Japan. In April 2001, she became a clinical psychologist at the Department of Psychiatry, and since 2009, she has been in the Department of Rehabilitation at Kawasaki Medical School Kawasaki Hospital. Her current research interests are dementia and clinical neuropsychology. In 2007, she received the Best Paper Award from the Japanese Association of Rehabilitation Medicine, and her team also received the 2nd Prize in the Talent Show at the 4th World Congress of the International Society of Physical and Rehabilitation Medicine.

Jinho Kim was born in 1984 in Busan, Korea and was raised in Seoul. After graduating from Seoul Science High School, Jinho entered KAIST, the Korea Advanced Institute of Science and Technology, Daejeon, in 2002. He graduated from the Department of Bio and Brain Engineering. His undergraduate research focused on the nonlinear analysis of EEG data from post-traumatic stress disorder patients. He continued his education in a graduate course of a computational cell biology laboratory in the same department; his master's thesis was on the role of mitochondria in oxidative stress-induced neuronal necrosis. Since 2008, he has been in the process of his PhD course in the laboratory for cognitive neuroscience and neuroimaging at KAIST. His research focuses on neurovascular coupling dysfunction in Alzheimer's disease.

Hikari Kirimoto was born in Osaka, Japan on February 22, 1968. He received a BA degree from Meiji University, Japan, in 1992 and an M.S. degree from the National Institute of Fitness and Sports in Kanoya, Japan, in 2005. He was an Assistant in the Department of Occupational Therapy, Faculty of Rehabilitation, International University of Health and Welfare in Fukuoka, Japan, from April 2005 to March 2007. Since April 2007, he has been an Assistant Professor in the Department of Occupational Therapy, Faculty of Medical Technology, Niigata University of Health and Welfare, Japan. His current research interests are neuro-rehabilitation and motor control in humans.

Noatsugu Kitayama graduated from the Graduate School of Natural Science and Technology, Okayama University, and studied the length perceptual characteristics in the sense of touch. The touch sense is one of the most important senses. It can be applied for virtual reality technology and remote medical fields. To research the length of perceptual characteristics on simultaneous touch by multiple fingers, Noatsugu developed a length display device that can adjust for subjects using 5 fingers and operated a length perceptual experiment. In addition, Noatsugu investigated the application for rehabilitation because the developed device is very useful. Noatsugu presented these studies at "The 2009 International Symposium on Early Detection and Rehabilitation Technology of Dementia". Noatsugu was employed by the NTN Corporation after graduation and focuses on manufacturing and design for Bearing.

Masayuki Kitazawa was born in Kochi, Japan on August 6, 1958. He received a BS in Mechanical Engineering from Meiji University, Japan in 1982, and a Doctorate in Engineering from Yamaguchi University, Japan in 2005. From April 1982 to March 1988, he worked for the design department of Imabari Shipbuilding Co., Ltd. as an engineer. From April 1988 to March 2008, he worked as a Technical Official in the Department of Mechanical Engineering, Faculty of Engineering, Yamaguchi University. Starting April 2008, he was an Associate Professor in the Department of Mechanical Engineering, Wakayama

National College of Technology. Since April 2010, he has been a Professor in the Department of Intelligent Mechanical Engineering, Wakayama National College of Technology. His current research interests are intelligent man-machine interfaces, constructing virtual realities using human characteristics, and brain science using functional magnetic resonance imaging. He is a member of the Japanese Society of Mechanical Engineering, the Japanese Society of Fuzzy Theory and Intelligent Informatics, and the Japanese Ergonomics Society.

Tetsuo Kobayashi was born in Hokkaido, Japan, in 1956. He received his BS, MS and PhD in electronic engineering in 1979, 1981 and 1984, respectively, from Hokkaido University, Sapporo, Japan. He was an associate professor in Hokkaido Institute of Technology and Hokkaido University, Sapporo, Japan. Since 2004, he has been a professor in the Department of Electrical Engineering, Kyoto University, Kyoto, Japan. He was a visiting scholar at the department of electrical engineering, University of Rochester, NY, USA, from 1987 to 1988 and at the Brain Behavior Laboratory, Simon Fraser University, BC, Canada, from 1996 to 1997. His research interests include biomedical engineering, functional neuroimaging and cognitive neuroscience. He is a councilor of the Institute of Complex Medical Engineering (ICME) and International Society for Brain Electromagnetic Topography (ISBET) and a member of the Institute of Electrical and Electronic Engineering (IEEE) and Organization for Human Brain Mapping (OHBM). In 2009, he organized, as a congress president, the 18th International Congress on Brain Electromagnetic Topography, Kyoto, Japan. Dr. Kobayashi has received several best paper awards, including the SCME2008 best paper award in 2008 and Kyoto Prize in ISBET2009 in 2009.

Eiji Kobayashi was born on April 13, 1967 in Japan. He graduated from Kagawa Medical University on March 31, 1997 and received a PhD from Kagawa Medical University in March 2007. He was an Otolaryngologist at Kagawa Medical University, Sakaide City Hospital and Eiko Hospital from May 1999 to March 2008. He has been an Otolaryngologist at Uchinomi Hospital since April 2008. His current research interest is objective olfactory tests using near-infrared spectroscopy.

Ryuichi Kobayashi was born on December 21, 1967 in Japan. He graduated from Kagawa Medical University on March 31, 1995. He was a Medical Doctor from July 1995 to September 1996 in the Department of Otolaryngology, Kagawa Medical University. He moved to the Department of Otolaryngology, Numakuma Hospital as a Medical Doctor from October 1996 to March 1998. He was a Medical Doctor from April 1998 to March 1999 and an Assistant Professor from April 1999 to March 2003 in the Department of Otolaryngology, Kagawa Medical University. He moved to the Department of Otolaryngology, Ritsurin Hospital as a Medical Doctor from April 2003 to March 2004. He moved to Sue Hospital as the Director of the Department of Otolaryngology in April 2004 (now referred to as the Department of Otorhinolaryngology and Allergy). He has held an additional post as the Director of the Sleep Disordered Breathing Center, Sue Hospital since March 2006. His current research interest is the evaluation of pediatric nasal airway patency by rhinomanometry.

Akiko Kobayashi completed the Physical Education major at Japan Women's Junior College of Physical Education, Japan in 1986. She joined Mizuho Bond Ltd. in 1986 and then joined the Business Design Laboratory Ltd. in 2003. She participated in the research and development of a communications robot and has now worked on dementia screening research and development since 2007. She was one of the founders of Ifcom Ltd. in 2009.

Toshiaki Kojima graduated from the Information Department of Hiroshima Institute of Technology in 1977. He joined Life Ltd. in 1977 where he became a project leader and developed a host computer system. He joined the Business Design Laboratory Ltd. in 2004 where he participated in the research and development of a communications robot and has worked on a dementia screening device since 2007. He was one of the founders of Ifcom Ltd. in 2009.

Yukitsuka Kudo was born in Aomori Prefecture, Japan on October 3, 1946. He received a Doctorate in Medicinal Science from Osaka University, Japan in 1991. He worked in research at Tanabe Pharmaceutical Co., Ltd., Japan, from April 1972 to March 2006. Since April 2006, he has been a Professor in the Innovation of New Biomedical Engineering Center, Tohoku University. His current research interest is the development of imaging probes for the diagnosis of Alzheimer's disease. Dr. Kudo received the Editor's Choice Award from the Journal of Nuclear Medicine in 2007.

Hiroshi Kusahara was born in Kagawa Prefecture, Japan, in 1980. He received a Bachelor of Engineering degree from the Department of Mechanical Engineering, Kagawa University, Takamatsu, Japan, and a Master of Engineering degree from the Graduate School of Faculty of Engineering, Kagawa University, Takamatsu, Japan, in 2004 and 2006, respectively. He has been working at the Toshiba Medical System Corporation, 1385 Shimoishigami, Otawara-shi, Tochigi-ken, Japan, from April 2006. He is working on magnetic resonance (MR) machine development for MR machines and MRI protocol design. From 2005 to 2010, he took part in CME 2005, where he presented his research.

Takashi Kusaka was born on August 13, 1964 in Japan. He graduated from the Medical Course of Kagawa Medical University in May 1991 and received a PhD from Kagawa Medical University in May 1995. He was an assistant professor from April 1995 to March 2001, a lecturer from April 2001 to September 2004 in The University Hospital, The Kagawa Medical University, and a lecturer from October 2004 to the present in The University Hospital, The Kagawa University. He is a pediatrician and neonatologist. He is very interested in neonatal neurology for the prevention of brain damage, especially assessments of cerebral hemodynamics using noninvasive optical devices.

Abdugheni Kutluk was born in Kashgar, Uyghur Autonomous Region of China, 1977. He received a B.E. degree in Textile Engineering and Computing from Xi'an Polytechnic University, Xi'an, China in 2001 and an M.E. in Electronics and Computer Engineering from Tokyo Denki University, Japan in 2005. Since April 2006, he has been a PhD student in Systems Engineering at Hiroshima University, Higashi-Hiroshima, Japan. His current research interests include monitoring autonomic nervous system activity, measurement of arterial elasticity, and biosignal analysis.

Chunlin Li was born in Henan Province, China, in 1981. He received the Bachelor of Engineering degree from Department of Mechanical Engineering, Okayama University of Science, Okayama, Japan, and the Master of Engineering degree both from Graduate School of Faculty of Engineering, Kagawa University, Takamatsu, Japan, in 2005 and 2007, respectively. He received the Doctor of Engineering degree from Okayama University, Okayama, Japan in 2010. He majored in fMRI study on human attention neural network. From 2005 to 2010, he took part in ICME2007, ICME2009, ICMA2009, DRD2009, and presented his research. At present, he is a researcher at Okayama University, Okayama, Japan. He is mainly engaging in the fMRI study on attention and dementia.

Xiujun Li was born on Sep 7, 1978 in China. He received a Bachelor of Science degree from the Graduate School of Technique of Education, Jilin Normal University, Siping, China in 2003. He then earned a Master of Engineering degree from the Graduate School of Technology, Kagawa University, Kagawa, Japan in 2009. He worked as a computer teacher in Zhengjing Yuanji Senior High School in China from 2003 to 2006. He research focuses on language study, utilizing neuroimaging technology, and his current research topic is "Chinese language processing mechanism and the effect of education on the functional organization of the adult brain." He has a good command of spoken and written English, has passed CET-4, and is skilled in the use of MS FrontPage, Win XP/2000/Vista, HTML, Photoshop, Illustrator, Visual Basic, Office 2003, Presentation, Premiere, and other software. He is currently a doctoral student in engineering at Okayama University, Okayama, Japan.

Qi Li was born in Huludao, China in 1977. He received a Bachelor of Engineering degree and a Master of Engineering degree from Changchun University of Science and Technology, Changchun, China in 2000 and 2003, respectively. He received a Doctor of Engineering degree from Okayama University, Okayama, Japan, in 2010. At present, he is a Lecturer in the Department of Computer Science and Technology, Changchun University of Science and Technology, China. He mainly conducts research in the fields of cognitive neuroscience, brain computer interface, and pattern recognition. He is a member of the program committee for the 2009 IEEE/ICME International Conference on Complex Medical Engineering and is a member of the Japanese Society of Clinical Neurophysiology.

Li Qinyun was born in Liaocheng, Shandong province in December 1966. After graduating from Jining Medical College in 1987, she worked in the Department of Neurology of a hospital affiliated with Jining Medical College in clinical teaching and medical research, and was promoted to attending neurologist in October of 1996. In 2005, she earned a Medical Master's degree from the Xiangya Medical School of Central Southern University. She engaged in pre-hospital emergency services for three months during the Olympic games in 2008. Currently, she works at the Beijing Geriatrics Hospital, focusing on the clinical and basic research of Alzheimer's disease. She has studied the effects of hypertension, hyperlipaemia and metabolic syndrome on cognitive functions, and her articles have been published in Chinese core periodicals.

Jun-Qian Liu is a PhD student in the Department of Anatomy and Neurobiology, Faculty of Medicine, Kagawa University. She graduated from Hebei Medical University in 2007, studied at Hebei University Hospital for 2 years, and then joined Kagawa University to study neurobiology. Her research uses Rab3A-siRNA and WGA *in vivo* to study the mechanism of transcytosis of proteins at synapses, with a particular focus on Amyloid-β.

Tingting Liu recently received her doctorate in Dehua Chui's lab at the Neuroscience Research Institute & Department of Neurobiology in Peking University Health Science Center. She did research on brain aging and cognitive impairment. At present, she is a postdoctoral fellow at the NorthShore University Health System. Prior to becoming a member of the Chui lab, Dr. Liu spent five years as a college student of Basic Medical Sciences in Peking University to lay the foundation for scientific research. Her research is focused on the effect of lipid metabolism on cognitive function. This research is highly relevant to human brain diseases, because it is becoming clear that lipids play important roles in learning and memory, brain aging, and cognitive impairment. Another major focus of her research is molecular imaging on lipid dysmetabolism, which is also a vigorous frontier science problem in the world.

Jiangyang Lu is Director and Chief Physician of the Department of Pathology at First Affiliated Hospital of General Hospital of PLA. He has spent 30 years on clinical work and scientific research. His expertise includes pathological diagnosis of diseases of the digestive and respiratory systems, soft-tissue tumors, and tumor drug resistance, application of targeted therapy for genetic testing, and ultrastructural pathological diagnosis by electron microscopy.

Shinichiro Maeshima is from Wakayama, Japan. He completed his medical training at the School of Medicine, Fujita Health University in 1986. He was a resident at Wakayama Medical University Hospital from 1986. He was a research fellow in the Department of Rehabilitation Medicine, University of Washington, and a Visiting Professor at the University of Sydney in 1996. He became the Chief of the Department of Neurosurgery at Hidaka General Hospital in 1997 and an Assistant Professor in the Department of Rehabilitation Medicine, Wakayama Medical University in 1999. He was a Professor in the Department of Sensory Science, Faculty of Health Science and Technology, Kawasaki University of Medical Welfare from 2004 to 2007. Since April 2007, he has been a Professor and the Chairman of the Department of Rehabilitation Medicine, International Medical Center, Saitama Medical University. His current research interests are stroke rehabilitation and clinical neuropsychology. He is a councilor at the Japanese Association of Higher Brain Function and a member of the Japanese Association of Rehabilitation Medicine and the Neuropsychological Association of Japan. In 2007, he received the Best Paper Award from the Japanese Association of Rehabilitation Medicine, and his team also received the 2nd Prize in the Talent Show at the International Society of Physical and Rehabilitation Medicine.

Keisuke Matsubara was born in Aichi, Japan, on January 9, 1983. He received a BS in applied chemistry from Ritsumeikan University, Japan, in 2005, a MS degree in Information Science from Nara Institute of Science and Technology, Japan, in 2007, and a doctorate in Information Science from Nara Institute of Science and Technology in 2010. Since April 2010, he has been a researcher in the Department of Radiology and Nuclear Medicine, Research Institute of Brain and Blood Vessels, Akita. His current research interest is PET pharmacokinetic analysis.

Yoshiki Matsumoto is an Assistant Professor in the Department of Anatomy and Neurobiology, Faculty of Medicine, Kagawa University. He graduated with a BSc from Nihon University in 1995, where he studied analytical methods used to create transgenic animals. After obtaining a MSc degree in 1997, he trained in molecular biological techniques at Tokyo University. To continue work on that project, he joined the Department of Veterinary Anatomy at Osaka Prefecture University as a PhD student. During this period, he studied the epigenetic effects of ectopic human growth hormone in transgenic animals, including the onset of puberty and modulation of the hypothalamo-pituitary axis. He completed his coursework at Osaka Prefecture University and became a Research Assistant at Kagawa University from 2001. He worked with Dr. Keiko Funa at Göteborg University in Sweden for 3 years as a Research fellow (utbildingsbidrag) beginning in 2004. He received a PhD degree from Kagawa University in 2007. His research interests include the mechanism of neuronal transcytosis, the remodeling of axon terminals by siRNA and lectins on the surface of neuronal membranes, and the effects of epigenetic molecules on developmental neuronal networks.

Kousuke Matsuzono was born in Kagoshima, Japan, on December 3, 1984. He graduated from the medical department of the Kagoshima University in March 2009. He has been a medical doctor at Kakunodate Hospital in Akita since April 2009. He focuses on functional neurological recovery after stroke and head injury. Here, Dr. Nishino, Dr. Dimitrijevvic, Dr. Simon, and he spent several weeks in April and March to establish a mesh glove stimulation team in their hospital in support of the 2nd International Motor Recovery Workshop in Kakunodate, Akita, Japan. He is interested in the correlation between functional recovery and underlying anatomical rearrangement.

Tiejun Miao graduated in 1983 from the Physics Department, Dalian University of Technology, obtained a MS in 1986 from the Physics Department, Jilin University, and obtained a PhD in 1995 in Ergonomics, University of Electro-Communications. He is currently working for CCI Corporation, conducting R&D on chaos and nonlinear analysis and applications.

Takanori Miki is an Associate Professor in the Department of Anatomy and Neurobiology at Kagawa University, Japan. He graduated from Kagawa Medical University, obtained his MD in 1991, and earned his PhD in 1995. He worked in Dr. Kuldip S. Bedi's lab at Queensland University, Australia as a postdoctoral follow for 3 years beginning in 1997. He conducts research in the field of developmental neuroscience, with a special interest in developmental disorders in the central nervous system (CNS) induced by various kinds of environmental insults (e.g., ethanol, mycotoxins, and X-irradiation). His research employs both morphological (e.g., immunohistochemistry and stereology) and molecular biological techniques (including real-time RT-PCR and western blotting). Among recent research projects, he is currently interested in CNS disorders induced by stressful events during brain development, i.e., the "molecular basis of brain vulnerability caused by nurturing environment (maternal deprivation) during early postnatal life." His research has been supported by a variety of grants from the Japanese government and from private funds. These research interests are related to serious social problems seen in news reports on parents who have difficulties nurturing their own children. Dr. Miki's research aims to clarify the etiological mechanisms behind this phenomenon using epigenetics-based molecular biological techniques.

Yuko Mizuno-Matsumoto received her MD from Shiga University of Medical Science, Japan, in 1991 and PhD's in Medical Science and Engineering from Osaka University, Japan, in 1996 and 2003, respectively. From 1999 to 2000, she was a post-doctoral research fellow in the Department of Neurology, Johns Hopkins University, Baltimore, USA. Since 2004, she has been an associate professor in the Graduate School of Applied Informatics, University of Hyogo, Kobe, Japan. She is a certifying physician of The Japanese Society of Psychiatry and Neurology and a certifying physician & electroencephalographer of the Japanese Society of Clinical Neurophysiology.

Hiroshi Mori was born in 1968. He received the BS degree in Biology and the MS degree in Biochemistry, both from Osaka University, Japan, in 1974 and 1976, respectively, and the doctorate in Biochemistry, from University of Tokyo, Graduate School of Science, Biochemistry, Japan, in 1979. He was an Associate Professor at Fukui Prefectural College, Fukui, Japan, from 1982 to 1986, a Chief Researcher in Department of Clinical Physiology, Tokyo Institute of Gerontology, Tokyo, Japan, from 1986 to 1988, a Research Associate at Harvard Medical School, Brighan & Women's Hospital, Boaton, U.S.A, from 1988-1990, a Chief Researcher in Department of Neurophysiology, Tokyo Institute of Gerontology, Tokyo, Japan, from 1990-1991, an Associate Professor in Department of Neuropathology, University of Tokyo, Medical School, Tokyo, Japan, from 1991-1992, a Head in Dept of Molecular Biology, Tokyo Institute of Psychiatry, Tokyo, Japan, from 1992-1998. Since 1998, he is Professor in the Department of Neuroscience, physiology, Osaka City University, Medical School, Osaka, Japan.

Nozomu Mori was born on February 19, 1950 in Japan. He graduated from the School of Medicine, Osaka University on March 31, 1974 and received a DMSc degree from Osaka University in 1986. He was a Medical Doctor from 1968 to 1974 in the Department of Otolaryngology, Osaka University. He moved to Kansai Rosai Hospital as a Medical Doctor in 1975. He moved to the Department of Otolaryngology, Nara Medical University as an Assistant Professor in 1978 and then to the Department of Otolaryngology, Osaka University, School of Medicine as an Assistant Professor in 1985. He moved to the Department of Otolaryngology, Kagawa Medical University as an Associate Professor in 1987 and has been a Professor in the Department since 1995 (now referred to as the Department of Otolaryngology, Head, and Neck Surgery, Faculty of Medicine, Kagawa University). His current research interest is Meniere's disease.

Shin Morita was born on August 18, 1974 in Japan. He graduated from the Department of Physical Therapy, Ehime Juzen School of Allied Medical Professions on May 31, 2000. Since then, he has been working in the Department of Rehabilitation, Kagawa Medical University Hospital, which changed its name to Kagawa University Hospital in October 2003. His current research interests are to evaluate changes in cerebral blood flow during isometric knee extension after knee arthroplasty using fNIRS and also to investigate the effect of the quadriceps femoris muscle weakness after the surgery on the central nervous system.

Koji Nagashima graduated from the Graduate School of Natural Science and Technology, Okayama University. He majored in Ergonomics in graduate school and studied the human auditory system, which provides a basic human sense and is very important in everyday life. His work elucidated the characteristics of the human auditory system and created new inspection machinery. He also studied differences in the characteristics of the auditory systems between AD patients and healthy senior citizens. His study aimed to perform early detection of dementia by quantitative measurement of the difference between these groups. Hearing characteristics were measured by performing a sound localization experiment in the vertical plane. His work has been published by academic societies such as the Japanese Society for Medical and Biological Engineering. After graduation, he joined JFE Mechanical Co., Ltd., where he is responsible for machine design and maintenance.

Hikaru Nakamura is a Professor in the Department of Welfare Systems and Health Science, Okayama Prefectural University, Japan. He was born in Kanagawa, Japan in 1962. He received a BA from Keio University, Japan in 1984. From 1992 to 2000, he worked in the Department of Audiology and Speech-Language Pathology at the College of Rehabilitation and Welfare in Nagoya, Japan where he was engaged in research and teaching on language and cognitive disorders. He completed his PhD at Nagoya City University, Japan in 2000. His doctoral research investigated characteristics of cognitive impairment in patients with Alzheimer's disease. Since April 2000, he has been at Okayama Prefectural University. His research focuses on assessment and intervention in acquired cognitive disorders, such as aphasia, memory disorders, and dementia. His current research interest is semantic deficits and communication disorders in brain damaged patients. He is a council member of the Japanese Association of Speech-Language-Hearing Therapists, the Neuropsychology Association of Japan, and the Japan Society for Higher Brain Dysfunction.

Naoya Nakamura was born in Okayama, Japan in 1988. He received a Bachelor of Engineering degree and a Master of Engineering degree in Mechanical Engineering from the Graduate School of Natural Science and Technology, Okayama University, Okayama, Japan in 2006 and 2010, respectively. He studies early detection of dementia by examining the cognitive characteristics of audiovisual integration in healthy elderly subjects, mild cognitive impairment patients, and Alzheimer's disease patients. This work characterizes subjects' responses to auditory, visual, and audiovisual stimuli and calculates their response times to examine their audiovisual integration ability. He believes that the early stage of dementia can be diagnosed by comparing audiovisual integration between subject groups.

Ryuji Nakamura was born in Fukuoka, Japan on December 16, 1973. He received a BA from Hiroshima University, Japan, in 1999 and a PhD from Hiroshima University, Japan, in 2010, both in Medical Science. He was a graduate student in Biomedical Sciences at Hiroshima University, Japan from April 2005 to March 2010. Since April 2010, he has been an Assistant Professor in the Department of Biomedical Sciences, Faculty of Medicine, Hiroshima University. His current research interests are the monitoring of autonomic nervous system function.

Tsunehiko Nishimura received his MD degree from KPUM, Japan, in 1972. He received his PhD from Osaka University. He served as the chairman of the Department of Nuclear Medicine at Osaka University from 1991 to 1999. He served as the chairman of Radiology at KPUM from 1999 to 2010.

Katsuhiro Nishino was born in Fukui Prefecture, Japan, on August 4, 1953. He received his MD from Akita University School of Medicine, Japan, and PhD Med Sci from Akita University School of Medicine, in 1978 and 1986, respectively. He was a lecturer at the Department of Neurosurgery, Akita University, from 1981 to 1990. He was a postdoctoral fellow at the Stroke Center (Prof. James Davis), Duke Medical Ctr., Durham, North Carolina, USA, from 1985 to 1988. He returned to Akita and was an assistant professor in the Department of Neurosurgery, Akita University, from April 1990 to March 1994. Since April 1994, he has been Director of the Department of Neurosurgery and Restorative Neurology, Kakunodate General Hospital, Sennboku City, Akita, Japan. Then in 1997, he was promoted to President of Kakunodate City General Hospital. He has been Adjunct Professor, Department of Systems of Life Engineering, Maebashi Institute of Technology, Gunmma, Japan. Since 2009, he has been in the International Working Group of Mesh Glove Stimulation, Department of Neurology, Vienna Medical University. Dr. Nishino received the Best Paper Award from the north-eastern district of the Japan Stroke Foundation in 1982.

Hiroki Nogawa was born in Osaka, Japan in 1966. He graduated from Osaka University Medical School and received his Medical License in 1990. He worked as a surgical resident at Osaka University Hospital from June 1990 to June 1991 and at Kure National Hospital from July 1991 to June 1993. He received a doctorate in Internal Medicine from Osaka University in 1997. He was an Assistant Professor at Sapporo Medical School from April 1997 to June 1999 and a Lecturer at Sapporo Medical School from July 1999 to July 2000. He was a Lecturer in the Cybermedia Center at Osaka University from August 2000 to June 2004 and a Visiting Professor at Tokyo Medical and Dental University from August 2004 to July 2008. Since August 2008, he has been a Fellowship Researcher at the Japanese Medical Information Network Association. He received the Kusumoto Award from Osaka University in 1990 and the Award of Advanced Infrastructure Technologies from the Award Committee of the Gigabit Network Symposium in 2004.His current research interests are internet security technology, public policy on information and communication technologies (including medical informatics), sociolegal and technological issues (including copyright issues), and the physiological effects of music on the brain.

Takashi Ogasa was born in Tokushima, Japan, in 1985. He received a Bachelor of Engineering degree from Kagawa University, Kagawa, Japan, in 2009 and will receive a Master of Engineering degree from the Graduate School of Natural Science and Technology, Okayama University, Okayama, Japan, in 2011. He majored in ergonomics and studied the relationship between the sense of touch and dementia. Some recent studies have reported that cognitive deficits in AD are related to a possible disconnection between cortical areas, and tactile object cognition is one of the major manual learning and memory skills that require extensive connections between cortical areas. Thus, he believes that the tactile cognitive deficit symptoms of AD can be detected using tactile cognitive tests. His overall aim is the development of a diagnostic test for dementia that uses the sense of touch.

Yasuyuki Ohta was born in Osaka, Japan on May 2, 1974. He received an M.D. from Okayama University, Japan in 2000 and a PhD from Okayama University, Japan in 2007. Since April 2010, he has been an Assistant Professor in the Department of Neurology, Graduate School of Medicine and Dentistry and Pharmaceutical Sciences, Okayama University, Japan. His current research interests are the molecular mechanisms of neurological disorders, especially of Alzheimer's disease and amyotrophic lateral sclerosis.

Nobuyuki Okamura was born in Sasayama City, Hyogo, Japan on May 9, 1969. He received an MD from Tohoku University School of Medicine, Japan in 1994 and a Doctorate in Medical Science from Tohoku University School of Medicine, Japan in 1998. He was a Researcher at the Cyclotron and Radioisotope Center, Tohoku University, Japan from April 1996 to March 1998, a Clinical Fellow in the Department of Geriatric Medicine, Tohoku University Hospital from April 1998 to March 2001, a Researcher at the BF Research Institute from April 2001 to March 2003, an Assistant Professor in the Department of Pharmacology, Tohoku University School of Medicine from April 2003 to January 2009, and a Research Fellow in the Mental Health Research Institute, University of Melbourne from

February 2009 to July 2009. Since August 2009, he has been an Associate Professor in the Department of Pharmacology, Tohoku University School of Medicine. His current research interests are molecular imaging and pharmacology. Dr. Okamura received the Best Paper Award from the Japanese Pharmacological Society in 2004, the Young Investigator Award from the Japanese Foundation for Aging and Health in 2005, the Silver Award from Tohoku University School of Medicine in 2005, the Sakisaka Memorial Award in 2006, the Encouraging Prize from the Japanese Society for Dementia Research in 2006, and the Best Paper Award from the International Symposium on Early Detection and Rehabilitation Technology of Dementia in 2009.

Yoshitsugu Omori was born in Kanagawa, Japan on December 12, 1970. He became a licensed Physical Therapist in 1995 and received an MS degree from Tsukuba University, Japan, in 2004. He was a Physical Therapist in the Department of Rehabilitation Medicine, St. Marianna University School of Medicine Hospital, Japan, from May 1995 to June 1997. Since July 1997, he has worked in the Department of Rehabilitation Medicine, St. Marianna University Yokohama City Seibu Hospital, Japan. His current research interest is in patient rehabilitation for practical locomotion by walking. He received the Presentation Award from the Human Ergology Society in 2004.

Aiko Osawa is from Osaka, Japan. She completed her medical training at the School of Medicine, Wakayama Medical University in 2002. She was a Research Fellow at the Royal Rehabilitation Centre, University of Sydney in 2007. She was a Resident at Wakayama Medical University from 2002 to 2004, and a Staff Physician in the Department of Rehabilitation Medicine at Kawasaki Medical School Hospital from 2004 to 2005 and at Kawasaki Medical School Kawasaki Hospital from 2005 to 2007. Since 2008, she has been an Assistant Professor in the Department of Rehabilitation Medicine, International Medical Center, Saitama Medical University. Her current research interests are brain injury rehabilitation and clinical neuropsychology. She received the Young Scientist Award from the 2nd World Congress of the International Society of Physical and Rehabilitation Medicine (ISPRM) in 2003. In 2007, she received the Best Paper Award from the Japanese Association of Rehabilitation Medicine, and her team also received the 2nd Prize in the Talent Show of the 4th World Congress of the ISPRM.

Nobuko Ota is from Okayama, Japan. She completed the Primary School Education program at the Department of Education of Okayama University, Japan, in 1986. She completed a speech therapist program in 1997 and received an M.Sc. degree in Sensory Science in 2008 from the Department of Sensory Science, Kawasaki University of Medical Welfare, Japan. Since April 2008, she has been a student in the Doctoral Course in Sensory Science, Graduate School of Health Science and Technology, Kawasaki University of Medical Welfare. She was a speech therapist at Kurashiki Heisei Hospital from 1997 to 2006 and at the Department of Rehabilitation at Kawasaki Medical School Kawasaki Hospital from 2006 to 2009. Since 2009, she has been a Teaching Assistant in the Department of Sensory Science, Kawasaki University of Medical Welfare. Her current research interests are prospective memory and clinical neuropsychology. In 2007, her team received the 2nd Prize in the Talent Show of the International Society of Physical and Rehabilitation Medicine. She received the Fukusako Award from the Japanese Language Disorder Clinical Research Association in 2009.

Mihoko Otake has been an Associate Professor of RACE (Research into Artifacts, Center for Engineering) at The University of Tokyo since 2006. She is also the Director of the Nonprofit Multisector Research Organization of the Fonobono Research Institute (FRI). She was an Assistant Professor with the Science Integration Program, Department of Frontier Science and Science Integration, The University of Tokyo starting in 2005. She was a Principal Investigator of the Precursory Research for the Embryonic Science and Technology Program of Japan Science and Technology Agency entitled "Development of Bilateral Multiscale Neural Simulator" from 2004 to 2008. Her research topics include simulating human sensorimotor algorithms utilizing a multiscale neural model, a musculoskeletal model, and a motion capture system, integration of neuroscience knowledge into simulation platforms and application of that knowledge to design, and dynamic computation by machines consisting of electroactive polymers. She is the author of the monograph, "Electroactive Polymer Gel Robots - Modeling and Control of Artificial Muscles," Springer-Verlag, (2009). She received her B.E., M.E., and PhD in Mechano-Informatics in 1998, 2000, and 2003, respectively, all from The University of Tokyo. She was recognized as a JSPS Research Fellow from 2001 to 2003. She is a member of the Institute of Electrical and Electronics Engineers, Inc. (IEEE), Society for Neuroscience (SfN), the Information Processing Society of Japan (IPSJ), and the Robotics Society of Japan (RSJ).

Mayumi Oyama-Higa was born in Hiratsuka, Japan, on February 11, 1941. She received a BE in quantum chemistry from Tohoku University, Sendai, Japan. She received a doctorate in information engineering in 1991 from Toyohashi University of Technology, Toyohashi, Japan. She was an assistant professor at the Information Processing Research Center, Kwansei Gakuin University, Nishinomiya, Japan, from April 1980 to March 1989 and was a professor from April 1989 to March 2000. She was an invited researcher of Computer Science at Columbia University, New York, NY, USA, from August 1992 to August 1993 and a professor from April 2000 to March 2009 in the Department of Psychological Science, Graduate School of Kwansei Gakuin University. She received the title of professor emeritus from Kwansei Gakuin University in 2009. She is an invited professor of the Osaka University Graduate School now. Her current research interests are non-linear analysis and fractal analysis of living body information. Dr. Oyama-Higa received the Franklin V. Taylor Memorial Award from the IEEE-SMC Society in 2009.

Kaechang Park was born in Osaka, Japan on June 3, 1956. He graduated and received a PhD from the Medical School of Osaka University, Japan in 1985 and 1992, respectively. He was a Lecturer from March 2000 to June 2007 and an Associate Professor in the Department of Neurosurgery, Medical School, Kochi University, Japan from July 2007 to August 2008. He has been the Director of the Brain Check-up Center, Kochi Kenshin Clinic, Japan, since September 2008. His current research interests are the diagnosis and treatment of mild cognitive impairment.

Noboru Saeki was born in Hiroshima, Japan on July 8, 1965. He received a BA in 1990 and a PhD in 2000, both in Medical Science from Hiroshima University, Japan. Since April 2000, he has been an Assistant Professor in the Graduate School of Biomedical Sciences, Hiroshima University. His current research interests are cardiovascular and brain monitoring during surgery and regulation of vascular permeability under inflammatory stimuli.

Yong Shen, is currently the Head and Senior Scientist of the Haldeman Laboratory of Molecular and Cellular Neurobiology at Banner Sun Health Research Institute, in Sun City, a suburb of Phoenix Arizona, and he is also an adjunct professor in the Molecular and Cellular Biology Program at Arizona State University and Psychiatry Department in University of Louisville Medical School. Much of Dr. Shen's scientific work has been conducted over the past 17 years in Cornell University, State University of New York, Rudolf Magnus Institute of Pharmacology, Dutch Royal Academy of Sciences, National Institute of Mental Health, National Institute of Neurological Disorders and Stroke, the Abbot Laboratories Neuroscience Division and Banner Sun Health Research Institute where he has made many contributions to the neuroscience area.

Zhibin Song received a BS from the College of Mechanical and Electrical Engineering from Harbin Engineering University (HEU), China, in 2006. He received a MS from Kagawa University, Japan, in 2009. Mr. Song is currently pursuing a PhD in intelligent machine systems at Kagawa University. Mr. Song has published approximately nine conference papers in recent years. He is an IEEE student member. His current research interests include upper-limb rehabilitation robotics and haptic robotics.

Miao Sun is a doctoral candidate researching brain aging and cognitive impairment in Dehua Chui's lab, Neuroscience Research Institute & Department of Neurobiology, Peking University Health Science Center. Prior to joining this lab, Sun Miao spent five years as a college student of medicine at Peking University, Department of Medicine center, to learn the foundation of basic medicine and scientific research. Today, his research is focused on the molecular regulation of hypoxia and abeta clearance. This research is highly relevant to human brain diseases because it is becoming clear that abeta plays important roles in learning and memory, brain aging and cognitive impairment. Another major focus of his research is molecular imaging on lipid dysmetabolism, which is also a vigorous frontier science problem in the world.

Makoto Suzuki was born in Kochi, Japan on May 12, 1972. He received a BA degree from Chuo University, Japan, in 1996, an M.S. degree from Tsukuba University, Japan, in 2004, and a doctorate in rehabilitation science from Nagoya University, Japan in 2008. He was an Occupational Therapist in the Department of Rehabilitation Medicine, St. Marianna University School of Medicine Hospital, Japan from April 1999 to March 2009. Since April 2009, he has been an Assistant Professor in the Faculty of Medical Technology, Niigata University of Health and Welfare. His current research interests are the relationship between strength and function in patients with dementia.

Toshihisa Takagi has been the Director and a Professor of the Database Center for Life Science (DBCLS) since 2007. He was an Associate Professor at Kyushu University since 1988, and an Associate Professor since 1992 and a Professor since 1994 at the Institute of Medical Science, The University of Tokyo. He was a Professor of the Graduate School of Frontier Science, The University of Tokyo since 2003. His main work includes "Biomedical knowledge navigation by literature clustering," Journal of Biomedical Informatics, 40(2), pp. 114-130, 2007, and "MetaGene: prokaryotic gene finding from environmental genome shotgun sequences," Nucleic Acids Res., Vol.34, No.19, pp. 5623-5630, 2006. He is a member of the Japanese Society for Bioinformatics (JSBI), the Information Processing Society of Japan (IPSJ), and the Biophysical Society of Japan.

Satoshi Takahashi was born in Hiroshima, Japan in 1966. He received B.Eng., M.Eng., and D.Eng. degrees from Okayama University, Japan in 1989, 1991, and 2001, respectively. He was an Associate Professor at Okayama University, Japan from April 2003 to March 2005. Since April 2005, he has been an Associate Professor in the Graduate School of Natural Science and Technology, Okayama University, Japan. He is a member of the Japan Society of Mechanical Engineers, the Society of Instrument and Control Engineers, and the Institute of Complex Medical Engineering. His current research interests are the development of instruments for rehabilitation and signal processing for brain-machine interfaces using electroencephalogram and electromyography and research on international social infrastructures around aging people and dementia patients.

Hajime Takechi was born in Shiga, Japan, on January 24, 1961. He graduated from the Faculty of Medicine, Kyoto University in 1986 and became a licensed Medical Doctor in Japan. He received a PhD in Medical Research from Kyoto University in 1993. From 1993 to 1996, he was a Research Fellow in the Division of Neuroscience, Osaka Bioscience Institute. From 1996 to 1999, he was a Postdoctoral Fellow in the Institute of Physiology, University of Saarland, Germany. He authored a paper in Nature regarding a new type of synaptic transmission. Since 1999, he has been an Assistant Professor in the Department of Geriatric Medicine, Kyoto University. Dr. Takechi is a specialist in dementia and a councilor of the Japan Geriatrics Society. He is also a member of the Japan Society for Dementia Research, the Japanese Psychogeriatric Society, the Japanese Society of Neurology, and the Japan Neuroscience Society. He is a certified physician of internal medicine.

Yoshiki Takeuchi is a Professor in the Department of Anatomy and Neurobiology, Faculty of Medicine, Kagawa University. He graduated from Mie Prefectural University in 1974 and received a PhD degree from Mie University in 1978. After studying neuroanatomy at Dalhousie University in Canada for 2 years as a Killam postdoctoral fellow, he worked at Hiroshima and Nagoya Universities and became a Professor at Kagawa University in 1989. His research interests include: neuronal networks between the forebrain and brain stem, particularly concerning the amygdaloid projections to the parabrachial and solitary nucleus, the study of the mechanism of transcytosis of proteins at synapses using Rab3A-siRNA and WGA-HRP, and the effects of alcohol on the central nervous system. He is a member of the Japanese Association of Anatomists and the Japan Neuroscience Society. He is also an editor of the International Journal "Current Neurobiology."

Hideaki Tanaka was born in Tokyo, Japan, on April 21, 1966. He received his MD and PhD from Dokkyo Medical University, Japan, both in clinical medicine, in 1991 and 1997, respectively. He has been an associate professor at Dokkyo Medical University from October 2006 to the present. His current research interests are the development of multichannel evoked ("ERP") and spontaneous ("EEG") brain electric field mapping and the spatial analysis of brain electric fields. He also conducts studies of human brain electric field properties in relation to normal and pathological cognition, especially neurodegenerative disorders such as Alzheimer's disease and Parkinson's disease, including the effects of medication.

Yuki Tanaka was born in Oita, Japan, on November 9, 1981. She received a Bachelor of Engineering degree from Tokai University, Japan, in 2005, and a Master of Engineering from Tokai University, Japan in 2007. Since April 2007, she has been a PhD student at Tokyo Medical and Dental University Graduate

School, Department of Medical Informatics. She studied piano in Japan under the pianist Toshie Nakashima since 1985, when she was 4 years old. She participated in piano contests, including the Student Music concourse of Japan, Tosu City Hupfer Memorial Piano Concourse, International Chopin Piano Competition in ASIA, the Oita Eisteddfod piano section, and the youth section of the Takahiro Sonoda Prize International Piano Contest. She has received several prizes, including a prize for encouragement at the An die Musik Piano contest in 2009. She is a part-time teacher at Nippon University (from 2008) and Kitazato University (from 2007). Her current research interests are "Music Therapy for Dementia Patients: Tuned for culture difference" and the "Effect of music upon awakening for comfortable awakening." She received the Nobuko Matsumae prize for encouragement of the Shigeyoshi Matsumae Memorial Fund from the Educational Foundation of Tokai University in 2005.

Hiroshi Tanaka was born in Tokyo, Japan in 1949. He received a Bachelor of Engineering degree from Tokyo University, Japan, in 1974 and a Master of Engineering degree from the Graduate School of Engineering, Tokyo University, Japan, in 1976. He received a Doctor in Medical Science degree from the Graduate School of Medicine, Tokyo University, Japan, in 1981 and a PhD from the Graduate School of Engineering, Tokyo University, Japan, in 1983. He was an Assistant Professor at the Institute for Medical Electronics in the School of Medicine of Tokyo University from 1982 to 1987, a Visiting Scientist at Uppsala University and Linkoping University in Sweden from 1982 to 1984, an Associate Professor at Hamamatsu University School of Medicine from 1987 to 1991, and a Visiting Scientist in the MIT Laboratory of Computer Science in 1990. He became a Full Professor of Bioinformatics at Tokyo Medical and Dental University in 1991 and has been the Dean of the Biomedical Science PhD Program of Tokyo Medical and Dental University since 2006. He received an award for his achievements in information and communication technology from the Ministry of Internal Affairs and Communications in 2008. His current research interests are medical informatics, systems biology, systems pathology, and clinical bioinformatics.

Jun Tanemura is from Tokyo, Japan. He completed the Educational Psychology program in the Department of Education of Waseda University, Japan, in 1975 and received an MA degree in Psychology from the Department of Literature Research of Waseda University in 1977. He received a PhD in Psychology from Meisei University, Japan, in 1995. He was the Chief Speech Therapist at Nirayama Rehabilitation Hospital, Japan from April 1982 to March 1996. Since April 1996, he has been a Professor in the Department of Sensory Science, Faculty of Health Science and Technology, Kawasaki University of Medical Welfare. His current research interests are aphasia and clinical neuropsychology. He has been a member of the Board of Directors of the Japanese Association of Higher Brain Function since April 2002. He received the Best Paper Award from the Japanese Association of Rehabilitation Medicine in 2007.

Manabu Tashiro was born in Matsumoto City, Nagano, Japan on December 31, 1966. He received an MD from Shinshu University School of Medicine, Japan in 1994 and a Doctorate in Medical Sciences from Tohoku University Graduate School of Medicine, Japan in 2000. He was a visiting researcher from July 1998 to March 2001 in the Division of Nuclear Medicine, Freiburg University Hospital, Germany, and an Assistant Professor in the Department of Pharmacology, Tohoku University Graduate School of Medicine, Japan from April 2001 to January 2005. He was then a Lecturer in the Division of Cyclotron Nuclear Medicine, Cyclotron and Radioisotope Center (CYRIC), Tohoku University, Japan from February 2005 to December 2007, where he has been an Associate Professor since January 2007. His current research interests are nuclear medicine, molecular imaging, and clinical pharmacology. Dr. Tashiro received the Inoue Research Aid Award for Young Scientists in 2001, the Poster Award of the Japanese Pharmacological Society in 2002, the New Investigator Award (Runner-Up) of the International Psycho-oncology Society in 2003, Encouragement Awards from the Japanese Society of Nuclear Medicine (JSNM) and the Japanese Society of Clinical Pharmacology and Therapeutics (JSCPT) in 2005, the JSNM Society Award in 2008, the Japanese Research Foundation for Clinical Pharmacology Award (JSCPT Society Award), and the Mitusi-Sumitomo Welfare Foundation Award in 2009.

Shozo Tobimatsu was born in Saga Prefecture, Japan, on February 2, 1955. He received a M.D. from the Faculty of Medicine, Kyushu University, Fukuoka, Japan, in 1979 and a doctorate in medicine from Kyushu University, Japan, in 1985. He was an assistant professor in the Department of Neurology, Faculty of Medicine, Kyushu University, from February 1982 to September 1985, a research associate in the Department of Neurology, Loyola University of Chicago (Prof. Gastone G. Celesia), Maywood, Illinois, USA, from October 1985 to October 1987, and a lecturer in the Department of Clinical Neurophysiology, Faculty of Medicine, Kyushu University, from November 1987 to November 1999. Since December 1999, he has been Professor and Chairman, Department of Clinical Neurophysiology, Neurological Institute, Faculty of Medicine, Graduate School of Medical Sciences, Kyushu University. He is now a Vice Dean of the Faculty of Medicine, Kyushu University. His current research interests are focused on higher brain functions and cognitive neuroscience in humans, using non-invasive methods such as EEG, ERP, and MEG. He is a member of the Editorial Board of *Clinical Neurophysiology*.

Tetsuo Touge was born on October 24, 1955 in Japan. He graduated from the Medical Course of Tokushima University on May 31, 1981, and received his PhD from Kagawa Medical University in June 1991. He was an assistant professor from December 1986 to November 1996 and a lecturer from December 1996 to June 2004 in the Third Department of Internal Medicine at Kagawa Medical University (changed to Department of Gastroenterology and Neurology, Faculty of Medicine, Kagawa University, in October 2003). He moved to Health Sciences, School of Nursing, Faculty of Medicine, Kagawa University as an associate professor in July 2004 and has been a professor in the department since June 2006. His current research interests are therapeutic application of magnetic brain stimulation, elucidation of the mechanism of multisensory cognitive processing using event-related potentials or NIRS, and the development of novel techniques to evaluate mental dysfunction.

Toshio Tsuji was born in Kyoto, Japan on October 17, 1956. He received a B.E. in Industrial Engineering and an M.E. and Doctorate of Engineering in Systems Engineering from Hiroshima University in 1982, 1985, and 1989, respectively. He was a Research Associate from 1985 to 1994 and an Associate Professor from 1994 to 2002 in the Faculty of Engineering, Hiroshima University. From 1992 to 1993, he was a Visiting Professor at the University of Genova, Genova, Italy. He is currently a Professor in the Department of Artificial Complex Systems Engineering, Hiroshima University. His research interests include human-machine interfaces and computational neural sciences, with a particular emphasis on biological motor control.

Teiji Ukawa was born in Mie, Japan on December 9, 1956. He received a Bachelor of Engineering degree from the Department of Applied Physics of Waseda University, Tokyo, Japan in 1980. He joined Nihon Kohden Corp., Tokyo, Japan, in April 1980. He has been a PhD student in Systems Engineering at Hiroshima University, Higashi-Hiroshima, Japan, since October 2009.

Takahiro Wada was born in Osaka, Japan, in 1971. He received a BS in Mechanical Engineering, an MS in Information Science and Systems Engineering, and a PhD in Robotics from Ritsumeikan University, Japan in 1994, 1996, and 1999, respectively. He was an Assistant Professor at Ritsumeikan University beginning in 1999. In 2000, he joined Kagawa University as an Assistant Professor in the Department of Intelligent Mechanical Systems Engineering, Faculty of Engineering, Kagawa University, Japan, where he is currently an Associate Professor. He spent a half a year in 2006 and 2007 as a Visiting Researcher at The University of Michigan Transportation Research Institute. His current research interests include human-machine systems, human modeling, and driver assistance systems for traffic safety. Dr. Wada is a member of the Society of Instrument and Control Engineers, the Society of Automotive Engineers of Japan (JSAE), the Japanese Society of Mechanical Engineers, the Robotics Society of Japan (RSJ), the Human Factors and Ergonomics Society, and SAE. Dr. Wada received the Young Investigator Excellence Award from RSJ in 1999 and the Best Paper Award from JSAE in 2008.

Shuoyu Wang was born in Heilongjiang, China on February 19, 1963. He received BE and ME degrees in Control Engineering from Shenyang University of Technology, China in 1983 and 1988, respectively, and a Doctorate in Electrical Engineering from Hokkaido University, Japan in 1993. He was an Associate Professor in the Electronic Information Engineering Department, Yamagata University from 1993 to 1997, and an Associate Professor in the Department of Intelligent Mechanical Systems Engineering, Kochi University of Technology from 1997 to 2002. Since January 2002, he has been a Professor in the Department of Intelligent Mechanical Systems Engineering, Kochi University of Technology. His current research interests are robotics, control, and fuzzy reasoning. Dr. Wang received the Best Paper Award from the Journal of Biomedical Fuzzy Systems Association in 1999, the Best Paper Award from the Virtual Reality Society of Japan in 2002, and the JSME Chugoku-Shikoku Branch Medal for New Technology in 2010.

Zhi-Yu Wang is a Clinical Doctor at Heibei Medical University Hospital in China. He graduated from Hebei Medical University in 2002 and completed the Master's degree in 2004. He worked at Hebei University Hospital from 2002 to 2005 as a Doctor of Orthopedics. He received a PhD degree from the Faculty of Medicine, Kagawa University in 2010. His research interests include the effects of alcohol on neurotrophic factors in the central nervous system and studying the mechanism of transcytosis of proteins at synapses using Rab3A-siRNA and WGA.

Haibo Wang was born September 3, 1980, in China. He received a Bachelor of Engineering degree from the Graduate School of Mechanical Engineering and Automation, Jilin University, Changchun, China, in 2003. He received a Master of Engineering degree from the Graduate School of Technology, Kagawa University, Kagawa, Japan, in March 2008. At present, he is under a doctoral course of engineering degree from Okayama University, Okayama, Japan. He is mainly engaged in tactile studies utilizing neuroimaging technology. His research topic is "Tactile shape perception mechanism and brain processing by precision gripping with five fingers". He has a good command of English and Japanese, both spoken and written. His research about length perception with two and three fingers was published in JSME, CME2009 and BI-AMT 2009.

Katsuhiko Warita is an Assistant Professor in the Department of Anatomy and Neurobiology, Faculty of Medicine, Kagawa University. He graduated from the School of Veterinary Medicine and Animal Sciences, Kitasato University in 2003 and received his PhD degree from the Graduate School of Science and Technology, Kobe University in 2008. Prior to attending graduate school at Kobe University, he worked for the Department of Histopathological Diagnosis for a contract research organization. His scientific interests include sex differentiation and impaired reproductive capacity. His research investigates reproductive disorders induced by exposure to estrogenic environmental pollutants during the early developmental period, as evaluated using morphological, endocrinological, and molecular-toxicological analyses. This research has a particular focus on the gene expression of the steroidogenic acute regulatory protein (StAR), which mediates the rate-limiting and acutely regulated step in steroidogenesis. His research interest areas also include bioinformatics and epigenetic alteration of steroidogenic genes.

Hiroshi Watabe was born in Shizuoka in 1967. He received a PhD in Nuclear Engineering from Tohoku University, Sendai in 1995. From 1995 to 2009, he conducted research in the Department of Investigative Radiology, National Cardiovascular Center, Osaka. Since October 2009, he has been an Associate Professor in the Department of Molecular Imaging in Medicine, Osaka University Graduate School of Medicine, Osaka. He is mainly interested in PET/SPECT physics, pharmacokinetics, and image analysis.

Shoichi Watanuki was born in Sapporo City, Hokkaido, Japan on November 5, 1957. He graduated from the College of Medical Technology, Hirosaki University, Japan in 1980. Following a period of clinical involvement, he has been working as a Research Associate in the Cyclotron and Radioisotope Center (CYRIC), Tohoku University, Japan since March 1983. His current research interest is in nuclear medicine technology, especially in the quality control of nuclear medicine imaging systems.

Weizhong Xiao is Professor and Deputy Director of the Neurology department in the Third Hospital of Peking University. He is also a contributing editor to Chinese Clinical Medicine, American Journal of Medical Progress and Journal of Practical Medicine. His expertise is in cerebrovascular disease, central nervous system infections, demyelinating and neurological diseases, clinical epidemiology, and evidence-based medicine. He has issued a "hypertensive thalamic hemorrhage and CT analysis", "high eosinophils increased damage to the nervous system disorder", "Clarantin and Chuan Qiong hydrochloride in the treatment of 60 patients with acute ischemic stroke", "migraine stroke", "watershed infarction of progress", "early intensive rehabilitation of stroke" and 10 more academic papers.

Tomiko Yakura entered Kagawa University as a PhD candidate student after graduating from Matsumoto Dental College in 2008. Since then, she has been engaged in research on neural network composition and nervous function. Her daily work is focused on learning fundamental neuroscience research techniques. Her research is focused the unusual structure of transmitting protein and phenomena of neuronal interaction and determined their intrinsic mechanisms. Her research fields include the mechanism of transcytosis of proteins, particularly at neuron-glia junction of satellite cells in the nodose ganglion of the vagus nerve. She has chosen to focus on the population of satellite cells and the transcytosis using Rab3A-siRNA and wheat germ agglutinin (WGA) conjugated horseradish peroxidase *in vivo*.

Kei Yamada was born in 1963 in Osaka, Japan. He received his MD degree from Kyoto Prefectural University of Medicine (KPUM), Japan, in 1989. He did his Radiology residency at KPUM and at St. Marianna's University of Medicine. He did his research fellowship in the field of neuroradiology at the University of Maryland. He then moved on to clinical fellowship programs at the University of Rochester and Massachusetts General Hospital (MGH). After a total of 4 years of training in the United States, he came back to KPUM, Japan and became a faculty member in 1999. He received the "Winthrop Fellow of the Year" from the University of Rochester in 1997. He also won a few awards from the Society of Magnetic Resonance in Medicine (1997, 2002, 2005) and the Japanese Society of Radiology. He serves as an editorial member of peer-reviewed international journals, such as Neuroradiology and the Neuroradiology Journal. He serves as a member of the publication committee for the Journal of Magnetic Resonance Imaging.

Sumio Yamada is a physical therapist who graduated from the School of Physical Therapy at the Kochi Rehabilitation Institute in 1978 and the School of Education of Aoyama Gakuin University in 1986. He was a research student in the Department of Rehabilitation Medicine at Fujita Health University from 1991 to 1994 and at Showa University from 1994 to 1999. He earned a doctoral degree at Showa University in 1999. He is the director of the Center for Elderly Fitness and Secondary Prevention Research and is a Professor in the School of Health Sciences, Nagoya University. Yamada's research interests include the role of exercise in patients with congestive heart failure, as well as exercise-based lifestyle modification in cardiac patients. He is currently directing a nationwide multi-center cohort trial that is being conducted in collaboration with cardiologists and physical therapists at 24 hospitals in Japan and that focuses on the time course of functioning in patients with congestive heart failure and the effect of exercise on that functioning. His current research also focuses on the prevention of stroke recurrence in mild stroke and lifestyle modification via the regional alliance path in patients with acute myocardial infarction. He has 20 years of clinical experience in cardiac rehabilitation at St. Marianna University Hospital and has been a Vice President of the Japanese Association of Cardiac Rehabilitation since 2006. He has authored or coauthored more than 100 scientific articles and books.

Eiji Yamada was born on December 12, 1970 in Japan. He graduated from the Department of Physical Therapy of Zentsuji Rehabilitation School attached to the National Zentsuji Hospital in 1993 and received a PhD from Kagawa Medical University in 2007. He was a physical therapist from April 1993 to May 1998 in the Department of Physical Therapy, Ishikawa Prefectural Central Hospital. He moved to the Department of Physical Therapy, Kagawa University Hospital as a Physical Therapist in April 1998, and he has been a chief physical therapist in the department since July 2005. His current research interest is about muscle metabolism during gait using electromyography and NIRS.

Suguru Yamaguchi graduated from Akita University, School of Medicine, Japan, in 2001 and completed the postgraduate course of the Department of Neurosurgery. He was a resident at several hospitals from 2001 to 2003 and a staff doctor in the Department of Neurosurgery, Akita University Hospital, from 2003 to 2005. From 2005 to 2006, he was a director in the Department of Neurosurgical Service, Kakunodate City Hospital, and in 2006 he became a staff doctor in the Department of Neurosurgery, Akita University Hospital. Since March 2007, he has been Director of the Department of Neurosurgical Service, Kakunodate City Hospital, Sennboku City, Akita, Japan. He is a member of the Japan Neurosurgical Board and the Japan Stroke Society Board.

Hiroyuki Yamamoto was born in Sapporo, Japan, on November 12, 1962. He received Bachelor's degree in civil engineering from Waseda University, Japan, in 1987. He received a BM from Kagawa University Medical School, Japan, 2009. He worked in the Nissan Motor Ltd Research & Development section from April 1987 to April 2004. His main specialized field at Nissan Motor was vehicle crash safety. His job at Nissan Motor was primarily in the development of new vehicles. He has been at Kakunodate Municipal Hospital as a junior resident since April 2009.

Hirotoshi Yamamoto was born in Hyogo, Japan, on May 23, 1951. He graduated from the Faculty of Engineering, Kyoto University, Japan, in 1975 and received a BS degree in mechanical engineering. He worked for ShinMaywa Ind. Ltd., Japan, from April 1975 to December 2007, where he participated in the development of industrial robots and high-performance direct drive motor systems. He was a visiting engineer at the Mechanical Engineering Research Laboratory, Hitachi Ltd., Japan, in 1980. From 1982 to 1983, he was a visiting research engineer at the Laboratory for Manufacturing and Productivity, Massachusetts Institute of Technology, MA, USA. He was a part-time Lecturer in the Department of Mechanical Engineering, Faculty of Engineering, Kyoto University from 2004 to 2007. Since April 2008, he has been a doctoral student in the Department of Mechanical Engineering and Science, Graduate School of Engineering, Kyoto University. His current research interests are dementia care and assistive technology for welfare engineering and rehabilitation engineering. Mr. Yamamoto received the Kinki Region Invention Award from the Japan Institute of Invention and Innovation in 1991 for a robotic sensor. He is a member of the Japanese Society for Dementia Care and the Japan Geriatrics Society.

Takao Yamasaki was born in Nagasaki, Japan, on October 29, 1972. He received his MD from Saga Medical School, Japan, in 1997. Afterwards, he joined the Department of Neurology (Prof. Jun-ichi Kira) at Kyushu University, Japan, and completed his residency at Kyushu University Hospital in 1999. In 2001, he entered the Graduate School of Medical Sciences at Kyushu University (Department of Clinical Neurophysiology, Prof. Shozo Tobimatsu). In 2002, he moved to the University of Tokyo, Japan, to study neuropsychology (Department of Cognitive Neuroscience, Prof. Morihiro Sugishita) for 6 months. He obtained his PhD from Kyushu University in 2005. After that, he worked at the Department of Clinical Neurophysiology, Kyushu University, as an assistant professor (2005-2007) and a research assistant professor (2007-present). Based on 13 years of clinical education and experience in the fields of neurology and clinical neurophysiology, his main interest has focused on non-invasive measurements of human brain function, especially higher visual recognition in healthy humans and various neurological disorders, by combining psychophysiological, electrophysiological (electroencephalogram, evoked potentials, event-related potentials) and neuroimaging (functional MRI, near-infrared spectroscopy) methods.

Tianyi Yan was born on June 17, 1981 in China. He received a Bachelor of Science degree from the Graduate School of Technique of Education, Chuangchun University of Science and Technology, Chang

Chun, China in 2005. He then received a Master of Engineering degree from the Graduate School of Technology, Kagawa University, Kagawa, Japan in 2008. He is mainly engaged in the study of vision, utilizing neuroimaging technology. His research topic is "Retinotopic Mapping of the Peripheral Visual Field to the Human Visual Cortex by Functional Magnetic Resonance Imaging." He has an excellent command of both spoken and written English, has passed CET-6 and JLPT-1, and he is skilled in using BrainVoyager, SPM, Win XP/Vista/Vin7, HTML, Photoshop, Illustrator, Visual Basic, Office 2003, Presentation, E-Prime, Premiere, and other software programs. He is currently a doctoral student in engineering at Okayama University, Okayama, Japan.

Kazuhiko Yanai was born in Yamanashi Pref., Japan on October 23, 1956. He received an MD from Tohoku University School of Medicine, Japan in 1981 and a Doctorate in Medical Sciences from Tohoku University, Japan in 1986. He was an Assistant Professor in the Department of Pharmacology, Tohoku University School of Medicine, Japan from June 1988 to March 1993, and an Associate Professor in the same department from April 1993 to October 1998. Since November 1998, he has been a Professor in the Department of Pharmacology, Tohoku University Graduate School of Medicine. His current research interests are molecular imaging and pharmacology.

Jiajia Yang is a Postdoctoral Fellow in the Biomedical lab of the Graduate School of Natural Science and Technology, Okayama University, Japan. His PhD was obtained in the Intelligent Mechanical System Engineering Department, Kagawa University, Japan, in 2009. His current research interests include cognitive and psychological neuroscience, neuroimaging, and early detection of Alzheimer's Disease (AD) using tactile and kinetic approaches. Dr. Yang received the Best Paper Award from the IEEE/ICME International Conference on Complex Medical Engineering and an International Exchange Grant from the TATEISI Science and Technology Foundation in 2009. He was also the Program Co-Chair of the 2010 IEEE/ICME International Conference on Complex Medical Engineering.

Yasuyoshi Yokokohji was born in Osaka, Japan, on August 4, 1961. He received BS and MS degrees in Precision Engineering in 1984 and 1986, respectively, and a Ph.D. in Mechanical Engineering in 1991, all from Kyoto University, Kyoto, Japan. From 1988 to 1989, he was a Research Associate in the Automation Research Laboratory, Kyoto University. From 1989 to 1992, he was a Research Associate in the Division of Applied Systems Science, Faculty of Engineering, Kyoto University. From 1992 to 2005, he was an Associate Professor in the Department of Mechanical Engineering, Kyoto University. From 2005 to 2009, he was an Associate Professor in the Department of Mechanical Engineering and Science, Graduate School of Engineering, Kyoto University. From 1994 to 1996, he was a visiting research scholar at the Robotics Institute, Carnegie Mellon University, Pittsburgh, PA. He is currently a Professor in the Department of Mechanical Engineering, Graduate School of Engineering, Kobe University. His current research interests are robotics, biomechanics, teleoperation systems, and haptic virtual reality systems. Dr. Yokokohji is a member of the Institute of Systems, Control, and Information Engineers (Japan), the Robotics Society of Japan, the Society of Instruments and Control Engineers (Japan), the Japanese Society of Mechanical Engineers, the Society of Biomechanisms Japan, the Virtual Reality Society of Japan, IEEE, and ACM.

Masao Yoshizumi was born in Okayama, Japan on October 17, 1956. He received a Doctor of Medicine degree from the University of Tokyo, Japan in 1981 and the PhD in Medical Science from the University of Tokyo, Japan in 1997. After completion of a fellowship in Cardiology and Molecular Cardiology research at the University of Tokyo, Japan, he was a Research Associate in Molecular Biology and an Instructor in Medicine at Harvard University, USA from January 1992 to April 1996. He was an Assistant Professor in the Department of Geriatric Medicine, Faculty of Medicine, University of Tokyo from August 1998 to March 2002. Since April 2002, he has been a Professor in the Department of Cardiovascular Physiology and Medicine, Faculty of Medicine, Hiroshima University. His current research interests are molecular mechanisms in cardiovascular diseases and biomedical engineering in cardiology.

Jia Yu is President Assistant of Beijing Geriatric Hospital and a Doctoral Candidate who does research on brain aging and cognitive impairment in Dehua Chui's lab at the Neuroscience Research Institute & Department of Neurobiology in Peking University Health Science Center, Beijing, China. Prior to becoming a member of this lab, Jia Yu spent five years as a college student of medicine at Peking University Health Science Center to learn the foundations of basic medicine and scientific research. Today, his research is focused on the molecular regulation of trace elements on APP processing and abeta metabolism. This research is highly relevant to human brain diseases because it is becoming clear that abeta plays important roles in learning and memory, brain aging and cognitive impairment. Another major focus of his research is lipid metabolism and cognitive function, which is also a vigorous frontier science problem in the world.

Zhang Shouzi was born in Shandong province, China, on May 21, 1968. He received a Master's degree from Shandong University, China. He is a neurologist working in Beijing Geriatric Hospital. He was a resident physician in Shandong province from September 1991 to September 2004, and doctor-in-charge from September 2004 to April 2007. He was an associate professor in the affiliated hospital of Weifang Medical College. He is currently a professor in the affiliated hospital of Beijing University of Chinese Medicine. His current research interests include Alzheimer's disease and other dementia. He has attended a series of projects of the National Natural Science Foundation of China.

Shuo Zhao was born in Nan Chang, China, in 1983. He received a Bachelor of Engineering degree and a Master of Engineering degree from the Graduate School of Natural Science and Technology, Okayama University, Okayama, Japan, in 2008 and 2010, respectively. He majored in the audiovisual attention of cognition. Spatial attention and temporal attention have been compared by brain-imaging data. He and his team developed a visual orienting attention task to compare an auditory stimulus while a visual target was presented. They also designed a control task in which subjects had to click a response key with a simultaneously presented spatial task. The effects of clicking the response key were removed by subtracting the brain activations elicited by the clicking of the response key from the results of the visual voluntary attention task. They measured brain activity in sixteen healthy volunteers using functional magnetic resonance imaging (fMRI). Shuo is mainly engaged in the design of human attention of cognition.

Liang Zhou is a doctoral candidate who does research on brain aging and cognitive impairment in Dehua Chui's lab, Neuroscience Research Institute & Department of Neurobiology, Peking University Health Science Center. Prior to becoming a member of this lab, Liang Zhou spent four years as a college student of life science in Nanjing Agricultural University to lay the foundation for scientific research. Today, his research is focused on the molecular regulation of hormones by lipids. This research is highly relevant to human brain diseases because it is becoming clear that lipids play important roles in learning and memory, brain aging and cognitive impairment. Another major focus of his research is molecular imaging of lipid dysmetabolism, which is also a vigorous frontier science problem in the world.

Index

C

D

E

F

G

H

I

J

K

L

M

N

O

P

T

U

V

W

Y

Z

CPSIA information can be obtained at www.ICGtesting.com
261352BV00007B/51-142/P

9 781609 605599